Current Progress in Pharmacology

Current Progress in Pharmacology

Editor: Phoenix McWilliams

FOSTER
ACADEMICS
www.fosteracademics.com

www.fosteracademics.com

FOSTER ACADEMICS

Cataloging-in-Publication Data

Current progress in pharmacology / edited by Phoenix McWilliams.
p. cm.
Includes bibliographical references and index.
ISBN 978-1-64646-150-9
1. Pharmacology. 2. Pharmacy. 3. Drugs. I. McWilliams, Phoenix.
RM301 .C87 2022
615.1--dc23

Foster Academics,
118-35 Queens Blvd., Suite 400,
Forest Hills, NY 11375, USA

ISBN 978-1-64646-150-9 (Hardback)

Contents

Preface

This book has been a concerted effort by a group of academicians, researchers and scientists, who have contributed their research works for the realization of the book. This book has materialized in the wake of emerging advancements and innovations in this field. Therefore, the need of the hour was to compile all the required researches and disseminate the knowledge to a broad spectrum of people comprising of students, researchers and specialists of the field.

Pharmacology is the branch of biomedical science that deals with the discovery, research and characterization of chemicals that show biological effects. It is concerned with the explanation of cellular and organismal functions in relation to these chemicals. It examines the interactions that occur between a living organism and chemicals that affect both normal and abnormal biochemical functions. It also includes drug composition, synthesis and drug design, cellular communication, molecular diagnostic, therapy, chemical biology and medical applications and antipathogenic capabilities. There are two main branches of pharmacology - pharmacodynamics and pharmacokinetics. Pharmacodynamics studies the chemicals with biological receptors and pharmacokinetics studies absorption, distribution, metabolism and excretion of chemicals from the biological systems. This book presents researches and studies performed by experts across the globe. It will also provide interesting topics for research which interested readers can take up. Students, researchers, experts and all associated with pharmaceutical science will benefit alike from this book.

At the end of the preface, I would like to thank the authors for their brilliant chapters and the publisher for guiding us all-through the making of the book till its final stage. Also, I would like to thank my family for providing the support and encouragement throughout my academic career and research projects.

Editor

1

Comparison of the Analgesic Effect of Diclofenac Sodium-Eudragit® RS100 Solid Dispersion and Nanoparticles Using Formalin Test in the Rats

Khosro Adibkia[1], Alireza Mohajjel Nayebi[2]*, Mohammad Barzegar-Jalali[1], Siavash Hosseinzadeh[3], Saeed Ghanbarzadeh[3], Afshin Shiva[1]

[1] *Drug Applied Research Center and Faculty of Pharmacy, Tabriz University of Medical Sciences, Tabriz, Iran.*
[2] *Clinical Psychiatry Research Center, Tabriz University of Medical Sciences, Tabriz, Iran.*
[3] *Students' Research Committee and Faculty of Pharmacy, Tabriz University of Medical Sciences, Tabriz, Iran.*

Article info

Keywords:
- Diclofenac sodium
- Eudragit® RS100
- Nanoparticles
- Solid dispersion
- Formalin test

Abstract

Purpose: In this study the intensity and duration of analgesic effect of diclofenac Na - Eudragit® RS100 solid dispersion and nanoparticles were evaluated by using formalin test in the rats.
Methods: The animals received different formulations of diclofenac Na and subsequently 50 µl of formalin solution (2.5%) was injected subcutaneously in the right paws after 1 h, 2 h and 3 h. The paw licking behavior was then evaluated in two phases. A dose of 20 mg/kg of pure diclofenac Na powder was determined as effective dose.
Results: In the first phase, in term of reduced paw licking time, no significant differences were found in any of the groups compared to the control group. However, in the second phase, the animals which received pure drug powder and the physical mixture of diclofenac Na with Eudragit® RS100 showed significant differences at the first and second hours. In the animals received the nanoparticles and solid dispersion, significant differences were observed in the third hour compared to the control group.
Conclusion: The analgesic effect of diclofenac Na could be improved by formulating its nanoparticles and solid dispersion with Eudragit® RS100. However, the nanoparticles revealed significantly higher analgesic effect than solid dispersion.

Introduction

Oral route is the most preferred route for drug administration due to greater convenience, less pain, high patient compliance and so on. However, oral drug delivery possesses some disadvantages like low drug solubility, poor gastrointestinal (GI) absorption, rapid metabolism, high fluctuation in the drug plasma concentration and variability in absorption due to food effects. Drug absorption from the intestine is the combination of some steps, including drug dissolution in the GI tract, uptake through the intestinal mucosa, and delivery into the systemic circulation.[1-3] Diclofenac Na is one of the most widely prescribed non-steroidal anti-inflammatory drug (NSAIDs) due to its analgesic and anti-inflammatory effects. It is administrated to relieve pain and inflammation in a wide range of musculoskeletal conditions, including various forms of arthritis, gout, back pain, dislocations, tendinitis and frozen shoulder.[4-6] Similar to other NSAIDs, diclofenac Na is associated with rare, but serious and sometimes fatal; GI tract side effects such as ulceration and hemorrhage. Therefore, this drug is an ideal candidate for taking with food and incorporation with different macromolecules to diminish its adverse effects after oral administration and also increase its bioavailability.[7-10] Eudragit® RS100, is a copolymer of poly (ethylacrylate, methylmethacrylate and chlorotrimethyl-ammonioethyl methacrylate) and contains 4.5–6.8% of quaternary ammonium groups which provide positive surface charge to the polymer. This property may cause to interact with negatively charged drugs or cellular surface of the target tissues.[10]
Solid dispersions and nanoparticles have frequently applied in order to improve physicochemical characteristics of the drugs as well as increase or decrease the drug release rate.[11-17] Our previously published study was revealed that both solid dispersions and nanoparticles of diclofenac Na – Eudragit® RS100 could considerably decrease the drug release rate.[10] In this study the solid dispersion and nanoparticles of diclofenac Na - Eudragit® RS100 with the drug: polymer ratio of 1:1 was prepared based on our previously published paper.
Subsequently, the intensity and duration of analgesic effect of the solid dispersion and nanoparticles were evaluated employing formalin test as an experimental model in male rats.

Materials and Methods

Materials

Acetone, ethanol, methanol, KH_2PO_4 and anhydrous sodium hydroxide were purchased from Merck Company (Germany). Diclofenac sodium was obtained from

***Corresponding author:** Alireza Mohajjel Nayebi, Email: nayebia@tbzmed.ac.ir

Shasun Chemicals and Drugs Company (India), Eudragit® RS100 was supplied from Boehringer Ingelheim Company (Germany).

Preparations of the nanoparticles, solid dispersion and physical mixture

Nanoparticles of diclofenac Na-Eudragit® RS100 were prepared via quasi-emulsion solvent diffusion method. Briefly, diclofenac Na and Eudragit® RS100 with the drug: polymer ratio of 1:1 were dissolved in 2 ml of ethanol at room temperature so that the total amount of drug and polymer was 100 mg. To evaporate the organic phase, the solution was stirred slowly in a shaker (MKV Orbital shaker Lh fermentation) at room temperature for 24 hrs. In order to separate the nanoparticles, the obtained suspension was centrifuged at 5 °C for 30 minutes in the 14000 rpm (Bekman: USA). The obtained nanoparticles were then lyophilized.

Coevaporation method was employed to prepare the solid dispersions of diclofenac Na-Eudragit® RS100. To this end, drug and polymer at the ratio of 1:1 with a total weight of 2 g was dissolved in 200 mL ethanol. To obtain the solid dispersions, ethanol was evaporated (Buchi® rotary evaporator, Germany) at 10 °C and 80 mmHg for an hour.

Physical mixture of diclofenac Na with Eudragit® RS100 was prepared by tumbling method (10 min) with the same drug: carrier ratio.

Animals and experimental protocol

Male Wistar rats (200 ± 20 g) were housed in the Animal House of Tabriz University of Medical Sciences at constant temperature (23 ± 2 °C) and relative humidity of 50 ± 10 % in standard polypropylene cages (four per cage), under a 12/12 hrs light/dark cycle. Animals were freely allowed food and water. This study was performed in accordance with the Guide for the Care and Use of Laboratory Animals of Tabriz University of Medical Sciences, Tabriz-Iran (National Institutes of Health publication No 85–23, revised 1985).

The rats were divided into a control group and 18 test groups, which consisted of 8 rats in each group. The animals were fed with standard laboratory food (rat chow) for one week.

To check the presence of any possible analgesic effect of normal saline, 2 mL of normal saline solution was gavaged in one group. In the control group only 50 µl of formalin solution 2.5 % (v: v) was injected subcutaneously into right foot of the animals and the rats did not receive any drug.

In the test groups, formulations were dispersed in 2 mL of normal saline solution and then were gavaged orally according to the following protocol: Four groups were received pure diclofenac Na powder (2.5, 5, 10, and 20 mg/Kg); three groups were received an effective dose of pure diclofenac Na powder (20 mg/Kg); three groups were received the nanoformulation; three groups were received the solid dispersion; and finally three groups were received the physical mixture (all equivalent to effective dose). All tests were performed between 8 am to 2 pm.

One hour (in the first group), two hours (in the second group) and three hours (in the third group) after the gavage, formalin solution was injected subcutaneously in the right foot. Immediately after injection, the animals were placed in the special glass chamber (20×25×40 cm) equipped with a mirror (with a 45 degree angle in the bottom) to evaluate the reaction to pain carefully. Reactions to injection of formalin solution was measured by stopwatch and recorded up to 5 minutes, in the first phase, and from 20 to 60 minutes, in the second phase.

Statistical analysis

One way ANOVA test followed by Tukey post test was used for comparisons between the treatment and control groups. Data were presented as Mean ± SEM. The P values <0.05 was considered as significance level during this study.

Results

Effect of different doses of formalin on licking time

In the animals which received formalin 2.5 % (v:v), paw licking time in the phase I (0-5 minutes) and phase II (20-60 min) were 79.0 ± 5.4 and 260.1 ± 6.7 seconds, respectively. Subcutaneous injection of 50 µl formalin solution 5 % (v:v) did not show any significant difference (p>0.05) in the duration of pain when compared with formalin 2.5% (Figure 1). Therefore, in order to avoid complications due to increased concentrations of formalin and tissue destruction, formalin 2.5 % (v: v) was applied to induce the inflammatory pain.

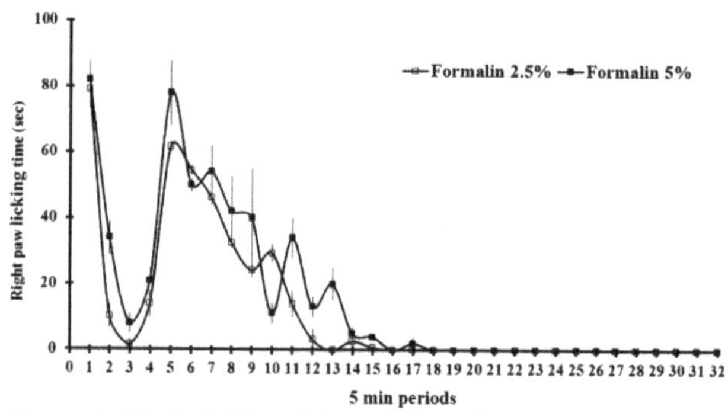

Figure 1. Effect of different doses of formalin on the licking time in the rats

Effect of different doses of pure diclofenac Na powder on the licking time

In order to investigate the effect of different doses of pure diclofenac Na on the licking time as well as to find the effective dose of the drug, four doses of pure drug powder (2.5, 5, 10, and 20 mg/Kg) were administered to the four groups of animals one hour before the injection of formalin.

In the first phase, no significant difference (p>0.05) was detected between the control group and the groups which received different doses of pure diclofenac Na. However, in the second phase, only the group which received a dose of 20 mg/kg of pure drug powder showed significant difference ($p<0.05$) in the licking time (220.25 ± 8.0 sec) compared to the control group (268.6 ± 9.4 sec) (Table 1). Therefore, the effective dose of pure diclofenac Na powder was determined as 20 mg/kg.

Table 1. Effect of different doses of pure diclofenac on licking time in phases I and II.

Group	Phase I (sec)	Phase II (sec)
Control	79.0 ± 5.4	268.6 ± 9.4
Normal Saline	81.0 ± 3.6	260.5± 8.9
Diclofenac 2.5 mg	74.8 ± 5.0	260.1±6.7
Diclofenac 5 mg	74.5 ± 3.2	251.2 ± 7.3
Diclofenac 10 mg	70.6 ± 6.1	246.3 ± 8.1
Diclofenac 20 mg	79.0 ± 5.4	220.2 ±8.1*

Results were expressed as mean ± SEM. (*: $p<0.05$ compared to the control group).

The animals which received 20 mg/mL of pure diclofenac Na powder did not show any significant difference ($p>0.05$) in phase I. On the other hand, following administration of the pure drug after one and two hours (phase II) the licking time was decreased significantly ($p<0.05$) from 268.6 ± 9.4 sec to 220.2 ± 8.0 sec and 218.8 ± 13.5 sec, respectively. However, after 3 h, decrease in licking time was not significant ($p>0.05$) (Table 2).

Table 2. Effect of different formulations on licking time in phases I and II at times 1h, 2h and 3h.

Group		Phase I (sec)	Phase II (sec)
Control		79.0 ±5.4	268.6 ±9.4
Pure Diclofenac	1 h	70.6 ±6.2	220.2 ±8.0*
	2 h	74.1 ±7.1	218.8 ±13.5*
	3 h	76.5 ±5.4	240.7 ±9.4
Physical mixture	1 h	75.0 ±8.6	224.2 ± 13.5*
	2 h	75.2 ±4.2	223.0 ±11.1*
	3 h	81.6 ±6.9	243.0 ±10.4
Solid dispersion	1 h	73.2 ±8.1	190.1 ±7.7***
	2 h	76.5 ±5.2	189.1 ±9.3***,#
	3 h	76.6 ±7.8	192.5 ±7.9***,##
Nanoparticles	1 h	70.0 ±5.9	166.7± 7.1***,a
	2 h	71.2 ±7.3	165.6 ±8.2***,###,a
	3 h	72.6 ±5.9	167.6 ±6.7***,###,a

Results were expressed as mean ±SEM. (*: $p<0.05$ and ***: $p<0.001$ compared to the control group,#: $p<0.05$, ##: $p<0.01$ and ###: $p<0.001$ compared to the pure diclofenac received groupand[a]: $p<0.05$) compared to the solid dispersionreceived group.

Effect of physical mixtures of diclofenac Na and Eudragit® RS100 on the licking time

In the phase I, there was no significant difference ($p>0.05$) between the control group and the group which received the physical mixture (Table 2). Nevertheless, the significant difference ($p<0.05$) was revealed between these groups only in times 1 h and 2 h of the phase II. However, the effects of physical mixtures did not significantly differ ($p>0.05$) from that of pure drug powder in the corresponding times.

Effect of the solid dispersion on licking time in phase I and II after different times

Similar to the previous groups, in the phase I, the licking times in the group which received the solid dispersion were not significantly ($p>0.05$) decreased compared to the control group (Table 2). However, in the phase II, difference in the licking time after all the three times was remarkably significant ($p<0.001$) compared to the control group. Then again, in comparison with pure diclofenac Na powder, the solid dispersion could significantly decrease the licking time after 2 h ($p<0.05$) and 3 h ($p<0.01$).

Effect of the nanoparticles on licking time

As it is shown in Table 2, the nanoparticles of diclofenac Na-Eudragit® RS100 could not decrease the licking time in phase I. However, in phase II, in all of the administered times, a significant difference was observed between the group which received the nanoparticles and the control group ($p<0.001$). Furthermore, the licking time in the nanoparticle administered animals was significantly less than the group which received pure drug powder ($p<0.001$) and the solid dispersion ($p<0.05$).

Discussion

The analgesic effects of pure diclofenac Na powder in the consecutive hours of pain are shown in Table 1. In the first phase, there was no significant difference ($p>0.05$) between pure diclofenac Na administered group and the control group demonstrating that diclofenac Na was not effective in the acute phase of pain. However, the analgesic effect was detected in the chronic phase of the pain. Lack of significant differences in the third hours of second phase, could be due to low half-life of drug in plasma (1-2 hr).

The analgesic effect of the physical mixture was not significantly ($p>0.05$) higher than that of pure drug powder, signifying that Eudragit® RS100 had no effect on pain reduction nevertheless the process and the type of formulation was important.

Table 2 also reveals that the analgesic effects of the solid dispersion and nanoparticles did not also show significant differences ($p>0.05$) in the first phase compared to the control group. However, the analgesic differences at the third hour (chronic phase) were noticeably significant ($p<0.05$) for the both formulations compared to the control group. Moreover, the results showed that these formulations had retained their analgesic effect which could be because of the slow release of diclofenac Na in the GI environments.

In the first phase, there was no significant difference ($p>0.05$) between the analgesic effect of the nanoparticles and solid dispersion, nevertheless the appropriate analgesic effect was observed by the nanoparticles in the chronic phase. This effect was interestingly superior than the solid dispersion associated analgesic effect which could be owing to the slow release of the drug from the nanoparticles as well as the increased absorption of the nanoparticles.

The comparison of the analgesic effects of the different formulations in the third hour after the pain experience indicated that unlike the pure drug powder and the physical mixture, the solid dispersion and nanoparticles prolonged the analgesic effect which could be as a result of slow drug release from these formulations.

According to our previously published findings, the mean particle size of diclofenac Na-Eudragit® RS100 nanoparticles with the drug/polymer ratio of 1:1 was 103±60 nm and the size distribution was relatively monodisperse (polydispersity index = 0.320 ± 0.083).[10] Due to sub-micron size of the nanoparticles, these particles can easily penetrate into the tissue, which lead to the reaching of the appropriate amount of drug into the targeted site of the body.[18] Other features of the nanoparticles are the delivery of drugs into the specific parts or organelles inside the cells making possible the increased bioavailability and reduced side effects of the drugs.[18]

Uptake of the particles can be take place by various processes such as phagocytosis, endocytosis or pinocytosis which are receptor-mediated.[19,20] Eudragit® RS100 with the zeta potential of 35 mV, produces positive charge on the surface of the nanoparticles and facilitate their uptake by the negatively charged cells.

Conclusion

According to the formalin test results, the nanoparticles and solid dispersion of diclofenac Na and Eudragit® RS100 showed higher intense and also duration of analgesic effects than pure drug which could be attributed to the improved physicochemical property and sustained release of the drug from these formulations. Physical mixture of diclofenac Na and Eudragit® RS100 showed similar analgesic effects with the pure drug powder. Nanoparticles also showed better analgesic effect than the solid dispersion which can be due to the higher absorption of the nanoparticles from GI tract and/or reduced drug removal by the phagocytic system. Because of the high risk of diclofenac Na toxicity which can initiate severe side effects in gastrointestinal track such as peptic ulceration and gastrointestinal bleeding, nanoparticles and solid dispersions of diclofenac Na could be considered as suitable candidates for drug delivery.

Acknowledgments

We wish to thank the Drug Applied Research Center, Tabriz University of Medical Sciences for supporting of this study. This article is based on a thesis submitted for Pharm. D degree (No. 3602) in Faculty of Pharmacy, Tabriz University of Medical Sciences, Tabriz, Iran.

Conflict of Interest

The authors declare no conflict of interests.

References

1. Di Maio S, Carrier RL. Gastrointestinal contents in fasted state and post-lipid ingestion: In vivo measurements and in vitro models for studying oral drug delivery. *J Control Release* 2011;151(2):110-22.
2. Keller J. Gastrointestinal Digestion and Absorption. In: Lennarz WJ, Lane MD, editors. Encyclopedia of Biological Chemistry. Waltham: Academic Press; 2013. P. 354-9.
3. Tao SL, Desai TA. Gastrointestinal patch systems for oral drug delivery. *Drug Discov Today* 2005;10(13):909-15.
4. Baraf HS, Gold MS, Petruschke RA, Wieman MS. Tolerability of topical diclofenac sodium 1% gel for osteoarthritis in seniors and patients with comorbidities. *Am J Geriatr Pharmacother* 2012;10(1):47-60.
5. De La Garza RII, Fabrizio KR, Radoi GE, Vlad T, Asnis GM. The non-steroidal anti-inflammatory drug diclofenac sodium attenuates lipopolysaccharide-induced alterations to reward behavior and corticosterone release. *Behav Brain Res* 2004;149(1):77-85.
6. Piao H, Kamiya N, Watanabe J, Yokoyama H, Hirata A, Fujii T, et al. Oral delivery of diclofenac sodium using a novel solid-in-oil suspension. *Int J Pharm* 2006;313(1–2):159-62.
7. Tawfeek HM. Evaluation of PEG and mPEG-co-(PGA-co-PDL) microparticles loaded with sodium diclofenac. *Saudi Pharm J* 2013;21(4):387-97.
8. Nayak AK, Pal D. Development of pH-sensitive tamarind seed polysaccharide-alginate composite beads for controlled diclofenac sodium delivery using response surface methodology. *Int J Biol Macromol* 2011;49(4):784-93.
9. Soares GA, De Castro AD, Cury BS, Evangelista RC. Blends of cross-linked high amylose starch/pectin loaded with diclofenac. *Carbohydr Polym* 2013;91(1):135-42.
10. Barzegar-Jalali M, Alaei-Beirami M, Javadzadeh Y, Mohammadi G, Hamidi A, Andalib S, et al. Comparison of physicochemical characteristics and drug release of diclofenac sodium–eudragit® RS100 nanoparticles and solid dispersions. *Powder Technol* 2012;219:211-6.

11. Adibkia K, Barzegar-Jalali M, Javadzadeh Y, Maheri-Esfanjani H. A review on the methods and applications of spray drying technology. *Pharmaceutical Sciences* 2012;18(2):119-32.
12. Adibkia K, Barzegar-Jalali M, Maheri-Esfanjani H, Ghanbarzadeh S, Shokri J, Sabzevari A, et al. Physicochemical characterization of naproxen solid dispersions prepared via spray drying technology. *Powder Technol* 2013;246:448-55.
13. Adibkia K, Barzegar-Jalali M, Mohammadi G, Ebrahimnejhad H, Alaei-Beirami M. Effect of sodium alginate chain length and Ca2+and Al 3+on the release of diltiazem from matrices. *Pharmaceutical Sciences* 2011;16(4):221-8.
14. Adibkia K, Barzegar-Jalali M, Nokhodchi A, Siahi Shadbad MR, Omidi Y, Javadzadeh Y, et al. A review on the methods of preparation of pharmaceutical nanoparticles. *Pharmaceutical Sciences* 2009;15(4):303-14.
15. Adibkia K, Javadzadeh Y, Dastmalchi S, Mohammadi G, Niri FK, Alaei-Beirami M. Naproxen-eudragit® RS100 nanoparticles: Preparation and physicochemical characterization. *Colloids Surf B Biointerfaces* 2011;83(1):155-9.
16. Barzegar-Jalali M, Dastmalchi S. Kinetic analysis of chlorpropamide dissolution from solid dispersions. *Drug Dev Ind Pharm* 2007;33(1):63-70.
17. Javadzadeh Y, Adibkia K, Bozorgmehr Z, Dastmalchi S. Evaluating retardation and physicochemical properties of co-ground mixture of Na- diclofenac with magnesium stearate Original Research Article. *Powder Technol* 2012;218:51-6.
18. Panyam J, Labhasetwar V. Biodegradable nanoparticles for drug and gene delivery to cells and tissue. *Adv Drug Deliv Rev* 2002;55(3):329-47.
19. Foster KA, Yazdanin M, Audus KL. Microparticulate uptake mechanisms of in-vitro cell culture models of the respiratory epithelium. *J Pharm Pharmacol* 2001;53(1):57-66.
20. Suh H, Jeong B, Rathi R, Kim SW. Regulation of smooth muscle cell proliferation using paclitaxel-loaded poly(ethylene oxide)-poly(lactide/glycolide) nanospheres. *J Biomed Mater Res* 1998;42(2):331-8.

Clofarabine Has Apoptotic Effect on T47D Breast Cancer Cell Line via P53R2 Gene Expression

Mohammad Rahmati-Yamchi[1,2*], Nosratollah Zarghami[2], Hojjatollah Nozad Charoudeh[3], Yasin Ahmadi[1,2], Behzad Baradaran[1], Mohammad Khalaj-Kondori[4], Morteza Milani[5], Abolfazl Akbarzadeh[5], Maghsud Shaker[6], Mohammad Pourhassan-Moghaddam[7]

[1] *Immunology Research Center, Tabriz University of Medical Sciences, Tabriz, Iran.*
[2] *Department of Clinical Biochemistry, Faculty of Medicine, Tabriz University of Medical Sciences, Tabriz, Iran.*
[3] *Stem Cell Research center, Tabriz University of Medical Sciences, Tabriz, Iran.*
[4] *Department of Biology, Faculty of Natural Science, University of Tabriz, Tabriz, Iran*
5 *Liver and Gastrointestinal disease research center, Tabriz University of Medical Sciences, Tabriz, Iran.*
[6] *Department of Clinical Biochemistry, Faculty of Medicine, Tabriz University of Medical Sciences, Tabriz, Iran.*
[7] *Department of Medical biotechnology, Tabriz University of Medical Sciences, Tabriz, Iran.*

Article info

Keywords:
· Apoptosis
· Breast Cancer
· DNA damage
· P53R2

Abstract

Purpose: Clofarabine, a purine nucleoside analogue and inhibitor of Ribonucleotide Reductase (RR), is used for treatment of leukemia. Clofarabine-induced defect in DNA replication, induces p53 and subsequently P53R2 genes as subunit of RR. clofarabine deregulated P53R2 gene expression leading to the elevated levels of P53R2 which impose resistance to DNA damaging drugs. In this study the apoptotic and cytotoxic effects of clofarabine has been investigated on breast cancer cell line.
Methods: Cofarabine cytotoxicity on T47D cells has been studied by MTT assay. T47D cells were exposed to the different concentrations of clofarabine for 24, 48 and 72 hours intervals. Relative expression of P53R2 gene has been studied using real-time PCR. Moreover, after treating with clofarabine the apoptotic and necrotic cells were detected using Annexin V and propodium iodide (PI) reagents by flowcytometry technique.
Results: MTT assay results showed that the clofarabine IC50 on T47D cell line were 3 and 2.5μM after 48 and 72 h exposure, respectively. Clofarabine did not show any significant cytotoxic effect after 24 h exposure. The analysis of qRT-PCR showed a significant increase in P53R2 gene expression in treated cells with both 2.5 and 3 μM doses and also, the results of flowcytometry revealed 26.91 and 74.46 percent apoptosis induction in 48 and 72h treatments respectively in comparison to the control groups.
Conclusion: Our results showed that apoptotic and cytotoxic effects of clofarabine on T47D cell line were in time and dose dependent manner; therefore it could be considered a new candidate in breast cancer therapy.

Introduction

After surgery, the standard procedure for treatment of breast cancer is chemotherapy. Clofarabin, one of the compounds that are used in chemotherapy, is a purine nucleoside analogue that has a strong inhibitory effect on wide-spread leukemia and some of solid tumors such as ovary, prostate, kidney and breast.[1-3] In the unphosphorylated form, clofarabine passes through the cell membrane using several transporting system including diffusion, facilitated diffusion and active transportation, and it is phosphorylates by intracellular kinases to its mono, di and three phosphates forms.[1] From these forms, only clolfarabine-3 phosphate is therapeutically active, and the remaining forms act as intracellular clofarabine reservoir.[2-4]

Clofarabine-3P plays its roles through different mechanisms including: a) it competes with dATP during DNA replication and repair. b) it binds to allostric site of regulatory subunits of Ribonucleotide Reductase (RR) enzyme and inhibts dCTP, dATP formation. Reducing the dCTP level limits DNA synthesis and reactivates deoxyCytidinekinase (dCK) and subsequently increases formation of clofarabine-3P. Also, high clofarabin - 3P/dATP concentration ratio results in priority of clofarabine-3P to dATP in competition for DNA-polymerase. c) It induces apoptosis through inhibition of DNA repair.[2-5]

P53R2, a p53-induced peptide, is a homologue of R2 subunit, which can substitute with R2 subunit in RR structure. RR is a tetramer composed of two different

***Corresponding author:** Mohammad Rahmati-Yamchi, Email: rahmatimo@tbzmed.ac.ir homodimers including hRRM1 (R1) and hRRM2 (R2).[6,7] P53, R1 and R2 are expressed in a cell cycle dependent manner. R1 and R2 expressed completely during the S-phase.[8,9] R2 gene is regulated by cell cycle-associated transcription factors, such as NF-Y and E2F;[10] however, P53R2 is regulated by p53 in response to genotoxic stresses such as irradiation.[11] After DNA damage, p53 not only causes to cell-cycle arrest in the G1 and G2 phases, but also induces P53R2 gene expression. Subsequently, P53R2 accumulates in cell nuclear and increases RR activity.[12,13] However, P53R2 activation may not be fast enough to provide dNTPs immidiatly, which can be completed during a few hours after DNA damage. It is shown that ATM phosphorylates P53R2 in response to genotoxic stress. This modification is essential for maintaining P53R2 protein stability against degradation by ubiquitylation.[14]

Because of the long half-life, R1 level is constant higher than R2 level throughout cell cycle.[6,15] In early G1-phase, R2, but not P53R2, is degraded by cadherin 1/anaphase promoting complex (Cdh1/APC).[12] Thus, in G1phase, P53R2 acts with R1 instead of R2 to provide dNTPs for DNA.[15-17] So there are two independent pathways in providing dNTPs: first, R2 provides dNTPs in S-phase and second, P53R2 provides dNTPs for DNA repair in G1 or G2-phase.[12]

The maximum level of P53R2 has been found at G1/S transition.[6] Furthermore, P53R2 up-regulates P21 and down-regulates cyclin D,[15] causing cell cycle arrest in G1 and providing both time and dNTP for the repair of damaged DNA.

Also, P53R2 plays an important role in mitochondrial veracity. Based on previous studies, mutations in P53R2 are associated with severe depletion of mitochondrial DNA in both human and mouse cell lines.[18,19] Moreover, P53R2 may plays a role in scavenging reactive oxygen species (ROS) and thereby protecting mitochondrial membrane from oxidative stress.[12] In addition, P53R2 down-regulates MEK-ERK signal pathway through direct interaction with ERK-Kinase2.[20] MEK-ERK signaling pathway regulates various cellular processes including cell cycle progression and cell survival, thus inhibition of this pathway is another anti-cancer property of P53R2.[21,22]

Since the P53R2 is critical molecule in dNTP formation and DNA repair, we hypothesizes that clofarabine might plays a role in apoptosis and cancer therapy by altering the expression levels of P53R2 gene. To evaluate this hypothesis, T47D breast cancer cell line was treated with several concentrations of clofarabine in different times. The MTT assay, flowcytometry, and qRT-PCR were used for evaluation of cytotoxicity, apoptosis and gene expression, respectively.

Materials and Methods

Human epithelial breast cancer cell line (T47D) was purchased from Pasteur Institute (Iran), RPMI1640 powdered cell culture medium was purchased from Gibco (England), Fetal Bovine Serum (FBS), Penicillin/ streptomycin 100X, Trypsin-EDTA 10X and Trypan-blue were acquired from Biosera (England); MTT reagent (3-(4,5-dimetylthiazol-2-yl)-2,5-diphenyltetrazolium bromide were obtained from Sigma (USA), PI was from CALBIOCHEM (Germany), cDNA synthesis kit and Real Time-PCR master mix were provided from Thermo Scientific (USA), RNX-Plus was purchased from Sinaclon (Iran). Clofarabine was obtained from Sigma (USA).

Cell culture

T47D cells were propagated in RPMI1640 media supplemented with 10% fetal bovine serum (FBS), 2mM of glutamine, penicillin (100 U/ml) and streptomycin (100 g/ml), at 37°C in a 5% CO_2 humidified atmosphere. Then, cells were seeded into plates for MTT assay and into flasks (25 cm^2) for gene expression and apoptosis studies, respectively.

Cytotoxicity assay

Before doing MTT assay, the count and viability of cultured cells were determined u8sing a hemocytometer. Then, for MTT assay, the cells were seeded at 5×10^3 cells per well in 96-well culture plates and were settled at 37°C for 24 h, followed by treatment with different concentrations of clofarabine (1.5 - 8μM). The concentration of clofarabine that inhibited cell proliferation by 50% (IC_{50}s) was determined from MTT assay data after 24, 48 and 72h treatments. Each experiment was done in triplicate manner.

P53R2 gene expression

The cells were seeded in 7 flasks with concentration of 1×10^6 cells/flask. Then 3 flasks were treated with IC_{50} of 48h exposure time for 24, 48 and 72h exposure, and other three flasks were treated with IC_{50} of 72h exposure time for 24, 48 and 72h exposure times; and last flask was served as control group. Total RNA was extracted from cultured cells using RNX Plus kit and 1μg of total RNA was used as substrate for reverse transcription using Thermo Scientific cDNA synthesis kit according to the manufacturer's protocols. Quantification of genes expression was performed with master mix from Thermo scientific company using thermo-cycler Corbet 2000 real-time PCR mashine. PCR primers were 5'-AGG CTC GCT TCT ATG GC-3' (forward) and5'-TCT GCT ATC CAT CGC AAG GC-3' (reverse) for P53R2. Gene expression levels in each cDNA sample were normalized to the internal β-actin gene expression level (Forward primer: 5′ACCGTGAAAAGATGACCCAG3′ and Reverse primer: 5′CCATACCCAAGAAGGAAGGC3′). The experiments were done in triplicate manner for each sample.

Apoptosis assay

T74D cells were seeded at concentration of 1×10^6 cells/ flask. One of these flasks was used as control and other two flasks were used for 48 and 72h treatment with clofarabine. The 24 h time exposure was not included in the experiments, because after treatments the 24 h exposure did not show significant cytotoxic effects on T47D cell line. After treatments, apoptosis detection kit (CALBIOCHEM, Germany) was used for apoptosis evaluation according to the manufacturer's protocol.

Statistical analysis

The alteration of P53R2 gene expression was analyzed by $\Delta\Delta$Ct method and version 16 of SPSS (with $p<0.05$) was used for statistical analyses. The results of apoptosis experiment were analyzed by Flowjo software.

Results

Clofarabine has cytotoxicity effect on T47D cell line

Clofarabine induces DNA damage and therefore it can impose cytotoxicity effect on T47D cells. After treatment of T47D cell line with different concentrations of clofarabine for 24, 48 and 72h, clofarabine IC_{50} was calculated as 3µM for 48h treatment and 2.5µM for 72h treatment. In this study, after 24h treatment, clofarabine did not show cytotoxic effect on T47D cell line (Figures 1 and 2). These results show that clofarabine at the longer treatment duration has a stronger cytotoxic effect on T47D cell line.

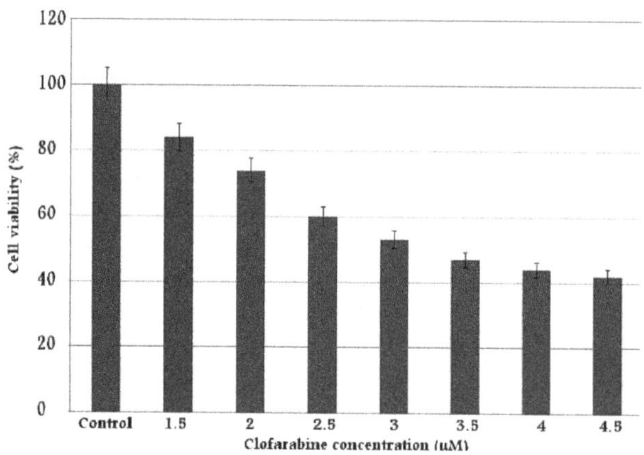

Figure 1. The results of MTT assay after 48h treatment with different concentrations of clofarabine. 3µM clofarabine is cytotoxic to half of cellular population (IC_{50} of 48h).

Clofarabine induces P53R2 gene expression

Clofarabine inhibits RR complex that results in gradual reduction of dNTPs pool. Low level of dNTPs inhibits or defects repair of damaged DNA which induces p53 and p53R2 proteins,subsequently. Upon binding of P53R2 to R1, they form an active RR complex that provides dNTPs for repair of DNA.

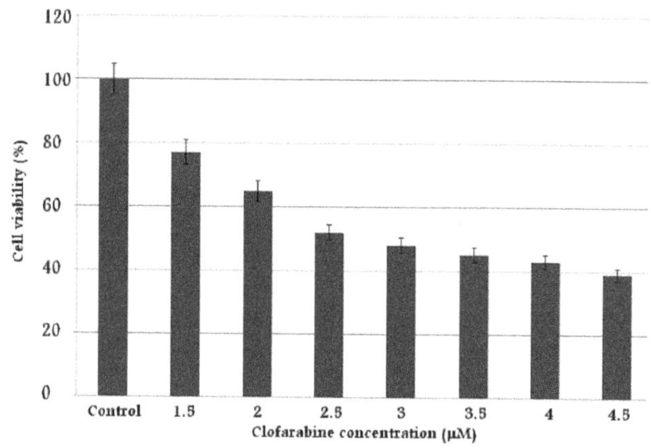

Figure 2. The results of MTT assay after 72h treatment with different concentrations of clofarabine. 2.5µM clofarabine induces cell death in half of cellular population (IC_{50} of 72h).

P53R2 expression after 24, 48 and 72h treatments with two clofarabine concentrations equal to acquired IC_{50}s (2.5 and 3µM) has shown in Table 1 and Figure 3. Based on the results, the higher concentration of clofarabine and longer treatment duration induce p53R2 gene expression more efficiently, but it seems that the effect of treatment duration is more significant than the effect of concentration (Figure 3). In other words, in longer treatment duration, the P53R2 gene expression was increased regularly.

Table 1. The effect of clofarabine on P53R2 gene expression in T47D cell line

samples	clofarabine concentration (µM)	P53R2 gene expression (fold change)
control	0	1
24h	3 µM	3.83
	2.5µM	8.39
48h	3 µM	28.24
	2.5µM	18.76
72h	3 µM	76.10
	2.5µM	61.39

The level of P53R2 gene expression after treatment with different clofarabine concentrations (3 µM and 2.5µM), shows that clofarabine induces P53R2 gene expression and it's level is directly related to treatment duration so that in treatment of 24h the gene expression is after the lowest level and after treatment of 72h is in the highest level .

Clofarabine induces apoptosis in T47D cell line

As mentioned earlier, clofarabine causes DNA damage by RR complex inhibition. And it can induce P53 gene expression that induces.

As shown in Table 2, after 48 and 72h treatments, clofarabine induced apoptosis in T47D cell line about 26.91% and 74.46%, respectively. These results show that treatment in longer duration is more effective for induction of apoptosis. The flowcytometry results for control, 48 and 72h treatments are shown in Figures 4-6.

Table 2. The apoptotic effect of clofarabine on T47D cell line

Cell situation (%)	Live cells (LL)	Apoptotic cells (LR)	Late apoptotic and necrotic cells (UR)	Necrotic cells (UL)
Control	97.24	0.09	0.68	1.99
After 48h treatment	63.52	7.73	19.18	9.57
After 72h treatment	21.15	7.59	66.87*	4.45

The results of flowcytometry (the percentage of live cell, early apoptotic, late apoptotic, and necrotic cells) after treatment of T47D cell line with 3µM clofarabine. The number of dead cells in the treated samples after 48 and 72h is remarkably more than the control sample. On the other hand, the number of apoptotic cells after 72h treatment is more than 48h treatment which suggests that clofarabine induces more apoptosis in longer duration treatment time. *: apoptosis induction in the treated cells is significant in comparison to the control group.

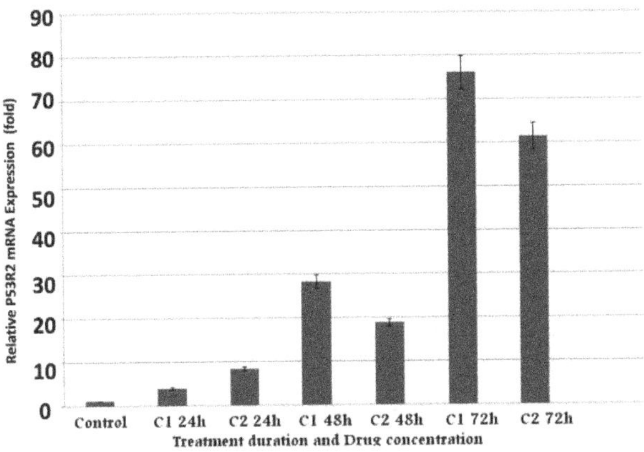

Figure 3. The clofarabine effect on P53R2 gene expression. As this figure shows, in higher clofarabine concentrations and treatment durations, the expression of P53R2 increases. P53R2 expression is more dependent on treatment duration than clofarabine concentration (C1=3µM amd C2=2.5µM). *: increasing in P53R2 gene expression is significant in comparison to the control group.

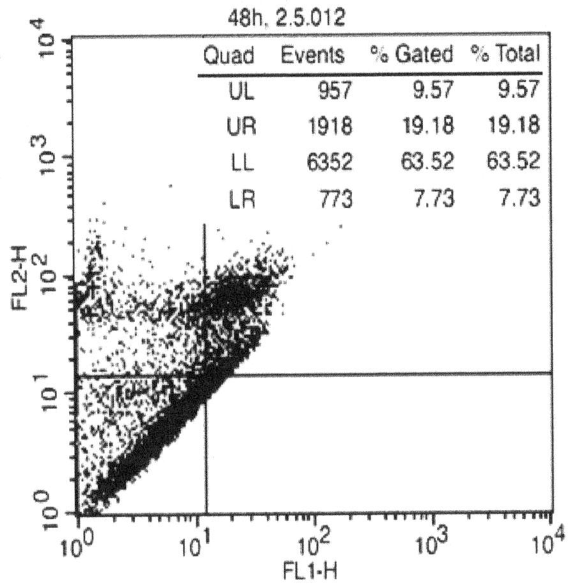

Figure 5. The flowcytometry result after 48h treatment with 3µM of clofarabine. After treatment there is a significant cell death.

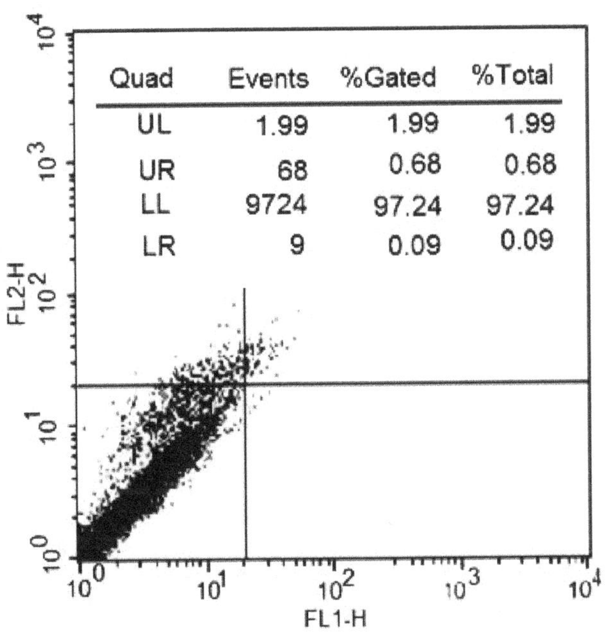

Figure 4. The flowcytometry result for the control sample. It shows there is an acceptable amount of alive cells in the control sample (%97.24), on the other hand the number of necrotic and apoptotic cell are not remarkable.

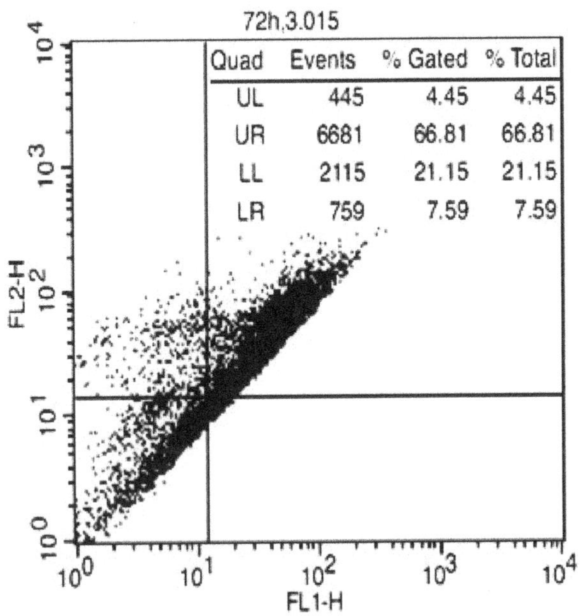

Figure 6. the flowcytometry result for 72h treatment with 3µM of clofarabine. The number of dead cells has increased significantly in comparison with control and treatment of 48h samples.

Discussion

Clofarabine is a therapeutic agent in treatment of leukemias, also, has a good inhibitory effect up on several solid tumors such as ovary and colon cancers.[23,24] The results of the present study show that clofarabine inhibits T47D cell growth. It means that clofarabine might have anti-cancer effects on breast cancer. It has been shown that clofarabine had anti-cancer effect by induction of p53 and P21 in MDA-MB-231 breast cancer cell line.[25] Considering the results of the present study, in T47D breast cancer cell line, clofarabine induces DNA damage and P53R2 gene expression. Therefore, clofarabine could plays cytotoxic effect by induction of DNA damage and gene expression on T47D cells line. Based on the results of flowcytometry, clofarabine can induces apoptosis in T47D cell line through induction of DNA damage and subsequent activation of internal apoptosis pathway. Deregulated expression of P53R2 has been shown in various cancer types.[20] P53R2 repairs DNA and acts as scavenger of ROS, maintaining cell survival of both cancerous and non-cancerous cells. Also, other studies showed apposite effects and in some cancers elevated P53R2 level can causes cancer progression through exerting resistance to DNA damaging therapies such as clofarabine and radiotherapy. Therefore, it is possible that clofarabine-induced P53R2 gene expression, attenuates cytotoxic effect of clofarabine on T47D cell and other solid cancer, and interesting neglable cytotoxic effect of clofarabine on T47D cells during 24 h exposure confirms anti-apoptotic behavior of P53R2 protein in breast cancer.

Conclusion

Clofarabine possess cytotoxic effect on T47D cell line and induces its apoptosis. On the other hand, it acts as an inducer for P53R2 gene expression. Some studies have reported that P53R2 can improve cancer cell response to therapy. Regarding to anti-growth effect of clofarabine on T47D cell line as in vitro model of breast cancer, further studies are required to study anti-cancer efficacy of clofarabine on breast cancer animal models, before using it in the clinical trial studies.

Acknowledgments

This study was supported by Immunology Research Center of Tabriz University of Medical Sciences, Tabriz, Iran.

Conflict of Interest

The authors declare that they have no conflict of interest.

References

1. Jeha S, Gaynon PS, Razzouk BI, Franklin J, Kadota R, Shen V, et al. Phase II study of clofarabine in pediatric patients with refractory or relapsed acute lymphoblastic leukemia. *J Clin Oncol* 2006;24(12):1917-23. doi: 10.1200/JCO.2005.03.8554
2. Zhenchuk A, Lotfi K, Juliusson G, Albertioni F. Mechanisms of anti-cancer action and pharmacology of clofarabine. *Biochem Pharmacol* 2009;78(11):1351-9. doi: 10.1016/j.bcp.2009.06.094
3. Nagai S, Takenaka K, Nachagari D, Rose C, Domoney K, Sun D, et al. Deoxycytidine kinase modulates the impact of the ABC transporter ABCG2 on clofarabine cytotoxicity. *Cancer Res* 2011;71(5):1781-91. doi: 10.1158/0008-5472.CAN-10-1919
4. Pui CH, Jeha S. Clofarabine. *Nat Rev Drug Discov* 2005;Suppl:S12-3.
5. Faderl S, Gandhi V, Keating MJ, Jeha S, Plunkett W, Kantarjian HM. The role of clofarabine in hematologic and solid malignancies--development of a next-generation nucleoside analog. *Cancer* 2005;103(10):1985-95. doi: 10.1002/cncr.21005
6. Wang X, Zhenchuk A, Wiman KG. Regulation of p53R2 and its role as potential target for cancer therapy. *Cancer Lett* 2009;276(1):1-7. doi: 10.1016/j.canlet.2008.07.019
7. Yanamoto S, Kawasaki G, Yoshitomi I, Mizuno A. Expression of p53R2, newly p53 target in oral normal epithelium, epithelial dysplasia and squamous cell carcinoma. *Cancer Lett* 2003;190(2):233-43. doi: 10.1016/s0304-3835(02)00588-8
8. Nakamura Y. Isolation of p53-target genes and their functional analysis. *Cancer Sci* 2004;95(1):7-11. doi: 10.1111/j.1349-7006.2004.tb03163.x
9. Zhou B, Liu X, Mo X, Xue L, Darwish D, Qiu W, et al. The human ribonucleotide reductase subunit hRRM2 complements p53R2 in response to UV-induced DNA repair in cells with mutant p53. *Cancer Res* 2003;63(20):6583-94.
10. Hakansson P, Hofer A, Thelander L. Regulation of mammalian ribonucleotide reduction and dNTP pools after DNA damage and in resting cells. J Biol Chem 2006;281(12):7834-41. doi: 10.1074/jbc.M512894200
11. Nakano K, Bálint E, Ashcroft M, Vousden KH. A ribonucleotide reductase gene is a transcriptional target of p53 and p73. *Oncogene* 2000;19(37):4283-9. doi: 10.1038/sj.onc.1203774
12. Xue L, Zhou B, Liu X, Heung Y, Chau J, Chu E, et al. Ribonucleotide reductase small subunit p53R2 facilitates p21 induction of G1 arrest under UV irradiation. *Cancer Res* 2007;67(1):16-21. doi: 10.1158/0008-5472.CAN-06-3200
13. Yamaguchi T, Matsuda K, Sagiya Y, Iwadate M, Fujino MA, Nakamura Y, et al. p53R2-dependent pathway for DNA synthesis in a p53-regulated cell cycle checkpoint. *Cancer Res* 2001;61(22):8256-62.
14. Chang L, Zhou B, Hu S, Guo R, Liu X, Jones SN, et al. ATM-mediated serine 72 phosphorylation stabilizes ribonucleotide reductase small subunit p53R2 protein against MDM2 to DNA damage. *Proc*

Natl Acad Sci U S A 2008;105(47):18519-24. doi: 10.1073/pnas.0803313105

15. Zhang K, Wu J, Wu X, Wang X, Wang Y, Zhou N, et al. P53R2 inhibits the proliferation of human cancer cells in association with cell-cycle arrest. *Mol Cancer Ther* 2011;10(2):269-78. doi: 10.1158/1535-7163.MCT-10-0728
16. Pontarin G, Ferraro P, Bee L, Reichard P, Bianchi V. Mammalian ribonucleotide reductase subunit p53R2 is required for mitochondrial DNA replication and DNA repair in quiescent cells. *Proc Natl Acad Sci U S A* 2012;109(33):13302-7. doi: 10.1073/pnas.1211289109
17. Morikawa T, Maeda D, Kume H, Homma Y, Fukayama M. Ribonucleotide reductase M2 subunit is a novel diagnostic marker and a potential therapeutic target in bladder cancer. *Histopathology* 2010;57(6):885-92. doi: 10.1111/j.1365-2559.2010.03725.x
18. Wang X, Liu X, Xue L, Zhang K, Kuo ML, Hu S, et al. Ribonucleotide reductase subunit p53R2 regulates mitochondria homeostasis and function in KB and PC-3 cancer cells. *Biochem Biophys Res Commun* 2011;410(1):102-7. doi: 10.1016/j.bbrc.2011.05.114
19. Thelander L. Ribonucleotide reductase and mitochondrial DNA synthesis. *Nat Genet* 2007;39(6):703-4. doi: 10.1038/ng0607-703
20. Piao C, Jin M, Kim HB, Lee SM, Amatya PN, Hyun JW, et al. Ribonucleotide reductase small subunit p53R2 suppresses MEK-ERK activity by binding to ERK kinase 2. *Oncogene* 2009;28(21):2173-84. doi: 10.1038/onc.2009.84
21. McCubrey JA, Steelman LS, Chappell WH, Abrams SL, Wong EW, Chang F, et al. Roles of the Raf/MEK/ERK pathway in cell growth, malignant transformation and drug resistance. *Biochim Biophys Acta* 2007;1773(8):1263-84. doi: 10.1016/j.bbamcr.2006.10.001
22. Peyssonnaux C, Eychene A. The Raf/MEK/ERK pathway: New concepts of activation. *Biol Cell* 2001;93(1-2):53-62. doi: 10.1016/s0248-4900(01)01125-x
23. Bonate PL, Arthaud L, Cantrell WR Jr, Stephenson K, Secrist JA 3rd, Weitman S. Discovery and development of clofarabine: A nucleoside analogue for treating cancer. *Nat Rev Drug Discov* 2006;5(10):855-63. doi: 10.1038/nrd2055
24. Kantarjian HM, Gandhi V, Kozuch P, Faderl S, Giles F, Cortes J, et al. Phase I clinical and pharmacology study of clofarabine in patients with solid and hematologic cancers. *J Clin Oncol* 2003;21(6):1167-73. doi: 10.1200/jco.2003.04.031
25. Lubecka-Pietruszewska K, Kaufman-Szymczyk A, Stefanska B, Cebula-Obrzut B, Smolewski P, Fabianowska-Majewska K. Clofarabine, a novel adenosine analogue, reactivates DNA methylation-silenced tumour suppressor genes and inhibits cell growth in breast cancer cells. *Eur J Pharmacol* 2014;723:276-87. doi: 10.1016/j.ejphar.2013.11.021

3

Evaluating the Anti-nociceptive and Anti-inflammatory Effects of Ketotifen and Fexofenadine in Rats

Mahdieh Anoush[1,2]*, Mohammad Reza Mohammad Khani[1]

[1] *Department of Pharmacology& Toxicology, School of Pharmacy, Zanjan University of Medical Sciences, Znjan, Iran.*
[2] *Applied Drug Research Center, Zanjan University of Medical Sciences, Znjan, Iran.*

Article info

Keywords:
- Ketotifen
- Fexofenadine
- Analgesic
- Anti-inflammatory
- Formalin test
- Carrageenan test

Abstract

Purpose: As H1 and H3 receptors' roles has been defined in peripheral pains in some papers and because histamine is known for its role in inflammatory responses; this study investigated the possible analgesic and anti-inflammatory effects of ketotifen and fexofenadine as relatively safe long acting anti histamines in both chronic chemical pain and acute inflammation in rats.
Methods: In this study, male Sprague-Dawley rats weighing 225-250 grams were used. In order to evaluate the chemical chronic pain, sub-plantar injection of formalin applied and the pain scores were recorded every 15 seconds during 60 minutes. Carrageenan injection to the right hind paw was used for induction of acute inflammation and the paw edema was measured every 60 minutes for 4 hours.
Results: Based on the results, both ketotifen and fexofenadine were able to significantly diminish chemical acute and chronic pain as well as inflammation in comparison with the control group and the effects were acceptable according to the standard treatment. Both effects for fexofenadine started later than those of ketotifen.
Conclusion: According to the outcomes of the study, ketotifen and fexofenadine demonstrated significant analgesic and anti-inflammatory characteristics in both models of chemical pain and acute inflammation in laboratory animals.

Introduction

The possible role of histamine in pain and inflammation was reported in 1958 for the first time,[1] but was under estimated till 1983.[2] Later on, lots of papers suggest different aspects of histamine as the main autocoid in allergic symptoms. Yet very few papers, suggest it as an inflammatory mediator until 2003 during which, a study on knockout mice represented the role of anti-histamines in inflammation.[3] Apparently the next step was to determine the role of different histamine blocking agents in the management of allergic reactions as well as pain and inflammation; While the role of H1 anti histamines in this area was neglected, may be because of their vast effects according to their CNS penetration property.

The major clinical treatment for allergic diseases at the present is suppression of inflammation symptoms.[4] Allergic reactions involve the release of histamine or other mediators from mast cells, cellular infiltration and inflammation respectively.[5] Allergy symptoms can be relieved effectively by suppressing any of these events.[6]

Fexofenadine, the active metabolite of terfenadine, is selective histaminic H1 receptor antagonist currently indicated for use in seasonal allergic rhinitis and chronic idiopathic urticaria worldwide,[7] which was believed not to cross the blood brain barrier (BBB) till 2009.[8] Fexofenadine is rapidly absorbed and has a long duration of action, making it suitable for once daily administration.[9] It undergoes minimal metabolism,[10] therefore is used as a probe substrate for the P-glycoprotein efflux transporter (P-gp). Fexofenadine has been shown to suppress eosinophil-induced inflammatory cytokine release from epithelial cells,[11] and to inhibit the release of chemotransmitters from basophils in vitro.[12]

Ketotifen also was suggested to improve allergic inflammation by decreasing lymphocytes in bronchial asthma[13] and later on known as a mast cell stabilizer.[14-15] There is no approved evidence for analgesic property of ketotifen except a controlled trial carried out in year 1994 in order to control neurofibroma-associated pain and itching using ketotifen again as a mast cell stabilizer.[16]

Despite the importance and high prevalence of conditions related to pain and inflammation, the number of new analgesics and anti-inflammations that have been introduced into clinical practice remains low.[17] Among the most widely used medications for inflammation, are non steroidal anti-inflammatory drugs (NSAIDs) which their world wide use is because of their demonstrated efficacy in reducing pain and inflammation.[18]

Although effective at relieving pain and inflammation, NSAIDs are associated with serious adverse events specially in chronic administration.[19] Thus, many pharmaceutical industries and researchers have dedicated

***Corresponding author:** Mahdieh Anoush, Email: anoushm@zums.ac.ir

their efforts to search for safer drugs representing the same effect or even less potencies but with less adverse effects.
Histaminic receptors especially H1[3,20] and H4[21-23] receptors have been shown to interfere with pain and inflammation. Therefore it can be deducted that their antagonists could possibly inhibit pain and inflammation.[24]
Based on the above mentioned evidences, we have investigated, for the first time, the anti-nociceptive and anti –inflammatory effects of fexofenadine and ketotifen in chronic pain induction model using formalin test; as well as an inflammation model of carrageenan induced paw edema in rats.

Materials and Methods

Animals

Male Sprague-Dawley rats (225-250g) were used in the present study. Animals were bred in animal department, School of Pharmacy, and were housed in the animal holding unit with a 12h light-darkness cycle and air-conditioning (22 ±2°C; 45-55% humidity), in Plexi-glass cages with free access to food and water.
The animals were handled and used according to the animal handling protocol of Zanjan University of Medical Sciences, Zanjan, Iran; which was approved by ethics committee. All animals were given a 3 day time to get acclimatized with laboratory conditions before experiments begin.

Chemicals

Chemicals include: Carrageenan lambda type I and formalin 35% obtained from Sigma-Aldrich. Fexofenadine (Batch No.ABEH000696) and ketotifen (Batch No.ABDH005217) powders purchased from Soha (Iran). Normal saline serum and diclofenac ampoules were bought from Abureihan (Iran), and Tolid Darou (Iran) Respectively.

Experimental design

All the experiments designed in a way that the number of animals decreases to an optimum level with the best result and reproducibility.
9 groups of animals received 3 different doses of ketotifen, fexofenadine and diclofenac in both formalin test and carrageenan induced inflammation in order to find the appropriate dose which has been reported in this study. The dose-response curves were omitted in order to abstracting the result section.

Carrageenan-induced Paw Edema in Rats

72 Male Sprague-Dawley (S.D) rats were rendered in nine groups of each 8. All animals received a sub-plantar injection of 50 µl 1% (w/v) solution of sterile carrageenan in saline to the right hind paw which caused acute inflammation.[24] Six groups of animals received 3 different doses of fexofenadine (10, 15, 20 mg/kg) and ketotifen (1, 1.5, 2 mg/kg), half an hour before carrageenan administration. Animals in the negative control group received normal saline (5ml/kg) and animals in the reference group received 25 mg/kg of Diclofenac, as the standard anti-inflammatory treatment.[25] The vehicle control group received carboxy methyl cellulose (5%), as the solvent for fexofenadine. It should be mentioned that ketotifen was dissolved in normal saline itself. According to the reference,[24] paw edema was measured before, and at the 1st, 2nd, 3rd and 4th hours after induction of inflammation, using a caliper vernier (scale.0.1mm). All treatments injected intraperitoneally (I.P).

Formalin Test and the Pain Score

In order to perform this test, 40 male S.D rats were rendered in 5 groups with 8 rats in each. Prior to injections, the animals were placed in a cone shaped chamber for 30 min. The experimental design is described below:
Negative control group received 5ml/kg of normal saline while positive control group treated with 25mg/kg of diclofenac as the standard drug. Animals in test groups received fexofenadine (15 mg/kg as the optimum dose) and ketotifen (1.5mg/kg as the optimum dose). The vehicle control group received CMC (5%). All treatments were administered I.P, followed by a sub-plantar injection of 50 µl formalin 2.5%.
The animals were then transferred to the mirror box (a plexi glass box with a 45 degree mirror at the bottom) in order to monitor the position of the animal in the chamber for accurate observation. They were observed by recording the reflexes every 15 seconds. The quantitative data was counted per 5 minutes and recorded based on the pain score on each time interval. The data gathered within 60 minutes. The first 5 minutes after injection for all groups was taken in account as acute phase, and 16-40 minutes as chronic phase.[25]

Statistical Analysis

In order to perform comparative statistical analysis SPSS 17.0 software was applied. The homogeneity of data was assessed using one way Analysis of Variances (ANOVA) while the possible differences between groups were reported using Tukey post-hoc test. All the results were expressed as (mean ± SEM) and P values less than 0.05 ($P < 0.05$) were determined as significant level of differences.

Results

Effects of Ketotifen on Carrageenan-induced Inflammation

After a sub-plantar injection of carrageenan the thickness of hind paw was measured in the rats received diclofenac, ketotifen and normal saline as positive control, test, and negative control groups respectively.
As it is shown in Figure 1, ketotifen (1.5 mg/kg) was able to decrease the hind-paw thickness significantly in comparison with negative control group ($P < 0.001$). The anti-inflammatory responses were weaker than that of diclofenac as the standard treatment, but not significantly ($P \geq 0.05$). The effects for ketotifen started after the second hour of inflammation (Figure 1).

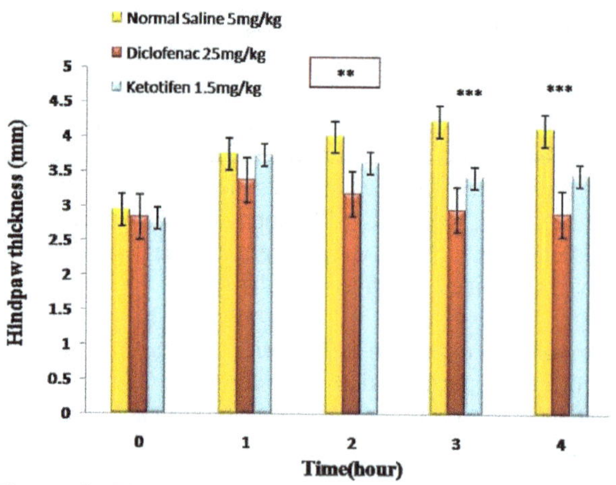

Figure 1. The anti-inflammatory effects of ketotifen and diclofenac towards hind paw edema. All values represent Mean ±S.E.M and are at least from 8 independent animals. ** (P <0.01), *** (P <0.001)

Effects of Fexofenadine on Carrageenan-induced Inflammation

In Figure 2 the anti-inflammatory effects of fexofenadine has been demonstrated. Fexofenadine (15 mg/kg) illustrated the best response in this test and showed a significant difference not only with negative control group but also with the vehicle control ($P < 0.001$). The anti-inflammatory effect started to be significant between second and third hour.

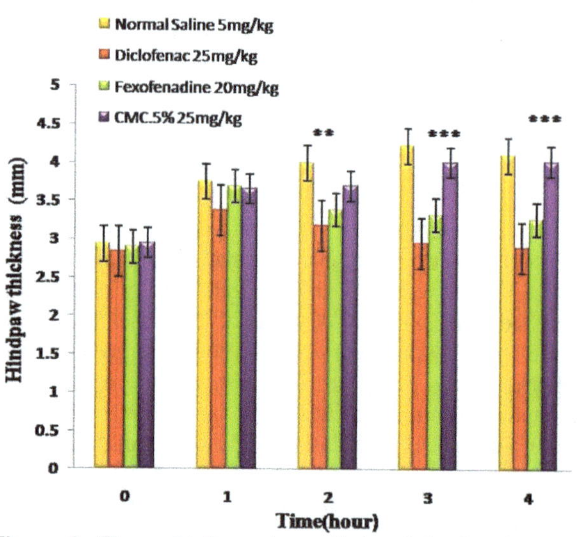

Figure 2. The anti-inflammatory effects of fexofenadine and diclofenac towards hind paw edema. All values represent Mean ±S.E.M and are at least from 8 independent animals. ** (P <0.05), *** (P <0.001)

Effects of Ketotifen on Formalin-induced Pain

In order to assess the analgesic effects of ketotifen, the pain score was calculated according to Dubuisson Dennis method[26] during 60 minutes. The results obtained from this method indicated that our treatments were effective in controlling both acute and chronic pain phases, but not when the animal experienced the maximum level of pain. As demonstrated in Figure 3, there has been reported no significant difference between diclofenac and ketotifen ($P \geq 0.05$) in both acute and chronic pain phases.

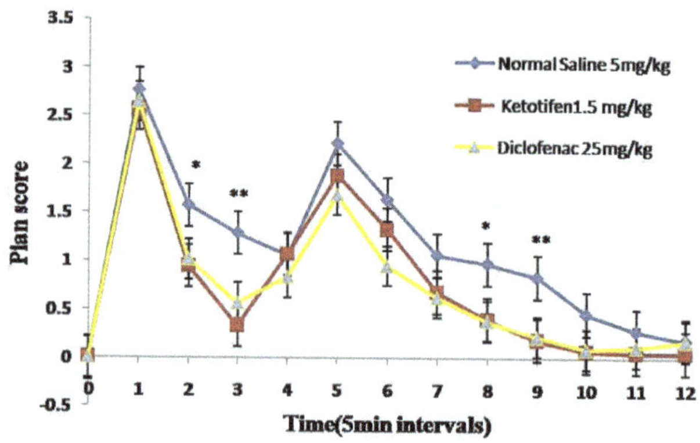

Figure 3. The effects of ketotifen and diclofenac on formaline induced hyper algesia. All values represent Mean ±S.E.M and are at least from 8 independent animals. * (P<0.05), ** (P <0.01)

Effects of Fexofenadine on Formalin-induced Pain

As it can be deducted from Figure 4, fexofenadine was not able to control acute phase of pain in comparison with negative control group ($P \geq 0.05$). Indeed, it was able to control the pain intensity in chronic phase. Besides, there were significant differences between groups received diclofenac and fexofenadine ($P < 0.05$) in acute pain phases (Figure 4).

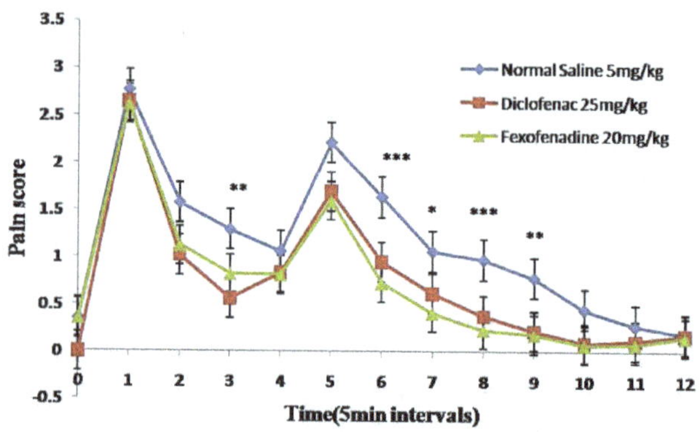

Figure 4. The effects of fexofenadine and diclofenac on formaline induced hyper algesia. All values represent Mean ±S.E.M and are at least from 8 independent animals. * (P <0.05), ** (P <0.01), *** (P <0.001)

Discussion

Based on the bibliographical searches, there were no studies carried out the assessment of both anti-inflammatory and anti nociceptive effects of two long acting H1 blocking agents ketotifen -with wide range of central effects- and fexofenadine (a safe H1 blocker with little central effects). This study reported these effects for the first time and suggested some possible related mechanisms.

In this study two different methods has been applied in order to identify the possible analgesic and anti-inflammatory effects of ketotifen and fexofenadine in rats.

Anti-inflammatory effects of ketotifen and fexofenadine

Results obtained from carrageenan test indicated a remarkable anti-inflammatory effect for ketotifen with a significant difference with the negative control group. This finding is in conformity with a research published in 2003 suggesting some novel mechanisms such as diminishing production of eotaxin and expression of CD29, in addition to the former well known mast-cell stabilizing effect of ketotifen, in management of inflammatory symptoms of allergy.[27] Besides it has been reported recently that ketotifen is able to decrease pro-inflammatory mediators, including nitric oxide, interleukin-1beta, and interleukin-6, production in rats with gouty inflammation.[28] The delay in responses to ketotifen might be because of its different mechanism with diclofenac in controlling the acute inflammation, but more studies needed to fulfill this claim. Fexofenadine also represented anti-inflammatory effects in this study. The first possible anti-inflammatory effect for fexofenadine was introduced by Abdelaziz who suggested that suggest that fexofenadine may reduce nasal inflammation by modulating the release of proinflammatory mediators and adhesion molecules from human nasal epithelial cell.[11] Later on, another study suggested that This study shows that terfenadine and fexofenadine exert a biologic effect directly on epithelial cells and fibroblasts reducing some adhesion molecules expression and release.[29]

Besides another research mentioned that fexofenadine is capable of modulating T-Cell functions which resulted in preventing airway inflanmmation.[30] Recently, other aspects of fexofenadine interfering with inflammation has been reported such as reducing methacholine-induced contractions of tracheal smooth muscle.[31] Fexofenadine's pro-drug has been suggested to use in chronically active ulcerative colitis in combination with sulfasalazine.[32] As this drug has a dose-dependent kinetics of penetrating into the CNS,[10] more studies needed to determine its central vs. peripheral effects. The most strong evidence in this field is a research in 2006 which has been proved that fexofenadine showed selective arachidonic acid-mediated COX-2 inhibitory enzyme activity and suggested that, the selective COX-2 inhibitor activity by fexofenadine may contribute to its anti-inflammatory properties.[33]

Anti nociceptive effects of ketotifen and fexofenadine

In 1989 two H1 blocking agents were introduced to have analgesic effects on acute surface pain while H2 blocker agents were proved to do nothing with pain.[34] Later on, an interaction between pain-relieving drugs and the brain histaminergic system was reported and multiple analgesic mechanisms suggested for antihistamines such as improgan and even cimetidine.[35] In addition, the role of histamine in different types of pain include central,[36] peripheral,[37] acute[38] chronic[39] or organ related pains such as muscle pain[40] was declared and the number of studies about antihistaminic agents administration as analgesic drugs have been augmented and hyper algesic role of H1 receptors have been proved strongly.[3,20]

In this study ketotifen was capable of inhibiting both acute and chronic phase in formalin induced pain model. The efficacy of ketotifen in pain managemen was suggested for the first time in 1993,[16] which was followed by very few researches but yet, the main emphasis was on its anti allergic with a few reports on its anti-inflammatory effects. Therefore no possible mechanisms for analgesic effects of ketotifen was released or reported yet. According to the results of this study and to this finding that ketotifen is able to penetrate BBB and interfere with paleospinothalamic pain transfer pathway; it can be deducted that this inhibition through unknown mediators might be the main mechanism for analgesic responses for ketotifen.

In the formalin test two phases of pain should be distinguished. The acute and the chronic pain phases which assumed as the first 5 minutes after formalin sub-plantar injection and the time period between 16-45 minutes, respectively; there is a gap between these two phases (minutes 5-16) with the least nociception responses. It has been assumed that these two stages represent two different type of pain related to direct nerve stimulation (acute pain) followed by an inflammatory process (chronic stage). In this study fexofenadine was able to inhibit both acute and chronic phases but its effects in acute phase were weaker than that of both diclofenac and ketotifen. This can be either because of systemic pharmacokinetics of fexofenadine resulted in a longer t-max time in comparison to ketotifen[10] or its special model for brain exposure which makes it difficult to penetrate from BBB.[41-42]

Even though there is a lack in documentary for analgesic properties of fexofenadine, this finding can be supported by a clinical finding of possible analgesic role of fexofenadine in incidence of myalgia while patients receive paclitaxel.[43]

According to the literature, a reduction in pain, inflammation and the signal transduction pathway(s) responsible for both above mentioned phenomenon in the acute stage results in a reduction in plasticity in dorsal root of spinal cord via deprivation in P substance [44] for ketotifen. In addition, some possible interactions between histaminic H1 receptor and opioid receptors have been suggested.[44-45]

Conclusion

It can be concluded that both ketotifen and fexofenadineis are capable of inhibiting pain and acute inflammation in rat models of sub-plantar injections of formalin and carrageenan respectively. The exact mechanism(s) for these effects need to be studied more, via receptor purification, using full antagonists, or Immuno histo chemistry assessments in the near future.

Acknowledgments

The authors wish to thank the Vice Chancellor's Office for Research Affairs because of the grant supporting this study (No. A-11-323-5).

Conflict of Interest

Authors declare no conflict of interest.

Abbreviations

IP (Intra Peritoneal), CNS (Central Nervous System), BBB (Blood Brain Barrier). P-gp (P-glycoprotein), NSAIDs (Non Steroidal Anti-Inflammatory Drugs)

References

1. Stern P. Inflammation & pain in histamine-free skin. *Acta Neuroveg (Wien)* 1958;18(1-4):237-41. doi: 10.1007/bf01234819
2. Galletti R, Chiarini P, Duranti R, Strazzulla G, Guazzelli R, Matassi L. Reactivation of the algogenic component in experimental inflammation induced by histamine administration. *Minerva Med* 1983;74(16):869-74.
3. Yanai K, Mobarakeh JI, Kuramasu A, Sakurada S. Roles of histamine receptors in pain perception: a study using receptors gene knockout mice. *Nihon Yakurigaku Zasshi* 2003;122(5):391-9. doi: 10.1254/fpj.122.391
4. Tiligada E. Editorial: is histamine the missing link in chronic inflammation? *J Leukoc Biol* 2012;92(1):4-6. doi: 10.1189/jlb.0212093
5. Somma T, Cinci L, Formicola G, Pini A, Thurmond R, Ennis M, et al. A selective antagonist of histamine H(4) receptors prevents antigen-induced airway inflammation and bronchoconstriction in guinea pigs: involvement of lipocortin-1. *Br J Pharmacol* 2013;170(1):200-13. doi: 10.1111/bph.12264
6. Neumann D, Schneider EH, Seifert R. Analysis of histamine receptor knockout mice in models of inflammation. *J Pharmacol Exp Ther* 2014;348(1):2-11. doi: 10.1124/jpet.113.204214
7. Simpson K, Jarvis B. Fexofenadine: a review of its use in the management of seasonal allergic rhinitis and chronic idiopathic urticaria. *Drugs* 2000;59(2):301-21. doi: 10.2165/00003495-200059020-00020
8. Tashiro M, Sakurada Y, Iwabuchi K, Mochizuki H, Kato M, Aoki M, et al. Central effects of fexofenadine and cetirizine: measurement of psychomotor performance, subjective sleepiness, and brain histamine H1-receptor occupancy using 11C-doxepin positron emission tomography. *J Clin Pharmacol* 2004;44(8):890-900. doi: 10.1177/0091270004267590
9. Craig-Mcfeely PM, Acharya NV, Shakir SA. Evaluation of the safety of fexofenadine from experience gained in general practice use in England in 1997. *Eur J Clin Pharmacol* 2001;57(4):313-20. doi: 10.1007/s002280100292
10. Chen C. Some pharmacokinetic aspects of the lipophilic terfenadine and zwitterionic fexofenadine in humans. *Drugs R D* 2007;8(5):301-14. doi: 10.2165/00126839-200708050-00004
11. Abdelaziz MM, Devalia JL, Khair OA, Bayram H, Prior AJ, Davies RJ. Effect of fexofenadine on eosinophil-induced changes in epithelial permeability and cytokine release from nasal epithelial cells of patients with seasonal allergic rhinitis. *J Allergy Clin Immunol* 1998;101(3):410-20. doi: 10.1016/s0091-6749(98)70256-8
12. Amon U, Amon S, Gibbs BF. In vitro studies with fexofenadine, a new nonsedating histamine H1 receptor antagonist, on isolated human basophils. *Inflamm Res* 2000;49 Suppl 1:S13-4. doi: 10.1007/pl00000160
13. Hoshino M. The effect of ketotifen on the inflammation of bronchial mucosa in atopic asthmatics. *Arerugi* 1994;43(6):689-95.
14. Klooker TK, Braak B, Koopman KE, Welting O, Wouters MM, Van Der Heide S, et al. The mast cell stabiliser ketotifen decreases visceral hypersensitivity and improves intestinal symptoms in patients with irritable bowel syndrome. *Gut* 2010;59(9):1213-21. doi: 10.1136/gut.2010.213108
15. Serna H, Porras M, Vergara P. Mast cell stabilizer ketotifen [4-(1-methyl-4-piperidylidene)-4h-benzo[4,5]cyclohepta[1,2-b]thiophen-10(9H)-one fumarate] prevents mucosal mast cell hyperplasia and intestinal dysmotility in experimental Trichinella spiralis inflammation in the rat. *J Pharmacol Exp Ther* 2006;319(3):1104-11. doi: 10.1124/jpet.106.104620
16. Riccardi VM. A controlled multiphase trial of ketotifen to minimize neurofibroma-associated pain and itching. *Arch Dermatol* 1993;129(5):577-81. doi: 10.1001/archderm.129.5.577
17. Parkitny L, Mcauley JH, Di Pietro F, Stanton TR, O'connell NE, Marinus J, et al. Inflammation in complex regional pain syndrome: a systematic review and meta-analysis. *Neurology* 2013;80(1):106-17. doi: 10.1212/wnl.0b013e31827b1aa1
18. Inflammation-induced pain. How rheumatism patients profit from the proper NSAID choice. *MMW Fortschr Med* 2012;154(8):74-5.
19. Scanzello CR, Moskowitz NK, Gibofsky A. The post-NSAID era: what to use now for the pharmacologic treatment of pain and inflammation in osteoarthritis. *Curr Rheumatol Rep* 2008;10(1):49-56. doi: 10.1007/s11926-008-0009-6
20. Mobarakeh JI, Sakurada S, Katsuyama S, Kutsuwa M, Kuramasu A, Lin ZY, et al. Role of histamine H(1) receptor in pain perception: a study of the receptor gene knockout mice. *Eur J Pharmacol* 2000;391(1-2):81-9. doi: 10.1016/s0014-2999(00)00060-1
21. Cowart MD, Altenbach RJ, Liu H, Hsieh GC, Drizin I, Milicic I, et al. Rotationally constrained 2,4-diamino-5,6-disubstituted pyrimidines: a new class of histamine H4 receptor antagonists with improved druglikeness and in vivo efficacy in pain and inflammation models. *J Med Chem* 2008;51(20):6547-57. doi: 10.1021/jm800670r
22. Kamo A, Negi O, Tengara S, Kamata Y, Noguchi A, Ogawa H, et al. Histamine H(4) receptor antagonists ineffective against itch and skin inflammation in atopic dermatitis mouse model. *J Invest Dermatol* 2014;134(2):546-8. doi: 10.1038/jid.2013.351

23. Cowden JM, Yu F, Banie H, Farahani M, Ling P, Nguyen S, et al. The histamine H4 receptor mediates inflammation and Th17 responses in preclinical models of arthritis. *Ann Rheum Dis* 2014;73(3):600-8. doi: 10.1136/annrheumdis-2013-203832
24. Coruzzi G, Adami M, Guaita E, De Esch IJ, Leurs R. Antiinflammatory and antinociceptive effects of the selective histamine H4-receptor antagonists JNJ7777120 and VUF6002 in a rat model of carrageenan-induced acute inflammation. *Eur J Pharmacol* 2007;563(1-3):240-4. doi: 10.1016/j.ejphar.2007.02.026
25. Nasri S, Anoush M, Khatmi N. Evaluation of analgesic and anti-inflammatory effects of fresh onion juice in experimental animals. *Afr J Pharm Pharmacol* 2012;6(23):1679-84. doi: 10.5897/ajpp12.179
26. Abbott FV, Franklin KB, Westbrook RF. The formalin test: scoring properties of the first and second phases of the pain response in rats. *Pain* 1995;60(1):91-102. doi: 10.1016/0304-3959(94)00095-v
27. Martin AP, Urrets-Zavalia J, Berra A, Mariani AL, Gallino N, Gomez Demel E, et al. The effect of ketotifen on inflammatory markers in allergic conjunctivitis: an open, uncontrolled study. *BMC Ophthalmol* 2003;3:2.
28. Hsu DZ, Chu PY, Chen SJ, Liu MY. Mast Cell Stabilizer Ketotifen Inhibits Gouty Inflammation in Rats. *Am J Ther* 2013. doi: 10.1097/MJT.0b013e31829ea238
29. Paolieri F, Battifora M, Riccio AM, Bertolini C, Cutolo M, Bloom M, et al. Terfenadine and fexofenadine reduce in vitro ICAM-1 expression on human continuous cell lines. *Ann Allergy Asthma Immunol* 1998;81(6):601-7. doi: 10.1016/s1081-1206(10)62712-3
30. Gelfand EW, Cui ZH, Takeda K, Kanehiro A, Joetham A. Fexofenadine modulates T-cell function, preventing allergen-induced airway inflammation and hyperresponsiveness. *J Allergy Clin Immunol* 2002;110(1):85-95. doi: 10.1067/mai.2002.124770a
31. Lai WS, Lin YY, Chu YH, Wang CH, Wang HW. Efficacy of fexofenadine in isolated rat tracheas. *Rhinology* 2013;51(4):376-80. doi: 10.4193/Rhin12.213
32. Dhaneshwar S, Gautam H. Exploring novel colon-targeting antihistaminic prodrug for colitis. *J Physiol Pharmacol* 2012;63(4):327-37.
33. Juergens UR, Gillissen A, Uen S, Racke K, Stober M, Darlath W, et al. New evidence of H1-receptor independent COX-2 inhibition by fexofenadine HCl in vitro. *Pharmacology* 2006;78(3):129-35. doi: 10.1159/000096016
34. Bjerring P. Effect of antihistamines on argon laser-induced cutaneous sensory and pain thresholds and on histamine-induced wheal and flare. *Skin Pharmacol* 1989;2(4):210-6. doi: 10.1159/000210822
35. Hough LB, Nalwalk JW, Svokos K, Leurs R, Timmermann H. Pain-relieving drugs and the brain histaminergic system: multiple analgesic mechanisms from histamine, improgan and cimetidine. *Inflamm Res* 2004;53 Suppl 1:S43-4. doi: 10.1007/s00011-003-0320-7
36. Erfanparast A, Tamaddonfard E, Farshid AA, Khalilzadeh E. Effect of microinjection of histamine into the dorsal hippocampus on the orofacial formalin-induced pain in rats. *Eur J Pharmacol* 2010;627(1-3):119-23. doi: 10.1016/j.ejphar.2009.10.063
37. Cannon KE, Leurs R, Hough LB. Activation of peripheral and spinal histamine H3 receptors inhibits formalin-induced inflammation and nociception, respectively. *Pharmacol Biochem Behav* 2007;88(1):122-9. doi: 10.1016/j.pbb.2007.07.014
38. Tamaddonfard E, Khalilzadeh E, Hamzeh-Gooshchi N, Seiednejhad-Yamchi S. Central effect of histamine in a rat model of acute trigeminal pain. *Pharmacol Rep* 2008;60(2):219-24.
39. Mobarakeh JI, Torkaman-Boutorabi A, Rahimi AA, Ghasri S, Nezhad RM, Hamzely A, et al. Interaction of histamine and calcitonin gene-related peptide in the formalin induced pain perception in rats. *Biomed Res* 2011;32(3):195-201. doi: 10.2220/biomedres.32.195
40. Wasner G, Schwarz K, Schattschneider J, Binder A, Jensen TS, Baron R. Interaction between histamine-induced itch and experimental muscle pain. *Eur J Pain* 2004;8(3):179-85. doi: 10.1016/s1090-3801(03)00099-5
41. Gundogdu E, Mangas-Sanjuan V, Gonzalez-Alvarez I, Bermejo M, Karasulu E. In vitro-in situ permeability and dissolution of fexofenadine with kinetic modeling in the presence of sodium dodecyl sulfate. *Eur J Drug Metab Pharmacokinet* 2012;37(1):65-75. doi: 10.1007/s13318-011-0059-4
42. Zhao R, Kalvass JC, Yanni SB, Bridges AS, Pollack GM. Fexofenadine brain exposure and the influence of blood-brain barrier P-glycoprotein after fexofenadine and terfenadine administration. *Drug Metab Dispos* 2009;37(3):529-35. doi: 10.1124/dmd.107.019893
43. Garrison JA, Mccune JS, Livingston RB, Linden HM, Gralow JR, Ellis GK, et al. Myalgias and arthralgias associated with paclitaxel. *Oncology (Williston Park)* 2003;17(2):271-7; discussion 81-2, 86-8.
44. Nakao K, Ikeda K, Kurokawa T, Togashi Y, Umeuchi H, Honda T, et al. Effect of TRK-820, a selective kappa opioid receptor agonist, on scratching behavior in an animal model of atopic dermatitis. *Nihon Shinkei Seishin Yakurigaku Zasshi* 2008;28(2):75-83.
45. Rehni AK, Singh TG, Singh N, Arora S. Tramadol-induced seizurogenic effect: a possible role of opioid-dependent histamine H1 receptor activation-linked mechanism. *Naunyn Schmiedebergs Arch Pharmacol* 2010;381(1):11-9. doi: 10.1007/s00210-009-0476-y

4

Doxorubicin Changes Bax/Bcl-x $_L$Ratio, Caspase-8 and 9 in Breast Cancer Cells

Simin Sharifi[1,2], Jaleh Barar[1,3], Mohammad Saeid Hejazi[1,4*], Nasser Samadi[3,4,5*]

[1]*Department of Pharmaceutical Biotechnology,* Faculty *of* Pharmacy, Tabriz University *of* Medical Sciences, *Tabriz, Iran.*
[2] *Students' Research Committee,* Tabriz University *of* Medical Sciences, *Tabriz, Iran.*
[3] *Research Center for Pharmaceutical Nanotechnology, Tabriz University of Medical Sciences, Tabriz, Iran.*
[4] *Faculty of Advanced Biomedical Sciences, Tabriz University of Medical Sciences, Tabriz, Iran.*
[5] *Department of Biochemistry and Medical Laboratories, Faculty of Medicine, Tabriz University of Medical Sciences, Tabriz, Iran.*

Article info

Keywords:
· MCF-7
· Apoptosis
· Doxorubicin
· Breast cancer
· *Bax /Bcl-x$_L$*
· Caspase-9

Abstract
Purpose: Doxorubicin is administrated as a single agent in first-line therapy of breast cancer to induce apoptosis in tumor cells. Bax, Bcl-xL, Caspase-8 and 9 proteins are involved in induction of apoptosis. The present study describes *Bax*, *Bcl-x$_L$* gene expression and Caspase-8 and 9 protein levels in MCF-7 cells incubated with doxorubicin at different doses an incubation times.
Methods: The cytotoxic effects of doxorubicin were studied using MTT assay. MCF-7 cells were treated with three concentrations of doxorubicin (0.1, 0.5, 1 μM) and incubated for 24, 48 and 72 hours then expression levels of *Bax* and *Bcl-x$_L$* genes were elucidated by Real-time RT-PCR technique and protein levels of caspase-8 and caspase-9 proteins were measured using ELISA method. Morphological modifications of the cells were also monitored via light microscopic images.
Results: Doxorubicin decreased the anti-apoptotic *Bcl-x$_L$* and increased pro-apoptotic *Bax* mRNA levels. Doxorubicin induced a significant increase in *Bax /Bcl-x$_L$* ratio in all doses and incubation times (p<0.05). Highest (more than 10 fold) increase in *Bax /Bcl-x$_L$* ratio was revealed after 48 h incubation of the cells with in all doses of doxorubicin. Doxorubicin also increased caspase-9 level in a time and dose-dependent manner, while caspase-8 level didn't follow time and dose dependency pattern.
Conclusion: Our results confirm that doxorubicin induces mitochondrial-dependent apoptosis by down-regulation of Bcl-xL and up- regulation of Bax and caspase-9 expressions.

Introduction

Apoptosis is the process of programmed cell death that occurs in response to environmental stimuli. Regulation of apoptosis is important for normal growth and homeostasis, during development, embryogenesis, and modification of normal tissues, also cancer treatment. Disorders of abnormal induction of apoptosis can cause severe outcomes.[1] Impaired regulation of apoptotic mechanisms provides an opportunity to growth cancerous cells and chemo-resistance. Apoptosis plays an important role in the treatment of cancer as it is the general goal of many treatment strategies.[2,3]

In mammalian cells, there are at least two main pathways that lead to apoptosis including extrinsic death-receptor dependent apoptosis and intrinsic mitochondrial dependent apoptosis.[4,5] In both extrinsic and intrinsic apoptotic pathways induction of cell death is associated with the activation of caspases.[6,7] Caspases are two types, initiator caspases (e.g. caspase-8 and -9) and effector caspases (e.g. caspase-3, -6, and -7). Caspase-8 is mainly activated in extrinsic apoptotic pathway, but caspase-9 activation is related to the mitochondrial or intrinsic pathway.[8] In anticancer chemotherapy, activation of caspases can be started through stimulating of the extrinsic pathway or by activation of intrinsic pathway at the mitochondria.[9,10]

One of the key regulators in the molecular mechanisms of apoptosis is the family of Bcl-2.[11] These proteins are attached to cell membrane or free in cytosol. They are operating in intracellular membranes of mitochondria that organize intrinsic apoptosis.[12,13] This family includes proapoptotic members including Bax, Bak and antiapoptotic members including Bcl-2, Bcl-x$_L$.[11,14-16] The localization of certain Bcl-2 family proteins changes when stimulation of apoptosis occurs. For example, Bax moves from cytosol to the membrane of mitochondria followed induction of apoptotic signals by an apoptotic stimulant.[17] The Bcl-2 gene is important in regulation of apoptosis that encodes variety of proteins that play key roles in regulation of cell apoptosis. *Bax* is another pro-apoptotic

***Corresponding authors:** Mohammad Saeid Hejazi, Email: msaeidhejazi@yahoo.com, Nasser Samadi, Email: drnsamadi@yahoo.com gene that meaningfully is homologous with Bcl-2.[14] However, Bax operates as an enhancer of apoptosis in contrast to Bcl-2 with antiapoptotic properties. Complex network of interactions between Bcl-2 family members both in the cytosol and on mitochondria determines the fate of the cell for death or survive.[13,18] Enhanced expression of *Bax* in breast cancer cells increases sensitivity to apoptotic stimuli and decreases tumour enlargement.[19] Bcl-x_L is another anti-apoptotic protein that inhibits apoptosis.[20] Progress of breast cancer has been associated with of Bcl-x_L expression.[21,22] Furthermore, it has been associated in advanced grade and development of metastatic cancer.[22] Since Bcl-x_L prevents apoptosis, this protein is considered as a key molecule to induce chemoresistance.[23]

A variety of stimuli and the molecular mechanisms of apoptosis are explained intensively.[24] Several chemotrapoetic agents have been identified to persuade apoptosis in cancer cells.[25] Doxorubicin is one of anthracycline drugs that used for treatment of variety of tumors especially solid tumors.[26] The mechanism for cytotoxic effects of doxorubicin is free radical production, DNA intercalating and blocking of topoisomerase II followed by preventing DNA replication and eventually DNA breakage.[27] Since doxorubicin is extensively utilized as a first line treatment of variety of different cancers including breast cancer, investigating the mechanisms of apoptosis induced by this chemotherapeutic agent is important.[27]

Breast cancer is second prevalent and deadly cancer in women worldwide.[28] Breast cancer treatment consists of radiotherapy, hormonal therapy and chemotherapy that stimulate apoptotic pathways followed by cancer cell death.[29] Different strategies have been developed for analysis and study of this cancer.[30-33] MCF-7 cell line is an excellent in vitro model for studying the mechanisms of chemoresistance as it is susceptible to apoptosis and applied for various investigations on apoptosis or survival of cancer cells.[34-36] Although the extensive clinical application of doxorubicin for cancer patients has been studied, its anti-proliferative and death-inducing signalling cascades are yet unclear. In this study, we investigated the molecular basis of induction of apoptosis by doxorubicin on MCF-7 cells. Cytotoxic effects of doxorubicin have been evaluated with MTT assay. Alteration in the expression of pro-apoptotic *Bax* and anti-apoptotic *Bcl-x_L* genes and *Bax/Bcl-x_L* ratio were investigated via Real-time RT-PCR method. Furthermore, the levels of caspase-8 and caspase-9 proteins have been evaluated with ELISA method.

Material and Methods

Cell culture

The human MCF-7 breast cancer cells were obtained from National Cell Bank of Iran (Pasteur Institute, Iran). The MCF-7 cells were cultivated in RPMI 1640 medium (Sigma, St Louis, MO, USA) enriched with 10% fetal bovine serum (FBS; Invitrogen), 100 mg/ml streptomycin and 100 units/ml penicillin G (Sigma, St Louis, MO, USA). Cells were incubated in a humidified atmosphere with 5% CO2 at 37°C.

Cell viability assessment using MTT assay

Cell proliferation and viability of doxorubicin treated MCF-7 cells determined using 3-(4,5-dimethylthiazol-2-yl)-2,5-diphenyl- tetrazolium bromide (MTT) which evaluates the percentage of viable cells. The MCF-7 cells with 70% confluency were detached from the dish with 0.05% trypsin/EDTA solution. Cells were seeded into 96-well plate with concentration of 4×10^4 cells/cm^2.

Cells with about 50% confluency were exposed with increasing concentrations of the doxorubicin (Ebewe, Unterach, Austria) 0.1-10 μM to induce cytotoxicity. Four wells were remained untreated as control. MTT assay was carried out 24, 48 and 72 hours after treatments. To prepare MTT (Sigma-Aldrich, St. Louis, MO) reagent, 2mg of MTT powder was dissolved in 1 ml PBS. The culture medium was exchanged with 150 μl fresh media plus 50 μl MTT reagent (2mg/ml in PBS); the cell-free wells were considered as blank controls. Cells were incubated in 37°C with 5% CO2 and humidified atmosphere for 4 hours. Then the MTT solution was removed and 200μl of DMSO were added to each well. The plate was maintained for 15 min at37 °C and then the optical density (OD) of the wells was determined at 570 nm through a spectrophotometric microplate reader (Biotek, EL x 800. USA).

RNA isolation and Assessment of mRNA expression via Real-time RT-PCR

Cultivated MCF-7 cells were treated with three concentrations of doxorubicin (0.1, 0.5, 1 μM) and incubated for 24, 48 and 72 hours. RNA extraction of treated cells was performed by RNX™-Plus Kit (CinnaGen, Iran) according to the protocol.

Quality of RNA was evaluated by agarose gel electrophoresis and concentration of extracted RNA was estimated by optical density measurement (A260/A280 ratio) with NanoDrop 1000 Spectrophotometer (Wilmington, DE, USA).

For synthesis of cDNA, reaction mixture was composed to 5μg extracted RNA, 1μg random hexonucleotides primersand 1μM deoxyribonucleotides (dNTP), 10 units RNase inhibitor and Moloney Murine Leukemia Virus SuperScript II® Reverse Transcriptase (M-MLV RT, Invitrogen). Then, the reaction tubes were maintained at 42°C for 60 min.

Real-time PCR technique was carried out using the SYBR *Green*-based PCR *Master Mix*. The iQ5 Optical System (Bio-Rad Laboratories, Inc., CA-USA) was used for performing all amplification reactions in a total volume of 25 μL. Each well in this experiment contained 1 μl of cDNA, 70-100 nM of each Primer (MWG Biotech, Ebersberg, Germany) and 12.5 μl of 2X Power SYBR green PCR Master Mix (Applied Biosystems, Warrington, UK). Applied Primer sequences and annealing temperature of them for Quantitative PCR showed in Table 1.

Table 1. Applied Primer sequences for Quantitative PCR of *Bax* and *Bcl-xL genes*.

Gene name	Primer sequence	Tm	Amplicon length (bp)
18S rRNA	F: 5'-CGATGCGGCGGCGTTATTC-3' R:5'-TCTGTCAATCCTGTCCGTGTCC-3'	59.4	198
Bcl-x_L	F: 5'- GTTCCCTTTCCTTCCATCC -3'(19) R: 5'- TAGCCAGTCCAGAGGTGAG -3'(19)	58	123
Bax	F: 5'- GATGCGTCCACCAAGAAG -3'(18) R: 5'- AGTTGAAGTTGCCGTCAG-3'(18)	56	163

For PCR thermal cycling program, the samples were included 10 min at 95 °C, 35 cycles of 30 s at 95 °C for denaturation step, 30 s at annealing temperature, and 30 s at 72°C for the extension respectively. Final 10 min incubation at 72°C was carried out to completion of amplicons. mRNA expressions were calculated in compare with 18S rRNA (housekeeping gene) expression. Melting-curve analysis was carried out after amplification to verification the validity of the amplicons. For reporting of gene expression level Pfaffl method was applied.

Analysis of Caspase-8 and Caspase-9 production
To measure Caspase-8 and Caspase-9 protein levels, MCF-7 cells were treated with various concentrations of doxorubicin (0.1, 0.5, 1 μM) and incubated for 24, 48 and 72 hours. Then Caspase-8 and Caspase-9 levels were measured using enzyme-linked immunosorbent assay (Platinum ELISA; eBioscience©) according to the instructions of the manufacturer.

Morphology of doxorubicin treated cells
To study the alteration in morphology of the cells, doxorubicin were applied with concentrations of 0.1, 0.5, 1 μM and the cells were incubated for 24, 48 and 72 h. Light Microscopy was applied to study the morphology of alive and dead cells.

Statistical analysis
All statistical analyses were performed using SPSS 16.0 software. Data obtained from three or more individual experiments were expressed as mean ± SD. Data were analyzed by One-Way ANOVA and Tukey post Hoc tests. *p-values* less than 0.05 were considered as statistically significant.

Results
Cell viability and IC50 values in doxorubicin treated MCF-7 cells
MCF-7 cells were treated with various concentrations of the doxorubicin ranging from 0.1-10 μM for 24, 48 and 72 hours, and cell viability was measured by MTT assay. MTT assay showed that increased concentrations of the doxorubicin decreased the viability of cells in a time and concentration dependent manner. IC_{50} values were 0.75 μM for the cells incubated for 24 h and 0.25 μM for the cells incubated for both 48 and 72 h (Figure 1).

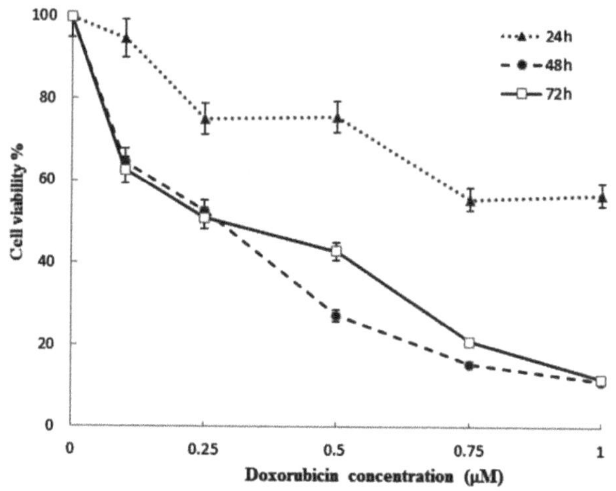

Figure 1.Column charts of MTT assay results of MCF-7 cell treated with different concentrations of doxorubicin.

Expression of Bax, Bcl-x_L genes and Bax /Bcl-$x_L$ratio in doxorubicin treated MCF-7 cells
Expression of *Bax* Gene significantly increased by increasing concentrations of doxorubicin (0.1, 0.5, 1 μM) after 24, 48 and 72 hours incubations ($p<0.05$) (Figur 2). Highest increase (4.5 fold) in expression of *Bax* revealed with 1μM doxorubicin after 72 h incubation. *Bcl-x_L* gene expression was decreased in 48 and 72 h (Figur 2. b). Highest decrease in *Bcl-x_L* mRNA level was shown after 48 h incubation. Change in *Bcl-x_L* gene expression was not dose dependent. Our results also revealed a significant increase in *Bax /Bcl-x_L* ratio in all doxorubicin concentrations ($p<0.05$). Highest increase in *Bax/Bcl-*x_L ratio (more than 10 fold) was revealed after 48 h incubation (Table 2).

Table 2.Bax/Bcl-x_L ratio was calculated and show that it was significantly increased in all of doxorubicin treated MCF-7 cells ($p<0.05$).

	doxorubicin concentration	*Bax/Bcl-x_L* ratio
24 h	0.1 μM	1.774
	0.5 μM	1.354
	1 μM	1.125
48 h	0.1 μM	13.445
	0.5 μM	14.976
	1 μM	11.950
72 h	0.1 μM	4.702
	0.5 μM	4.884
	1 μM	5.484

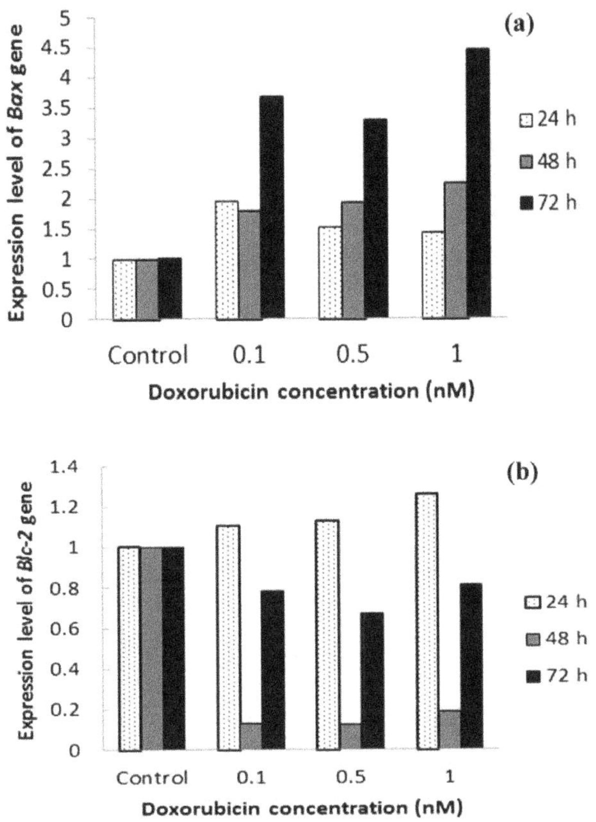

Figure 2. Expression of $Bcl\text{-}x_L$ and *Bax* genes in apoptosis pathway were investigated to demonstrate the induction of apoptosis by doxorubicin. Cultivated MCF-7 cells were treated with three concentrations of doxorubicin (0.1, 0.5, 1 μM) and incubated for 24, 48 and 72 hours.

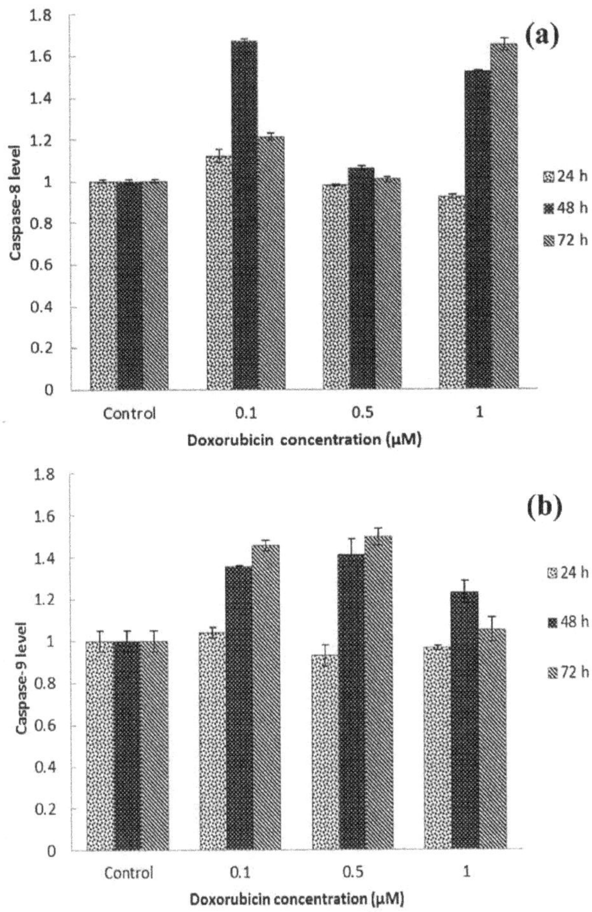

Figure 3. For evaluation of Caspase-8 and 9 was used from ELISA method. MCF-7 cell was treated with various concentrations of doxorubicin (0.1, 0.5, 1 μM) for 24, 48 and 72 hours. **a:** level of Caspase-8 and **b**: level of Caspase-9 in MCF-7 cell was treated with various concentrations of doxorubicin (0.1, 0.5, 1 μM) for 24, 48 72 hours compare with untreated MCF-7 cell.

Caspase-8 and 9 proteins level in doxorubicin treated MCF-7 cells

Caspase-8 levels in the cells exposed to doxorubicin (0.1, 0.5 and 1 μM) didn't show any significant increase after 24 h incubation ($p>0.05$). Caspase-8 levels increased with 0.1 and 1 μM concentrations of doxorubicin after 48 and 72 h incubation ($p<0.05$) (Figure. 3a).

Caspase-9 level showed no significant increase when we incubated the cells with different concentrations of doxorubicin after 24 h incubation ($p>0.05$). Doxorubicin (0.1 μM, 0.5 μM) also caused a significant increase in caspase-9 after 48 h and 72 h incubations ($p<0.05$) (Figure. 3b).

Alteration in morphology of MCF-7 cells by doxorubicin

Doxorubicin displayed morphological alterations in MCF-7 cells. Adherent cells after treated with doxorubicin became rounded, condensed and detached from the dish. Number of detached and rounded cells was increased by increase in the dose of doxorubicin and incubation time. Doxorubicin (0.1 μM) after 24 h incubation showed least and 1 μM doxorubicin with 72 h incubation showed the most rounded and detached cells in comparison with other doxorubicin concentrations and incubation times (Figure. 4 a-j).

Discussion

Cytotoxic agents induce apoptosis by initiating death signalling pathways in susceptible target cells.[37] Activating of apoptosis by chemotherapeutic agents is involved in simultaneous or consequent activation of death receptor systems, disturbance in mitochondrial function and proteolytic processing of caspases.[38] Thus, the cell death pathway may occur in several locations; however the accurate molecular mechanisms for each particular drug and special target cell have not been determined completely. In this study, the alteration in $Bcl\text{-}x_L$(anti-apoptotic), *Bax* (pro-apoptotic) genes' expression, *Bax* /$Bcl\text{-}x_L$ ratio and caspase 8 and 9 proteins' level following the stimulation of apoptosis by doxorubicin in MCF-7 cells were reported.

For evaluation of cytotoxicity induced by doxorubicin MTT assay was applied. The results demonstrated that the viability of MCF-7 cells was clearly decreased in a time and dose-dependent manner. IC50 values were 0.75, 0.25 and 0.25 μM for 24, 48 h and 72 h incubations respectively. Based on Lukyanova study, the IC50 of doxorubicin on MCF-7 was about 0.5 μM which is consistent with our findings.[39] Moreover, the reported IC50 of doxorubicin on MCF-7 were approximately 0.1 μM and 1.19 μM using MTT assay based on Fornari et al. and Taherian et al. studies, respectively. The mentioned differences can be explained regarding different brands of doxorubicin or technical strategies.[40,41]

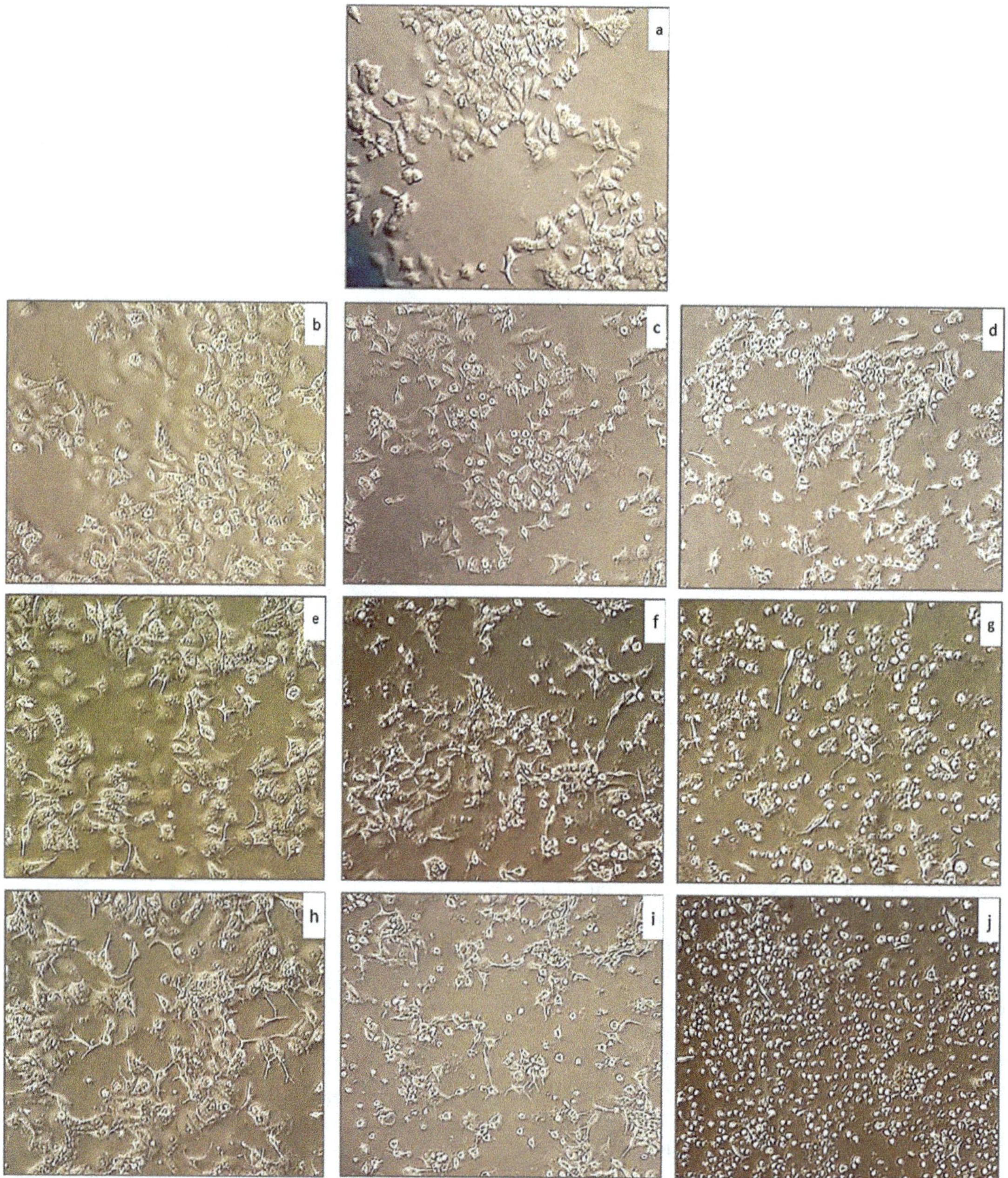

Figure 4. Morphology and cell death of doxorubicin treated MCF-7 cells was investigated via light Microscopic image. **a**: untreated MCF-7 cell line, **b**: MCF-7 cells treated with 0.1 μM for 24 h, **c**: cells treated with 0.5 μM for 24 h, **d**: cells treated with 1 μM for 24 h, **e**: treated with 0.1 μM for 48 h, **f**: cells treated with 0.5 μM for 48 h, **g**: cells treated with 1 μM for 48 h, **h**:cells treated with 0.1 μM for 72 h, **i**: cells treated with 0.5 μM for 72 h, **j**: cells treated with 1 μM for 72 h.

Members of the Bcl-2 family are main regulators of cell death or cell survival. Chemotherapeutic drugs apply their effects in part by controlling the expression of numerous members of the Bcl-2 family in MCF-7 cells. The Bcl-2 family proteins play a significant role in apoptosis, either as apoptotic activators (Bax) or as apoptotic inhibitors (Bcl-x_L).[42,43]

Bax and Bak are the effectors of the Bcl-2 family as upon activation, they change conformation, insert into the outer mitochondrial membrane, oligomerize, and induce mitochondrial outer membrane permeabilization (MOMP).[11,18] On the other hand, Bcl-x_L is a strong inhibitor of apoptosis that heterodimerize with Bax and neutralizes the effects of the latter. When Bcl-x_L is present in excess, cells are protected against apoptosis. In contrast, when Bax is in excess and the homodimers of Bax dominate, cells are susceptible to programmed death.

High expression of *Bax* gene in the cells incubated with doxorubicin demonstrated that doxorubicin has *Bax* enhancer effects followed by induction in intrinsic apoptosis pathway on MCF-7 breast cancer cells. April measured *Bax* in rats and declared that *Bax* declined markedly in the cells after treatment with doxorubicin.[44]

Our data showed that doxorubicin was reduced expression of Bcl-x_L protein, suggesting the importance of Bcl-2 family proteins for breast cancer cell survival. Clinical studies have showed that increased level of *Bcl-x_L* is related to a poor response to chemotherapy in breast cancer.[22,45]

In this study, expression of *Bcl-x_L* gene in doxorubicin treated MCF-7 cells was not time and dose dependent. The most decrease in expression of this gene was in the treated cells with 0.1, 0.5, 1 µM doxorubicin for 48 h which showed more than 5 fold decrease compared with non-treated MCF-7 cells ($p<0.05$).

Several apoptosis regulators have been associated with various human malignancies. For example, studies on human tumors have demonstrated an overall positive correlation between increased expression of *Bcl-x_L*, decreased expression of *Bax* and uncontrolled tumour cell growth (due to suppressed apoptosis). A wide range of experimental and clinical reports have demonstrated biological effects for doxorubicin. Similar results were shown with doxorubicin, which causes a decrease in *Bcl-2* expression and increase in *Bax* expression.[46] Other chemotherapeutic agents such as paclitaxel and thiotepa up-regulate several proapoptotic Bcl-2 proteins and down-regulate antiapoptotic Bcl-2 proteins.[47] Additionally, the present study evaluated the effects of doxorubicin on *Bcl-x_L* and *Bax* expression ratio in induction of apoptosis *in vitro*. The *Bax/Bcl-x_L* ratios determine the fate of a cell rather than the absolute concentration of either.[48] The treatment of MCF-7 cells with doxorubicin originate a significant percentage in the *Bax/Bcl-x_L* ratios ($p<0.05$). Thus, the imbalance between *Bcl-x_L* and *Bax* expressions during doxorubicin treatment is believed to play important role in doxorubicin-induced apoptosis as observed in this study and in other investigation.[49]

Mariana and Gonzalez suggest that *Bax/Bcl-x_L* expression ratio may be a sensitive monitor of cancer progression and an early predictor for cancer patients.[50]

In this study, we investigated at least three distinct parameters: absolute expression levels of *Bax* and *Bcl-x_L* genes and the ratio of these pro and antiapoptotic proteins. Our results support the existence of a specific apoptotic mechanism in MCF-7 cells that increasing in *Bax/Bcl-x_L* ratio causes the loss of cell viability and enhanced apoptosis.

Doxorubicin-induced apoptosis is regulated by the Bcl-2 family of proteins upstream of caspase activation. The *Bax* gene expression is known to cause the activation of caspases followed by apoptosis.[51-53] Caspases are members of a family of cysteine proteases that are divided into initiator caspases, such as caspase-8 and -9 and executioner caspases such as caspase-3 or -7.[54] Initiator caspase-8 is known to be activated through extrinsic pathway, whereas caspase-9 is activated in the event of mitochondrial cytochrome c leakage.[54,55]

In our study, treatment of the cells with doxorubicin caused a time dependent increase in caspase-9 levels, while caspase-8 level didn't follow time and dose dependency pattern. Liang *et al.*[56] showed that MCF-7 cells can undergo apoptosis by the sequential activation of caspases-9, -7, and -6. An increased level of caspase-9 is similar to Bax gene expression, therefore, both of these proteins increased with increase in doxorubicin dose and incubation time. Up regulation of caspase-9 takes place in doxorubicin treated MCF-7 cells. Bcl-x_L interacts with Apafl to prevent apoptosis by inhibiting Apafl dependent activation of caspase-9.[57] These results suggest that doxorubicin induced apoptosis via mitochondrial dependent intrinsic pathway.

In this study, decreased level of *Bcl-x_L* caused increase in caspase-9 levels consequently in apoptotic cells. These results are compatible with our other findings for the *Bax/Bcl-x_L*ratio, since BCL-2 family controls the intrinsic apoptotic pathway in doxorubicin treated MCF-7 breast cancer cells.

MCF7 cells are deficient in capase-3 expression because of a deletion mutation in their *caspase-3* gene, suggesting the existence of caspase-3-independent apoptotic pathways.[58,59] Participation of activated caspase-3 is crucial for activation of caspase-8 which explains our results on caspase 8 protein level in the cells with lack of caspase-3 protein level.[60] Therefore, increased level of caspase-8 couldn't trigger extrinsic apoptosis pathway in MCF-7 cells. This is compatible with other studies on a disabled Fas pathway in this cell line.[61]

The presence of caspase-3 can increase cell sensitivity to apoptosis-inducing agents. MCF-7 cells, which are relatively insensitive to many chemotherapeutic agents, acquire greater sensitivity to doxorubicin and etoposide-induced apoptosis when caspase-3 is reconstituted.[62] Future research may show whether maximizing cross-talk between the intrinsic and extrinsic pathways of apoptosis and up-regulation of caspase-3 are potential targets for breast cancer therapy.

In conclusion, our data suggest that increase in the *Bax/Bcl-x_L* ratio and caspase-9 level can play a key role in doxorubicin-induced apoptosis in MCF-7 cells, however further studies are warranted to validate these findings.

Acknowledgments

Authors would like to thank Research Center for Pharmaceutical Nanotechnology (RCPN) and Faculty of Advanced Biomedical Sciences for supporting this project (which was a part of PhD thesis No: 76).

Conflict of Interest

The authors report no conflicts of interest.

References

1. Jacobson MD, Weil M, Raff MC. Programmed cell death in animal development. *Cell* 1997;88(3):347-54. doi: 10.1016/s0092-8674(00)81873-5
2. Wong RS. Apoptosis in cancer: from pathogenesis to treatment. *J Exp Clin Cancer Res* 2011;30(1):87. doi: 10.1186/1756-9966-30-87
3. Johnstone RW, Ruefli AA, Lowe SW. Apoptosis: a link between cancer genetics and chemotherapy. *Cell* 2002;108(2):153-64. doi: 10.1016/s0092-8674(02)00625-6
4. Ashkenazi A, Dixit VM. Death receptors: signaling and modulation. *Science* 1998;281(5381):1305-8. doi: 10.1126/science.281.5381.1305
5. Harris MH, Thompson CB. The role of the Bcl-2 family in the regulation of outer mitochondrial membrane permeability. *Cell Death Differ* 2000;7(12):1182-91. doi: 10.1038/sj.cdd.4400781
6. Fulda S, Debatin KM. Extrinsic versus intrinsic apoptosis pathways in anticancer chemotherapy. *Oncogene* 2006;25(34):4798-811. doi: 10.1038/sj.onc.1209608
7. Degterev A, Boyce M, Yuan J. A decade of caspases. *Oncogene* 2003;22(53):8543-67. doi: 10.1038/sj.onc.1207107
8. Cryns V, Yuan J. Proteases to die for. *Genes Dev* 1998;12(11):1551-70. doi: 10.1101/gad.12.11.1551
9. Olsson M, Zhivotovsky B. Caspases and cancer. *Cell Death Differ* 2011;18(9):1441-9. doi: 10.1038/cdd.2011.30
10. Fulda S, Debatin KM. Targeting apoptosis pathways in cancer therapy. *Curr Cancer Drug Targets* 2004;4(7):569-76. doi: 10.2174/1568009043332763
11. Chipuk JE, Moldoveanu T, Llambi F, Parsons MJ, Green DR. The BCL-2 family reunion. *Mol Cell* 2010;37(3):299-310. doi: 10.1016/j.molcel.2010.01.025
12. Krajewski S, Tanaka S, Takayama S, Schibler MJ, Fenton W, Reed JC. Investigation of the subcellular distribution of the bcl-2 oncoprotein: residence in the nuclear envelope, endoplasmic reticulum, and outer mitochondrial membranes. *Cancer Res* 1993;53(19):4701-14.
13. Ola MS, Nawaz M, Ahsan H. Role of Bcl-2 family proteins and caspases in the regulation of apoptosis. *Mol Cell Biochem* 2011;351(1-2):41-58. doi: 10.1007/s11010-010-0709-x
14. Oltvai ZN, Milliman CL, Korsmeyer SJ. Bcl-2 heterodimerizes in vivo with a conserved homolog, Bax, that accelerates programmed cell death. *Cell* 1993;74(4):609-19. doi: 10.1016/0092-8674(93)90509-o
15. Kelly PN, Strasser A. The role of Bcl-2 and its pro-survival relatives in tumourigenesis and cancer therapy. *Cell Death Differ* 2011;18(9):1414-24. doi: 10.1038/cdd.2011.17
16. Reed JC. Bcl-2 family proteins. *Oncogene* 1998;17(25):3225-36. doi: 10.1038/sj.onc.1202591
17. Zhang H, Heim J, Meyhack B. Redistribution of Bax from cytosol to membranes is induced by apoptotic stimuli and is an early step in the apoptotic pathway. *Biochem Biophys Res Commun* 1998;251(2):454-9. doi: 10.1006/bbrc.1998.9485
18. Lindsay J, Esposti MD, Gilmore AP. Bcl-2 proteins and mitochondria--specificity in membrane targeting for death. *Biochim Biophys Acta* 2011;1813(4):532-9. doi: 10.1016/j.bbamcr.2010.10.017
19. Bargou RC, Wagener C, Bommert K, Mapara MY, Daniel PT, Arnold W, et al. Overexpression of the death-promoting gene bax-alpha which is downregulated in breast cancer restores sensitivity to different apoptotic stimuli and reduces tumor growth in SCID mice. *J Clin Invest* 1996;97(11):2651-9. doi: 10.1172/jci118715
20. Simonian PL, Grillot DaM, Nunez G. Bcl-2 and Bcl-XL can differentially block chemotherapy-induced cell death. *Blood* 1997;90(3):1208-16.
21. Zapata JM, Krajewska M, Krajewski S, Huang RP, Takayama S, Wang HG, et al. Expression of multiple apoptosis-regulatory genes in human breast cancer cell lines and primary tumors. *Breast Cancer Res Treat* 1998;47(2):129-40. doi: 10.1023/a:1005940832123
22. Olopade OI, Adeyanju MO, Safa AR, Hagos F, Mick R, Thompson CB, et al. Overexpression of BCL-x protein in primary breast cancer is associated with high tumor grade and nodal metastases. *Cancer J Sci Am* 1997;3(4):230-7.
23. Kojima H, Endo K, Moriyama H, Tanaka Y, Alnemri ES, Slapak CA, et al. Abrogation of mitochondrial cytochrome c release and caspase-3 activation in acquired multidrug resistance. *J Biol Chem* 1998;273(27):16647-50. doi: 10.1074/jbc.273.27.16647
24. Rodriguez-Nieto S, Zhivotovsky B. Role of alterations in the apoptotic machinery in sensitivity of cancer cells to treatment. *Curr Pharm Des* 2006;12(34):4411-25. doi: 10.2174/138161206779010495
25. Adjei AA, Rowinsky EK. Novel anticancer agents in clinical development. *Cancer Biol Ther* 2003;2(4 Suppl 1):S5-15. doi: 10.4161/cbt.218
26. Hortobagyi GN. Anthracyclines in the treatment of cancer. An overview. *Drugs* 1997;54 Suppl 4:1-7.
27. Gewirtz DA. A critical evaluation of the mechanisms of action proposed for the antitumor effects of the anthracycline antibiotics adriamycin and daunorubicin. *Biochem Pharmacol* 1999;57(7):727-41. doi: 10.1016/s0006-2952(98)00307-4
28. Moulder S, Hortobagyi GN. Advances in the treatment of breast cancer. *Clin Pharmacol Ther* 2008;83(1):26-36. doi: 10.1038/sj.clpt.6100449
29. Makin G, Dive C. Apoptosis and cancer chemotherapy. *Trends Cell Biol* 2001;11(11):S22-6. doi: 10.1016/S0962-8924(01)02124-9
30. Ghanbari P, Mohseni M, Tabasinezhad M, Yousefi B, Saei AA, Sharifi S, et al. Inhibition of survivin

restores the sensitivity of breast cancer cells to docetaxel and vinblastine. *Appl Biochem Biotechnol* 2014;174(2):667-81. doi: 10.1007/s12010-014-1125-6

31. Sabzichi M, Hamishehkar H, Ramezani F, Sharifi S, Tabasinezhad M, Pirouzpanah M, et al. Luteolin-loaded phytosomes sensitize human breast carcinoma MDA-MB 231 cells to doxorubicin by suppressing Nrf2 mediated signalling. *Asian Pac J Cancer Prev* 2014;15(13):5311-6. doi: 10.7314/apjcp.2014.15.13.5311
32. Samadi N, Ghanbari P, Mohseni M, Tabasinezhad M, Sharifi S, Nazemieh H, et al. Combination therapy increases the efficacy of docetaxel, vinblastine and tamoxifen in cancer cells. *J Cancer Res Ther* 2014;10(3):715-21. doi: 10.4103/0973-1482.139152
33. Sharifi S, Barar J, Hejazi MS, Samadi N. Roles of the Bcl-2/Bax ratio, caspase-8 and 9 in resistance of breast cancer cells to paclitaxel. *Asian Pac J Cancer Prev* 2014;15(20):8617-22. doi: 10.7314/apjcp.2014.15.20.8617
34. Levenson AS, Jordan VC. MCF-7: the first hormone-responsive breast cancer cell line. *Cancer Res* 1997;57(15):3071-8.
35. Hamedeyazdan S, Fathiazad F, Sharifi S, Nazemiyeh H. Antiproliferative activity of Marrubium persicum extract in the MCF-7 human breast cancer cell line. *Asian Pac J Cancer Prev* 2012;13(11):5843-8. doi: 10.7314/apjcp.2012.13.11.5843
36. Simstein R, Burow M, Parker A, Weldon C, Beckman B. Apoptosis, chemoresistance, and breast cancer: insights from the MCF-7 cell model system. *Exp Biol Med (Maywood)* 2003;228(9):995-1003.
37. Fisher DE. Apoptosis in cancer therapy: crossing the threshold. *Cell* 1994;78(4):539-42. doi: 10.1016/0092-8674(94)90518-5
38. Debatin KM. Cytotoxic drugs, programmed cell death, and the immune system: defining new roles in an old play. *J Natl Cancer Inst* 1997;89(11):750-1. doi: 10.1093/jnci/89.11.750
39. Lukyanova NY, Rusetskya NV, Tregubova NA, Chekhun VF. Molecular profile and cell cycle in MCF-7 cells resistant to cisplatin and doxorubicin. *Exp Oncol* 2009;31(2):87-91.
40. Taherian A, Mazoochi T. Different Expression of Extracellular Signal-Regulated Kinases (ERK) 1/2 and Phospho-Erk Proteins in MBA-MB-231 and MCF-7 Cells after Chemotherapy with Doxorubicin or Docetaxel. *Iran J Basic Med Sci* 2012;15(1):669-77.
41. Fornari FA, Randolph JK, Yalowich JC, Ritke MK, Gewirtz DA. Interference by doxorubicin with DNA unwinding in MCF-7 breast tumor cells. *Mol Pharmacol* 1994;45(4):649-56.
42. Green DR, Reed JC. Mitochondria and apoptosis. *Science* 1998;281(5381):1309-12. doi: 10.1126/science.281.5381.1309
43. Rao L, White E. Bcl-2 and the ICE family of apoptotic regulators: making a connection. *Curr Opin Genet Dev* 1997;7(1):52-8. doi: 10.1016/s0959-437x(97)80109-8
44. Childs AC, Phaneuf SL, Dirks AJ, Phillips T, Leeuwenburgh C. Doxorubicin treatment in vivo causes cytochrome C release and cardiomyocyte apoptosis, as well as increased mitochondrial efficiency, superoxide dismutase activity, and Bcl-2:Bax ratio. *Cancer Res* 2002;62(16):4592-8.
45. Campos L, Rouault JP, Sabido O, Oriol P, Roubi N, Vasselon C, et al. High expression of bcl-2 protein in acute myeloid leukemia cells is associated with poor response to chemotherapy. *Blood* 1993;81(11):3091-6.
46. Leung LK, Wang TT. Differential effects of chemotherapeutic agents on the Bcl-2/Bax apoptosis pathway in human breast cancer cell line MCF-7. *Breast Cancer Res Treat* 1999;55(1):73-83. doi: 10.1023/a:1006190802590
47. Tudor G, Aguilera A, Halverson DO, Laing ND, Sausville EA. Susceptibility to drug-induced apoptosis correlates with differential modulation of Bad, Bcl-2 and Bcl-xL protein levels. *Cell Death Differ* 2000;7(6):574-86. doi: 10.1038/sj.cdd.4400688
48. Gross A. BCL-2 proteins: regulators of the mitochondrial apoptotic program. *IUBMB life* 2001;52(3-5):231-6. doi: 10.1080/15216540152846046
49. Huynh H. Induction of apoptosis in rat ventral prostate by finasteride is associated with alteration in MAP kinase pathways and Bcl-2 related family of proteins. *Int J Oncol* 2002;20(6):1297-303. doi: 10.3892/ijo.20.6.1297
50. Gonzalez MS, De Brasi CD, Bianchini M, Gargallo P, Moiraghi B, Bengio R, et al. BAX/BCL-XL gene expression ratio inversely correlates with disease progression in chronic myeloid leukemia. *Blood Cells Mol Dis* 2010;45(3):192-6. doi: 10.1016/j.bcmd.2010.07.011
51. Rosse T, Olivier R, Monney L, Rager M, Conus S, Fellay I, et al. Bcl-2 prolongs cell survival after Bax-induced release of cytochrome c. *Nature* 1998;391(6666):496-9. doi: 10.1038/35160
52. Jurgensmeier JM, Xie Z, Deveraux Q, Ellerby L, Bredesen D, Reed JC. Bax directly induces release of cytochrome c from isolated mitochondria. *Proc Natl Acad Sci U S A* 1998;95(9):4997-5002. doi: 10.1073/pnas.95.9.4997
53. Kagawa S, Pearson SA, Ji L, Xu K, Mcdonnell TJ, Swisher SG, et al. A binary adenoviral vector system for expressing high levels of the proapoptotic gene bax. *Gene Ther* 2000;7(1):75-9. doi: 10.1038/sj.gt.3301048
54. Kumar S. Regulation of caspase activation in apoptosis: implications in pathogenesis and treatment of disease. *Clin Exp Pharmacol Physiol* 1999;26(4):295-303. doi: 10.1046/j.1440-1681.1999.03031.x
55. Ouyang L, Shi Z, Zhao S, Wang FT, Zhou TT, Liu B, et al. Programmed cell death pathways in cancer: a

review of apoptosis, autophagy and programmed necrosis. *Cell Prolif* 2012;45(6):487-98. doi: 10.1111/j.1365-2184.2012.00845.x

56. Liang Y, Yan C, Schor NF. Apoptosis in the absence of caspase 3. *Oncogene* 2001;20(45):6570-8. doi: 10.1038/sj.onc.1204815
57. Hu Y, Benedict MA, Wu D, Inohara N, Nunez G. Bcl-XL interacts with Apaf-1 and inhibits Apaf-1-dependent caspase-9 activation. *Proc Natl Acad Sci U S A* 1998;95(8):4386-91. doi: 10.1073/pnas.95.8.4386
58. Kurokawa H, Nishio K, Fukumoto H, Tomonari A, Suzuki T, Saijo N. Alteration of caspase-3 (CPP32/Yama/apopain) in wild-type MCF-7, breast cancer cells. *Oncol Rep* 1999;6(1):33-7. doi: 10.3892/or.6.1.33
59. Janicke RU, Sprengart ML, Wati MR, Porter AG. Caspase-3 is required for DNA fragmentation and morphological changes associated with apoptosis. *J Biol Chem* 1998;273(16):9357-60. doi: 10.1074/jbc.273.16.9357
60. Ferreira KS, Kreutz C, Macnelly S, Neubert K, Haber A, Bogyo M, et al. Caspase-3 feeds back on caspase-8, Bid and XIAP in type I Fas signaling in primary mouse hepatocytes. *Apoptosis* 2012;17(5):503-15. doi: 10.1007/s10495-011-0691-0
61. Scaffidi C, Fulda S, Srinivasan A, Friesen C, Li F, Tomaselli KJ, et al. Two CD95 (APO-1/Fas) signaling pathways. *EMBO J* 1998;17(6):1675-87. doi: 10.1093/emboj/17.6.1675
62. Yang XH, Sladek TL, Liu X, Butler BR, Froelich CJ, Thor AD. Reconstitution of caspase 3 sensitizes MCF-7 breast cancer cells to doxorubicin- and etoposide-induced apoptosis. *Cancer Res* 2001;61(1):348-54.

The Effect of Tween 20, 60, and 80 on Dissolution Behavior of Sprionolactone in Solid Dispersions Prepared by PEG 6000

Jafar Akbari[1,2]*, Majid Saeedi[1,2], Katayoun Morteza-Semnani[3], Hamid Reza Kelidari[2], Farshad Sadegh Moghanlou[1], Gity Zareh[1], Sohrab Rostamkalaei[1]

[1] *Department of Pharmaceutics, Faculty of Pharmacy, Mazandaran University of Medical Sciences, Sari, Iran.*

[2] *Pharmaceutical Sciences Research Centre, Mazandaran University of Medical Sciences, Sari, Iran.*

[3] *Department of Medicinal Chemistry, Faculty of Pharmacy, Mazandaran University of Medical Sciences, Sari, Iran.*

Article info

Keywords:
- Solid dispersion
- Spironolactone
- PEG 6000
- Tweens
- Dissolution

Abstract

Purpose: Solid dispersions have been efficient in improving the dissolution rate and bioavailability of hydrophobic drugs. The aim of the present study was enhancement of the dissolution profile of Spironolactone using solid dispersion.

Methods: Spironolactone solid dispersions (1:1, 1:2 and 2:1 drug: carrier weight ratio) were prepared by polyethylene glycol (PEG) 6000 as a carrier by hot melt method. The influence of several amounts of Tween 20, 60, and 80 were also studied. The dissolution profile was evaluated by USP Apparatus II.

Results: The results showed that solid dispersions were efficacious to enhance the dissolution rate of Spironolactone in water; and the procedure indicated that there was an increase in dissolution rate for solid dispersions containing the surfactant Tweens. The solid dispersions were evaluated using Fourier-transform infrared (FTIR) spectroscopy, X-ray diffraction (XRD) and Differential Scanning Calorimetry (DSC) studies; and the results showed no complex formation or change in crystal shape of drug.

Conclusion: It is concluded that solid dispersion technique can be successfully used for improvement of dissolution of Spironolactone.

Introduction

Solid dispersion (SD) refers to a group of solid products consisting of at least two different components, generally a hydrophilic matrix and a hydrophobic drug.[1] The matrix can be either crystalline or amorphous. The drug can be dispersed molecularly, in amorphous particles or in crystalline particles.[2] In other words, SD involved a dispersion of one or more active ingredients in an inner carrier in solid state.[3]

Some of these carriers are PEGs, Gelucires, Poloxamers, PVP, Sugar or Urea. PEG polymers are used widely because of their low melting point, low toxicity, wide drug compatibility and hydrophilicity.[4] A water-soluble carrier results in a faster release of the drug from the matrix.[5] Many methods like spray drying, co-precipitation, co-evaporation and freeze dying are used for solid dispersion manufacturing. Apart from these techniques, fusion method is a method of choice because it is environmentally friendly, cost effective, represents no stability nor toxicity problems and can be easily scaled up for commercial purpose.[6]

Spironolactone is a synthetic steroid that acts as a competitive antagonist to aldosterone. Potassium-sparing diuretics are most useful in states of mineralocorticoid excess or hyperaldosteronism (also called aldosteronism), due either to primary hypersecretion (Crohn's syndrome, ectopic adrenocorticotropic hormone production) or secondary hyperaldosteronism (evoked by heart failure, hepatic cirrhosis, nephrotic syndrome, or other conditions associated with diminished effective intravascular volume).[7] Spironolactone has a low water solubility (0.028 mg/ml, at 25°C) and slow dissolution rate.[8] Solubility and dissolution rate are key determinant of oral bioavailability of a drug and dissolution may be rate determining step for appearance of medicinal effect, therefore efforts to increase dissolution of drug with limited water solubility is often needed. Various methods used for the improvement of the dissolution rate of poorly water-soluble drugs. SD is one of these techniques. Surface-active agents (surfactants) are substances that at low concentrations adsorb onto the surfaces or interfaces of a system and alter the surface or interfacial free energy and the surface and the interfacial tension. Surface-active agents have a characteristic structure, possessing both polar (hydrophilic) and non-polar (hydrophobic) regions in the same molecule. The surface active carriers are said to be amphipathic in nature.[9] Surfactants are used to enhance solubility.

The aim of this study was to prepare different solid dispersions of Spironolactone by fusion method with PEG and several types of Tweens, and evaluate the effect of them on solubility profile of the drug.

***Corresponding author:** Jafar Akbari, Email: jafakbari@gmail.com

Materials and Methods

Materials

Spironolactone was obtained from Behdasht-Kar Co. (Behdasht-Kar Co., Iran). PEG 6000, Tween 20, 60, and 80 were purchased from Merck (Merck, Germany). All other chemicals and solvents used were of pharmaceutical grade.

Preparation of solid dispersion

Fusion (hot melt) method was used for the preparation of Spironolactone SD. Several formulations were prepared by adding required amount of PEG 6000 to accurately weighed drug with the drug: carrier weight ratio of 1:1, 1:2 and 2:1; and several amounts of Tween 20, 60, and 80 (Table 1). The formulations were heated on a water bath (Behdad, Iran) at the temperature of 70°C to melt the carrier and stirred to make homogenous mixing. The combination was cooled rapidly, and grinded to obtain the SDs as powder that is easy to handle.[10] Finally the preparations were passed through 50-mesh sieve and stored in desiccators for next evaluations.

Table 1. Drug –carrier and Tween (20, 60, 80) weight ratio in prepared formulations.F_0 is pure spironolactone,F_1 to F_{12} are solid dispersions,F_{13} to F_{16} are physical mixtures.

Formulation code	Drug :Carrier ratio	Tween 80	Tween 60	Tween 20
F0	1: 0	-	-	-
F1	1:1	-	-	-
F2	1:2	-	-	-
F3	2:1	-	-	-
F4	1:1	1%	-	-
F5	1:1	0.5%	-	-
F6	1:1	1.5%	-	-
F7	1:1	-	1%	-
F8	1:1	-	0.5%	-
F9	1:1	-	1.5%	-
F10	1:1	-	-	1%
F11	1:1	-	-	0.5%
F12	1:1		-	1.5%
F13*	1:1	1%	-	-
F14*	1:1	-	1%	-
F15*	1:1	-	-	1%
F16*	1:1	-	-	-

* Physical mixture

Preparation of Physical mixture

The physical mixtures were prepared by weighing Spironolactone and PEG accurately in the ratio of 1:1 w/w of drug to carrier and mixing them with determined amount of Tween. The formulations were obtained by mixing the components using spatula in a mortar for 3 minutes. They were passed through 50-mesh sieve and kept in desiccators for other studies.[4]

Release studies of Solid Dispersions

In vitro dissolution of samples equivalent to 25 mg of pure drug was carried out in a USP apparatus No. II (Erweka, Germany) in 900ml of distilled water as medium at 37±0.5°C for 8 hours and at a rotational speed of 100 rpm, the system was allowed to equilibrate for 60 minutes. Dissolution samples (5ml) were withdrawn at predetermined intervals of 5, 10, 15, 20, 30, 45, 60 then every 30 minutes up to 8 hours , and were filtered through Whatmann number 41 filter papers. The samples withdrawn were replaced by distilled water to maintain the constant volume of dissolution medium. The samples were analyzed at 239.8 nm in UV spectrophotometer (Varian, Italy). Each preparation was tested three times and the mean values were figured out. Percentage of drug release was calculated using the equation obtained from the standard curve prepared in the media.[11,12]

The percent dissolution efficiency (%DE) was computed to compare the relative performance of various type and concentrations of surfactant in the investigated formulations. The %DE of a solid dispersion is defined as the area under the dissolution curve up to a certain time, t, expressed as a percentage of the area of the rectangle described by 100% dissolution at the same time. The %DE can be calculated from %DE.

$$\%DE = \frac{\int_0^t Ydt}{Y_{100}t}$$

where Y is the percent drug dissolved at time t.

To understand the extent of dissolution-rate increase from its solid dispersion, the dissolution data were used to calculate the mean dissolution time (MDT). The MDT can be calculated as follow:

$$MDT_{in-vitro} = \frac{\sum_{i=1}^{n} T_{mid}\Delta M}{\sum_{i=1}^{n}\Delta M}$$

Where, i is the dissolution sample number, n is the number of dissolution sampling times, T_{mid} is the midpoint between times Ti and Ti-1, and DM is the amount of dissolved drug between times Ti and Ti-1.[13]

Fourier-Transform Infrared Spectroscopy

IR spectroscopy is used to assess the interaction between carrier or complexing agent and guest molecule in solid state. Because of their high structural resolution this technique is valuable for characterization of an amorphous system.[14] The samples were previously ground and mixed thoroughly with potassium bromide, an infrared transparent matrix, at 1:5 (Sample: KBr) ratio, respectively. The KBr discs were prepared by compressing the powder at a pressure of 5 tons for 5 min in a hydraulic press. Scans were obtained at a resolution of 4 cm^{-1}, from 4000 to 500 cm^{-1}.[14] FT-IR spectra were obtained by using an FT-IR spectrometer (Perkin Elmer , Spectrum One , USA).

X-ray diffraction

Powder X-ray diffraction can be used to qualitatively detect material with long range order. Sharper diffraction peaks indicate more crystalline material.[15]

X-ray powder diffraction patterns were obtained at room temperature using a D8 ADVANCE X-ray diffractometer (Bruker, Germany) with Cu as anode material and graphite monochromator, operated at a voltage of 40 kV and 20 mA current. The samples were analyzed in the 2θ angle range of 4°–40° and the process parameters were set as: scan step size of 0.02° (2θ), and scan step time of 0.5 degree/min.[15]

Differential scanning calorimetry (DSC)

In DSC, samples are heated with a constant heating rate and the amount of energy necessary for that is detected. With DSC the temperatures at which thermal events occur can be detected. Thermal events can be a glass to rubber transition, (re)crystallization, melting or degradation. Furthermore, the melting- and (re)crystallization energy can be quantified. The melting energy can be used to detect the amount of crystalline material.[16]

The DSC thermograms of pure drug, physical mixtures and solid dispersions were recorded using Differential scanning calorimeter (Perkin Elmer Pyris 6). About 5 mg of each sample was weighed and hermitically sealed in aluminum pans prior to analysis, and the thermal behavior of each sample was investigated at a scanning rate of 10°C/min, from 0 to 300°C. Dry nitrogen at a flow rate of 50 ml/min was used to purge the DSC cell.

Statistical Analysis

ANOVA followed Tukey test was used to determine significant differences between groups and "$P<0.05$" was considered significant.

Results and Discussion

Dissolution profiles

Comparison of release behaviour of The various formulations are shown in Figure 1-4. The Spironolactone solid dispersions were prepared employing hot melt method. Drug –carrier and Tween (20, 60, 80) weight ratio applied in prepared formulations is shown in Table 1. The dissolution study showed that the release percentage of pure Spironolactone after one hour was only 55.06% (Figure 1). During dissolution studies, it was noted that drug carrier systems sink immediately, whereas pure drug keeps floating on the surface for a longer time interval. There was an appeal difference between the release rate of pure Spironolactone and solid dispersions (F1, F2, and F3) ($P<0.001$). Comparative dissolution profile showed that an increase in the percentage of PEG 6000 from (formulation F1 to F3) resulted in an increase in the release rate of Spironolactone ($P<0.01$). Chaulang et al. showed that the solid dispersion (SD) technique has improved the dissolution rate of Furosemide to a great extent. The release percentage of drug was increased when the concentrations of carrier increased.[8] *In vitro* dissolution in Islam et al. studies indicated that drug release from SDs was faster from their pure drug. Drug release from SDs was found to depend on the nature and amount of carrier.[15] Bolourchian et al. evaluated the effect of several PEG (6000, 12000, and 20000) as solid dispersion carriers on the dissolution behavior of simvastatin. The results showed that the kind of carrier had effect on drug dissolution. This study revealed that release rate was increased by increase in ratio of carrier to drug.[17]

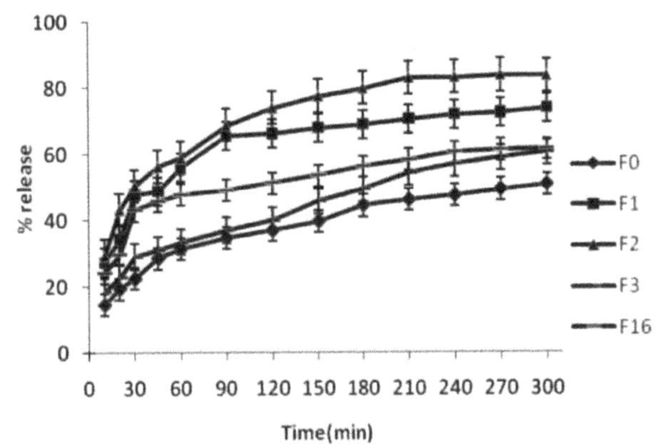

Figure 1. Release percentage of prepared formulations, dissolution condition: distilled water; RPM: 100; 37°C ± 0.5°C (n=3).

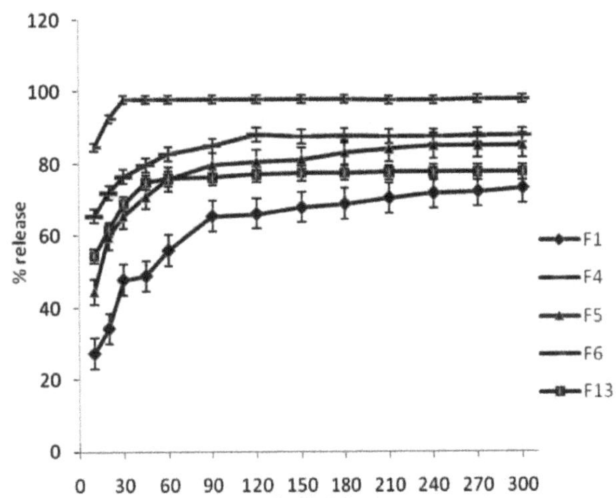

Figure 2. Release percentage of prepared formulations, dissolution condition: distilled water; RPM: 100; 37°C ± 0.5°C (n=3).

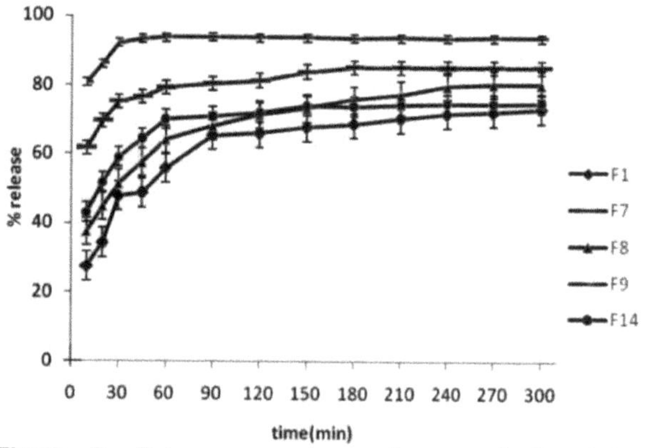

Figure 3. Release percentage of prepared formulations, dissolution condition: distilled water; RPM: 100; 37°C±0.5°C (n=3).

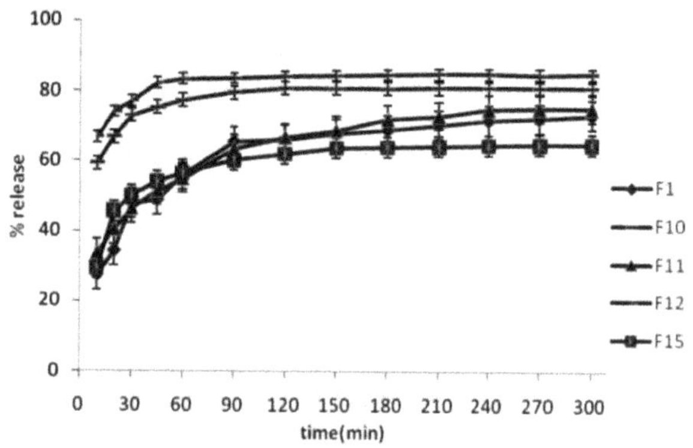

Figure 4. Release percentage of prepared formulations, dissolution condition: distilled water; RPM: 100; 37°C±0.5°C (n=3).

Solid dispersions containing Spironolactone with both PEG 6000 and Tween 60 or 80 provided higher release rate than the release rate of pure Spironolactone and SD preparations containing PEG ($P<0.01$). The release profile showed that release rate was increased by increasing in amount of Tween 60 or 80 ($P<0.05$). The drug release in SD formulation containing 0.5% Tween 20 (F11) was similar to SD preparation containing drug and PEG 6000 (F1) ($P>0.05$). The drug release increased by increasing in amount of Tween 20 to 1 and 1.5% ($P<0.05$). Comparing the dissolution profile of SDs with other preparations at similar ratios of Tween revealed that, the release rates of SDs containing Tween 80 was higher than release rates in formulations containing Tween 60 and 20 ($P<0.05$ for all investigations).

DE% and MDT of investigated solid dispersions are shown in Table 2. The DE% of F0 (drug powder) was significantly lower than solid dispersions. The onset of release was faster than drug powder in all of formulations. The most DE% was observed in F6 containing 1.5% of tween 80.

The MDT of F0 was 131.17 min. This time was decreased in investigated solid dispersions significantly. This proved the increase in release rate by solid dispersion preparation.

Table 2. Dissolution parameters of spironolactone solid dispersions

Formulation code	%DE	MDT(min)
F0	43.69	131.17
F1	67.11	94.69
F2	75.47	74.42
F3	50.77	146.57
F4	84.39	46.38
F5	79.80	52.18
F6	95.50	22.62
F7	81.41	51.50
F8	73.07	77.46
F9	91.37	25.45
F10	78.04	37.81
F11	68.30	81.99
F12	82.18	35.82
F13*	75.11	49.97
F14*	71.05	51.00
F15*	61.00	50.98
F16*	55.15	89.55

In one study, solid dispersions of Meloxicam containing PEG 6000 and SLS showed a significant increase in dissolution rate with an increase in PEG 6000 and the surfactant sodium lauryl sulphate.[12] In another research the effect of sucrose laurate as surfactant was evaluated in gemfibrosil solid dispersions containing PEG 6000 as carrier. Drug released increased significantly in solid dispersions containing this surfactant.[18]

Possible mechanisms of increased dissolution rates of solid dispersions have been proposed by Craig, and include: reduction of drug crystallite size, a solubilisation effect of the carrier, absence of aggregation of drug crystallites, improved wettability and dispersibility of a drug from the dispersion, dissolution of the drug in the hydrophilic carrier, conversion of the drug to the amorphous state and finally the combination of the above mentioned methods. Dry mixing of Spironolactone with PEG and Tween brings drug in close contact with the hydrophilic carrier. The increased dissolution rate in this study can thus be contributed by several factors such as a solubilisation effect of the carrier, conversion of drug to amorphous state, improved wettability and dispersibility of the drug.[19]

The dissolution of the physical mixtures was higher compared to pure Spironolactone. SDs of Spironolactone in hydrophilic carrier considerably enhanced dissolution compared to the physical mixtures (Figure 1). Dehghan et al. study showed the solid dispersions of Meloxicam with PEG 6000 improved dissolution when compared with physical mixtures and pure drug.[12]

FTIR analysis

Figure 5 represents the FTIR spectra of the samples. PEG 6000 spectrum showed characteristic peaks at 1107(–C-O stretching), 2890(–C-H stretching), 3445(–O-H stretching). Pure Spironolactone spectrum showed sharp peaks at wave numbers 1617 (-C=C stretching of α, β-unsaturated ring), 1673(-C=O stretching of α, β-unsaturated ring), 1768(-C=O stretching of the thioacetyl group), 1791 (-C=O stretching of the lactone ring), 2950cm^{-1}(-C=H stretching). In the spectra of all physical mixture and SD formulations, major characteristic peaks of both drug individually and polymer were retained. This confirms that there were no physical or chemical interactions amongst the components of the formulation and compatibility of the drug with the carrier.[20]

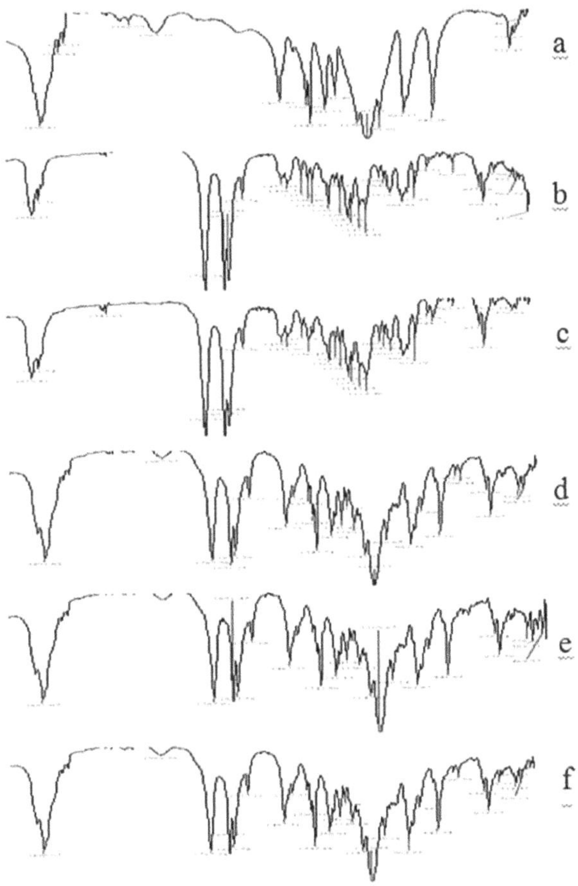

Figure 5. FTIR spectra of PEG and Spironolactone preparations
a: PEG, b: Spironolactone, c: Physical mixture (1:1 Drug-carrier), d: Solid dispersion (1:1 Drug carrier), e: Solid dispersion (1:1 Drug-carrier and 1.5% Tween 80), f: Solid dispersion (1:1 Drug-carrier and 1.5% Tween 60)

Powder X-Ray diffraction

Powder X-ray diffraction patterns of pure spironolactone, polymer, physical mixtures and solid dispersions of spironolactone are displayed in Figure 6. The X-ray diffraction spectrum of Spironolactone showed numerous distinct lines (9.21, 11.5, 12.5, 16.3,17, 17.5, 18.8, 20.21) indicating that it is present in highly crystalline state. XRD spectrum of formulation 1, 6 and 9 showed peaks at 9.1, 11.5, 12.5, 16.3, 17.1, 17.5, 18.8, 19.2, 20.21, and 23.1. The position of characteristic peaks was not changed in physical mixtures which suggest absence of change in the polymorph.[4,16] These peaks were observed in solid dispersions too, but intensity of them was decreased which proved changing from crystalline to amorphous form.

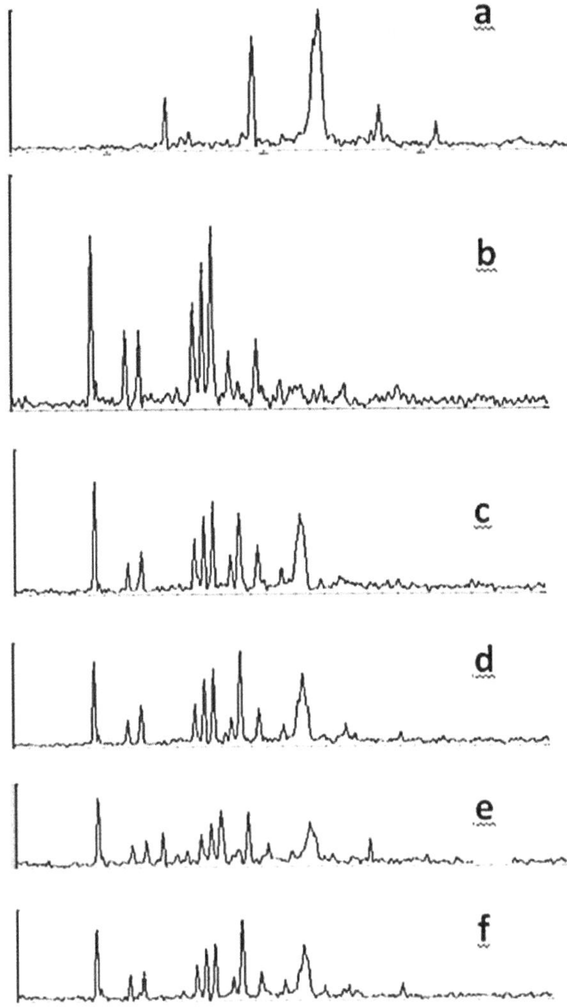

Figure 6. X-ray diffraction (XRD) patterns of PEG and Spironolactone preparations
a: PEG, b: Spironolactone, c: Physical mixture (1:1 Drug-carrier), d: Solid dispersion (1:1 Drug-carrier), e: Solid dispersion (1:1 Drug-carrier and 1.5% Tween 80), f: Solid dispersion (1:1 Drug-carrier and 1.5% Tween 60)

DSC analysis

The DSC thermograms of Spironolactone and PEG as well as their solid dispersions and physical mixtures are shown in Figure 7. The DSC thermogram of pure Spironolactone showed sharp endothermic peak at 208.7°C, with a melting enthalpy of 47.2 J/g, which is associated with melting point of the drug and indicates the crystalline nature of the drug. There is also a broad peak at 267.7°C with an enthalpy of 182.0 J/g, which may be suggestive of Spironolactone decomposition at this high temperature. From the thermograms of SDs and physical mixtures the endothermic peak of spironolactone was shifted to a lower temperature, around 198 to 202°C, and the calorimetric enthalpy was markedly reduced from 47.2 J/g (for pure drug) to 0.65±0.08 J/g. This signifies that most of the drug has dissolved in the liquid vehicle, and there is reduced number of drug crystal particles. A broadened peak with markedly reduced intensity was observed at approximately 250°C. The broad peak at about 250°C in

SD formulations might indicate that Spironolactone decomposition was minimized as the decomposition enthalpy was reduced from 182.0 J/g at 267.7°C to 38.35±5.41 J/g and some of crystalline form was changed to amorphous form. DSC thermograms of solid dispersion and physical mixture formulations after storage at 25°C and 76% relative humidity for 4 weeks revealed that there are no significant changes in thermal properties of the formulations compared to fresh formulations.[3,4,8]

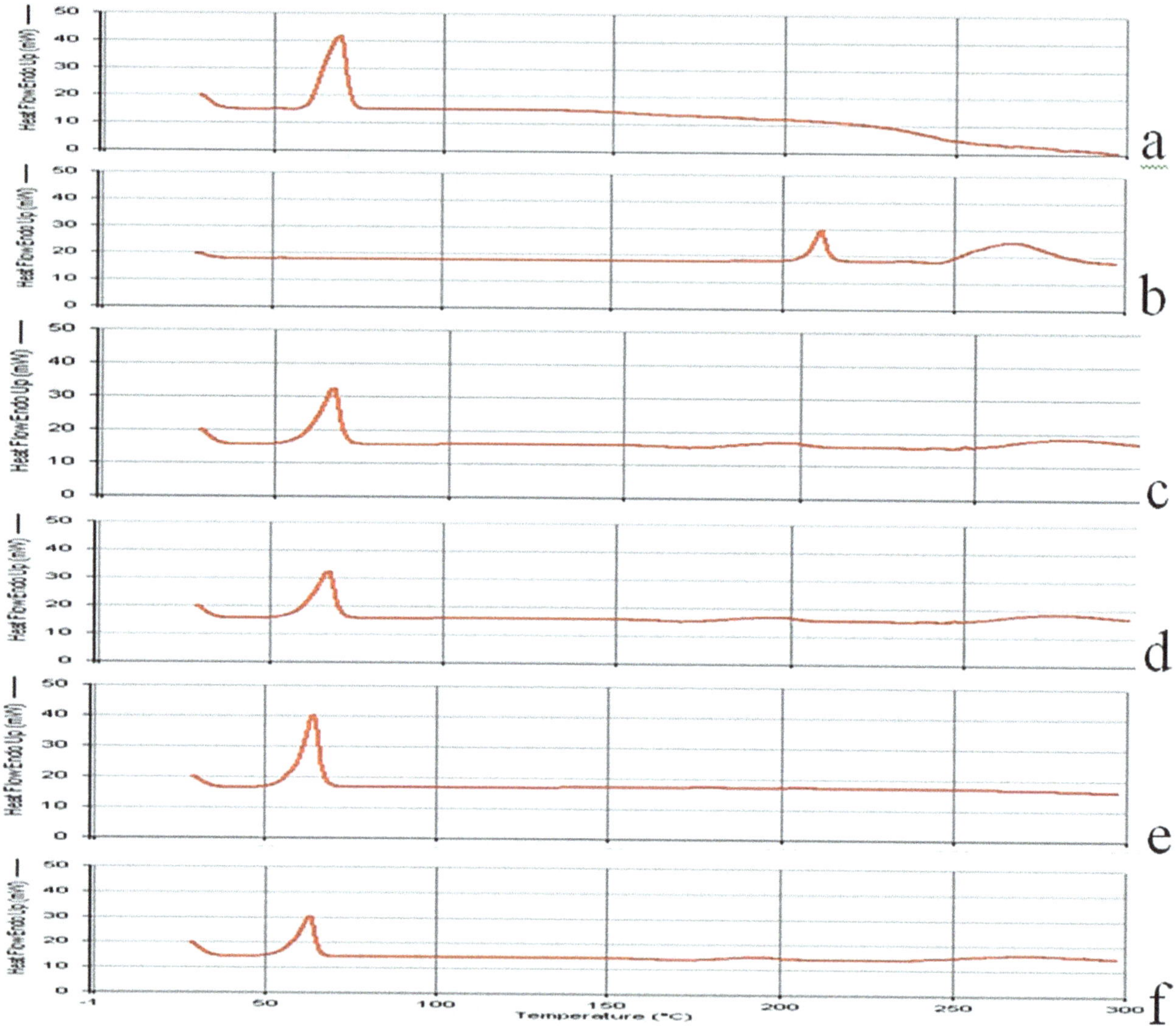

Figure 7. DSC thermograms of PEG and Spironolactone preparations
a: PEG, b: Spironolactone, c: Physical mixture (1:1 Drug-carrier), d: Solid dispersion (1:1 Drug-carrier), e: Solid dispersion (1:1 Drug-carrier and 1.5% Tween 80), f: Solid dispersion (1:1 Drug-carrier and 1.5% Tween 60)

Conclusion

In this experiment an attempt has been taken to evaluate Spironolactone release from the different polymer-drug concentrations loaded formulation of Solid dispersions. Observations of In-vitro dissolution of the solid dispersion of Spironolactone using distilled water as the media to study the drug release efficiency from the solid dispersion. These distorted solid dispersions may cause a wide variation in drug release pattern. Spironolactone is a potassium-sparing diuretic, acts as a competitive antagonist to aldosterone and is poorly water soluble drug. The present study was aimed to enhance the dissolution property of Spironolactone. So this study was endeavored to observe release pattern of drug from the solid dispersion of Spironolactone by using different concentrations of PEG as a carrier and Tween as a surfactant. The variables affecting drug dissolution was matrix property, hydrophilic excipients loading from the solid dispersion and also depend on the physicochemical property of the drug molecule. The major problem of poorly water soluble drugs especially for new molecules is bioavailability. Thus the main target is to increase the solubility of poorly water soluble drugs. So the present study reveals that solid dispersion may be an ideal means of drug delivery system for poorly water soluble drugs. Further study in this field is required to establish these drug delivery systems so that in future it can be used effectively in commercial basis.

Acknowledgments
This work was supported by a grant from the Research Council of the Mazandaran University of Medical Sciences.

Conflict of Interest
The authors report no conflicts of interest.

References
1. Ford JL. The current status of solid dispersions. *Pharm Acta Helv* 1986;61(3):69-88.
2. Nokhodchi A, Talari R, Valizadeh H, Jalali MB. An investigation on the solid dispersions of chlordiazepoxide. *Int J Biomed Sci* 2007;3(3):211-6.
3. Chaulang G, Patil K, Ghodke D, Khan S, Yeole P. Preparation and characterization of solid dispersion tablet of Furosemide with crospovidone. *Res J Pharm Tech* 2008;1(4):386-89.
4. Kshirsagar SJ, Ubhe A, Malshe J, Sengaokar V. A Modified Solvent Method for Preparation of Solid Dispersions. *Iran J Pharm Sci* 2011:8(1):287-98.
5. Arunachalam A, Karthikeyan M, Konam K, Prasad P, Sethuraman S, Ashutoshkumar S. Solid Dispersions: A Review. *Curr Pharm Res* 2010;1:82-90.
6. Saffoon N, Jhanker YM, Huda NH. Dissolution profile of Ibuprofen solid dispersion prepared with cellulosic polymers and sugar by fusion method. *Stamford J Pharm Sci* 2011;4(1): 31-7. doi: 10.3329/sjps.v4i1.8864
7. Katzung BG. Introduction to autonomic pharmacology. In: Katzung BG, Masters SB, Trevor AJ, editors. Basic and Clinical Pharmacology. 11th ed. New York: McGraw-Hill Companies Inc; 2009.
8. Elkordy AA, Tan XN, Essa EA. Spironolactone release from liquisolid formulations prepared with Capryol 90, Solutol(R) HS-15 and Kollicoat(R) SR 30 D as non-volatile liquid vehicles. *Eur J Pharm Biopharm* 2013;83(2):203-23. doi: 10.1016/j.ejpb.2012.08.004
9. Patidar K, Kshirsagar MD, Saini V, Joshi PB, Soni M. Solid dispersion technology: a boon for poor water soluble drugs. *Indian J Novel Drug Deliv* 2011;3(2):83-90.
10. Dhirendra K, Lewis S, Udupa N, Atin K. Solid dispersions: a review. *Pak J Pharm Sci* 2009;22(2):234-46.
11. Dewan I, Islam SM, Shahriar M. Dissolution study of Spironolactone by using solid dispersion technique. *Stamford J Pharm Sci* 2011;4(2):42-7. doi: 10.3329/sjps.v4i2.7776
12. Dehghan MH, Jafar M. Improving dissolution of Meloxicam using solid dispersions. *Iran J Pharm Res* 2006;4(5):231-38.
13. Sruti J, Patra CN, Swain S, Panigrahi KC, Patro AP, Beg S, et al. Improvement in the dissolution rate and tableting properties of cefuroxime axetil by melt-granulated dispersion and surface adsorption. *Acta Pharm Sinica B* 2013;3(2):113-22. doi: 10.1016/j.apsb.2013.01.001
14. Saindane DS, Kulkarni AS, Khade TS, Patil MD. Enhancing drug solubility and oral bioavailability using solid dispersions: A review. *Int J Biopharm* 2011:2(1):22-30.
15. Kumar P, Mohan C, Kanamsrinivasan Uma Shankar M, Gulati M. Physiochemical Characterization and Release Rate Studies of SolidDispersions of Ketoconazole with Pluronic F127 and PVP K-30. *Iran J Pharm Res* 2011;10(4):685-94.
16. Rani KS, Poornima G, Krishnaveni A, Brahmaiah B, Nama S. A review on solid dispersions. *Asian J Pharm Res* 2013;3(2):93-8.
17. Bolourchian N, Mahboobian MM, Dadashzadeh S. The effect of PEG molecular weights on dissolution behavior of simvastatin in solid dispersions. *Iran J Pharm Res* 2013;12(Suppl):11-20.
18. Szuts A, Lang P, Ambrus R, Kiss L, Deli MA, Szabo-Revesz P. Applicability of sucrose laurate as surfactant in solid dispersions prepared by melt technology. *Int J Pharm* 2011;410(1-2):107-10. doi: 10.1016/j.ijpharm.2011.03.033
19. Craig DQ. The mechanisms of drug release from solid dispersions in water-soluble polymers. *Int J Pharm* 2002;231(2):131-44. Doi: 10.1016/s0378-5173(01)00891-2
20. Shah S, Joshi S, Lin S, Madan PL. Preparation and characterization of Spironolactone solid dispersions using hydrophilic carrier. *Asian J Pharm Sci* 2012;7(1):40-9.

6

Solid Lipid Nanoparticles as Efficient Drug and Gene Delivery Systems

Jafar Ezzati Nazhad Dolatabadi[1,2], Hadi Valizadeh[3,4]*, Hamed Hamishehkar[3]

[1] *Research Center for Pharmaceutical Nanotechnology, Tabriz University of Medical Sciences, Tabriz, Iran.*
[2] *Student Research Committee, Tabriz University of Medical Sciences, Tabriz, Iran.*
[3] *Drug Applied Research Center, Tabriz University of Medical Sciences, Tabriz, Iran.*
[4] *Faculty of Pharmacy, Tabriz University of Medical Sciences, Tabriz, Iran.*

Article info

Keywords:
· Solid lipid nanoparticles
· Colloidal carrier
· Drug delivery
· Gene delivery

Abstract
In recent years, nanomaterials have been widely applied as advanced drug and gene delivery nanosystems. Among them, solid lipid nanoparticles (SLNs) have attracted great attention as colloidal drug delivery systems for incorporating hydrophilic or lipophilic drugs and various macromolecules as well as proteins and nucleic acids. Therefore, SLNs offer great promise for controlled and site specific drug and gene delivery. This article includes general information about SLN structures and properties, production procedures, characterization. In addition, recent progress on development of drug and gene delivery systems using SLNs was reviewed.

Introduction

Recently, nanotechnological sciences brought considerable progresses in the diagnosis and treatment of disease. Drug and gene delivery, production of improved biocompatible materials and *in vitro* and *in vivo* diagnostics are examples of nanotechnology application.[1-3] Nanoparticles can improve drug efficacy in cancer and other diseases, while simultaneously diminishing side effects, due to features such as more targeted localization in tumors and active cellular uptake.[4-6] The reason why nanomaterials are excellent candidates for medical purposes is based on their unique properties, such as their surface to mass ratio that is much larger than that of other colloidal particles, high chemical reactivity, tunable properties, and their ability to carry other compounds. The relatively large surface of nanoparticles provides the possibility of binding and carrying of other compounds such as drugs, probes and proteins.[7-9] The main purposes for nanomaterials application in drug and gene delivery consist of: a) Biocompatibility and safety, b) Specific drug targeting and delivery, c) Toxicity decreasing while maintaining therapeutic effects, and d) Development of safe medicines.[7]

In order to omit limitations associated with traditional formulations, lipid based drug delivery systems are introduced.[10] In comparison to liposomes, solid particles have some advantages as well as prevention of incorporated active compounds from chemical degradation and more flexibility in modulating the release of the compound.[11]

Solid lipid nanoparticles (SLNs) as example of lipid based drug delivery system have distinctive property such as high drug loading, large surface area and can protect the drug from the environment, while increasing its bioavailability. Consequently, two noticeable advantages can be attained; first, less active drug consumption during the formulation process owing to the enhanced encapsulation efficiency. Second, the preferred effects of the drug are accelerated owing to the initial release increasing, which is because of the homogenization production process of SLNs.

Drug incorporation models of SLNs including solid solution model and core-shell model (drug-enriched shell and drug-enriched core) has been shown in Figure 1. Drug is molecularly dispersed in the lipid matrix in solid solution model when the particles are formed by application of neither any surfactant nor drug-solubilizing surfactant using cold homogenization technique. The drug has robustly distinct interactions with the lipid. In the drug-enriched shell model, a solid lipid core forms once the recrystallization temperature of the lipid is achieved and the drug concentrates in the still liquid outer shell of the SLN due to the dispersion temperature reduction.[12,13] Finally, in the drug-enriched core model, cooling the nanoemulsion results in a super-saturation of the drug which is dissolved in the melted lipid at or close to its saturation solubility and the drug

***Corresponding author:** Hadi Valizadeh, Email: valizadeh@tbzmed.ac.ir precipitation occurs before lipid recrystallization. Extra cooling ultimately leads to the recrystallization of the lipid surrounding the drug as a membrane.[13]

This review presents the preparation and characterization methods of SLNs and the recent advances in application of them as drug/gene delivery system are discussed in more details.

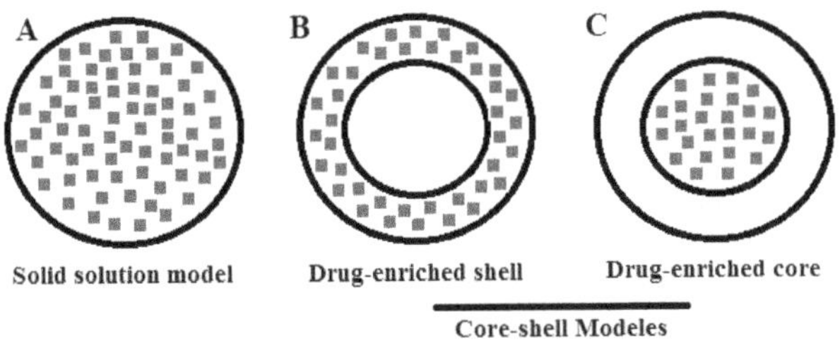

Figure 1. Drug incorporation models into SLN: A) homogeneous matrix of solid solution, B) drug-free core with drug-enriched shell and C) drug-enriched core with lipid shell.

SLN preparation

Solid lipid, emulsifier and water/solvent have been used in preparation of SLNs. The lipids used may be triglycerides (compritol), partial glycerides, fatty acids (stearic acid, palmitic acid), steroids (cholesterol) and waxes (cetyl palmitate). In order to stabilize the lipid dispersion, a variety of emulsifiers and their combination have been utilized. The particle agglomeration can be avoided by application of mixture of emulsifiers.[14] There are numerous methods of SLN preparation like high shear homogenization, hot homogenization, cold homogenization, ultrasonication or high speed homogenization, micro emulsion based SLN preparations, SLN preparation by using supercritical fluid, SLN prepared by solvent emulsification/evaporation, double emulsion method, spray drying method.

High shear homogenization

High shear homogenization techniques were initially applied for the preparation of SLNs. Dispersion quality is often compromised by the presence of micro particles. Olbrich et al investigated different process parameters, which affect the particle size and zeta potential as well as stirring rate, emulsification time and cooling condition. The particle size has not been influenced by higher stirring rates, but slightly improved the polydispersity index.[15,16]

Hot homogenization

Hot homogenization method is performed at higher temperature than the melting point of the lipid and it is similar to homogenization of emulsion. It can be performed by both high pressure homogenizers and high intensity ultrasound. A pre-emulsion of the drug incorporated lipid melt and the aqueous emulsifier phase is attained by high-shear mixing device at the same temperature. High pressure homogenization of the pre-emulsion is done above the lipid melting point. The quality of the final product to a great extent has been affected by the quality of the pre-emulsion and it is desirable to achieve droplets in the size range of a few micrometers. Lower particle sizes are acquired because of lower viscosity of the lipid phase at higher processing temperatures, which results in drug and carrier degradation acceleration. Good product is acquired due to several passes through the high-pressure homogenizer, typically 3-5 passes. Increasing the homogenization period, results in particle size enlarging due to particle coalescence, which occurs because of the high kinetic energy of the particles. Degradation of active compound and metal contamination due to high intensity ultrasound is disadvantage of this method.[3,17]

Cold homogenization

Cold homogenization method has been carried out to omit the following problems of the hot homogenization technique like temperature mediated drug and carrier degradation acceleration and consequently release of drug into the aqueous phase during homogenization. First stage in cold homogenization is the same with hot homogenization method but the next steps are different. The drug loaded lipid melt is cooled quickly by ice or liquid nitrogen for distribution of drug in the lipid matrix. The acquired particle sizes are in the range 50-100 microns for this method. Disadvantages of cold homogenized samples are larger particle sizes and a broader size distribution. However, this method reduces the thermal exposure of the sample.[17]

Ultrasonication or high speed homogenization

Sonication or high speed stirring method can be used for production of SLNs as well. It is very simple and the applied equipment in this technique is very common in every lab. Large particle size and metal contamination due to ultrasonication are examples of this method disadvantage.[18]

Microemulsion based SLN preparations

This technique is based on the dilution of microemulsions in which SLNs are produced by stirring an optically transparent mixture at 65-70° which is normally composed of a low melting fatty acid (stearic acid), an emulsifier (polysorbate 20, polysorbate 60, soy phosphatidylcholine, and sodium taurodeoxycholate), co-emulsifiers (sodium monooctylphosphate) and water. After that, the hot micro-emulsion is dispersed in cold water under stirring.[19] The volume ratios of the hot micro emulsion to cold water usually are in the range of 1:25 to 1:50. The dilution process is verified by the composition of the micro emulsion. As reported previously, the droplet structure is already contained in the microemulsion and as a result, no energy is needed to get submicron particle sizes.[19]

Supercritical fluid technique

This novel technique has the advantage of solvent-less processing for SLN preparation. SLN preparation is based on the fast expansion of supercritical carbon dioxide solutions (RESS) method. Carbon dioxide (99.99%) was the fine candidate as a solvent for this method.[20,21]

Solvent emulsification/evaporation method

This technique is based on SLN dispersions by precipitation in oil/water emulsions. The lipophilic compound is dissolved in water immiscible organic solvent such as cyclohexane, which is emulsified in an aqueous phase. SLN dispersion is formed by precipitation of the lipid in the aqueous medium after evaporation of the solvent. The mean diameter of 25 nm with cholesterol acetate as model drug and lecithin/sodium glycocholate mixture as emulsifier has been reported for the prepared SLN. The reproducibility of the result was verified by Siekmann and Westesen, who produced the cholesterol acetate SLN with mean size of 29 nm.[22,23]

Double emulsion method

This procedure is based on solvent emulsification evaporation for incorporating hydrophilic drug into SLNs. In order to avoid drug partitioning to outer water phase during solvent evaporation in the external water phase of w/o/w double emulsion, the drug is encapsulated with a stabilizer. After evaporation of organic solvent by rotary, SLNs were recovered by centrifugation at 12000 ×g for 30 min at 4°C.[24]

Spray drying technique

This method leads in particle aggregation because of high temperature, shear forces and partial melting of the particle. The most favorable result was acquired in SLN concentration of 1% in a solution of trehalose in water or 20% trehalose in ethanol water mixtures (10/90 v/v).[25]

Characterization of SLNs

The prepared SLNs should be evaluated to distinguish if they are appropriate for the intended type of administration or not. Particle size and the (solid) state of the particle matrix are the main factors to be considered. Other important characteristics of SLNs are its shape, surface characteristics, and in particular, its interaction with incorporated drugs. Application of various characterization techniques is the most promising approach to attain a practical image of the sample properties due to the complexity of the systems.[26]

Particle size distribution is one of the most widely employed physical characteristic methods of SLNs, which is affected by numerous factors like lipid matrix, surfactant blend, lipid viscosity, drug to lipid ratio and aqueous phase and production parameters. Photon correlation spectroscopy and laser diffraction are main techniques which have been used for measurement of particle size.[3,17]

The zeta potential is a measurement of surface charge and is important factor in preventing aggregation and imparts the physical stability to formulation. Due to electrical repulsion at higher zeta potential, particle aggregation is less likely to occur.[3]

To study the morphology like sphericity and aggregation of SLNs, Scanning Electron Microscopy (SEM), Transmission Electron Microscopy (TEM) and Atomic Force Microscopy (AFM) have been performed.[3,27]

Drug encapsulation and release rate strongly has been affected by the cristallinity and the polymorphic behavior of lipids. The application of emulsifiers, the preparation procedure, and the high dispersity such as the small particle size of the colloidal system affected crystallinity of lipids in the SLNs. Differential scanning calorimetry and X-Ray diffractometry is basic techniques, which is used to investigate behavior of the lipids.[28]

There are three basic models for the drug and ingredients loading into SLNs: homogeneous matrix model, drug-enriched shell model and drug-enriched core model. The obtained construction of SLNs is depend on the formulation combination (lipid, active compound, surfactant) and of the fabrication conditions and methods.[29]

SLNs have capability for encapsulation of enormous amount of lipophilic compounds like steroids, retinol, and sunscreens but for hydrophilic ones, the payload amount is low. The low solubility of hydrophilic compounds into lipidic phase and crystalline structure of the lipid matrix can be reason of this effect. Two methods were reported to increase the payload of hydrophilic drugs. The first approach was the development of oil loaded SLN and the second strategy is modification of the lipid matrix by incorporation of amphiphilic compounds as well as phosphatydilcholine, polyglyceryl-3-diisostearate and sorbitan.[29]

The SLN suspension's ability to retain homogeneity (suspension stability), particle size and the lipid crystalline state are perspectives that should be considered in SLNs stability. The instability of the above processes results in disturbing the uniform suspension and increase of size. Besides, the recrystallization process causes cross-linking of crystallized particles, thereby changing the suspension into the gel.[3,30]

Biocompatibility and safety of prepared SLNs should be assessed using various *in vitro* cyto/genotoxicity assays such as with MTT, DAPI staining and DNA fragmentation assays and flow cytometry analysis.[3,31]

Dolatabadi et al (2014) confirmed the safety and lack of toxicity of alendronate sodium loaded SLNs to A549 cells by various cytotoxicity methods[3]. In order to identify non toxic concentration of SLN suspension, Perugini et al (2010) determined the EC50 values of aqueous suspension that can to be use in topical formulation.[32]

SLNs application in drug and gene delivery systems

SLNs have been considered as an efficient and non-toxic alternative lipophilic colloidal carrier for delivery of various drugs and other biological macromolecules like DNA and peptides. SLNs are biodegradable and are stable for a long period of time and easy to scale up compared to other colloidal systems. Drug delivery by SLNs to the liver cells has been reported, which are actively phagocytic. Their colloidal dimensions and the controlled release actions facilitate drug protection and administration by both parenteral and non-parenteral routes. The application of lipid nanoparticles by parenteral routes as well as biodistribution and pharmacokinetic studies upon intravenous administration has been described in literature.[33-36]

Drug delivery using SLNs

SLNs have been reported to be useful as drug carriers to treat various diseases as well as cancer. They offer a distinctive drug delivery system to prevent rapid clearance by the immune system. Stealth SLNs can be utilized to target specific tissues in accessible cells. Fluorescent markers together with drugs (Fluorescent SLNs) have been successfully evaluated in animal models. Methotrexate, paclitaxel and camptothecin- loaded SLNs have been reported for tumor targeting. Longer circulation times have been achieved by paclitaxel.[37-40]

SLNs can penetrate the blood–brain barrier (BBB) owing to adsorption of blood proteins such as apolipoproteins on their surface which can facilitate the adherence to endothelial cells. This effect was studied for the drugs like tobramycin, doxorubicin and idarubicin.[41-44]

Various administration routes such as oral, topical, parenteral and pulmonary have been reported for drug delivery using SLNs.[5]

Oral administration of SLNs

Oral administration of SLNs is feasible as aqueous dispersion or after transforming into dosage form i.e. tablets, pellets, capsules or powder in sachets. Antitubercular drugs like rifampicin, isonizide, pyrazinamide-loaded SLN systems have been reported for oral administration, which were able to reduce the dose amount and improve patient compliance. Formulation of poor orally bioavailable drug lopinavir into SLNs were reported using hot self nano-emulsification technique by Negi et al. They demonstrated that the oral bioavailability of lopinavir was improved due to higher intestinal lymphatic uptake of lopinavir-loaded SLNs.[45] In another study, Silva et al formulated a risperidone (an atypical antipsychotic drug) into SLNs and investigated its long-term stability, biocompatibility and drug transport. They believed that the prepared drug delivery system has potential for the oral delivery of poorly water-soluble drugs like risperidone.[46] In order to prevent rifampicin from hydrolyzes at the acidic pH of the stomach; Singh et al. encapsulated it into SLNs and reduced the risk of failure of therapy.[47] In addition, various anticancer drugs loaded SLNs such as camptothecin and tamoxifen were reported for this administration route as well.[48]

Parenteral administration of SLNs

Because of SLNs small size, they can be administered intravenously, intramuscularly, subcutaneously or to the target organ. Miao et al reported that SLN drug delivery system can enhance the transport of standard anticancer drugs like paclitaxel and doxorubicin into cancer cells and improve the cytotoxicity effect against sensitive cancer cells and their multi-drug resistant variant cells, compared to free drug solutions.[49] Also pharmacokinetic studies of doxorubicin loaded SLNs showed higher blood levels compared to a commercial drug solution after intravenous injection in rats. SLN loaded with the cationic amphiphilic doxorubicin and the anionic lipophilic docosahexaenoic acid (DHA), a polyunsaturated fatty acid that enhances the activity of anticancer drugs, has been developed with Mussi et al. They reported higher cytotoxicity and improved cellular uptake of doxorubicin-DHA-loaded SLN on human lung tumor cell line compared to free doxorubicin and DHA and suggested that DHA-doxorubicin-loaded SLN is a promising alternative for the treatment of cancer.[50] Regarding to the body distribution, SLNs showed high drug concentrations in lung, spleen and brain, whilst the solution causes a distribution more into liver and kidneys.[51] The distribution of camptothecin incorporated SLNs showed increased uptake in some organ especially in brain following intravenous administration.[12,52]

Topical administration of SLNS

Topical applications of SLNs have been reported with promising results for therapeutic purposes. It has a potential advantage of direct drug delivery to the site of action, which will generate higher tissue concentrations. Development and evaluation of SLNs of terbinafine hydrochloride for sustained release and skin targeting has been carried out by Vaghasiya et al. *In vivo* pharmacodynamic investigation indicated that the SLNs based gel decreased fungal burden of *Candida albicans* in rats as compared to commercial product in shorter duration of time.[53] Carbopol gels of aceclofenac SLNs have been prepared by Chawla et al. They demonstrated that the prepared gel could preserve the concentration of bioactives such as aceclofenac in desirable levels at sites of inflammation and injury.[54] A variety of drug such as anticancers, vitamin-A, isotretinoin, flurbiprofen has been incorporated in SLNs for topical applications as well.[55-57]

Pulmonary administration of SLNS

Pulmonary administration of drugs has some exclusive characteristics as well as large surface area, avoidance of the first-pass effect, high capacity for solute exchange, excellent vascularisation, and ultra-thinness of the alveolar epithelium (0.1-0.5 mm) that can facilitate systemic delivery. Moreover, degradation of drugs in the lung is slow because of low extracellular and intracellular enzyme activity. Thus, even compounds with low absorption rates can be absorbed to a relative high amount after pulmonary application. For the local treatment of airway diseases, the pulmonary application stands out by direct reaching the lung epithelium and thus the site of action which indicates that there is a fast onset of action and the necessary dose is reduced compared with traditional administration routes like the oral route. Furthermore, after local delivery of poorly absorbed drugs, high-dose exposures to the systemic circulation and therefore systemic adverse effects are minimized or avoided.[58-61]

One of the proposed strategies that can decrease both doses and the side effects of drugs is administration of them through dry powder aerosol form. Insulin-loaded SLN by micelle-double-emulsion method has been prepared by Liu et al. they demonstrated the stability of SLN during nebulization, the deposition properties and the hypoglycaemic effect after intrapulmonary application and showed higher bioavailability of insulin in lungs due to deposition of insulin-SLN.[62] Paclitaxel-loaded SLNs has been delivered to the lung lymphatics through the pulmonary route in experimental mouse mammary carcinoma. Paclitaxel-loaded SLNs was 20-fold more effective than a paclitaxel-solution on MXT-B2 cells, which was related to a higher internalization rate of paclitaxel-loaded SLNs than of free paclitaxel.[63] Budesonide-loaded SLNs were prepared by Zhang et al. for asthma therapy.[64] Also, SLNs of glucocorticoids, beclomethasone, dipropionate and alendronate sodium (bone resorption inhibitor) are examples of drugs, which have been developed for administration through this method.[5,65-67]

The published data show that SLNs could offer an extensive advantage for the local treatment for severe airway diseases as well as for the systemic drug delivery. Table 1 shows the application of SLNs in delivery of various drugs.

Table 1. Examples of SLNs based drug delivery systems.

Drug	Disease type	Lipid Type	Preparation technique	Ref
Stavudine, delavirdine & saquinavir	Human immunodeficiency virus (HIV)	Compritol 888 ATO, tripalmitin & cacao butter	Microemulsion	68
Lopinavir	HIV infections	Stearic acid	Hot self nano-emulsification	45
Aceclofenac	Inflammation in rheumatoid arthritis	Compritol & precirol	Ultrasonication	54
Norfloxacin	Bacterial infection	Stearic acid	Hot homogenization and ultrasonication	69
Rifampicin	Bacterial infection	Compritol 888 ATO	Microemulsion	47
Doxorubicin	Cancer	Docosahexaenoic acid	Hot homogenization	50
Gemcitabine	Solid tumors	4-(N)-stearoyl	Solvent emulsification	70
Paclitaxel & doxorubicin	Solid tumors	Glyceryl monostearate	Solvent diffusion	49
Terbinafine hydrochloride	Skin infections	Compritol & precirol	Solvent injection	53
Alendronate sodium	Bone diseases	Compritol & precirol	Hot homogenization	3
Risperidone	Schizophrenia	Compritol 888 ATO	Hot high pressure homogenization	46
Insulin	Diabetes mellitus	Phosphatidylcholine	Micelle-double-emulsion method	62

Gene delivery using SLNs

Successful gene therapy is defined as expression of the therapeutic gene in the target organ or tissue. Viral gene delivery (or viral vector) and non-viral gene delivery (or non-viral vector) are two types of gene therapy technique. In first type, the genes are transferred by a virus into the cells because of virus ability in penetrating cells.[71-76] Even though high levels of gene expression reported with viral gene delivery but it can have oncogenic and immunogenic effects, and induce inflammation that render transgene expression transient.[71-73] Non-viral vectors can overcome some of these concerns and compared to viral vectors they have considerable manufacturing and safety advantages. A variety of non-viral delivery systems have been demonstrated for efficient delivery of small-interfering RNAs (siRNAs) and DNA including cationic polymers, liposomes, cationic lipids, cell-penetrating peptide, carbon nanotubes and so on.[72,73,77]

SLNs as gene delivery systems have attracted increasing attention in recent years. Cationic SLNs usually have been used for gene delivery due to the possible electrostatic interaction between the negative charges of the DNA and the positive charges of the lipid, which allow the formation of a complex called lipoplex. These lipoplexes can form a structure that protects the DNA and direct it towards the target cells (Figure 2).[36,78] Carrillo et al. demonstrated cationic SLNs capable of forming a complex with DNA plasmids.[36] Jin et al. developed the siRNA-PEG/SLN, which can cross the BBB to the tumor site with no apparent systemic toxicity.[79] In another study, Montana et al. utilized cationically modified SLN as *Paracentrotus lividus bep3* RNA carriers and evaluated their potential as a nonviral vector for gene delivery.[80]

Future gene expression study definitely will open a new horizon for the achievement of rational design approaches in the development of cationic SLNs as effective gene delivery systems due to remarkable capability of them such as penetrating into cells, capability to achieve spatially- and temporally-controlled release for targeted gene silencing.

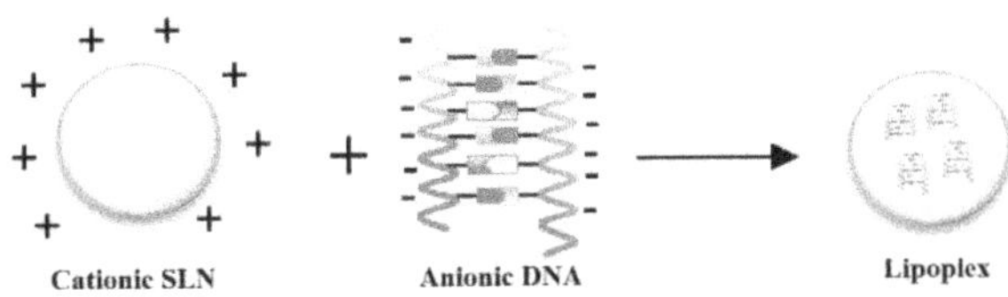

Figure 2. Lipoplexes complex formation due to the interaction between the negative charges of the DNA and the positive charges of the SLN.

Conclusion

SLNs are a novel and biocompatible colloidal drug and gene carrier system that merges the advantages of both liposomes and polymeric nanoparticles and simultaneously avoid some of their disadvantages. SLNs as an advanced drug and gene delivery nanosystems present significant opportunities for improving medical therapeutics. This article has reviewed various aspects of SLNs and their application in the encapsulation of various drugs and genes. Because of the SLN potential for facilitating controlled drug delivery to a target tissue and its biocompatibility, there will be much investigation in improvement of quality, efficacy, and safety profile of drugs using them in the future.

Acknowledgments

Authors would like to thank Research Center for Pharmaceutical Nanotechnology (RCPN), Tabriz University of Medical Sciences for supporting this project (which was a part of PhD thesis No: 90/014/104/2).

Conflict of Interest

The authors report no conflicts of interest.

References

1. Ezzati Nazhad Dolatabadi J, de la Guardia M. Nanomaterial-based electrochemical immunosensors as advanced diagnostic tools. *Anal Methods* 2014;6(12):3891-900. doi: 10.1039/c3ay41749b
2. Jamali AA, Pourhassan-Moghaddam M, Dolatabadi JEN, Omidi Y. Nanomaterials on the road to microRNA detection with optical and electrochemical nanobiosensors. *Trac-Trend Anal Chem* 2014;55:24-42. doi: 10.1016/j.trac.2013.10.008
3. Ezzati Nazhad Dolatabadi J, Hamishehkar H, Eskandani M, Valizadeh H. Formulation, characterization and cytotoxicity studies of alendronate sodium-loaded solid lipid nanoparticles. *Colloids Surf B Biointerfaces* 2014;117:21-8. doi: 10.1016/j.colsurfb.2014.01.055
4. Rostami E, Kashanian S, Azandaryani AH, Faramarzi H, Dolatabadi JEN, Omidfar K. Drug targeting using solid lipid nanoparticles. *Chem Phys Lipids* 2014;181:56-61. doi: 10.1016/j.chemphyslip.2014.03.006
5. Ezzati Nazhad Dolatabadi J, Hamishehkar H, Valizadeh H. Development of dry powder inhaler formulation loaded with alendronate solid lipid nanoparticles: Solid-state characterization and aerosol dispersion performance. *Drug Dev Ind Pharm* 2014:1-7. doi: 10.3109/03639045.2014.956111
6. Ezzati Nazhad Dolatabadi J, Jamali AA, Hasanzadeh M, Omidi Y. Quercetin Delivery into Cancer Cells with Single Walled Carbon Nanotubes. *Int J Biosci Biochem Bioinform* 2011;1:21-5. doi: 10.7763/ijbbb.2011.v1.4
7. Ezzati Nazhad Dolatabadi J, Omidi Y, Losic D. Carbon Nanotubes as an Advanced Drug and Gene Delivery Nanosystem. *Curr Nanosci* 2011;7(3):297-314. doi: 10.2174/157341311795542444
8. Dolatabadi JEN, Mashinchian O, Ayoubi B, Jamali AA, Mobed A, Losic D, et al. Optical and electrochemical DNA nanobiosensors. *TrAC, Trends Anal Chem* 2011;30(3):459-72. doi: 10.1016/j.trac.2010.11.010
9. Saei AA, Dolatabadi JEN, Najafi-Marandi P, Abhari A, de la Guardia M. Electrochemical biosensors for glucose based on metal nanoparticles. *TrAC, Trends Anal Chem* 2013;42:216-27. doi: 10.1016/j.trac.2012.09.011
10. Pouton CW. Lipid formulations for oral administration of drugs: non-emulsifying, self-emulsifying and 'self-microemulsifying' drug delivery systems. *Eur J Pharm Sci* 2000;11 Suppl 2:S93-8. doi: 10.1016/s0928-0987(00)00167-6
11. Muller RH, Radtke M, Wissing SA. Solid lipid nanoparticles (SLN) and nanostructured lipid carriers (NLC) in cosmetic and dermatological preparations. *Adv Drug Deliv Rev* 2002;54 Suppl 1:S131-55. doi: 10.1016/s0169-409x(02)00118-7
12. Muller RH, Mader K, Gohla S. Solid lipid nanoparticles (SLN) for controlled drug delivery - a review of the state of the art. *Eur J Pharm Biopharm* 2000;50(1):161-77. doi: 10.1016/s0939-6411(00)00087-4
13. Uner M, Yener G. Importance of solid lipid nanoparticles (SLN) in various administration routes and future perspectives. *Int J Nanomedicine* 2007;2(3):289-300.
14. Manjunath K, Reddy JS, Venkateswarlu V. Solid lipid nanoparticles as drug delivery systems. *Methods Find Exp Clin Pharmacol* 2005;27(2):127-44.
15. Ahlin Grabnar PKJSm-KJ. Optimization of procedure parameters and physical stability of solid lipid nanoparticles in dispersions. *Acta Pharmaceut* 1998;48no:259-67.
16. Olbrich C, Gessner A, Kayser O, Muller RH. Lipid-drug-conjugate (LDC) nanoparticles as novel carrier system for the hydrophilic antitrypanosomal drug

diminazenediaceturate. *J Drug Target* 2002;10(5):387-96. doi: 10.1080/1061186021000001832
17. Kamble VA, Jagdale DM, Kadam VJ. Solid lipid nanoparticles as drug delivery system. *Int J Pharm Biol Sci* 2010;1:1-9.
18. Alda Jusceline L, Hulda Noemi Mamani C, Daniel B-A, Heloise Oliveira P, Carlos Raimundo Ferreira G. Production and characterization of lipid microparticles produced by spray cooling encapsulating a low molar mass hydrophilic compound. *Food Sci Technol* 2010;30(1):276-81. doi: 10.1590/s0101-20612010005000014
19. Mukherjee S, Ray S, Thakur RS. Solid lipid nanoparticles: a modern formulation approach in drug delivery system. *Indian J Pharm Sci* 2009;71(4):349-58. doi: 10.4103/0250-474x.57282
20. Kaiser CS, Rompp H, Schmidt PC. Pharmaceutical applications of supercritical carbon dioxide. *Pharmazie* 2001;56(12):907-26.
21. Gosselin PM, Thibert R, Preda M, Mcmullen JN. Polymorphic properties of micronized carbamazepine produced by RESS. *Int J Pharm* 2003;252(1-2):225-33. doi: 10.1016/s0378-5173(02)00649-x
22. Sjostrom B, Bergenstahl B. Preparation of submicron drug particles in lecithin-stabilized o/w emulsions I. Model studies of the precipitation of cholesteryl acetate. *Int J Pharm* 1992;88(1-3):53-62. doi: 10.1016/0378-5173(92)90303-j
23. Siekmann B, Westesen K. Investigations on solid lipid nanoparticles prepared by precipitation in O/W emulsions. *Eur J Pharm Biopharm* 1996;42:104-9.
24. Qi C, Chen Y, Jing QZ, Wang XG. Preparation and characterization of catalase-loaded solid lipid nanoparticles protecting enzyme against proteolysis. *Int J Mol Sci* 2011;12(7):4282-93. doi: 10.3390/ijms12074282
25. Freitas C, Mullera RH. Spray-drying of solid lipid nanoparticles (SLN TM). *Eur J Pharm Biopharm* 1998;46(2):145-51. doi: 10.1016/s0939-6411(97)00172-0
26. Pardeike J, Hommoss A, Muller RH. Lipid nanoparticles (SLN, NLC) in cosmetic and pharmaceutical dermal products. *Int J Pharm* 2009;366(1-2):170-84. doi: 10.1016/j.ijpharm.2008.10.003
27. Yoon G, Park J, Yoon IS. Solid lipid nanoparticles (SLNs) and nanostructured lipid carriers (NLCs): recent advances in drug delivery. *J Pharm Invest* 2013;43(5):353-62. doi: 10.1007/s40005-013-0087-y
28. Rizwan M, Aqil M, Talegaonkar S, Azeem A, Sultana Y, Ali A. Enhanced transdermal drug delivery techniques: an extensive review of patents. *Recent Pat Drug Deliv Formul* 2009;3(2):105-24. doi: 10.2174/187221109788452285
29. Mehnert W, Mader K. Solid lipid nanoparticles: production, characterization and applications. *Adv Drug Deliv Rev* 2001;47(2-3):165-96. doi: 10.1016/s0169-409x(01)00105-3
30. Taratula O, Kuzmov A, Shah M, Garbuzenko OB, Minko T. Nanostructured lipid carriers as multifunctional nanomedicine platform for pulmonary co-delivery of anticancer drugs and siRNA. *J Control Release* 2013;171(3):349-57. doi: 10.1016/j.jconrel.2013.04.018
31. Weyenberg W, Filev P, Van Den Plas D, Vandervoort J, De Smet K, Sollie P, et al. Cytotoxicity of submicron emulsions and solid lipid nanoparticles for dermal application. *Int J Pharm* 2007;337(1-2):291-8. doi: 10.1016/j.ijpharm.2006.12.045
32. Perugini P, Tomasi C, Vettor M, Dazio V, Conti B, Genta I, et al. Influence of SLN matrix modification on"in vitro" and "in vivo" nanoparticle performances. *Int J Pharm Pharm Sci* 2010;2:37-42.
33. Fundaro A, Cavalli R, Bargoni A, Vighetto D, Zara GP, Gasco MR. Non-stealth and stealth solid lipid nanoparticles (SLN) carrying doxorubicin: pharmacokinetics and tissue distribution after i.v. administration to rats. *Pharmacol Res* 2000;42(4):337-43. doi: 10.1006/phrs.2000.0695
34. Zara GP, Cavalli R, Bargoni A, Fundaro A, Vighetto D, Gasco MR. Intravenous administration to rabbits of non-stealth and stealth doxorubicin-loaded solid lipid nanoparticles at increasing concentrations of stealth agent: pharmacokinetics and distribution of doxorubicin in brain and other tissues. *J Drug Target* 2002;10(4):327-35. doi: 10.1080/10611860290031868
35. Almeida AJ, Souto E. Solid lipid nanoparticles as a drug delivery system for peptides and proteins. *Adv Drug Deliv Rev* 2007;59(6):478-90. doi: 10.1016/j.addr.2007.04.007
36. Carrillo C, Sanchez-Hernandez N, Garcia-Montoya E, Perez-Lozano P, Sune-Negre JM, Tico JR, et al. DNA delivery via cationic solid lipid nanoparticles (SLNs). *Eur J Pharm Sci* 2013;49(2):157-65. doi: 10.1016/j.ejps.2013.02.011
37. Wang Y, Wu W. In situ evading of phagocytic uptake of stealth solid lipid nanoparticles by mouse peritoneal macrophages. *Drug Deliv* 2006;13(3):189-92. doi: 10.1080/10717540500315930
38. Ruckmani K, Sivakumar M, Ganeshkumar PA. Methotrexate loaded solid lipid nanoparticles (SLN) for effective treatment of carcinoma. *J Nanosci Nanotechnol* 2006;6(9-10):2991-5. doi: 10.1166/jnn.2006.457
39. Yang SC, Lu LF, Cai Y, Zhu JB, Liang BW, Yang CZ. Body distribution in mice of intravenously injected camptothecin solid lipid nanoparticles and targeting effect on brain. *J Control Release* 1999;59(3):299-307. doi: 10.1016/s0168-3659(99)00007-3
40. Chen DB, Yang TZ, Lu WL, Zhang Q. In vitro and in vivo study of two types of long-circulating solid lipid nanoparticles containing paclitaxel. *Chem Pharm Bull (Tokyo)* 2001;49(11):1444-7. doi: 10.1248/cpb.49.1444

41. Bargoni A, Cavalli R, Zara GP, Fundaro A, Caputo O, Gasco MR. Transmucosal transport of tobramycin incorporated in solid lipid nanoparticles (SLN) after duodenal administration to rats. Part II--tissue distribution. *Pharmacol Res* 2001;43(5):497-502. doi: 10.1006/phrs.2001.0813
42. Zara GP, Cavalli R, Fundaro A, Bargoni A, Caputo O, Gasco MR. Pharmacokinetics of doxorubicin incorporated in solid lipid nanospheres (SLN). *Pharmacol Res* 1999;40(3):281-6. doi: 10.1006/phrs.1999.0509
43. Zara GP, Bargoni A, Cavalli R, Fundaro A, Vighetto D, Gasco MR. Pharmacokinetics and tissue distribution of idarubicin-loaded solid lipid nanoparticles after duodenal administration to rats. *J Pharm Sci* 2002;91(5):1324-33. doi: 10.1002/jps.10129
44. Solaro R, Chiellini F, Battisti A. Targeted Delivery of Protein Drugs by Nanocarriers. *Materials* 2010;3(3):1928-80. doi: 10.3390/ma3031928
45. Negi JS, Chattopadhyay P, Sharma AK, Ram V. Development of solid lipid nanoparticles (SLNs) of lopinavir using hot self nano-emulsification (SNE) technique. *Eur J Pharm Sci* 2013;48(1-2):231-9. doi: 10.1016/j.ejps.2012.10.022
46. Silva AC, Kumar A, Wild W, Ferreira D, Santos D, Forbes B. Long-term stability, biocompatibility and oral delivery potential of risperidone-loaded solid lipid nanoparticles. *Int J Pharm* 2012;436(1-2):798-805. doi: 10.1016/j.ijpharm.2012.07.058
47. Singh H, Bhandari R, Kaur IP. Encapsulation of Rifampicin in a solid lipid nanoparticulate system to limit its degradation and interaction with Isoniazid at acidic pH. *Int J Pharm* 2013;446(1-2):106-11. doi: 10.1016/j.ijpharm.2013.02.012
48. Kamboj S, Bala S, Nair AB. Solid Lipid Nanoparticles: An effective lipid based technology for poorly water soluble drugs. *Int J Pharm Sci Rev Res* 2010;5(2):78-90.
49. Miao J, Du YZ, Yuan H, Zhang XG, Hu FQ. Drug resistance reversal activity of anticancer drug loaded solid lipid nanoparticles in multi-drug resistant cancer cells. *Colloids Surf B Biointerfaces* 2013;110:74-80. doi: 10.1016/j.colsurfb.2013.03.037
50. Mussi SV, Silva RC, Oliveira MC, Lucci CM, Azevedo RB, Ferreira LA. New approach to improve encapsulation and antitumor activity of doxorubicin loaded in solid lipid nanoparticles. *Eur J Pharm Sci* 2013;48(1-2):282-90. doi: 10.1016/j.ejps.2012.10.025
51. Goppert TM, Muller RH. Polysorbate-stabilized solid lipid nanoparticles as colloidal carriers for intravenous targeting of drugs to the brain: comparison of plasma protein adsorption patterns. *J Drug Target* 2005;13(3):179-87. doi: 10.1080/10611860500071292
52. Cavalli R, Caputo O, Gasco MR. Preparation and characterization of solid lipid nanospheres containing paclitaxel. *Eur J Pharm Sci* 2000;10(4):305-9. doi: 10.1016/s0928-0987(00)00081-6
53. Vaghasiya H, Kumar A, Sawant K. Development of solid lipid nanoparticles based controlled release system for topical delivery of terbinafine hydrochloride. *Eur J Pharm Sci* 2013;49(2):311-22. doi: 10.1016/j.ejps.2013.03.013
54. Chawla V, Saraf SA. Rheological studies on solid lipid nanoparticle based carbopol gels of aceclofenac. *Colloids Surf B Biointerfaces* 2012;92:293-8. doi: 10.1016/j.colsurfb.2011.12.006
55. Chen H, Chang X, Du D, Liu W, Liu J, Weng T, et al. Podophyllotoxin-loaded solid lipid nanoparticles for epidermal targeting. *J Control Release* 2006;110(2):296-306. doi: 10.1016/j.jconrel.2005.09.052
56. Jenning V, Schafer-Korting M, Gohla S. Vitamin A-loaded solid lipid nanoparticles for topical use: drug release properties. *J Control Release* 2000;66(2-3):115-26. doi: 10.1016/s0168-3659(99)00223-0
57. Santos Maia C, Mehnert W, Schaller M, Korting HC, Gysler A, Haberland A, et al. Drug targeting by solid lipid nanoparticles for dermal use. *J Drug Target* 2002;10(6):489-95. doi: 10.1080/1061186021000038364
58. Weber S, Zimmer A, Pardeike J. Solid Lipid Nanoparticles (SLN) and Nanostructured Lipid Carriers (NLC) for pulmonary application: a review of the state of the art. *Eur J Pharm Biopharm* 2014;86(1):7-22. doi: 10.1016/j.ejpb.2013.08.013
59. Yang W, Peters JI, Williams RO 3rd. Inhaled nanoparticles--a current review. *Int J Pharm* 2008;356(1-2):239-47. doi: 10.1016/j.ijpharm.2008.02.011
60. Gehr P, Bachofen M, Weibel ER. The normal human lung: ultrastructure and morphometric estimation of diffusion capacity. *Respir Physiol* 1978;32(2):121-40. doi: 10.1016/0034-5687(78)90104-4
61. Cryan SA, Sivadas N, Garcia-Contreras L. In vivo animal models for drug delivery across the lung mucosal barrier. *Adv Drug Deliv Rev* 2007;59(11):1133-51. doi: 10.1016/j.addr.2007.08.023
62. Liu J, Gong T, Fu H, Wang C, Wang X, Chen Q, et al. Solid lipid nanoparticles for pulmonary delivery of insulin. *Int J Pharm* 2008;356(1-2):333-44. doi: 10.1016/j.ijpharm.2008.01.008
63. Videira M, Almeida AJ, Fabra A. Preclinical evaluation of a pulmonary delivered paclitaxel-loaded lipid nanocarrier antitumor effect. *Nanomedicine* 2012;8(7):1208-15. doi: 10.1016/j.nano.2011.12.007
64. Zhang PR, Tu YF, Wang S, Wang YH, Xie Y, Li M, et al. Preparation and characterization of budesonide-loaded solid lipid nanoparticles for pulmonary delivery. *J Chin Pharm Sci* 2011;20(4):390-6. doi: 10.5246/jcps.2011.04.049
65. Zeng XM, MacRitchie HB, Marriott C, Martin GP. Correlation between inertial impaction and laser diffraction sizing data for aerosolized carrier-based

dry powder formulations. *Pharm Res* 2006;23(9):2200-9. doi: 10.1007/s11095-006-9055-9

66. Jaafar-Maalej C, Andrieu V, Elaissari A, Fessi H. Beclomethasone-loaded lipidic nanocarriers for pulmonary drug delivery: preparation, characterization and in vitro drug release. *J Nanosci Nanotechnol* 2011;11(3):1841-51. doi: 10.1166/jnn.2011.3119
67. Ezzati Nazhad Dolatabadi J, Hamishehkar H, De La Guardia M, Valizadeh H. A fast and simple spectrofluorometric method for the determination of alendronate sodium in pharmaceuticals. *BioImpacts* 2014;4(1):39-42. doi: 10.5681/bi.2014.005
68. Kuo YC, Chung CY. Solid lipid nanoparticles comprising internal Compritol 888 ATO, tripalmitin and cacao butter for encapsulating and releasing stavudine, delavirdine and saquinavir. *Colloids Surf B Biointerfaces* 2011;88(2):682-90. doi: 10.1016/j.colsurfb.2011.07.060
69. Wang Y, Zhu L, Dong Z, Xie S, Chen X, Lu M, et al. Preparation and stability study of norfloxacin-loaded solid lipid nanoparticle suspensions. *Colloids Surf B Biointerfaces* 2012;98:105-11. doi: 10.1016/j.colsurfb.2012.05.006
70. Wonganan P, Lansakara PD, Zhu S, Holzer M, Sandoval MA, Warthaka M, et al. Just getting into cells is not enough: mechanisms underlying 4-(N)-stearoyl gemcitabine solid lipid nanoparticle's ability to overcome gemcitabine resistance caused by RRM1 overexpression. *J Control Release* 2013;169(1-2):17-27. doi: 10.1016/j.jconrel.2013.03.033
71. Tran PA, Zhang L, Webster TJ. Carbon nanofibers and carbon nanotubes in regenerative medicine. *Adv Drug Deliv Rev* 2009;61(12):1097-114. doi: 10.1016/j.addr.2009.07.010
72. Singh R, Pantarotto D, Mccarthy D, Chaloin O, Hoebeke J, Partidos CD, et al. Binding and condensation of plasmid DNA onto functionalized carbon nanotubes: toward the construction of nanotube-based gene delivery vectors. *J Am Chem Soc* 2005;127(12):4388-96. doi: 10.1021/ja0441561
73. Ji SR, Liu C, Zhang B, Yang F, Xu J, Long J, et al. Carbon nanotubes in cancer diagnosis and therapy. *Biochim Biophys Acta* 2010;1806(1):29-35. doi: 10.1016/j.bbcan.2010.02.004
74. Singh S. Nanomaterials as Non-viral siRNA Delivery Agents for Cancer Therapy. *BioImpacts* 2013;3(2):53-65.
75. Barar J, Omidi Y. Targeted Gene Therapy of Cancer: Second Amendment toward Holistic Therapy. *BioImpacts* 2013;3(2):49-51. doi: 10.5681/bi.2013.014
76. Razi Soofiyani S, Baradaran B, Lotfipour F, Kazemi T, Mohammadnejad L. Gene therapy, early promises, subsequent problems, and recent breakthroughs. *Adv Pharm Bull* 2013;3(2):249-55. doi: 10.5681/apb.2013.041
77. Elfinger M, Üzgün S, Rudolph C. Nanocarriers for gene delivery - polymer structure, targeting ligands and controlled-release devices. *Curr Nanosci* 2008;4(4):322-53. doi: 10.2174/157341308786306062
78. Goncalves C, Berchel M, Gosselin MP, Malard V, Cheradame H, Jaffres PA, et al. Lipopolyplexes comprising imidazole/imidazolium lipophosphoramidate, histidinylated polyethyleneimine and siRNA as efficient formulation for siRNA transfection. *Int J Pharm* 2014;460(1-2):264-72. doi: 10.1016/j.ijpharm.2013.11.005
79. Jin J, Bae KH, Yang H, Lee SJ, Kim H, Kim Y, et al. In vivo specific delivery of c-Met siRNA to glioblastoma using cationic solid lipid nanoparticles. *Bioconjug Chem* 2011;22(12):2568-72. doi: 10.1021/bc200406n
80. Montana G, Bondi ML, Carrotta R, Picone P, Craparo EF, San Biagio PL, et al. Employment of cationic solid-lipid nanoparticles as RNA carriers. *Bioconjug Chem* 2007;18(2):302-8. doi: 10.1021/bc0601166

Effect of Buspirone, Fluoxetine and 8-OH-DPAT on Striatal Expression of Bax, Caspase-3 and Bcl-2 Proteins in 6-Hydroxydopamine-Induced Hemi-Parkinsonian Rats

Hamdollah Sharifi[1], Alireza Mohajjel Nayebi[2,3]*, Safar Farajnia[2], Rasool Haddadi[4]

[1] *Department of Pharmacology, Faculty of Pharmacy, Urmia University of Medical Sciences, Urmia, Iran.*
[2] *Drug Applied Research Center, Tabriz University of Medical Sciences, Tabriz, Iran.*
[3] *Department of Pharmacology and Toxicology, Faculty of Pharmacy, Tabriz University of Medical Sciences, Tabriz, Iran.*
[4] *Department of Pharmacology and Toxicology, Faculty of Pharmacy, Hamadan University of Medical Science, Hamadan, Iran.*

Article info

Keywords:
- Fluoxetine
- Buspirone
- 8-OH-DPAT
- Apoptosis
- Parkinson's disease

Abstract

Purpose: The exact pathogenesis of sporadic parkinson's disease (PD) is still unclear. Numerous evidences suggest involvement of apoptosis in the death of dopaminergic neurons. In this study we investigated the effect of sub-chronic administration of buspirone, fluoxetine and 8-hydroxy-2-[di-n-propylamino]tetralin (8-OH-DPAT) in 6-hydroxydopamine (6-OHDA)-lesioned rats and assayed striatal concentrations of apoptotic (Bax, Caspase3) and anti-apoptotic (Bcl-2) proteins.

Methods: 6-OHDA (8μg/2μl/rat) was injected unilaterally into the central region of the substantia nigra pars copmacta (SNc) of male Wistar rats and then, after 21 days lesioned rats were treated with intraperitonel (i.p) 1 mg/kg injections of buspirone, fluoxetine and 8-OH-DPAT for 10 consecutive days. Striatum of rats was removed at tenth day of drugs administration and were analyzed by western blotting method to measure Bax, caspase3 and Bcl-2 expression.

Results: The results showed that the expression of Bax and caspase3 proteins was increased three weeks after 6-OHDA injection while they were decreased significantly in parkinsonian rats which were treated by buspirone, fluoxetine and 8-OH-DPAT. Bcl-2 was decreased and increased in parkinsonian rats and parkinsonian rats treated with buspirone, fluoxetine and 8-OH-DPAT, respectively.

Conclusion: Our study indicates that sub-chronic administration of serotonergic drugs such as buspirone, fluoxetine and 8-OH-DPAT restores striatal concentration of apoptotic and anti-apoptotic factors to the basal levels of normal non-lesioned rats. We suggest that these drugs can be used as a potential adjunctive therapy in PD through attenuating neuronal apoptotic process.

Introduction

The pathogenesis of sporadic Parkinson disease (PD) is still enigmatic; many factors are speculated to operate in the mechanism of cell death of the nigrostriatal dopaminergic neurons in PD. Recent studies have been focused on the factors of the pathways of programmed cell death, i.e., apoptosis, that might be involved in the neurodegeneration in PD.[1] By end-stage disease in PD there is 80–95% loss of neurons in the substantia nigra.[2] Increased levels of proteins that signal for apoptosis have been demonstrated not only in neurons of postmortem PD but also in experimental models of PD strongly suggested involvement of apoptosis in the death of nigrostriatal neurons.[3] The major anti-apoptotic family members, Bcl-2 and Bcl-xL, which are thought to exert their effect at the mitochondrial outer membrane contribute to maintenance of membrane integrity. In contrast, one of the major pro-apoptotic family members, Bax, exerts its effects by compromising the membrane integrity leading to leakage of apoptogenic factors such as cytochrome c into the cytosol, resulting in caspase-3 activation and demise of the cell.[4] Altered expressional levels of Bcl-2, Bax and increased caspase 1 and 3 activity have been reported in dopaminergic neurons of PD patients[5,6] and in 6-OHDA-lesioned rats[7] but the effect of serotonergic drugs on these proteins in PD have not studied. The stimulation of $5HT_{1A}$ receptors induces a variable level of neuroprotection in different animal models of CNS injury.[8] In vitro evidence indicates that $5HT_{1A}$ agonists are able to protect neurons from apoptosis.[9] Thus in this study we attempted to investigate the effect of chronic administration of serotonergic drugs (8-OH-DPAT, buspirone and fluoxetine) on 6-OHDA-induced PD in rats and possible involvement of Bax, Bcl-2 and Caspase-3 in this context.

***Corresponding author:** Alireza Mohajjel Nayebi, Email: nayebia@tbzmed.ac.ir

Materials and Methods

Chemicals

All chemicals were obtained from Sigma Chemical Co. except for antibodies used for western blotting technique which were purchased from Abcam Co. Drugs and 6-OHDA were dissolved in physiological saline (0.9% NaCl) and 0.9% saline containing 0.2% (w/v) ascorbic acid respectively.

Animals and Treatment Protocol

The experiments were carried out on male Wistar rats weighing 270-300 g. The animals were given food and water ad libitum and were housed in standard polypropylene cages, four per cage at an ambient temperature of 25±2 °C under a 12-h light/12-h dark cycle. Animals were habituated to the testing conditions including being transferred to the experimental environment, handled, weighed, and restrained on the test platform for 10 min; 2 days before the investigations were conducted. The present study was carried out in accordance with the ethical guidelines for the Care and Use of Laboratory Animals of Tabriz University of Medical Sciences, Tabriz, Iran (National Institutes of Health Publication No. 85-23, revised 1985).

The parkinsonian rats were randomly allocated to equal groups (six rats per group) and were treated with 8-OH-DPAT (1mg/kg, i.p), fluoxetine (1mg/kg, i.p) and buspirone (1 mg/kg, i.p) for ten days. According to our previous study[10-12] 1mg/kg dose of these drugs had more profound anti-cataleptic effect in 6-OHDA-induced hemiparkinsonian rats. Then their striatal apoptotic proteins (Bcl-2, Bax and Caspase 3) were assessed by western blotting technique.

6-OHDA-Induced SNc Lesion

Animals were anesthetized with an intraperitoneal (i.p) injection of ketamine (50 mg/kg) and xylazine (5 mg/kg) and were mounted in a stereotaxic frame in the flat skull position. A central incision made to expose the skull. 6-OHDA was injected thorough a guide cannula (23 gauge stainless steel) implanted in the SNc. The coordinates for this site were based on the rat brain atlas[13] anteroposterior (AP): –5.0 mm from the bregma; mediolateral (ML): –2.1 mm from the midline and dorsoventral (DV): –7.7 from the skull. Desipramine (25 mg/kg, i.p) was injected 30 min before the intra-SNc injection of 6-OHDA to avoid the destruction of noradrenergic neurons. Then, 6-OHDA (8 µg/per rat in 2 µl saline with 0.2% ascorbic acid) was infused with an infusion pump at a constant flow rate of 0.2 µl/min into the left SNc.

Western Blot Analysis

Animals were sacrificed after ten days administration of drugs and their striatum was dissected and homogenized in lysis buffer (Cocktail Protease Inhibitor 10 µl/ml and Phenyl Methane Sulfonyl Fluoride 10 µl/ml). Lysates (30 µg protein) were resolved by SDS-PAGE for Bax, Caspase3 and Bcl-2 assay; then were transferred to polyvinylidene difluoride filters (PVDF) which were blocked with 5% milk and were incubated overnight at 4°C with the following primary antibodies: Bax, Bcl-2 and GAPDH, 1:1000 , Caspase-3, 1:500. Subsequently, PVDF membranes were incubated for 1 hr at room temperature with an HRP-conjugated secondary antibody (1:3000); incubated with the chemiluminescent substrate for 90 s; and exposed for 30 s to 5 min, to Hyperfilm. Finally the developed films were scanned, and density of immonoreactive bands was measured using "Image J" software and was normalized to the internal control bands (GAPDH was the loading control).

Statistical Analysis

Statistical analysis of each data set was performed by use of SPSS software (version 16.0). Data were expressed as the mean±SEM, and were analyzed by one-way ANOVA in behavioral and biochemical experiments. In the case of significant variation ($p<0.05$), the values were compared by Tukey test.

Results

The Effects of Buspirone, Fluoxetine and 8-OH-DPAT on Bax Expression

The Expression of striatal Bax protein in 6-OHDA-lesioned rats increased significantly ($p<0.001$) when compared to non-lesioned (control) rats. The amount of this protein in buspirone, fluoxetine and 8-OH-DPAT-treated parkinsonian rats was almost same as the control level. On the other hand, these drugs decreased expression of Bax protein in 6-OHDA-lesioned rats (Figure 1).

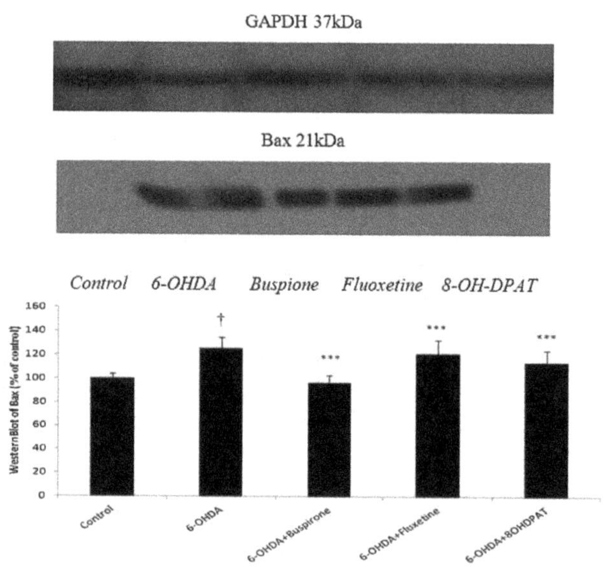

Figure 1. Effect of sub-chronically(10 days) administered buspirone,fluoxetine and 8-OH-DPAT (1 mg/kg, i.p) on SNcbax expression analyzed by Western Blot. Data represent the mean percentage of controls (±SEM) for 6 animals in each group. Data were analyzed by ANOVA followed by tukey's-test. † $p<0.001$ when compared with normal group (control), *** $p<0.001$ when compared with 6-OHDA-lesioned group .GAPDH was loading control.

The Effects of Buspirone, Fluoxetine and 8-OH-DPAT on Caspase-3 Expression

The striatum of aforementioned groups was investigated for evaluation of pro-apoptotic Caspase-3 protein activity. Results showed that in 6-OHDA-lesioned rats expression of this protein was more than control group ($p<0.001$), while in 6-OHDA-lesioned rats which were treated with buspirone, fluoxetine and 8-OH-DPAT expression of Caspase-3 protein was reduced to control level (Figure 2).

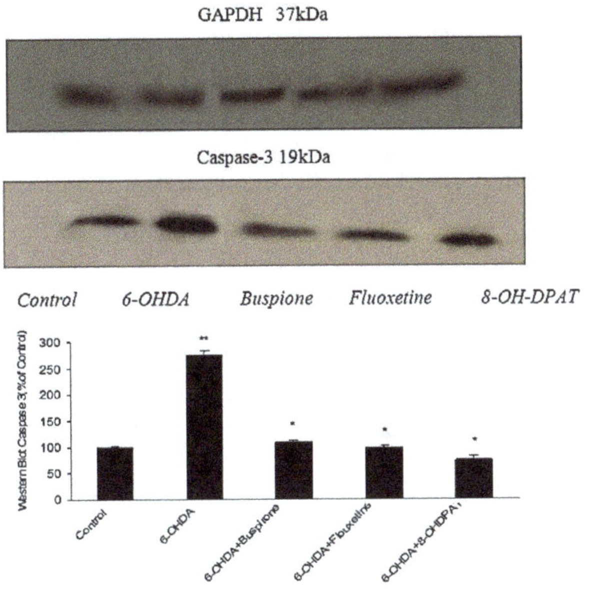

Figure 2. Effect of chronically (10 days) administered buspirone,fluoxetine and 8-OH-DPAT (1 mg/kg, i.p) on SNc Caspase-3 activity analyzed byWestern Blot. Data represent the mean percentage of controls (±SEM) for 6 animals in each group. Data were analyzed by ANOVA followed by tukey's-test. **$p<0.001$ when compared with normal group (control), *$p<0.001$ when compared with 6-OHDA-lesioned group .GAPDH was loading control.

The Effects of Buspirone, Fluoxetine and 8-OH-DPAT on Bcl-2 Expression

As it has been shown in Figure 3, the expression of anti-apoptotic Bcl-2 protein in the striatum of 6-OHDA-lesioned rats was less than ($p<0.001$) control group. In 6-OHDA-lesioned rats which were treated with buspirone, fluoxetine and 8-OH-DPAT, expression of Bcl-2 protein was greater ($p<0.001$) than 6-OHDA-lesioned rats.

Discussion

In our previous studies we have shown that 6-OHDA (8 μg/2 μl/rat) could induce significant catalepsy in bar test when compared with control (normal) and sham-operated animals.[10-12, 14-17] Furthermore, 8-OH-DPAT (1 mg/kg, i.p),[10] fluoxetine (1 mg/kg, i.p)[11] and buspirone (1 mg/kg, i.p)[12] attenuated 6-OHDA-induced catalepsy in hemiparkinsonian rats. Thus, in this study we attempted to assess the effect of these drugs on expression of pro-apoptotic proteins, Bax and Caspase-3 as well as anti-apoptotic Bcl-2 protein in 6-OHDA-lesioned rats. Our results showed that expression of Bax protein was increased significantly in 6-OHDA-lesioned rats. This is in agreement with previous studies showing an over expression of Bax protein in parkinsonian patients[18] and 6-OHDA-treated rats.[19-20] In those groups of parkinsonian rats which were treated sub-chronically by buspirone, fluoxetine and 8-OH-DPAT, striatal expression of Bax protein was dropped markedly to the level of control group. The attenuating effect of buspirone and 8-OH-DPAT on expression of Bax Protein was greater than fluoxetine.

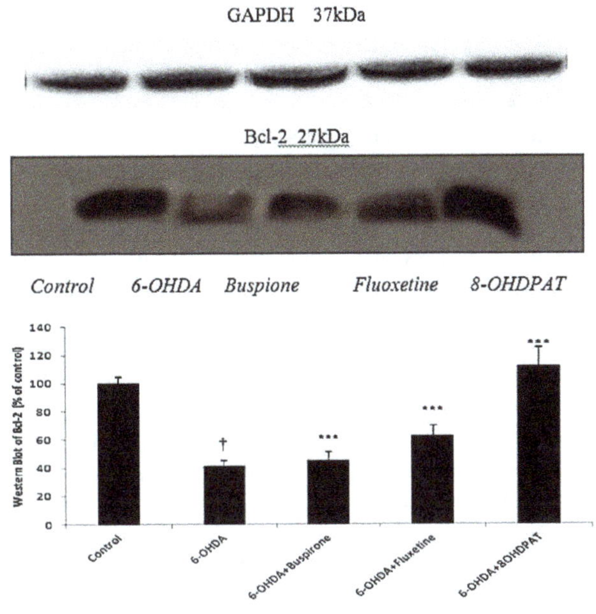

Figure 3. Effect of chronically (10 days) administered buspirone,fluoxetine and 8-OH-DPAT (1 mg/kg, i.p) on SNc Bcl-2 expression analyzed byWestern Blot. Data represent the mean percentage of controls (±SEM) for 6 animals in each group. Data were analyzed by ANOVA followed by tukey's-test. †$p<0.001$ when compared with normal group (control); ***$p<0.001$ when compared with 6-OHDA-lesioned group .GAPDH was loading control.

Caspase family has 14 members that many of these proteases have been implicated in neuronal apoptosis. The first evidence that caspase activity is required for neuronal apoptosis came from experiments using pharmacological inhibitors of caspases. Moreover caspases may play pivotal roles in a number of acute and chronic neurologic disorders including stroke, Amyotrophic lateral sclerosis (ALS), PD and Huntington's disease.[21] For example, mice transgenic for a dominant negative mutant of caspase-1 exhibit reduced sensitivity to ischemia as well as trophic factor deprivation. Accordingly, inhibition of caspase-3 expression plays a crucial neuroprotective role in a number of animal and human models of neurodegenerative disease such as Alzheimer disease (AD) and PD.[22] Our data demonstrate that in 6-OHDA-lesioned rats there was a significant increase in striatal Caspase-3 level when compared to control group. This is in accordance with previous studies reporting an increase of in 6-OHDA, Methyl-4-phenyl-1,2,3,6-tetrahydropyridine (MPTP) and lipopolysaccharide (LPS)-treated rats.[3,23] Additionally we assessed Caspase-3 activity in striatum of buspirone, fluoxetine and 8-OH-DPAT-treated parkinsonian rats. In parkinsonian rats which were treated with these drugs Caspase-3 expression diminished to the level of non-lesioned (control) animals. The effect of 8-OH-DPAT on Caspase-3 expression was more profound than buspirone and fluoxetine. In a previous study it has been shown that 8-OH-DPAT can reduce morphine-induced apoptosis in hippocampus of rats.[24] Since 8-OH-DPAT is a pure agonist of 5-HT_{1A} receptors, therefore we may suggest possible involvement of these receptors in apoptosis process of PD.

Bcl-2 is specifically considered as an important anti-apoptotic protein and is thus classified as an oncogene. Many members of the Bcl-2 family have been implicated in the regulation of neuronal cell death. The exact mechanism by which the Bcl-2 proteins control apoptosis is still not entirely clear but studies have shown that it's over expression in cell culture and in transgenic mice increases resistance of neurons to death during development and protects from apoptosis induced by excitotoxic, metabolic and oxidative insults relevant to AD, stroke and other disorder.[22,25] In this study, Bcl-2 level was decreased in 6-OHDA-lesioned rats.[26] Following treatment with buspirone, fluoxetine and 8-OH-DPAT, striatal level of this protein was elevated significantly in comparison to 6-OHDA-lesioned rats. The effect of 8-OH-DPAT and buspirone (as a partial agonist of 5-HT_{1A} receptors) was greater than fluoxetine. Previous studies suggested that 5-HT_{1A} receptors have neuroprotective effect.[27-30] We have shown that these drugs via stimulation of 5-HT_{1A} receptors, can improve 6-OHDA-induced catalepsy in rats.[10-12] The stimulation of 5HT_{1A} receptors induces a variable level of neuroprotection in different animal models of CNS injury such as ischemia, *N*-methyl-d-aspartate (NMDA) excitotoxicity, acute subdural hematoma, and traumatic brain injury. Furthermore, in vitro evidence indicates that 5HT_{1A} agonists are able to protect neurons from apoptosis.[24] There are different hypotheses on the mechanisms involved in 5HT_{1A}-mediated neuroprotection, including neuronal membrane hyperpolarization that reduces excitability, reduced glutamate release, and blockade of voltage-sensitive Na+ channels.[24] Other neuroprotective mechanisms have also been proposed for 5HT_{1A} agonists such as stimulation of the BCL-2 expression through the MAPK/ERK signaling pathway and suppression of the pro-apoptotic protein caspase-3 in a MAPK- and protein kinase C-α dependent manner.[31,32] Thus, we may suggest that the observed anti-apoptotic effects of serotonergic drugs i.e. buspirone, fluoxetine and 8-OH-DPAT is exerted through 5-HT_{1A} receptors.

According to the obtained results buspirone, fluoxetine and 8-OH-DPAT diminished striatal expression of Bax and Caspase-3 proteines in parkinsonian rats, whereas they increased Bcl-2 level. On the other hand, these drugs could attenuate apoptotic process in 6-OHDA-induced experimental model of PD. This correlates well with the results of our previous behavioral studies[10-12] reporting an anti-cataleptic effect for buspirone, fluoxetine and 8-OH-DPAT in 6-OHDA-lesioned rats.

Conclusion

In conclusion, we suggest that serotonergic agents may have beneficial effect in preventing the progression of PD through attenuating apoptotic events. However, further clinical investigations should be carried out to prove this.

Conflict of Interest

The authors report no conflicts of interest.

References

1. Nagatsu T. Parkinson's disease: Changes in apoptosis-related factors suggesting possible gene therapy. *J Neural Transm* 2002;109(5-6):731-45. doi: 10.1007/s007020200061
2. Double KL, Reyes S, Werry EL, Halliday GM. Selective cell death in neurodegeneration: Why are some neurons spared in vulnerable regions? *Prog Neurobiol* 2010;92(3):316-29. doi: 10.1016/j.pneurobio.2010.06.001
3. Singh S, Dikshit M. Apoptotic neuronal death in parkinson's disease: Involvement of nitric oxide. *Brain Res Rev* 2007;54(2):233-50. doi: 10.1016/j.brainresrev.2007.02.001
4. Zaldana M, Bonastre M, Aguilar E, Marin C. Differential nigral expression of bcl-2 protein family in chronically haloperidol and clozapine-treated rats: Role in neurotoxicity and stereotyped behavior. *Exp Neurol* 2007;203(2):302-8. doi: 10.1016/j.expneurol.2006.08.009
5. Hartmann A, Troadec JD, Hunot S, Kikly K, Faucheux BA, Mouatt-Prigent A, et al. Caspase-8 is an effector in apoptotic death of dopaminergic neurons in parkinson's disease, but pathway inhibition results in neuronal necrosis. *J Neurosci* 2001;21(7):2247-55.
6. Hartmann A, Mouatt-Prigent A, Vila M, Abbas N, Perier C, Faucheux BA, et al. Increased expression and redistribution of the antiapoptotic molecule bcl-xl in parkinson's disease. *Neurobiol Dis* 2002;10(1):28-32.
7. Kramer BC, Mytilineou C. Alterations in the cellular distribution of bcl-2, bcl-x and bax in the adult rat substantia nigra following striatal 6-hydroxydopamine lesions. *J Neurocytol* 2004;33(2):213-23.
8. Oosterink BJ, Harkany T, Luiten PG. Post-lesion administration of 5-ht1a receptor agonist 8-oh-dpat protects cholinergic nucleus basalis neurons against nmda excitotoxicity. *Neuroreport* 2003;14(1):57-60. doi: 10.1097/01.wnr.0000051543.96524.3c

9. Ahlemeyer B, Glaser A, Schaper C, Semkova I, Krieglstein J. The 5-ht1a receptor agonist bay x 3702 inhibits apoptosis induced by serum deprivation in cultured neurons. *Eur J Pharmacol* 1999;370(2):211-6.
10. Sharifi H, Nayebi AM, Farajnia S. Chronic administration of 8-OH-DPAT attenuates catlepsy in 6-hydroxydopamine-lesioned rats through modulation of inflammatory cytokines. *Iran J Basic Med Sci* 2013;16(12):1270–75.
11. Sharifi H, Mohajjel Nayebia A, Farajnia S. Dose-dependent effect of flouxetine on 6-ohda-induced catalepsy in male rats: A possible involvement of 5-ht1a receptors. *Advanced pharmaceutical bulletin* 2013;3(1):203-6. doi: 10.5681/apb.2013.033
12. Sharifi H, Mohajjel Nayebia A, Farajnia S. The effect of chronic administration of buspirone on 6-hydroxydopamine-induced catalepsy in rats. *Adv Pharm Bull* 2012;2(1):127-31. doi: 10.5681/apb.2012.019
13. Paxinos G, Watson C. The rat brain in stereotaxic coordinates. 6th ed. Sydney: Academic Press; 1982.
14. Mahmoudi J, Mohajjel Nayebi A, Reyhani-Rad S, Samini M. Fluoxetine improves the effect of levodopa on 6-hydroxy dopamine-induced motor impairments in rats. *Adv Pharm Bull* 2012;2(2):149-55. doi: 10.5681/apb.2012.023
15. Javad Mahmoudi, Alireza Mohajjel Nayebi, Morteza Samini, Siamak Reyhani-Rad, Vahab Babapour. Buspirone improves the anti-cataleptic effect of levodopa in 6-hydroxydopamine-lesioned rats. *Pharmacolo Rep* 2011; 63 (4): 908-914.
16. Mahmoudi J, Mohajjel Nayebi A, Samini M, Reyhani-Rad S, Babapour V. 5-ht(1a) receptor activation improves anti-cataleptic effects of levodopa in 6-hydroxydopamine-lesioned rats. *Daru* 2011;19(5):338-43.
17. Nayebi AM. Hypothesis: A promising effect of 5-HT1A receptor agonists in alleviating motor symptoms of Parkinsons disease. *Afr J Pharm Pharmaco* 2010;4(6):289-90.
18. Levy OA, Malagelada C, Greene LA. Cell death pathways in parkinson's disease: Proximal triggers, distal effectors, and final steps. *Apoptosis* 2009;14(4):478-500. doi: 10.1007/s10495-008-0309-3
19. Ayllon V, Cayla X, Garcia A, Roncal F, Fernandez R, Albar JP, et al. Bcl-2 targets protein phosphatase 1 alpha to bad. *J Immunol* 2001;166(12):7345-52.
20. Djordjevic A, Djordjevic J, Elakovic I, Adzic M, Matic G, Radojcic MB. Fluoxetine affects hippocampal plasticity, apoptosis and depressive-like behavior of chronically isolated rats. *Prog Neuropsychopharmacol Biol Psychiatry* 2012;36(1):92-100. doi: 10.1016/j.pnpbp.2011.10.006
21. Yuan J, Yankner BA. Apoptosis in the nervous system. *Nature* 2000;407(6805):802-9. doi: 10.1038/35037739
22. Becker EB, Bonni A. Cell cycle regulation of neuronal apoptosis in development and disease. *Prog Neurobiol* 2004;72(1):1-25. doi: 10.1016/j.pneurobio.2003.12.005
23. Han BS, Hong HS, Choi WS, Markelonis GJ, Oh TH, Oh YJ. Caspase-dependent and -independent cell death pathways in primary cultures of mesencephalic dopaminergic neurons after neurotoxin treatment. *J Neurosci* 2003;23(12):5069-78.
24. Charkhpour M, Nayebi AR, Doustar Y, Hassanzadeh K. 8-oh-dpat prevents morphine-induced apoptosis in rat dorsal raphe nucleus: A possible mechanism for attenuating morphine tolerance. *Anesth Analg* 2010;111(5):1316-21. doi: 10.1213/ANE.0b013e3181f1bb9a
25. Mattson MP. Apoptosis in neurodegenerative disorders. *Nat Rev Mol Cell Biol* 2000;1(2):120-9. doi: 10.1038/35040009
26. Guo DJ, Li F, Yu PH, Chan SW. Neuroprotective effects of luteolin against apoptosis induced by 6-hydroxydopamine on rat pheochromocytoma pc12 cells. *Pharm Biol* 2013;51(2):190-6. doi: 10.3109/13880209.2012.716852
27. Berends AC, Luiten PG, Nyakas C. A review of the neuroprotective properties of the 5-ht1a receptor agonist repinotan hcl (bayx3702) in ischemic stroke. *CNS drug reviews* 2005;11(4):379-402.
28. Ohman J, Braakman R, Legout V, Traumatic Brain Injury Study G. Repinotan (bay x 3702): A 5ht1a agonist in traumatically brain injured patients. *J Neurotrauma* 2001;18(12):1313-21. doi: 10.1089/08977150152725614
29. Meller E. 5-ht1a receptor-mediated apoptosis: Death by jnk? *Biochim Biophys Acta* 2007;1773(6):691-3. doi: 10.1016/j.bbamcr.2007.01.003
30. Cowen DS, Johnson-Farley NN, Travkina T. 5-ht receptors couple to activation of akt, but not extracellular-regulated kinase (erk), in cultured hippocampal neurons. *J Neurochem* 2005;93(4):910-7. doi: 10.1111/j.1471-4159.2005.03107.x
31. Kukley M, Schaper C, Becker A, Rose K, Krieglstein J. Effect of 5- hydroxytryptamine 1A receptor agonist BAY X 3702 on BCL-2 and BAX proteins level in the ipsilateral cerebral cortex of rats after transient focal ischemia. *Neuroscience* 2001;107(3):405-13.
32. Adayev T, Ray I, Sondhi R, Sobocki T, Banerjee P. The g protein-coupled 5-ht1a receptor causes suppression of caspase-3 through mapk and protein kinase calpha. *Biochim Biophys Acta* 2003;1640(1):85-96.

8

Aberrant Wnt/β-Catenin Signaling Pathway in Testis of Azoospermic Men

Marefat Ghaffari Novin[1,2], Reza Mirfakhraie[3], Hamid Nazarian[1]*

[1] *Department of Biology and Anatomical Sciences, School of Medicine, Shahid Beheshti University of Medical Sciences, Tehran, Iran.*
[2] *Shahid Beheshti University of Medical Sciences, Infertility and Reproductive Health Research Center (IRHRC), Tehran, Iran.*
[3] *Department of Medical Genetics, School of Medicine, Shahid Beheshti University of Medical Sciences, Tehran, Iran.*

Article info

Keywords:
- β-catenin
- Male infertility
- Obstructive and non-obstructive azoospermia
- Leydig cells

Abstract

Purpose: The Importance and key role of Wnt/β-catenin signaling pathway in spermatogenesis is known. Abnormalities of this pathway in Sertoli and germ cells leads to infertility. Leydig cells play an important role in spermatogenesis and male reproduction. As of now, exact position of the Wnt/β-catenin signaling pathway disorders in the tissue and possible involvement of Leydig cells has not been investigated.
Methods: Samples of our previous study were used for common Y chromosome microdeletions screening and common CFTR gene mutations.[1] β-catenin gene expression were evaluated and compared between testicular tissue obtained by testicular sperm extraction (TESE) in two groups of obstructive (n=10) and non-obstructive (n=10) azoospermic infertile men. Location of β-catenin accumulation was detected by immunofluorescence technic and quantitatively compared in the tissue followed by counterstaining with anti-vimentin antibody. It was used as specific marker of leydig cells to determine and confirm the cells in which this gathering was occurred.
Results: β-catenin gene expression does not have a significant difference between the obstructive azoospermia (0.998) and non-obstructive azoospermia group (0.891). β-catenin was abnormally aggregated in leydig cell of non-obstructive azoospermic men.
Conclusion: Gathering β-catenin in cytoplasm of leydig cells can disrupt spermatogenesis and cause infertility in men.

Introduction

Male sex hormone testosterone is made by leydig cells in the interstitial tissue of the testes form about 20 percent of the adult testes weight. Function of these cells is controlled by LH (Luteinizing hormone) and it is secreted from the pituitary gland in the brain. Leydig cells in childhood are almost absent and there is no secretion of testosterone from the testes. Many of these cells during the first three months after birth in boys and adult men are present, thus; the large amount of testosterone secretion happen by the testes during childhood. Testosterone inhibits the formation of the female sexual organs in contrast it increases the formation of the prostate gland, seminal bags, and male genital tract.

Azoospermia is the most important factor for male infertility. It can be divided into two categories; Obstructive and non-obstructive azoospermia. Spermatogenesis is normally done in obstructive azoospermia, however; produced spermatozoa are not found in seminal fluid for various reasons. The good example is, anatomical abnormalities or infections.[2] On the other hand, spermatogenesis is impaired in non-obstructive azoospermia and no spermatozoa is made in seminiferous tubules. Non-obstructive azoospermia happens mainly due to congenital genetic and metabolic reasons. Intercellular communications andintracellular signaling pathways play an important role in spermatogenesis. Their abnormalities can affect this process with various intensities from low (Oligospermia) to high (Azoospermia).

Wnt/β-catenin signaling pathway is one of the major cellular signaling pathways which plays a key role in the lives of humans and animals. This pathway involves in cell polarization, migration, early differentiation, neurogenesis and somitogenesis during embryonal development. On the other hand, in adulthood cell proliferation and differentiation is deeply under control of Wnt/β-catenin signaling pathway. In which impairments causes many pathological diseases most notably cancers. Wnt/β-catenin signaling pathway role in reproductive processes has been demonstrated.[3] In general, two routes are defined for Wnt/β-catenin signaling pathway: canonical and non-canonical. In canonical pathway Wnt molecules connect to the Frizzled (FZD) receptors caused inhibition in β-catenin phosphorylation by GSK3-β (a serine/threonine protein kinase with two isoforms of GSK3-α and GSK3-β), caused migration of b-catenin into the nucleus and expression of specific target genes. In contrast, in the absence of activating Wnt signal, β-catenin is phosphorylated by GSK3-β-Axin (a cell scaffold protein)-APC (Adenomatous polyposis coli) complex. It

***Corresponding author:** Hamid Nazarian, Email:h.nazarian@sbmu.ac.ir

is ubiquinated and degraded by proteasome. This chain reaction causes repression of target gene.[4-7] Non-canonical pathway acts through alternative molecules other than β-catenin.[8]
Several types of Wnt proteins including 1, 3, 4, 5a and 7a in the testes of fetal and adult rodents and humans have been reported.[9-13] Some components of the Wnt/β-catenin signaling pathway such as Fz9, Nkd1 and β-catenin have been identified in the testis.[14] β-catenin has a high level expression in mice germ and sertoli cells.[15] Impaired β-catenin signaling in Sertoli cells of the mouse embryo results in the destruction of the testicular cord and Mullerian duct.[16] The aberrant activity of Wnt/β-catenin signaling pathway leads to abnormal differentiation of the PGCs.[17]
Wnt/β-catenin signaling pathway and androgen receptors have direct effect each other in many aspects. β-catenin binds to the ligand-receptor complex and serves as transcription co-activator. Canonical Wnt/β-catenin signaling pathway leads increase in expression of the androgen receptors.[18] GSK3-β phosphorylates the androgen receptors and regulates its ability to activate gene transcription.[19] Altogether, interaction between Wnt/β-catenin signaling pathway and androgen receptors is very complex, it depends on the conditions of the cell. During early development, estrogen injection in newborn rats increased expression of Wnt5a; the increase in expression could be an indirect response because promoter of the Wnt5a gene has no response factor for estrogen.[20,21]
The removal of β-catenin in the mouse spermatid increases apoptosis, acrosome defects, abnormal chromatin condensation, and degradation of Sertoli-germ cell junctions in which can lead to infertility.[22] Overexpression of β-catenin leads to uncontrolled proliferation, inhibition of differentiation in Sertoli cells and their function to support germ cells in mice.[23]
As a result, relationship of Wnt/β-catenin signaling dysfunction in sertoli, germ cell, and infertility has been confirmed. Leydig cells have not been studied in this regard. Therefore, this study was aimed to investigate the probability of disruption of Wnt/β-catenin signaling pathway in leydig cells of azoospermic men.

Materials and Methods

Human subjects

Human subjects, sample size, sampling technique, and screening were described completely in the previous article.[1] Briefly, the test group included 10 patients with non-obstructive azoospermia. Samples were prepared by testicular sperm extraction (TESE) aseptically by an urologist and local anesthesia. 10 men with obstructive azoospermia were considered as the control group (n=10). Non-obstructive azoospermia subjects were screened for Y chromosome microdeletions and obstructive azoospermia patients were checked for CFTR mutations before the study. Samples were transferred to the laboratory within an hour in Dulbecco's modified Eagle's medium (DMEM) (Invitrogen, Carlsbad, U.S.A.).

Realtime-PCR

Expression of β-catenin was quantitatively evaluated using Realtime-PCR method. cDNA was made from extracted RNA by Revert Aid First Strand cDNA Synthesis Kit (Thermo, USA), according to the manufacturer's instructions. Realtime-PCR were done using the Power SYBR green kit and Step one device manufactured by Applied biosystems (Applied biosystems, USA). 20 microliter reactions were made including 10 ml of Power SYBR green master mix, 500 micrograms per microliter of cDNA, 0.5 microliter of forward primer, 0.5 microliter of reverse primer, and 8 microliter of water (*β-catenin* forward: 3'-CAGCAGCAATTTGTGGAGGG-5', reverse: 3'-GCAGCTGCACAAACAATG GA-3' and *GAPDH* forward: 5'-ACAGTCAGCCGCATCTTCTT-3', reverse: 5'-ACGACC AAATCCGTTGACTC-3'). Results were analyzed by Rest 2009 software following normalization using LinRegPCR software.[24]

Immunofluorescence

Immunofluorescence analysis was performed to determine the location of β-catenin accumulation. The samples were first rinsed with phosphate buffered saline (PBS) and fixed with %10 formalin. In the second step they were dehydrated using ascending grades of ethanol and 5 micron sections were made using microtome (Thermo scientific, USA). Samples were placed on glass slides and hematoxylin-eosin staining was performed. Photomicrographs were taken by Nikon TS-100 microscope (Nikon, Japan). Some samples were placed on poly L-lysine coated glass slides and were deparaffinised with xylol and rehydrated with descending grades of ethanol. Following 3 times rinse with deionized water unspecific antigens were blocked with 10% goat serum. Incubation in 4°C with primary antibody (Mouse anti human β-catenin; SC-7963, Santa Cruz biotechnology, USA) was done overnight after 3 times with deionized water. Secondary antibody exposure was performed in 4°C and dark following 3 times rinse with deionized water. Slides were mounted by mounting fluid. Fluorescent photomicrographs were immediately taken with TS-100 microscope (Nikon, Japan). Leydig cells were labeled by specific primary antibody (Mouse anti human Vimentin; V6389, Sigma, USA) against vimentin in a similar manner. Finally, the taken photomicrographs were analyzed and quantitatively compared using Image J (version 1.40g) software.

Results

Realtime-PCR

Samples were quantitatively analyzed regarding the expression level of β-catenin gene. The gene expression of β-catenin did not have significant difference between the obstructive azoospermia (0.998) and non-obstructive azoospermia group (0.891). (Table 1 and Figure 1).

Table 1. Realtime-PCR results analysed by Rest software. β-catenin (NO: Non-obstructive azoospermia) sample group is not different to control group. P(H1)=0.139 β-catenin (O: Obstructive azoospermia) sample group is not different to control group. P(H1)=0.924P(H1) - Probability of alternate hypothesis that difference between sample and control groups is due only to chance. TRG– Target, REF– Reference.

Gene	Type	Reaction Efficiency	Expression	Std. Error	95% C.I.	P(H1)	Result
GAPDH (NO)	REF	1.0244	0.999	-	-	-	-
β-catenin (NO)	TRG	0.8538	0.891	0.712 - 1.131	0.618 - 1.353	0.139	-
β-catenin (O)	TRG	0.8288	0.998	0.848 - 1.166	0.715 - 1.220	0.969	-
GAPDH (O)	REF	1.0244	1.001	-	-	-	-

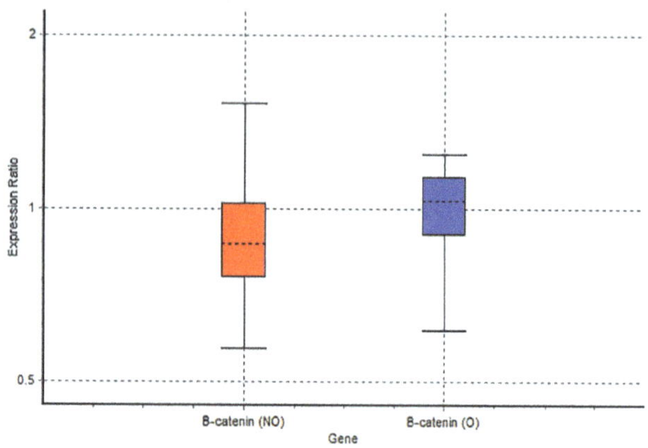

Figure 1. β-catenin gene expression has no significant difference between the obstructive azoospermia (O) (0.998) and non-obstructive azoospermia (NO) group (0.891).

Immunofluorescence

The Location of β-catenin accumulation in the tissue were detected using immunofluorescence technique. As it is shown in the images, β-catenin was aggregated in interstitial tissue. Counterstaining with vimentin antibody revealed that this accumulation was done specifically in leydig cells. Comparison of fluorescence intensity by Image J software displayed, accumulation of β-catenin was significantly more in non-obstructive azoospermia than obstructive azoospermia samples (Figure 2).

Discussion

In this experiment, the Wnt/β-catenin signaling pathway was examined in testicular tissue and compared between obstructive and non-obstructive azoospermic men. The result of realtime-PCR showed β-catenin gene expression in both groups were not significantly different. According to our previous study, expression of GSK3-β gene was down regulated in non-obstructive azoospermic men significantly. The data showed that over expression of β-catenin gene is not obligatory for its increasing and accumulation in cytoplasm, but down regulation of GSK3-β could lead to aberration gathering of β-catenin in cytoplasm. Tanwar et al. reported that overexpression of β-catenin leads to uncontrolled proliferation, inhibition of differentiation of Sertoli cells, and their function in protecting spermatogonia. It leads to cessation of spermatogenesis in mice. They used mutant mices which their β-catenin gene was manipulated in a way that GSK3-β could not phosphorylate and degrade it. In this situation AMH (Anti mullerian hormone) and GDNF (glial cell-derived neurotrophic factor) is only expressed in immature Sertoli cells which continue to express at a high level. Their results showed that the accumulation of β-catenin in Sertoli cells and spermatogonia increased apoptosis in the cells.[23] These researchers studied only Sertoli cells and the importance of other cells especially leydig cells were not considered. Leydig cells play a crucial role in spermatogenesis and fertility. Immunofluorescence test was performed to identify the accumulation of β-catenin. Results showed that β-catenin unusually accumulated in interstitial tissue of non-obstructive azoospermic samples. Counterstaining with anti vimentin antibody (a marker of leydig cells) revealed this aberrant accumulation of β-catenin was done in leydig cells. The results confirmed the similar study of Boyer et al used mutant mice whose sertoli and leydig cells Wnt/β-catenin signaling pathway was continuously active which confirmed the results. These mice lack germ cells with testicular atrophy and became infertile from fifth week.[25]

Conclusion

Overall, aberrant accumulation of β-catenin in leydig cell cytoplasm can cause impaired spermatogenesis and lead to non-obstructive azoospermia and infertility.

Acknowledgments

This research was supported by Shahid Beheshti University of Medical Sciences and Iran National Science foundation (INSF) (project number 91000914). The authors thank Mr.Ramin Pouriran for literary and grammatical edit.

Conflict of Interest

The authors report no conflicts of interest.

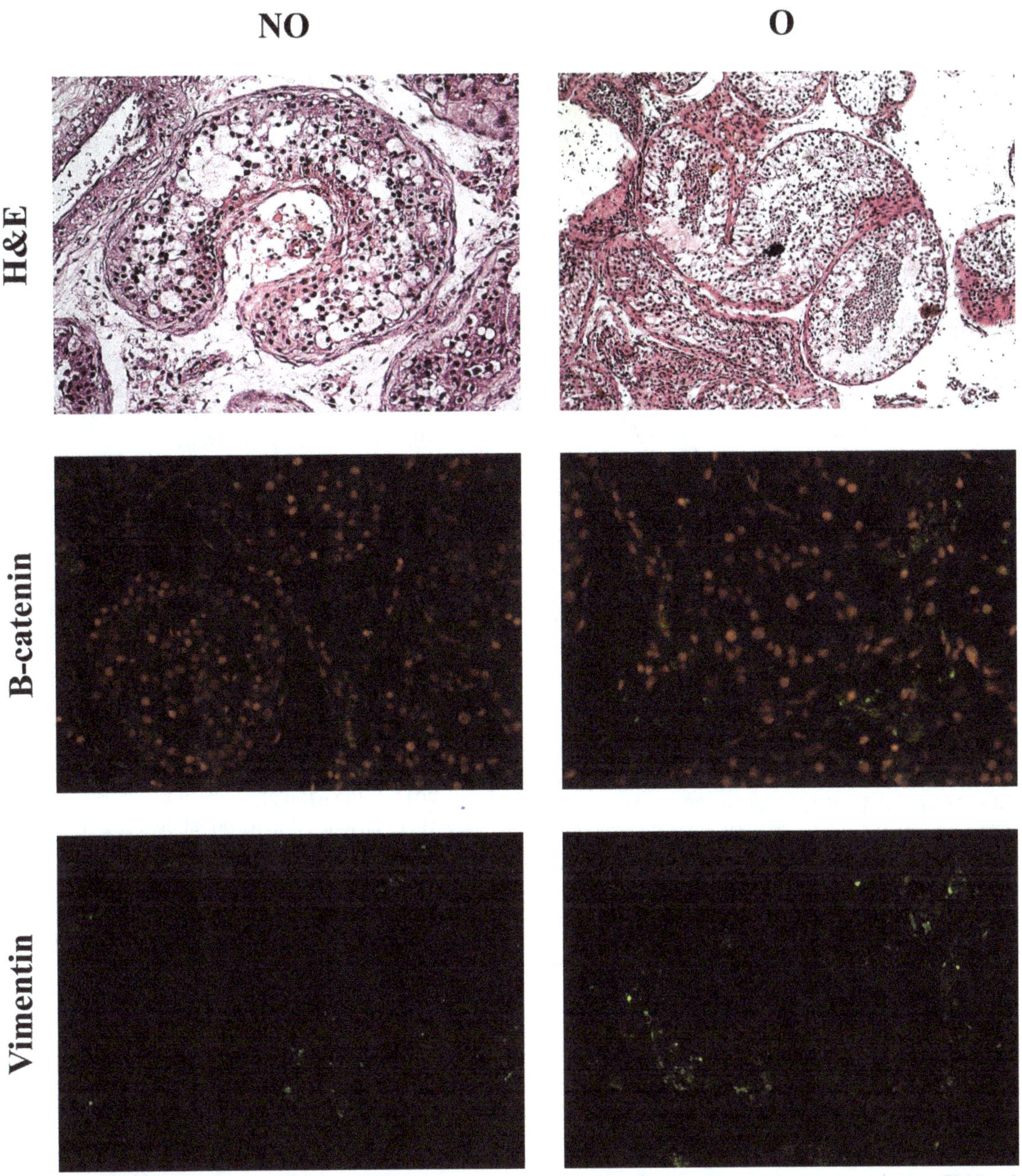

Figure 2. Histologic and Immunofluorescence microscopy. *Left column:* Non-obstructive azoospermic samples. *Right column:* Obstructive azoospermic samples. *First row:* 5μ sections and H&E staining. *Second row:* Detection of β-catenin accumulation site in the tissue by anti β-catenin antibody. Comparison of fluorescence intensity by Image J software revealed that β-catenin has significantly more accumulation in interstitial tissue of testis in non-obstructive azoospermic men. *Third row:* Immunofluorescence staining of leydig cells by specific anti-vimentin antibody. β-catenin was accumulated in leydig cells.

References

1. Nazarian H, Ghaffari Novin M, Jalili MR, Mirfakhraie R, Heidari MH, Hosseini SJ, et al. Expression of Glycogen synthase kinase 3-beta (GSK3-beta) gene in azoospermic men. *Iran J Reprod Med* 2014;12(5):313-20.
2. World Health Organization. Laboratory manual of the WHO for the examination of human semen and sperm-cervical mucus interaction. *Ann Ist Super Sanita* 2001;37(1):I-XII, 1-123.
3. Carreau S, Bouraima-Lelong H, Delalande C. Estrogens in male germ cells. *Spermatogenesis* 2011;1(2):90-4. doi: 10.4161/spmg.1.2.16766
4. Clevers H, Nusse R. Wnt/beta-catenin signaling and disease. *Cell* 2012;149(6):1192-205. doi: 10.1016/j.cell.2012.05.012
5. Chang H, Guillou F, Taketo MM, Behringer RR. Overactive beta-catenin signaling causes testicular sertoli cell tumor development in the mouse. *Biol*

Reprod 2009;81(5):842-9. doi: 10.1095/biolreprod.109.077446

6. Boyer A, Paquet M, Lague MN, Hermo L, Boerboom D. Dysregulation of WNT/CTNNB1 and PI3K/AKT signaling in testicular stromal cells causes granulosa cell tumor of the testis. *Carcinogenesis* 2009;30(5):869-78. doi: 10.1093/carcin/bgp051
7. Kypta RM, Waxman J. Wnt/beta-catenin signalling in prostate cancer. *Nat Rev Urol* 2012;9(8):418-28. doi: 10.1038/nrurol.2012.116
8. Lombardi AP, Royer C, Pisolato R, Cavalcanti FN, Lucas TF, Lazari MF, et al. Physiopathological aspects of the Wnt/beta-catenin signaling pathway in the male reproductive system. *Spermatogenesis* 2013;3(1):e23181. doi: 10.4161/spmg.23181
9. Erickson RP, Lai LW, Grimes J. Creating a conditional mutation of Wnt-1 by antisense transgenesis provides evidence that Wnt-1 is not essential for spermatogenesis. *Dev Genet* 1993;14(4):274-81. doi: 10.1002/dvg.1020140405
10. Katoh M. Molecular cloning and characterization of human WNT3. *Int J Oncol* 2001;19(5):977-82. doi: 10.3892/ijo.19.5.977
11. Jeays-Ward K, Dandonneau M, Swain A. Wnt4 is required for proper male as well as female sexual development. *Dev Biol* 2004;276(2):431-40. doi: 10.1016/j.ydbio.2004.08.049
12. Yeh JR, Zhang X, Nagano MC. Wnt5a is a cell-extrinsic factor that supports self-renewal of mouse spermatogonial stem cells. *J Cell Sci* 2011;124(Pt 14):2357-66. doi: 10.1242/jcs.080903
13. Ikegawa S, Kumano Y, Okui K, Fujiwara T, Takahashi E, Nakamura Y. Isolation, characterization and chromosomal assignment of the human WNT7A gene. *Cytogenet Cell Genet* 1996;74(1-2):149-52. doi: 10.1159/000134404
14. Wang YK, Sporle R, Paperna T, Schughart K, Francke U. Characterization and expression pattern of the frizzled gene Fzd9, the mouse homolog of FZD9 which is deleted in Williams-Beuren syndrome. *Genomics* 1999;57(2):235-48. doi: 10.1006/geno.1999.5773
15. Chang H, Gao F, Guillou F, Taketo MM, Huff V, Behringer RR. Wt1 negatively regulates beta-catenin signaling during testis development. *Development* 2008;135(10):1875-85. doi: 10.1242/dev.018572
16. Kobayashi A, Stewart CA, Wang Y, Fujioka K, Thomas NC, Jamin SP, et al. beta-Catenin is essential for Mullerian duct regression during male sexual differentiation. *Development* 2011;138(10):1967-75. doi: 10.1242/dev.056143
17. Kimura T, Nakamura T, Murayama K, Umehara H, Yamano N, Watanabe S, et al. The stabilization of beta-catenin leads to impaired primordial germ cell development via aberrant cell cycle progression. *Dev Biol* 2006;300(2):545-53. doi: 10.1016/j.ydbio.2006.06.038
18. Mulholland DJ, Dedhar S, Coetzee GA, Nelson CC. Interaction of nuclear receptors with the Wnt/beta-catenin/Tcf signaling axis: Wnt you like to know? *Endocr Rev* 2005;26(7):898-915. doi: 10.1210/er.2003-0034
19. Macdonald BT, Tamai K, He X. Wnt/beta-catenin signaling: components, mechanisms, and diseases. *Dev Cell* 2009;17(1):9-26. doi: 10.1016/j.devcel.2009.06.016
20. Huang L, Pu Y, Hu WY, Birch L, Luccio-Camelo D, Yamaguchi T, et al. The role of Wnt5a in prostate gland development. *Dev Biol* 2009;328(2):188-99. doi: 10.1016/j.ydbio.2009.01.003
21. Bourdeau V, Deschenes J, Metivier R, Nagai Y, Nguyen D, Bretschneider N, et al. Genome-wide identification of high-affinity estrogen response elements in human and mouse. *Mol Endocrinol* 2004;18(6):1411-27. doi: 10.1210/me.2003-0441
22. Chang YF, Lee-Chang JS, Harris KY, Sinha-Hikim AP, Rao MK. Role of beta-catenin in post-meiotic male germ cell differentiation. *PloS one* 2011;6(11):e28039. doi: 10.1371/journal.pone.0028039
23. Tanwar PS, Kaneko-Tarui T, Zhang L, Rani P, Taketo MM, Teixeira J. Constitutive WNT/beta-catenin signaling in murine Sertoli cells disrupts their differentiation and ability to support spermatogenesis. *Biol Reprod* 2010;82(2):422-32. doi: 10.1095/biolreprod.109.079335
24. Ruijter JM, Ramakers C, Hoogaars WM, Karlen Y, Bakker O, Van Den Hoff MJ, et al. Amplification efficiency: linking baseline and bias in the analysis of quantitative PCR data. *Nucleic Acids Res* 2009;37(6):e45. doi: 10.1093/nar/gkp045
25. Boyer A, Hermo L, Paquet M, Robaire B, Boerboom D. Seminiferous tubule degeneration and infertility in mice with sustained activation of WNT/CTNNB1 signaling in sertoli cells. *Biol Reprod* 2008;79(3):475-85. doi: 10.1095/biolreprod.108.068627

A Combination of Prebiotic Inulin and Oligofructose Improve Some of Cardiovascular Disease Risk Factors in Women with Type 2 Diabetes

Akbar Aliasgharzadeh[1], Mohammad Khalili[2], Elham Mirtaheri[3], Bahram Pourghassem Gargari[3], Farnaz Tavakoli[1], Mahdieh Abbasalizad Farhangi[4], Hossein Babaei[5] Parvin Dehghan[6]*

[1] *Faculty of Medicine, Bone Research Center, Tabriz University of Medical Sciences, Tabriz, Iran.*
[2] *Neurosciences Research Center Tabriz University of Medical Sciences, Tabriz, Iran.*
[3] *Department of Biochemistry and Nutrition, Faculty of Nutrition, Tabriz University of Medical Sciences, Tabriz, Iran.*
[4] *Department of Community Nutrition, Faculty of Nutrition, Tabriz University of Medical Sciences, Tabriz, Iran.*
[5] *Drug Applied Research Center and Faculty of Pharmacy, Tabriz University of Medical Sciences, Tabriz, Iran.*
[6] *Nutrition research center, Department of Food Science and Technology, Student Research committee, Faculty of Nutrition, Tabriz University of Medical Sciences, Tabriz, Iran.*

Article info

Keywords:
- MDA
- Antioxidants
- Lipid profile
- Prebiotic
- Type 2 diabetes

Abstract
Purpose: This trial was conducted to evaluate the effects of oligofructose-enriched inulin on some of cardiovascular disease risk factors in women with type 2 diabetes.
Methods: 52 females (25<BMI<35 kg/m^2) with type 2 diabetes were randomly assigned to two groups. Participants received 10g/d oligofructose-enriched inulin (n=27) or 10g/d placebo (n=25) for 8 weeks. Fasting blood samples were taken to measure metabolic profiles, malondialdehyd and antioxidant enzymes at baseline and after the 8 weeks intervention. Paired, unpaired sample t-test and analysis of covariance were used to comparison of quantitative variables.
Results: After 8 weeks, in the oligofructose-enriched inulin group there was a significant increase in total antioxidant capacity (0.2 mmol/l, 20.0%) and a significant decrease in fasting plasma glucose (19.2 mg/dL, 9.4%) HbA1c (0.5%, 8.4%), total cholesterol (TC) (28.0 mg/dL, 14.1%), low-density lipoprotein cholesterol (LDL-c) (22.0 mg/dL, 21.7%), TC/HDL-c ratio (0.73, 20.7%), LDL-c/HDL-c ratio (0.55, 27.5%) and malondialdehyd (1.7 nmol/ml, 39.7%) compared to the placebo group. Changes in concentrations of triglycerides, high-density lipoprotein cholesterol (HDLc), superoxide dismutase, catalase and glutathione peroxidase were not significant in oligofructose-enriched inulin group compared to the placebo group.
Conclusion: Oligofructose-enriched inulin may improve glycemic indices, lipid profile, antioxidant status and malondialdehyd in women with type 2 diabetes.

Introduction

Diabetes mellitus (DM) is a common health problem in developing and developed countries. The prevalence of DM in the world is estimated to be 8.3% in US.[1] In Iran, the prevalence of DM and its health expenditure were 8% and 600 million US dollars in 2010, respectively.[2] DM is a metabolic disease that is characterized by hyperglycemia together with biochemical alterations of lipid profile, insulin resistance and oxidative stress.[3] Increased oxidative stress plays a key role in the initiation, propagation and development of diabetes complications such as retinopathy, neuropathy and nephropathy.[4] Improvement of serum lipids and oxidative stress are associated with better glycemic control. Dietary intervention can alter the potential consequence of oxidative stress and lipid abnormalities.

Inulin–type fructan belong to indigestible carbohydrates which its chain contains a variable number of fructose units, linked by β-(1→2) D-fructosyl-fructose bonds, usually terminates with only one glucose. It is a substitute for sugar or fat having a very low caloric value, arranged as nonviscous, soluble and fermentable fibers. Oligofructose-enriched inulin is a mixture of oligofructose and inulin. Oligofructoses and inulin are metabolised in the proximal colon and distal colon, respectively. Oligofructose-enriched inulin is fermented in the colon throughout; hence it can produce different effects than inulin and oligofructose alone.[5] Oligofructose-enriched inulin can change composition of the gut microflora toward bifidobacteria and lactobacilli.[6]

***Corresponding author:** Parvin Dehghan, Email:dehghan.nut@gmail.com

Some animal studies had shown the specific effects of inulin-type fructans on lipid profile[7] and oxidative stress.[8,9] The results of reviews have shown beneficial effect of inulin-type fructans on the blood glucose[10] and lipid profiles[11] in human, limited data are available assessing the effects of inulin-type fructans on metabolic profiles and oxidative stress biomarkers in diabetic patients. Review of the related literature in this area shows a need for further research of the inulin-type fructans effects in diabetic patients. Animal studies have shown that degree of polymerization of inulin-type fructans differentially affects metabolic status.[12,13] A randomized clinical trial to compare inulin and oligofructose-enriched inulin effect on glycemic indices and blood pressure in women with type 2 diabetes showed that inulin is effective than oligofructose-enriched inulin on food intake, glycemic indices and blood pressure in type 2 diabetes patients.[14] Recently, we have reported that supplementation of diabetic patients with inulin (10g/d for 2 months) improves glycemic status and oxidative stress biomarkers.[15] The present study is a part of recent clinical trial that was designed to assess the efficacy of oligofructose-enriched inulin on some of cardiovascular disease risk factors including glycemic indices, lipid profile and oxidative stress biomarkers in women with type 2 diabetes.

Materials and Methods

Study design

In this randomized, triple-blind, placebo-controlled trail, conducted from December 2011 to February 2012, 70 diabetic female volunteers from Iran Diabetes Society and Endocrinology and Metabolism Clinics of Tabriz University of Medical Sciences participated. This study is part of a large clinical trial that was approved by the Ethics Committee of the Tabriz University of Medical Sciences and it was registered on the Iranian Registry of Clinical Trials website (www.irct.ir/,IRCT201110293253N4).

Participant

In this trial, seventy females with type 2 diabetes who were between 20 and 65 y old were participated. Inclusion criteria were as follows: having type 2 diabetic for>6 months; taking oral anti-diabetic drugs and maintaining them throughout the trial; normal diet; and Body Mass Index (BMI)>25 kg/m^2 for the past 3 months. Type 2 diabetic was defined as having a fasting glucose level of ≥126 mg/dl.[16] Subjects recorded their daily physical activity on a calendar. These recordings were reviewed to ensure subjects maintained a consistent level of physical activity throughout the study. Patients were excluded if they had a history of gastrointestinal, cardiovascular diseases; if they had renal, thyroid, liver, or pancreatic diseases; if they were smoker, pregnant, lactating; if they are currently taking prebiotics, probiotics, antibiotics, antacids, alcohol, anti-diarrheal, anti-inflammatory, laxatives drugs; if they had taken lipid-lowering medications within 2 weeks before the intervention or during the intervention; if they had a daily fiber intake of >30g; or if they changed their oral antidiabetic medication during the intervention. The diagram of study is shown in Figure 1.

Intervention

Before the intervention, an appointment was made for each patient to provide trial information, to fill a questionnaire, and to provide written informed consent. Participants were randomly assigned to either an intervention group, in which participants received 10 g/d oligofructose- enriched inulin (Frutafit, Sensus, Borchwef 3, 4704 RG Roosendaal the Netherlands), or to a control group, in which participants received similar amounts of maltodextrin as the placebo (JiujiangHurirong Trade CO., LTD, China) for 8 weeks. Daily supplements were divided into two packages of 5 g each to be eaten during breakfast and dinner with a cup of water. Both the maltodextrin and the oligofructose-enriched inulin had a similar taste and appearance, and they were given to the volunteers in similar opaque packages. Supplements divided between participants in accordance with the allocation code after randomization. Participants received half of packages at the beginning and the remainder in the middle of the trial. In order to minimize dropout, assurance of supplements consumption and monitor of supplements compliance, the participants received a phone call once per week. Subjects were recommended to return all packets (full and empty) to assess consumption status.

Measurements

At baseline, information including age, menopausal status, diabetes duration (years) and drugs was collected using a general questionnaire. Measurement of anthropometric indices, food intake and serological tests were performed at baseline and after 8 weeks. Weight and height were measured to the nearest 0.1 kg and 0.1 cm, respectively. BMI was calculated as weight in kilograms divided by the square of height in meters. Dietary intakes were evaluated using a 3-day food dairy (two usual and one weekend). Dietary intakes were analyzed using the nutritionist 4 software (First Databank Inc., Hearst Corp., San Bruno, CA) containing the database from tables of content and nutritional value.

At baseline and at the end of trial, 10 ml venous blood samples were collected between 7-9 a.m. after an overnight fasting. Fasting plasma glucose (FPG) concentration was measured by the enzymatic method using an Abbot ModelAclyon 300, USA autoanalyzer with Pars-Azmone kit (Tehran, Iran). HbA1c in whole blood was determined using an automated high performance liquid chromatography analyzer with commercially Bio-Rad D-10 Laboratories, Schiltigheim, France kit. The concentrations of TC, TG and HDL-c were measured by enzymatic colorimetric method (Cholesterol CHOD-PAP and Triglycerides GPO-PAP, Pars-Azmone, IRI) on an automatic analyzer (Abbott, model Alcyon300, USA). Serum LDL-c was calculated according to the Friedewald equation.[17] Since the TC/HDL-c and LDL-c/HDL-c ratios determine the relative risk of coronary artery disease, they were also calculated. The levels of glutathione peroxidase (GSH-Px) and superoxide dismutase (SOD) and total antioxidant capacity (TAC) were measured by colorimetric method (TAS: RANDOX kits, SOD: RANSOD kits and GSH-Px: RANSEL kits; RANDOX Laboratory, UK), on an automatic analyzer (Abbott model Alcyon 300, USA). Malondialdehyde (MDA), as a marker of lipid peroxidation and oxidative stress was measured through reaction with thiobarbituric acid (TBA) as a TBARS to produce a pink colored complex. Then, its fluorescence intensity was measured at 547 nm with excitation at 525 nm by a spectrofluorimeter (Kontron, model SFM 25A, Italy).[18] The levels of catalase were estimated by the method of Aebi.[19] Catalase degrades hydrogen peroxide which can be measured directly by the decrease in the absorbance at 240 nm. One unit of catalase activity was defined as the amount of catalase which absorbed in 30 seconds at 25°C. The catalase was expressed as units per milliliter and TAC was expressed as mmol/l.

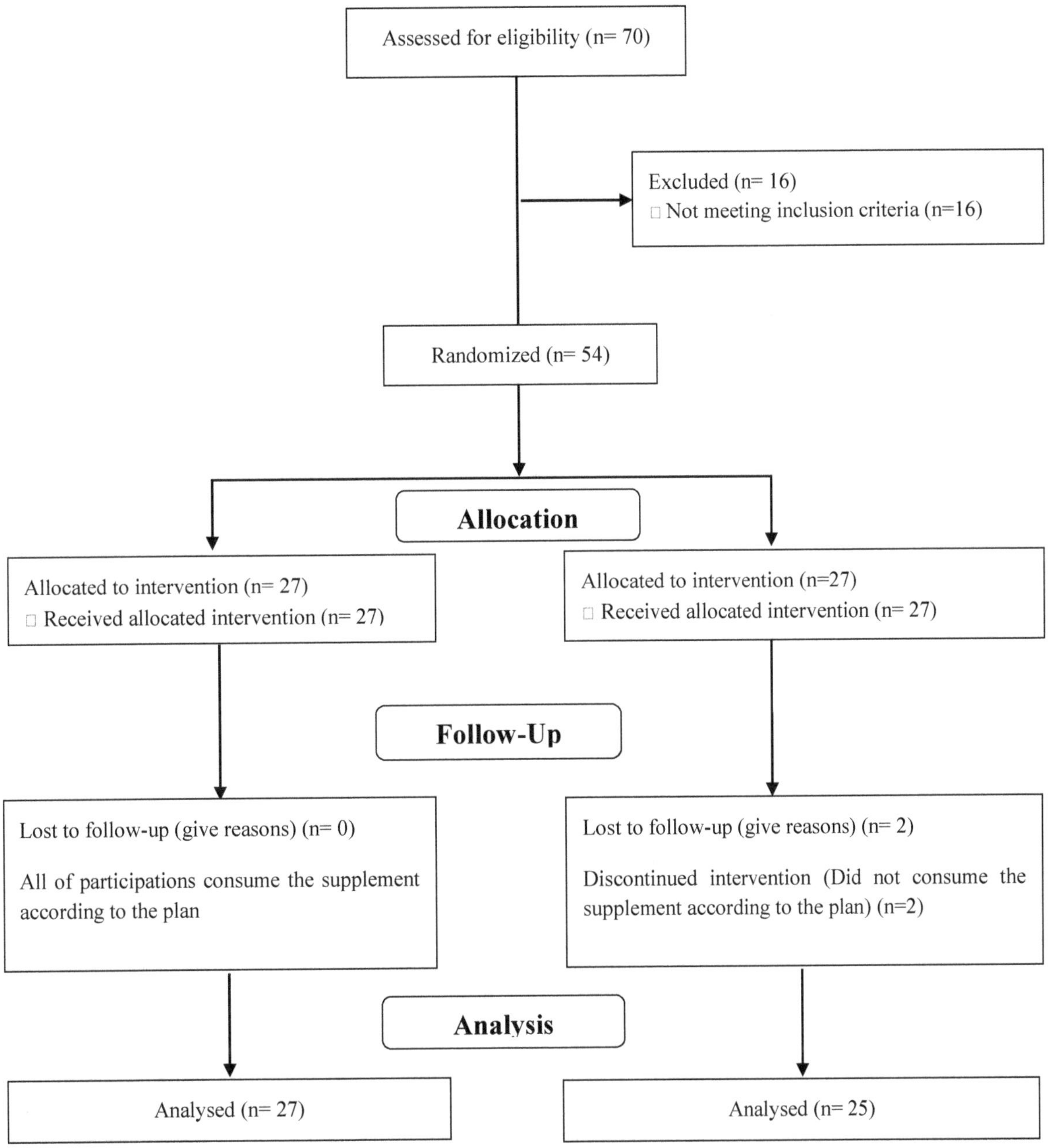

Figure 1. Flow diagram.

Statistical analyses

Data were analyzed using SPSS software (version 13). All statistical analyses were performed based on intention to treat analysis. The Sample size was determined based on information obtained from the study by Sheu and colleagues[20] for LDL-c. For an anticipated change of 28.3mg/dL between experimental and control groups with a confidence level of 95% and, a power of 90%. The sample size was estimated at least 19 per group. To cover an anticipated dropout of 25%, the sample size was increased to 27 in each group. In this trial, participants were randomly assigned in to one of two groups by using a block randomization procedure, which matched subjects to each block based on BMI and age. In every block of participants, five subjects allocated to each arm of the trial. The allocation sequence was randomly generated by random allocation software (RAS). To maintain blinding, the allocation was performed by an investigator with no clinical involvement in the study, whereas main investigator and statistician remained blind until the end of analysis. All data were kept according to code until the end of study. The results were expressed as mean (SD). The normality of the distributions was evaluated by the one-sample Kolmogorov-Smirnov test. Paired and unpaired sample t-tests were used to compare comparison of quantitative variables. Medications used in two groups were compared using the Mann-Whitney U test. ANCOVA was used to identify any differences between the two groups after intervention, adjusting for baseline values and covariates including diabetes duration, weight and energy intake changes. Mean changes of markers between groups were calculated by [(intervention values-control values)/control values)]. $P<0.05$ were considered to be statistically significant.

The primary outcomes of the study were FPG, HbA1c, TC, TG, LDL-c, HDL-c, TC/ HDL-c ratio, LDL-c/HDL-c ratio, MDA, TAC, SOD, GSH-Px, catalase while the secondary outcomes were weight and energy changes. In addition, diabetes duration, energy intake and weight changes for glycemic parameters, lipid profile, MDA and related antioxidant enzymes were considered as covariates variables in this study.

Results

Participants flow

Out of 70 participants assigned to the trial, 52 participants completed the study (intervention group, 27; placebo group, 25; Figure 1). Participants had good compliance with oligofructose-enriched inulin and no adverse effects or symptoms were reported following supplementation.

Baseline characteristics

Table 1 shows the baseline characteristics of participants in the two groups. The two groups were similar in initial characteristics expecting diabetes duration. To take this difference into consideration, duration of diabetes was included as covariate in analyses of efficacy outcomes.

Table 1. Baseline characteristics of the study participants

Characteristics	Placebo group (n=25)	Intervention group (n=27)
Age (year) (range)	48.40 (9.70) (40-65)	48.45(8.40) (40-60)
Pre / Postmenopause n (%)	5(20.00) / 20 (80.00)	4 (14.80)/ 23 (85.20)
Weight (kg)	70.50(11.00)	76.00 (12.20)
Height (cm)	153.50 (6.50)	154.10 (5.30)
Body mass index (kg/m^2)	29.90 (4.10)	31.90(4.00)
Diabetes duration (y)	5.30 (4.60)	8.50 (5.00)^a
Metformin, 500mg (tablets/d)	2.70 (0.90)	2.70 (0.92)
Glibenclamide, 5mg (tablets/d)	1.90 (1.20)	2.40(1.10)

Data are presented as mean (SD) excepting menopause status that is presented n (%). $^aP<0.05$, unpaired *t* test.

Dietary intake of energy and macronutrients was reported previously.[21] There were no significant differences between the baseline dietary intakes of the two groups in energy, carbohydrate, protein, fat, saturated fat, monounsaturated fat, polyunsaturated fat, cholesterol and dietary fiber. Participants' dietary composition -with the exception of energy and total fat, which significantly decreased in the intervention group-did not significantly change during the study period. In the intervention group, energy and total fat intake decreased significantly, while in the placebo group they remained unchanged.

Efficacy results

Anthropometric indices, glycemic control and lipid profile

The comparison between two groups showed that there were no significant differences at baseline anthropometric indices; FPG, HbA1c and lipid profile. Change in glycemic status including fasting blood glucose and serum HbA1c has been reported elsewhere.[21] After 8 weeks supplementation, body weight, BMI, FPG and HbA1c remained unchanged in the placebo group, while body weight and BMI were significantly decreased in the intervention group (76.0 ± 12.4 to 72.9 ± 12.4 kg, 31.9 ± 4.5 to 30.6 ± 4.6 kg/m^2, respectively; $P<0.05$).

Significant reductions were observed in FPG (19.2 mg/dL; 9.5%) and HbA1c (1.0%; 8.4%) in the intervention group as compared with the placebo group. These changes were significant compared to the placebo group (P<0.05, ANCOVA adjusted for diabetes duration, weight and energy intake changes and baseline values).
Oligofructose–enriched inulin decreased significantly, serum TC (28.0 mg,dL, 14.1%), LDL-c (22.0 mg/dL, 21.7%), TC/HDL-c ratio (0.7, 20.7%), LDL-c/HDL-c ratio (0.5, 27.5%). We observed a nonsignificant decrease in TG (38.8 mg/dL, 16.2 %) and a nonsignificant increase in HDL-c (1.9 mg/dL, 8.9%) compared with the placebo group after adjusting for diabetes duration, weight and energy intake changes and baseline values. In the placebo group changes for TC, TG, LDL-c, HDL-c, TC/HDL-c ratio and LDL-c /HDL-c ratio were not significant (Table 2).

Table 2. Changes in lipid profile of patients at baseline and at the end of the study

Variables	Period	Placebo group (n=25)	Intervention group(n=27)
TC (mg/dL)	Initial	197.9 (37.7)	198.6 (38.7)
	End	203.1 (45.6)	175.0 (36.3) [a, b]
TG (mg/dL)	Initial	213.0 (68.0)	211.2 (80.0)
	End	216.8 (59.8)	176.9 (61.2) [a]
HDL-c (mg/dL)	Initial	40.6 (5.6)	38.8 (5.9)
	End	43.4 (4.2)	45.4 (6.5) [a]
LDL-c (mg/dL)	Initial	114.6 (35.3)	117.4 (36.7)
	End	116.3 (42.9)	94.3 (34.3) [a, b]
TC /HDL-c	Initial	4.9 (0.8)	5.2 (1.3)
	End	4.7 (0.9)	3.9 (0.9) [a, b]
LDL-c /HDL-c	Initial	2.8 (0.7)	3.1 (1.0)
	End	2.7 (0.9)	2.1 (0.8) [a, b]

TC, total cholesterol; TG, triglyceride; HDL-C, high-density lipoprotein cholesterol; LDL-C, low-density lipoprotein. Values are presented as the mean (SD). [a] *P<0.05*, paired t test. [b] *P<0.05*, ANCOVA adjusted for diabetes duration, weight and energy intake changes and baseline values.

MDA and antioxidant markers

Comparison between the two groups showed that there were no significant differences with regard to baseline TAC, SOD, GSH-Px, catalase and MDA (Table 3). After 8 weeks, no statistically significant difference existed in TAC, MDA, SOD, GSH-Px and catalase in the placebo group. Significant increase in the levels of TAC (0.2 mmol/l, 20.0%) and significant decrease in the levels of MDA (1.7 nmol/ml, 39.7%) were observed in the intervention group compared to the placebo group (P<0.05, ANCOVA adjusted for diabetes duration, weight and energy intake changes and baseline values). No significant increase was observed in the levels of SOD, GSH-Px and catalase in the intervention group compared to the placebo group (P>0.05, ANCOVA adjusted for diabetes duration, weight and energy intake changes andbaseline values). The levels of SOD and catalase increased in the intervention group (P<0.05, paired *t* test) but glutathione peroxidase was not changed significantly (P>0.05, paired *t* test). In the placebo group changes for TAC, MDA, SOD, GSH-Px and catalase were not significant.

Table 3. Changes in oxidative stress biomarkers of patients at baseline and at the end of the study

Variables	Period	Placebo group (n=25)	Intervention group(n=27)
TAC (mmol/L)	Initial	0.9 (0.1)	0.9 (0.1)
	End	0.8 (0.2)	1.0 (0.2) [a, b]
SOD (U/mg Hb)	Initial	1599.6 (138.1)	1633.9 (237.3)
	End	1580.0 (144.5)	1684.7 (254.2) [a]
GSH-Px (U/g Hb)	Initial	33.4 (2.6)	33.7 (5.1)
	End	33.3 (2.8)	34.4 (5.4)
Catalase (U/g Hb)	Initial	66.5 (17.7)	57.2 (16.0)
	End	65.0 (18.4)	69.5 (20.2) [a]
MDA (nmol/ml)	Initial	3.8 (1.2)	3.4 (1.0)
	End	4.3 (1.9)	2.6 (1.2) [a, b]

TAC, total antioxidant capacity; SOD, superoxide dismutase; GSH-Px, glutathione peroxidase; MDA, malondialdehyde. Data are presented as the mean (SD).
[a] *P<0.05*, paired *t* test.
[b] *P<0.05*, ANCOVA adjusted for diabetes duration, weight and energy intake changes and baseline values

Discussion

This clinical trial, showed that the oligofructose-enriched inulin supplementation for 8 weeks in diabetic patients decreased significantly body weight, BMI, the levels of FPG, HbA1c, TC, LDL-c, TC/ HDL-c ratio, LDL-c/HDL-c ratio and MDA, however, we could not find any significant effect on TG, SOD, GSH-Px and catalase compared to the placebo group.
Increased body weight and BMI are associated with diabetes. We demonstrated that supplementation with oligofructose-enriched inulin resulted in a significant decrease in body weight and BMI. Similar results have been reported with oligofructose supplementation in a systematic review.[22]
In our study, energy intake of the oligofructose–enriched inulin group was significantly decreased. The exact mechanism(s) of weight reduction by oligofructose–enriched inulin remains unclear. Some gut satiety hormones that is released as response to diet composition, including glucagon-like peptide-1 (GLP-1), Peptide YY (PYY), and ghrelin, are proposed for weight reduction.[22]
In this study, we showed that oligofructose–enriched inulin supplementation for 8 weeks reduced FPG, HbA1c, TC, LDL-c, TC/ HDL-c ratio and LDL-c/ HDL-c ratio, but could not significantly affect TG and HDL-c levels compared to maltodextrin group. Nassar and colleagues[7] reported that inulin resulted in significant decrease in serum glucose, insulin, insulin resistance,

TC, TG, LDL-c and significant increase in HDL-c. Garcia and colleagues[23] reported that 5 weeks supplementation with inulin was resulted in 8% decrease in LDL-c. Bonsu and colleagues[24] did not find significant effect of inulin on serum lipid and serum glucose concentrations. We have already reported that inulin can improve lipid profile.[25] Beneficial effects of oligofructose–enriched inulin on lipid profile mainly mediated by short chain fatty acid (SCFA). Butyrate inhibits liver cholesterol synthesis and provides a source of energy for human colon epithelial cells. Acetate may act as a precursor for cholesterol synthesis, while propionate could inhibit hepatic cholesterol synthesis by decreasing the use of acetate as a precursor of cholesterol.[26] Also, inulin-type fructans may contribute to cholesterol reduction by increasing fecal bile acid excretion, reducing intestinal cholesterol absorption, as well as increasing of the expression of 3-hydroxy-3-methylglutaryl-COA reductase (HMG-COA reductase).[27] Their impact on TLR4 signaling and proinflammatory cytokines might be explaining the role of their lipid lowering.[28] Prebiotics might also improve glycemic status via increasing insulin sensitivity with their impact on gene expression which involved in reduction of inflammatory activity and adiposity.[29]

The current study showed that oligofructose–enriched inulin (10 g/day for 8 weeks) in diabetic patients significantly increased plasma TAC levels and significantly decreased plasma MDA levels, but did not significantly affect SOD, catalase and GSH-Px activities. Because antioxidant micronutrients and kind of fat remained unchanged in throughout study, it suggests oligofructose–enriched inulin supplementation might be the main factor affecting the oxidativestress in this study. In a study by Wang and colleagues[29] increased activity of catalase, SOD and GSH-Px enzymes and decreased levels of MDA were observed by the use of 5% wheat bran xylooligosaccharides in rats. Similar results had been shown in treated mice with Lactobacillus acidophilus in conjunction with inulin.[30] In a study by Nikniaz and colleagues,[31] supplementation of lactating mothers with symbiotic (lactobacillus + bifidobacterium + fructooligosaccharide for 30 days) resulted in a significant increase in plasma TAC levels and a nonsignificant decrease in levels of MDA. We have already reported that supplementation of diabetic patients with inulin (10g/day for 2 months) improves oxidative stress and antioxidants (TAC, SOD).[15] These results are in agreement with our results. Despite these, some studies reported conflicting findings. In rat model, supplementation with inulin and FOS did not affect serum TAC, GSH-Px and SOD activities, while the concentration of TBARS was decreased.[8] In another study, dietary supplementation with dextrin or oligofructose led to a 20% decrease in total and reduced glutathione. The activities of glutathione dependent antioxidant enzymes, SOD, catalase, and MDA remained unchanged in dextrin or oligofructose groups.[9] Asemi and colleagues[32] reported that symbiotic food (lactobacillus + inulin for 6 weeks) consumption in diabetic patients led to a significant increase in plasma total GSH and serum uric acid levels. No significant change was observed in plasma TAC levels.

These discrepancies may be due to differences between species, different study designs, the dosage and kind of supplementation used, variation in diet, basal antioxidant and glycemic status, duration of supplementation, basal gut microflora as well as the patients under investigation.

The underlying mechanism(s) of the modulation of oxidative stress by inulin-type fructans have remained obscures. Inulin-type fructans exerts antioxidant effects in biological systems through direct and indirect pathways. The fructans may act as antioxidant themselves; they could act directly as reactive oxygen species (ROS) scavenger and indirectly through modulation of SCFA production,[33] cytokine[34] as well as gene expression.[35] Butyrate as SCFA, leads to reduction in colonic myeloperoxidase activity, restoration of glutathione concentration and reduction in ROS-mediated p 42/44 mitogen-activated protein kinase (MAPK) phosphorylation.[33] We have already reported that Oligofructose-enriched inulin and resistant dextrin, as prebiotic, improve some inflammatory markers and metabolic endotoxemia in women with type 2 diabetes mellitus.[21,36] Furthermore, the inulin-type fructans may improve oxidative stress status through modulation of cytokine-induced oxidative stress, down-regulation of genes involved in oxidative stress and TLR pathways,[34] modification of antioxidant enzymes gene expression.[35] Moreover, modification of microflora toward lactobacilli containing antioxidants in the gastrointestinal tract and releasing their intracellular antioxidants upon lyses of lactobacilli resident[30] might be other mechanism.

Some aspects need to be considered in the interpretation of our results, including short interventional time, lack of assessment serum fatty acids, glucose clamp, lack of define gut microflora changes and other oxidative stress indices, such as F (2)-isoprostanes. Also, the sample size was determined on the basis of changes in LDL-c, in the case of this particular variable, the power obtained was sufficient to produce significant results. However, for some other variables, it seems that a larger sample size and a higher power are needed to attain statistical significance. Despite these limitations, this is the first triple blind study to investigate the effect of oligofructose-enriched inulin on lipid profile and oxidative stress in diabetic patients.

Conclusion

Based on the results of this trial, oligofructose-enriched inulin supplementation may improve glycemic indices, lipid profile, antioxidant status and decrease MDA concentrations in type 2 diabetic patients. These finding propose a safe and effective therapy in diabetes management and its complications. Obviously, more investigations are needed for confirmation of positive effects of oligofructose-enriched inulin on metabolic status, antioxidant indices in diabetic patients and clarify its underlying mechanism(s).

Acknowledgments
The authors would like to thank all of the participants. The present study was financially supported by Nutrition Faculty, Nutrition Research Center and Vice Chancellor for Research of Tabriz University of Medical Sciences, Iran. This article was written on the basis of data obtained for a Ph.D. thesis about nutrition, which was registered at the Tabriz University of Medical Sciences.

Conflict of Interest
The authors declare that they have no conflict of interest.

References

1. Amrican Diabetes Association. Diagnosis and classification of diabetes mellitus. *Diabetes Care* 2012;35(Suppl 1):S64-71. doi: 10.2337/dc12-s064
2. Golozar A, Khademi H, Kamangar F, Poutschi H, Islami F, Abnet CC, et al. Diabetes mellitus and its correlates in an Iranian adult population. *PLOS One* 2011;6(10):e26725. doi: 10.1371/journal.pone.0026725
3. Tripathi BK, Srivastava AK. Diabetes mellitus: complications and therapeutics. *Med Sci Monit* 2006;12(7):RA130-47.
4. Pitocco D, Tesauro M, Alessandro R, Ghirlanda G, Cardillo C. Oxidative stress in diabetes: implications for vascular and other complications. *Int J Mol Sci* 2013;14(11):21525-50. doi: 10.3390/ijms141121525
5. Roberfroid MB. Inulin-type fructans: functional food ingredients. *J Nutr* 2007;137(11 Suppl):2493S-502S.
6. Langlands SJ, Hopkins MJ, Coleman N, Cummings JH. Prebiotic carbohydrates modify the mucosa associated microflora of the human large bowel. *Gut* 2004;53(11):1610-6. doi: 10.1136/gut.2003.037580
7. Nassar SE, Ismail GM, El-Damarawi MA, Alam El-Din AA. Effect of inulin on metabolic changes produced by fructose rich diet. *Life Science J* 2013;10:1807-14.
8. Kozmus CE, Moura E, Serrao MP, Real H, Guimaraes JT, Guedes-de-Pinho P, et al. Influence of dietary supplementation with dextrin or oligofructose on the hepatic redox balance in rats. *Mol Nutr Food Res* 2011;55(11):1735-9. doi: 10.1002/mnfr.201100287
9. Zary-Sikorska E, Juskiewicz J. Effect of fructans with different degrees of polymerization on bacterial enzyme activity, lipid profile and antioxidant status in rats. *Pol J Food Nutr Sci* 2008;58:269-72.
10. Bonsu NKA, Johnson CS, Mcleod KM. Can dietary fructans lower serum glucose? *J Diabetes* 2011;3(1):58-66. doi: 10.1111/j.1753-0407.2010.00099.x
11. Guo Z, Liu XM, Zhang QX, Tian FW, Zhang H, Zhang HP, et al. Effects of inulin on the plasma lipid profile of normolipidemic and hyperlipidemic subjects: a meta-analysis of randomized controlled trials. *Clin Lipidol* 2012;7(2):215-22. doi: 10.2217/clp.12.8
12. Han KH, Tsuchihira H, Nakamura Y, Shimada K, Ohba K, Aritsuka T, et al. Inulin-type fructans with different degrees of polymerization improve lipid metabolism but not glucose metabolism in rats fed a high-fat diet under energy restriction. *Dig Dis Sci* 2013;58(8):2177-86. doi: 10.1007/s10620-013-2631-z
13. Ito H, Takemura N, Sonoyama K, Kawagishi H, Topping DL, Conlon MA, et al. Degree of polymerization of inulin-type fructans differentially affects number of lactic acid bacteria, intestinal immune functions, and immunoglobulin A secretion in the rat cecum. *J Agric Food Chem* 2011;59(10):5771-8. doi: 10.1021/jf200859z
14. Dehghan P, Pourghassem Gargari B, Faghfoori Z, Salekzamani S, Jafarabadi M. Comparative effect of inulin and oligofructose-enriched inulin on glycemic indices and blood pressure in women with type 2 diabetes: a randomized clinical trial. *ZUMS J* 2014;22(91):25-38.
15. Pourghassem Gargari B, Dehghan P, Aliasgharzadeh A, Asghari Jafar-Abadi M. Effects of high performance inulin supplementation on glycemic control and antioxidant status in women with type 2 diabetes. *Diabetes Metab J* 2013;37(2):140-8. doi: 10.4093/dmj.2013.37.2.140
16. Association Diabetes Association. Diagnosis and classification of diabetes mellitus. *Diabetes Care* 2004;27 Suppl 1:S5-S10.
17. Friedewald WT, Levy RI, Fredrickson DS. Estimation of the concentration of low-density lipoprotein cholesterol in plasma, without use of the preparative ultracentrifuge. *Clin Chem* 1972;18(6):499-502.
16. Del Rio D, Pellegrini N, Colombi B, Bianchi M, Serafini M, Torta F, et al. Rapid fluorimetric method to detect total plasma malondialdehyde with mild derivatization conditions. *Clin Chem* 2003;49(4):690-2. doi: 10.1373/49.4.690
19. Aebi H. Catalase in vitro. *Methods Enzymol* 1984;105:121-6. doi: 10.1016/s0076-6879(84)05016-3
20. Sheu WH, Lee IT, Chen W, Chan YC. Effects of xylooligosaccharides in type 2 diabetes mellitus. *J Nutr Sci Vitaminol (Tokyo)* 2008;54(5):396-401. doi: 10.3177/jnsv.54.396
21. Dehghan P, Pourghassem Gargari B, Asghari Jafar-abadi M. Oligofructose-enriched inulin improves some inflammatory markers and metabolic endotoxemia in women with type 2 diabetes mellitus: a randomized controlled clinical trial. *Nutrition* 2014;30(4):418-23. doi: 10.1016/j.nut.2013.09.005
22. Liber A, Szajewska H. Effects of inulin-type fructans on appetite, energy intake, and body weight in children and adults: systematic review of

randomized controlled trials. *Ann Nutr Metab* 2013;63(1-2):42-54. doi: 10.1159/000350312
23. Garcia-Garcia E, Narbona E, Carbonell-Barrachina AA, Sanchez-Soriano J, Roche E. The effect of consumption of inulin-enriched Turron upon blood serum lipids over a 5-week period. *Int J Food Sci Technol* 2013;48(2):405-11. doi: 10.1111/j.1365-2621.2012.03202.x
24. Bonsu NKA, Johnson S. Effects of inulin fiber supplementation on serum glucose and lipid concentration in patients with type 2 diabetes. *Int J Diabetes & Metab* 2012;21:80-6.
25. Dehghan P, Pourghassem Gargari B, Asgharijafarabadi M. Effects of high performance inulin supplementation on glycemic status and lipid profile in women with type 2 diabetes: a randomized, placebo-controlled clinical trial. *Health Promot Perspect* 2013;3(1):55-63. doi: 10.5681/hpp.2013.007
26. Ooi LG, Liong MT. Cholesterol-lowering effects of probiotics and prebiotics: a review of in vivo and in vitro findings. *Int J Mol Sci* 2010;11(6):2499-522. doi: 10.3390/ijms11062499
27. Ouwehand AC, Tiihonen K, Saarinen M, Putaala H, Rautonen N. Influence of a combination of Lactobacillus acidophilus NCFM and lactitol on healthy elderly: intestinal and immune parameters. *Br J Nutr* 2009;101(3):367-75. doi: 10.1017/S0007114508003097
28. Esteve E, Ricart W, Fernandez-Real JM. Gut microbiota interactions with obesity, insulin resistance and type 2 diabetes: Did gut microbiote co-evolve with insulin resistance? *Curr Opin Clin Nutr Metab Care* 2011;14(5):483-90. doi: 10.1097/MCO.0b013e328348c06d
29. Wang J, Cao Y, Wang C, Sun B. Wheat bran xylooligosaccharides improve blood lipid metabolism and antioxidant status in rats fed a high-fat diet. *Carbohydr Polym* 2011;86:1192-7. doi: 10.1016/j.carbpol.2011.06.014
30. Rishi P, Mavi SK, Bharrhan S, Shukla G, Tewari R. Protective efficacy of probiotic alone or in conjunction with a prebiotic in Salmonella-induced liver damage. *FEMS Microbiol Ecol* 2009;69(2):222-30. doi: 10.1111/j.1574-6941.2009.00703.x
31. Nikniaz L, Mahdavi R, Ostadrahimi A, Hejazi MA, Vatankhah AM. Effects of synbiotic supplementation on total antioxidant capacity of human breastmilk. *Breastfeed Med* 2013;8:217-22. doi: 10.1089/bfm.2012.0078
32. Asemi Z, Khorrami-Rad A, Alizadeh SA, Shakeri H, Esmaillzadeh A. Effects of synbiotic food consumption on metabolic status of diabetic patients: A double-blind randomized cross-over controlled clinical trial. *Clin Nutr* 2014;33(2):198-203. doi: 10.1016/j.clnu.2013.05.015
33. Russo I, Luciani A, De Cicco P, Troncone E, Ciacci C. Butyrate attenuates lipopolysaccharide-induced inflammation in intestinal cells and Crohn's mucosa through modulation of antioxidant defense machinery. *PLoS One* 2012;7(3):e32841. doi: 10.1371/journal.pone.0032841
34. D'Souza A, Cai CL, Kumar D, Cai F, Fordjour L, Ahmad A, et al. Cytokines and Toll-like receptor signaling pathways in the terminal ileum of hypoxic/hyperoxic neonatal rats: benefits of probiotics supplementation. *Am J Transl Res* 2012;4(2):187-97.
35. Hassan HA, Yousef MI. Ameliorating effect of chicory (Cichorium intybus L.)-supplemented diet against nitrosamine precursors-induced liver injury and oxidative stress in male rats. *Food Chem Toxicol* 2010;48(8-9):2163-9. doi: 10.1016/j.fct.2010.05.023
36. Aliasgharzadeh A, Dehghan P, Pourghassem Gargari B, Asghari-Jafarabadi M. Resistant dextrin, as a prebiotic, improves insulin resistance and inflammation in women with type 2 diabetes: a randomised controlled clinical trial. *Br J Nutr* 2015;113(02):321-30. doi: 10.1017/S0007114514003675

Involvement of Glycogen Synthase Kinase-3β and Oxidation Status in the Loss of Cardioprotection by Postconditioning in Chronic Diabetic Male Rats

Reza Badalzadeh[1], **Mustafa Mohammadi**[1]*, **Bahman Yousefi**[2], **Safar Faranjia**[3], **Moslem Najafi**[4], **Shima Mohammadi**[2]

[1] *Department of Physiology, Faculty of Medicine, Tabriz University of Medical Sciences, Tabriz, Iran.*
[2] *Students' Research Committee, Tabriz University of Medical Sciences, Tabriz, Iran.*
[3] *Biotechnology Research Center, Tabriz University of Medical Sciences, Tabriz, Iran.*
[4] *Department of Pharmacology, Faculty of Pharmacy, Tabriz University of Medical Sciences, Tabriz, Iran.*

Article info

Keywords:
- Reperfusion injury
- Postconditioning
- GSK-3β, Diabetes
- Cardioprotection

Abstract
Purpose: Diabetes mellitus as a main risk-factor of ischemic heart disease may interfere with postconditioning'scardioprotective effects. This study aimed to investigate the involvement of glycogen synthase kinase-3β (GSK-3β) and oxidation status in chronic diabetes-induced loss of cardioprotective effect of ischemic-postconditioning (IPostC) in Wistar rats.
Methods: After 8 weeks of induction of diabetes by streptozotocin (50mg/kg), hearts of control and diabetic rats were isolated and mounted on a constant-pressure Langendorff system. All hearts were subjected to 30min regional ischemia followed by 60min reperfusion (by occluding and re-opening of left anterior descending coronary artery, respectively). IPostC was applied immediately at the onset of reperfusion. At the end of reperfusion, the infarct size of myocardium was measured via computerized planimetry. Myocardial contents of malondealdehyde and glutathione as indices of oxidative status were assayed spectrophotometrically and the total and phosphorylated forms of myocardial GSK-3β were quantified through western blotting.
Results: IPostC reduced the infarct size of control hearts from 41±2.9% to 28±1.9% ($P<0.05$), whereas it could not induce significant changes in infarct size of diabetic animals (35±1.8% vs. 39±3.1%). IPostC-induced reduction in malondealdehyde and elevation in glutathione contents were significant only in control not in diabetic hearts. The total forms of GSK-3β were similar in all groups; however, the phosphorylation of GSK-3β (at Ser9) by IPostC was greater in control hearts than diabetics ($P<0.01$).
Conclusion: The failure of cardioprotection by IPostC in diabetic hearts may be attributed to the loss of phosphorylation of GSK-3β and thereby increase in oxidative stress in diabetic states.

Introduction

Ischemic heart disease (IHD) is the main cause of mortality in human societies and cardioprotection against ischemia is a matter of life and death in clinics.[1,2] Ischemic postconditioning (IPostC) is one of the cardioprotective strategies introduced in recent years which had significant effect on reduction of infarct size and improvement of cardiac function after ischemia-reperfusion (IR) injury.[3-5] In IPostC strategy, short episodes of reperfusion and ischemia are applied to the heart exactly after a long term ischemia.[6] According to previous studies, the protective effect of this therapeutic strategy is decreased in pathologic conditions like diabetes mellitus, metabolic syndrome, arthrosclerosis, and hypertension.[7,8]

Diabetes mellitus is one of the main risk factors of cardiovascular diseases and there are evidences that diabetes intensify the myocardial ischemic damages. Considering the progressive increase of diabetes prevalence in different societies and the high rate of mortality among diabetic patients due to myocardial infarction, cardioprotection against IR injuries in diabetic patients is very important.[9,10]

IPostC shows its protective effects through different mechanisms, including activation of certain ion channels and receptors, phosphorylation of intracellular protein kinases, opening/closing of mitochondrial pores, and inhibiting cell necrosis and apoptosis.[4,11] Pathologic conditions like diabetes, especially in chronic phases, may interfere with IPostC in cardioprotection, by changing any one of these mechanisms.

Glycogen synthase kinase-3β (GSK-3β) is a protein kinase plays an important role in most pathologic cellular processes like apoptosis, oxidative stress and

***Corresponding author:** Mustafa Mohammadi, Email: m.mohammadin@yahoo.com mitochondrial dysfunction and is active in several disease conditions like diabetes, Alzheimer, ischemia, so forth.[12-14] GSK-3β, in the case of activation, may open mitochondrial permeability transition pores (mPTP), leading to the activation of apoptotic factors and oxidative stress mediators.[15] Oxidative stress is another main cause in the pathophysiology of IR injuries.[16] There is a direct link between the activity of GSK-3β, opening of mPTP and production of reactive oxygen species and oxidative stress in the cell.[17] According to direct involvement of GSK-3β and oxidative stress in the pathology of diabetes and myocardial ischemia, it is probable that these same factors are of the main mechanisms in interference of chronic diabetes with protective effect of IPostC in ischemic heart. As a result, the present study aimed to investigate the involvement of GSK-3β as well as glutathione and lipid peroxidation in the failure of IPostC on cardioprotection of diabetic hearts against IR injury.

Materials and Methods

Animals

Male Wistar rats (250–300 g body weight) were used in this study and had free access to food and water at all times before the start of the experiments. They were housed in laboratory room with a 12-h dark and 12-h light cycle. This study was performed in accordance with the Guide for the Care and Use of Laboratory Animals published by the US National Institutes of Health (NIH publication No 85-23, revised 1996) and was approved by the local Animal Care Committee.

Induction of Diabetes

Diabetes was induced by a single injection of streptozotocin (50 mg/kgbody weight, i.p.) in diabetic groups. Development of the diabetes was confirmed 72h later by measuring blood glucose levels using a glucometer device through the sampling of blood with small scratching of tail of rats. The animals with blood glucose levels higher than 300 mg/dl were considered as diabetic. After 8 weeks of the disease, the diabetic animals as well as the controls were sacrificed and all experiments were performed in isolated perfused hearts.[18]

Surgical Preparation and Isolated Heart Perfusion

Surgical preparation was performed as described previously.[18] All animals were heparinized (500 IU) and anesthetized with a mixture of ketamine (60 mg/kg) and xylosine (10 mg/kg). The hearts were rapidly excised, then mounted on the Langendorff perfusion apparatus and retrogradely perfused via the aorta with a Krebs–Henseleit solution (in mM/l: NaCl 118; KCl 4.7; $CaCl_2$ 2.5; $MgSO_4$. 1.2; $NaHCO_3$ 25; KH_2PO_4 1.2; glucose 11.1) at a constant perfusion pressure of 75 mmHg and pH 7.4. The perfusion solution was gassed with a mixture of 95% O2, 5% CO2 at 37°C.

Induction of Regional Ischemia and Reperfusion

At the onset of experiment, a 5-0 silk thread was placed around the left anterior descending (LAD) coronary artery, close to its origin. After stabilization period of 15 min, all hearts were subjected to regional ischemia for 30 min followed by reperfusion for 60 min. Regional ischemia and reperfusion were induced by occluding and re-opening of LAD, respectively. An immediate fall in coronary flow at the onset of index ischemia (to about 30-40% of its baseline value) and its recovery upon reperfusion served as evidences of effective coronary occlusion and reperfusion.[18] Ischemic postconditioning (IPostC) strategy in this study was three cycles of 30s reperfusion and ischemia (3 cycles of 30s R/I), respectively, immediately at the onset of reperfusion.

Experimental Protocol

The animals were divided into six groups (n=7/each) as following (the experiment was done in two series; one for infarct size study and another for biochemical assays):

1) Control (C); in which after surgical preparation and stabilization period, the isolated hearts of non-diabetic animals were subjected to 30 min ischemia and 60 min reperfusion.

2) Control with ischemic postconditioning (C+IPostC); in which the condition was similar to control group except that at the onset of reperfusion, the hearts were received 3 cycles of 30s R/I.

3) Diabetic (D); in which after surgical preparation and stabilization period, the isolated hearts of 8-week diabetic animals were subjected to 30 min ischemia and 45 min reperfusion.

4) Diabetic with ischemic postconditioning (D+IPostC); in which the condition was similar to diabetic group except that at the onset of reperfusion, the hearts were received 3 cycles of 30s R/I.

Infarct Size Measurement

After the end of reperfusion period, the coronary ligature was retightened at the same site and 0.25% Evance blue dye was infused via the side arm of aortic cannula into the coronary system to identify the risk zone as unstained from intact part of myocardium. The hearts were then frozen at -20°C and thereafter cut into thin slices (1 mm) from the apex to the base. The slices were incubated in 1% triphenyltetrazolium chloride (TTC) in phosphate buffer solution, pH 7.4 for 10 min at 37°C. The heart slices were immersed in 10% formalin for 24h to identify viable myocardium as red stained while necrotic tissue remains pale gray. The risk zone and the infarct area were determined by the computerized planimetry (Summa Sketch III, LandCalc). Infarct and risk area volumes were expressed in cubic millimeters and the percent of infarct to risk zone ratio was calculated.[18]

Preparation of Tissue Homogenates for Western Blot and Biochemical Analysis

At the end of the second series of experiment, the hearts from the ischemic part of left ventricle were sampled and immediately frozen in liquid nitrogen and stored at -80°C. The ventricular tissue was weighted and cut into pieces in ice-cold lysis buffer containing (in mmol) 1 KH_2PO_4, 1 KCL, 50 Tris-HCl pH 7.4, 1 EDTA, 1 NaF, 1 Na_3VO_4, and triton X100 and protease inhibitor cocktail and then homogenized with a Polytron PT-10/ST homogenizer. The homogenate was centrifuged at 10000 g for 10 min at 4°C. The supernatants were removed from the homogenates and quickly frozen at -80°C until western blot and biochemical analysis. The amount of proteins of supernatants was detected spectrophotometrically using Bradford metho.[13,18]

Myocardial Malondealdehyde Content

Myocardial malondealdehyde (MDA) as a marker of lipid peroxidation was estimated by measuring thiobarbituric acid-reactive substances (TBARS) in heart homogenates. Briefly, the samples were mixed with 1 mL 10% trichloroacetic acid and 1 mL 0.67% thiobarbituric acid. Then, the samples were heated in boiling water for 15 min, and N-butanol (2:1, v:v) were added to the solution. After centrifugation (900g, 5 min), TBARS were determined from the solution absorbance at 532 nm.[19]

Myocardial Glutathione Content

Myocardial tissue glutathione (GSH) concentration was quantified using a glutathione reductase-5, 5′-dithiobis (2-nitrobenzoic acid)-based enzymatic recycling assay. To each well of a 96-well plate, 25 μl of standards or supernatant of samples, 25 μl of sample buffer (143 mM NaH2PO4, and 6.3 mM EDTA-Na), and 200 μl of working solution [10 mM glutathione reductase-5,5′-dithiobis (2-nitrobenzoic acid) and 2 mM NADPH in sample buffer] were added. The reaction was initiated by adding 50 μl of 7.2 IU of oxidized glutathione-reductase (Cayman, USA) to each well, and the absorbance change at 405 nm was continuously monitored for 2 min at 9-s intervals with a microplate spectrophotometer. Myocardial GSH concentration was expressed as nanomoles per milligram of protein.

Western Blotting

After electrophoresis of samples, proteins in SDS-gels were transferred to a polyvinylidene fluoride (PVDF) membrane (Millipore). The transfer was carried out at about 70 mA for 1 hour. Thereafter, the membranes were blocked in 5% skim milk buffer containing 0.1% Tween-20 for 1 hour and then incubated with primary antibodies against the total form of glycogen synthase kinase-3β (GSK-3β), phosphorylated form of GSK-3β at serine-9 (phospho$^{(Ser9)}$GSK-3β), and β-actin (all antibodies from Cell Signaling, USA) overnight at 4 °C on a shaker. After 3 x 10 min washes with tris buffer saline containing 0.1% Tween-20, membranes were incubated with horseradish peroxidase conjugated (HRP) secondary antibody (Cell Signaling, USA) for 1 hour at RTon a shaker. The membranes were then rinsed at least 3 x 10 min with wash buffer before detection. Blots were then developed using the enhanced chemiluminescence (ECL) method. Following incubation with the ECL reagents, the membranes were exposed to an X-ray hyperfilm inside a hypercassette in darkroom and then the chemiluminescenceof antibody binding was visualized by a visualizing machine.The intensity of protein bands in the blots was digitally quantified using densitometric analysis. To analyze the amount of phosphorylation of GSK-3β in each sample, the ratio of the intensity of phospho$^{(Ser9)}$GSK-3β to total GSK-3β was calculated and expressed in arbitrary unit (AU).[13]

Statistical Analysis

All values were expressed as means±SEM. The data were analyzed using *one-way ANOVA* followed by *Tukey's* post hoc test. Differences were considered statistically significant when *P<0.05*.

Results

Risk zone and infarct size

Thirty minutes occlusion of LAD coronary artery produced a similar risk zone in all isolated hearts, so that there were no significant differences in the risk zone among all groups of control or diabetic animals, indicating similarity in induction of ischemia in all hearts (Figure 1). On the other hand, this 30 minutes occlusion and 60 minutes reopening of LAD coronary artery produced an infarct size approximately 41±2.9% of the risk zone in control and 39±3.1% in diabetic groups (Figure 2). The differences between infarct size values of control and diabetic animals was not statistically significant. IPostC significantly reduced the infarct size of non-diabetic control animals to 28±1.9% (*P*<0.01). However, IPostC could not significantly influence the infarct size in the diabetic rats (35±1.8% vs. 39±3.1%).

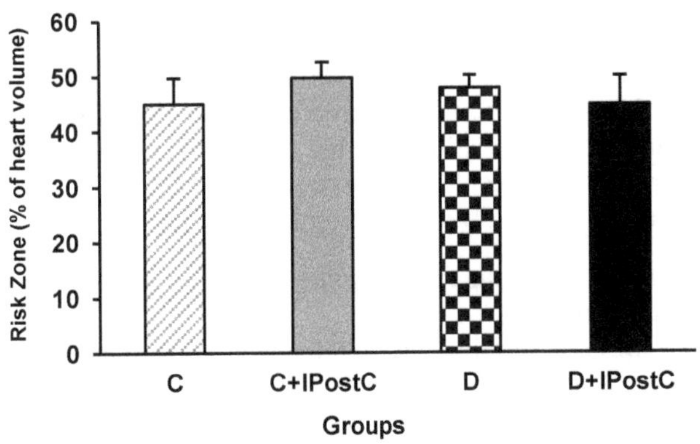

Figure 1. Risk zone (in percent of left ventricle) in control (C) and diabetic (D) animals. IPostC: ischemic postconditioning.

Lipid peroxidation index: MDA level

The level of MDA was measured as an index of lipid peroxidation. The MDA level were significantly reduced by application of IPostC in control animals (*P*<0.05) whereas, the effect of IPostC was not statistically significant in diabetic animals (Figure 3).

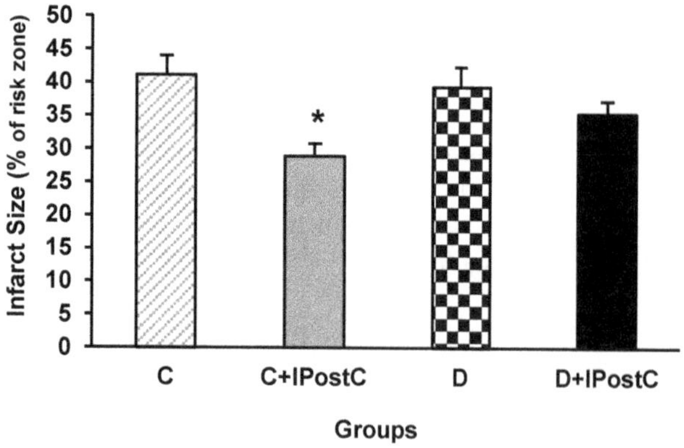

Figure 2. Infarct size (in percent of risk zone) in control (C) and diabetic (D) animals. IPostC: ischemic postconditioning. *$P<0.01$ *vs.* group C.

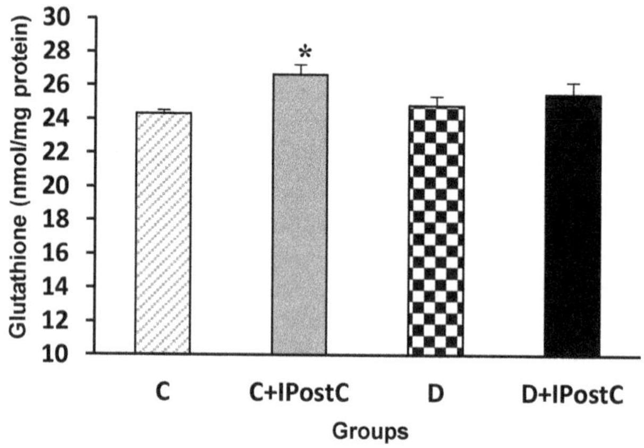

Figure 4. Myocardial glutathione content in control (C) and diabetic (D) animals. IPostC: ischemic postconditioning. *$P<0.05$ *vs.* group C.

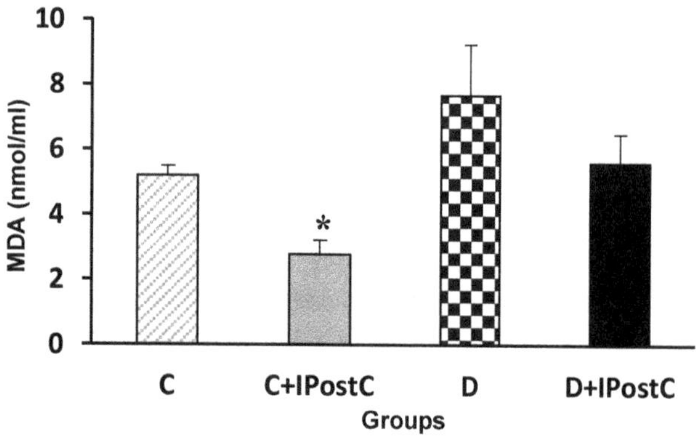

Figure 3. Myocardial MDA activity in control (C) and diabetic (D) animals. IPostC: ischemic postconditioning. *$P<0.05$ *vs.* group C.

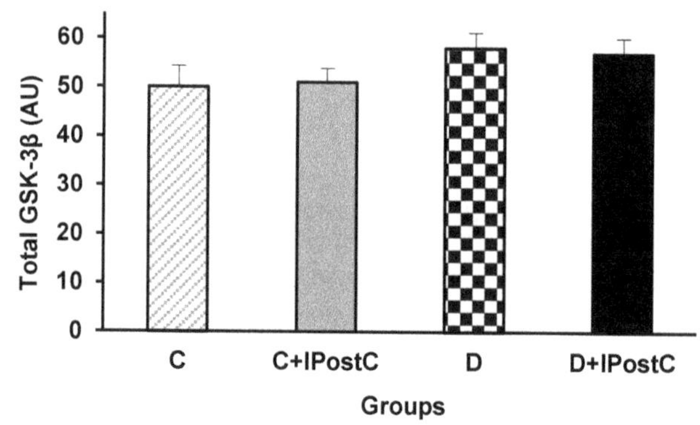

Figure 5. The total form of the GSK-3β (AU; arbitrary unit) in the myocardium of control (C) and diabetic (D) animals. GSK-3β: Glycogen Synthase Kinase-3beta, IPostC: ischemic postconditioning.

Glutathione

To determine whether IPostC in control and diabetic hearts may change myocardial GSH, we measured myocardial GSH contents in all experimental groups (Figure 4). IPostC in nondiabetic hearts resulted in a statistically significant elevation in GSH content (27±0.6 vs. 24±0.2 nmol/mg of protein, $P<0.05$). However, administration of IPostC at the onset of reperfusion in diabetic hearts could not increase GSH content in this condition (26±0.7 vs. 25±0.5 nmol/mg of protein).

Total form and the ratio of phosphorylated (at Ser 9) to total form of GSK-3β

For western blotting, the total and phosphorylated (at serine 9) form of GSK-3β were investigated. According to the densitometric analysis, there were no changes in the level of the total form of GSK-3β in control or diabetic animals (Figure 5). Nevertheless, in non-diabetic control animals, the IPostC intervention significantly increased the phosphorylated form of the GSK-3β as compared to those of the control group ($P<0.01$). However, in diabetic animals, IPostC failed to increase significantly the amount of phosphorylated form of GSK-3β and therefore, there was no difference in the ratio of phosphorylated to total form of GSK-3β between diabetic and diabetic plus IPostC groups (Figure 6).

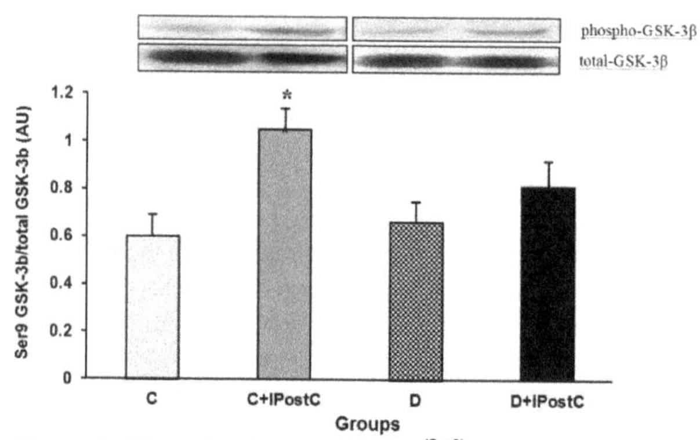

Figure 6. The ratio of phosphorylated$^{(Ser9)}$ to total form of GSK-3β (AU; arbitrary unit) in the myocardium of control (C) and diabetic (D) animals. GSK-3β: Glycogen Synthase Kinase-3beta, Ser9: Serine 9, IPostC: ischemic postconditioning. *$P<0.01$ *vs.* group C.

Discussion

In the present study, IPostC, as an effective method of cardioprotection in normal condition without any cardiac risk factors, was failed to induce protection in diabetic hearts. In other words, chronic diabetes (for 8 weeks) prevented the infarct size limiting and protective effect of IPostC in ischemic hearts. The phosphorylation of GSK-3β by IPostC in diabetic hearts was much less than controls one (although this difference was not statistically significant). In addition, IPostC significantly increased tissue content of glutathione and decreased the MDA level in control and healthy hearts; however, it failed to alter the amount of these markers in diabetic group.

IPostC, applied in the protocols of 3 cycles of 30-second reperfusion-ischemia or 6 cycles of 10-second reperfusion-ischemia immediately at the onset of reperfusion, have been showed appropriate protective effects on ischemic heart and caused significant reduction in infarct size.[4,11] IPostC is an effective therapeutic strategy which may be used in clinic through inflating and deflating the balloon during angioplasty, and therefore, can be used in patients.[5,19] Despite the fact that the most studies in the field of IPostC are performed on healthy animals, ischemic heart disease (IHD) in human patients are mainly resulted from other underlying co-morbidities like diabetes, arthrosclerosis, and hypertension. Diabetes is the most important cardiovascular risk factor that may increase the rate of IHD and prevent cardioprotective effects of therapeutic approaches.[2,4]

In the present study, chronic diabetes for 8 weeks totally prevented the positive effects of IPostC on reduction of infraction. There are a few studies in this regard; all of them show similar results. Przyklenk reported that 2-week diabetes (although it is not accord with chronic disease as in our study) demolishes the IPostC effects.[20] Similarly, it was reported that the protective effect of morphine or sevoflurane are diminished in diabetic and hyperglycemic conditions.[21,22] However, why this loss of cardioprotection occurs in diabetic state, is poorly understood yet.

There is not enough study on the mechanisms of interference of diabetes with protective effects of IPostC. Hyperglycemia, increase of oxidative stress and inflammation, and change in the activity of intracellular protein kinases might be considered as the interfering mechanisms, all of which are produced in diabetic conditions[23] and may prevent postconditioning effects. GSK-3β is a protein kinase that is active in normal and non-phosphorylated state and can open the mPTP, leading to the release of cytochrome C into the cytosol and starting the apoptosis and oxidative reactions.[14]

By activating PI3K-Akt signaling pathway, IPostC causes phosphorylation of GSK-3β and inactivates it and therefore, protects the ischemic heart by this way.[4,11] In the present study, protective effects of IPostC on non-diabetic hearts accompanied with significant phosphorylation of GSK-3β; however, IPostC failed to phosphorylate and inactivate GSK-3β in diabetic hearts, significantly. Another finding of this study is that the total amount of GSK-3β was the same in diabetic and non-diabetic groups and there were no significant changes among different groups. This result indicates that the chronic diabetes diminishes the power of IPostC to phosphorylate GSK-3β and thus, large quantities of this detrimental protein kinase are remained in its active form in diabetic conditions. Previous studies indicated that the activity of cellular protein kinases changes in diabetic and hyperglycemic conditions. For example, Drenger et al, reported that diabetes causes significant decrease in the amount of phosphorylation and activity of PI3K.[22] Therefore, these intracellular changes induced by chronic diabetes act as the interfering factor in the effect of IPostC on phosphorylation of GSK-3β and cardioprotection. As a result, IPostC in diabetic conditions can't phosphorylate and inactivate this protein kinase in a more effective way.

Keeping the GSK-3β in its active form may compromise the processes of cellular damage through the activation of apoptosis and oxidative stress which are mediated by mitochondrial pathways such as mPTP and ATP-sensitive potassium channels or other relative mediators.[13,14] In the present study, the amount of glutathione was measured as a strong antioxidant factor and the level of MDA as an index of lipid peroxidation in cardiac tissue of experimental groups. IPostC significantly increased the amount of glutathione and decreased the lipid peroxidation in non-diabetic hearts, however such effects were not observed in diabetic hearts. Postconditioning may attenuate myocardial injury by reducing oxidative stress in vivo in rats and in humans.[24-26] It has also been indicated that using exogenous antioxidants or activation of intrinsic antioxidants by postconditioning strategies may cause cardioprotection.[27-30] IPostC may decrease the activity of GSK-3β or inactivate it by its phosphorylation, and thereby, increase the cell tolerance to oxidative insult. Therefore, the inability of IPostC to exert cardioprotection in diabetic conditions may be attributed somehow to low activity of antioxidants and/or high peroxidative status which are resulted from diabetes.[23] For the better clarification of the postconditioning effects in diabetic hearts, it is suggested to investigate the expression levels of other proteins involved in oxidative stress such as Nrf or eNOS or proteins involved in apoptosis such as BAD/BAX in the future studies.

Conclusion

According to the findings of the present study, chronic diabetes impedes the protective effect of IPostC in diabetic hearts. The low phosphorylation (or low inactivation) of GSK-3β by IPostC, low production of glutathione and high lipid-peroxidation level in diabetic hearts may play the important roles in this loss of cardioprotection.

Acknowledgments

This work was supported by a grant from Research Deputy of Tabriz University of Medical Sciences, Tabriz-Iran.

Conflict of Interest

The authors have no conflicts of interest in regard to this research or its funding.

References

1. Go AS, Mozaffarian D, Roger VL, Benjamin EJ, Berry JD, Borden WB, et al. Heart disease and stroke statistics--2013 update: a report from the American Heart Association. *Circulation* 2013;127(1):e6-e245.
2. Whittington HJ, Babu GG, Mocanu MM, Yellon DM, Hausenloy DJ. The diabetic heart: too sweet for its own good? *Cardiol Res Pract* 2012;2012:845698. doi: 10.1155/2012/845698
3. Zhao ZQ, Corvera JS, Halkos ME, Kerendi F, Wang NP, Guyton RA, et al. Inhibition of myocardial injury by ischemic postconditioning during reperfusion: comparison with ischemic preconditioning. *Am J Physiol Heart Circ Physiol* 2003;285(2):H579-88. doi: 10.1152/ajpheart.01064.2002
4. Ferdinandy P, Schulz R, Baxter GF. Interaction of cardiovascular risk factors with myocardial ischemia/reperfusion injury, preconditioning, and postconditioning. *Pharmacol Rev* 2007;59(4):418-58. doi: 10.1124/pr.107.06002
5. Kharbanda RK. Cardiac conditioning: a review of evolving strategies to reduce ischaemia-reperfusion injury. *Heart* 2010;96(15):1179-86. doi: 10.1136/hrt.2009.179101
6. Lacerda L, Somers S, Opie LH, Lecour S. Ischaemic postconditioning protects against reperfusion injury via the SAFE pathway. *Cardiovasc Res* 2009;84(2):201-8. doi: 10.1093/cvr/cvp274
7. Wagner C, Kloeting I, Strasser RH, Weinbrenner C. Cardioprotection by postconditioning is lost in WOKW rats with metabolic syndrome: role of glycogen synthase kinase 3beta. *J Cardiovasc Pharmacol* 2008;52(5):430-7. doi: 10.1097/fjc.0b013e31818c12a7
8. Miki T, Itoh T, Sunaga D, Miura T. Effects of diabetes on myocardial infarct size and cardioprotection by preconditioning and postconditioning. *Cardiovasc Diabetol* 2012;11:67. doi: 10.1186/1475-2840-11-67
9. Grundy SM, Benjamin IJ, Burke GL, Chait A, Eckel RH, Howard BV, et al. Diabetes and cardiovascular disease: a statement for healthcare professionals from the American Heart Association. *Circulation* 1999;100(10):1134-46. doi: 10.1161/01.cir.100.10.1134
10. Sowers JR, Epstein M, Frohlich ED. Diabetes, hypertension, and cardiovascular disease: an update. *Hypertension* 2001;37(4):1053-9. doi: 10.1161/01.hyp.37.4.1053
11. Sanada S, Komuro I, Kitakaze M. Pathophysiology of myocardial reperfusion injury: preconditioning, postconditioning, and translational aspects of protective measures. *Am J Physiol Heart Circ Physiol* 2011;301(5):H1723-41. Doi: 10.1152/ajpheart.00553.2011
12. Gomez L, Paillard M, Thibault H, Derumeaux G, Ovize M. Inhibition of GSK3beta by postconditioning is required to prevent opening of the mitochondrial permeability transition pore during reperfusion. *Circulation* 2008;117(21):2761-8. doi: 10.1161/circulationaha.107.755066
13. Xi J, Wang H, Mueller RA, Norfleet EA, Xu Z. Mechanism for resveratrol-induced cardioprotection against reperfusion injury involves glycogen synthase kinase 3beta and mitochondrial permeability transition pore. *Eur J Pharmacol* 2009;604(1-3):111-6. doi: 10.1016/j.ejphar.2008.12.024
14. Juhaszova M, Zorov DB, Yaniv Y, Nuss HB, Wang S, Sollott SJ. Role of glycogen synthase kinase-3beta in cardioprotection. *Circ Res* 2009;104(11):1240-52. doi: 10.1161/circresaha.109.197996
15. Nishihara M, Miura T, Miki T, Tanno M, Yano T, Naitoh K, et al. Modulation of the mitochondrial permeability transition pore complex in GSK-3beta-mediated myocardial protection. *J Mol Cell Cardiol* 2007;43(5):564-70. doi: 10.1016/j.yjmcc.2007.08.010
16. Kaminski KA, Bonda TA, Korecki J, Musial WJ. Oxidative stress and neutrophil activation--the two keystones of ischemia/reperfusion injury. *Int J Cardiol* 2002;86(1):41-59. doi: 10.1016/s0167-5273(02)00189-4
17. Zhai P, Sciarretta S, Galeotti J, Volpe M, Sadoshima J. Differential roles of GSK-3beta during myocardial ischemia and ischemia/reperfusion. *Circ Res* 2011;109(5):502-11. doi: 10.1161/circresaha.111.249532
18. Badalzadeh R, Mohammadi M, Najafi M, Ahmadiasl N, Farajnia S, Ebrahimi H. The additive effects of ischemic postconditioning and cyclosporine-A on nitric oxide activity and functions of diabetic myocardium injured by ischemia/reperfusion. *J Cardiovasc Pharmacol Ther* 2012;17(2):181-9. doi: 10.1177/1074248411416118
19. Yun Y, Duan WG, Chen P, Wu HX, Shen ZQ, Qian ZY, et al. Ischemic postconditioning modified renal oxidative stress and lipid peroxidation caused by ischemic reperfusion injury in rats. *Transplant Proc* 2009;41(9):3597-602. doi: 10.1016/j.transproceed.2009.06.203
20. Przyklenk K, Maynard M, Greiner DL, Whittaker P. Cardioprotection with postconditioning: loss of efficacy in murine models of type-2 and type-1 diabetes. *Antioxid Redox Signal* 2011;14(5):781-90. doi: 10.1089/ars.2010.3343
21. Gross ER, Hsu AK, Gross GJ. Diabetes abolishes morphine-induced cardioprotection via multiple pathways upstream of glycogen synthase kinase-

3beta. *Diabetes* 2007;56(1):127-36. doi: 10.2337/db06-0907

22. Drenger B, Ostrovsky IA, Barak M, Nechemia-Arbely Y, Ziv E, Axelrod JH. Diabetes blockade of sevoflurane postconditioning is not restored by insulin in the rat heart: phosphorylated signal transducer and activator of transcription 3- and phosphatidylinositol 3-kinase-mediated inhibition. *Anesthesiology* 2011;114(6):1364-72. doi: 10.1097/ALN.0b013e31820efafd
23. Ansley DM, Wang B. Oxidative stress and myocardial injury in the diabetic heart. *J Pathol* 2013;229(2):232-41. doi: 10.1002/path.4113
24. Fan Q, Yang XC, Liu Y, Wang LF, Liu SH, Ge YG, et al. Postconditioning attenuates myocardial injury by reducing nitro-oxidative stress in vivo in rats and in humans. *Clin Sci (Lond)* 2011;120(6):251-61. doi: 10.1042/CS20100369
25. Zhao ZQ, Vinten-Johansen J. Postconditioning: reduction of reperfusion-induced injury. *Cardiovasc Res* 2006;70(2):200-11. doi: 10.1016/j.cardiores.2006.01.024
26. Vaez H, Samadzadeh M, Zahednezhad F, Najafi M. Resistance to reperfusion injury following short term postischemic administration of natural honey in globally ischemic isolated rat heart. *Adv Pharm Bull* 2012;2(2):189-96. doi: 10.5681/apb.2012.029
27. Badalzadeh R, Yousefi B, Majidinia M, Ebrahimi H. Anti-arrhythmic effect of diosgenin in reperfusion-induced myocardial injury in a rat model: activation of nitric oxide system and mitochondrial KATP channel. *J Physiol Sci* 2014;64(6):393-400. doi: 10.1007/s12576-014-0333-8
28. Rodrigo R, Prieto JC, Castillo R. Cardioprotection against ischaemia/reperfusion by vitamins C and E plus n-3 fatty acids: molecular mechanisms and potential clinical applications. *Clin Sci (Lond)* 2013;124(1):1-15. doi: 10.1042/cs20110663
29. Ebrahimi H, Badalzadeh R, Mohammadi M, Yousefi B. Diosgenin attenuates inflammatory response induced by myocardial reperfusion injury: role of mitochondrial ATP-sensitive potassium channels. *J Physiol Biochem* 2014;70(2):425-32. doi: 10.1007/s13105-014-0320-9
30. Kumar M, Sharma S, Vasudeva N. In vivo assessment of antihyperglycemic and antioxidant activity from oil of seeds of brassica nigra in streptozotocin induced diabetic rats. *Adv Pharm Bull* 2013;3(2):359-65. doi: 10.5681/apb.2013.058

Vasorelaxant Effect of 17α-Ethynylestradiol on Human Saphenous Vein

Ahmad Reza Jodati[1], Hossein Babaei[2,3]*, Yadollah Azarmi[3], Sahar Fallah[3], Afsaneh Gharebageri[2], Danial Fadaei Fouladi[2], Naser Safaei[1]

[1] *Cardiovascular Research Center, Tabriz University of Medical Sciences, Tabriz, Iran.*
[2] *Drug Applied Research Center, Tabriz University of Medical Sciences, Tabriz, Iran.*
[3] *School of Pharmacy, Tabriz University of Medical Sciences, Tabriz, Iran.*

Article info

Keywords:
- 17α- Ethynylestradiol
- Vasorelaxation
- Saphenous Vein
- Estrogen

Abstract

Purpose: A protective effect for estrogens against cardiovascular problems has long been known. The aim of this study was to investigate the vasorelaxant effect of 17α-Ethynylestradiol (17α-EE) on human saphenous vein.
Methods: The veins were suspended horizontally between two triangular stainless steel hooks for the measurement of isometric tension in individual organ baths containing 10ml Krebs solution, at 37°C and gassed with carbogen under 3gr optimum tension. The effect of different concentrations of 17α-EE (2-40 μM) on vascular tone was investigated in veins precontracted with $PGF_{2\alpha}$. Relaxation was measured after 40min and expressed as the percent decrease of initial contraction. To determine the involvement of potassium channels, endothelium, nitric oxide synthase, guanylylcyclase and prostaglandins in the vasorelaxant effect of estrogen, the veins were incubated with tetraethyl ammonium, N-nitro-L-arginine methyl ester, methylene blue or indomethacin, respectively for 20min prior to experimentation. Responses to 17α-EE were directly compared to those obtained in the same tissues in the absence of the inhibitors.
Results: The mean relaxations induced by 17α-EE with concentrations of 2, 5, 10, 20 and 40μM in tissues precontracted with $PGF_{2\alpha}$ were 19.8 ±5.5%, 26.1±10.8%, 32.2±7.4%, 48.6±10.8%and56±7.6%, respectively. The results of the inhibition of potassium channels, nitric oxide synthase, guanylylcyclase, cyclooxygenase and removing endothelium in relaxation induced by 17α-EE on precontracted veins with $PGF_{2\alpha}$ proved no significant differences.
Conclusion: This study showed that 17α-EE has significant vasorelaxant effect on human saphenous vein in a concentration-dependent manner. This effect is probably independent of potassium channels, nitric oxide synthase, guanylylcyclase, prostaglandin synthesis and endothelium functions.

Introduction

Estrogens are known for their cardiovascular protective properties through direct vasorelaxing mechanisms. Despite extensive research, however, the exact mechanisms underlying estrogen-induced vasorelaxation are unclear.[1] In addition, the underlying mechanism(s) of vasorelaxation by estrogens varies from type to type.[2-4]
Actions of estrogenic compounds on the vascular wall include alteration/ modulation of ion influxes, receptors on smooth muscle cells, and endothelium-derived factors production and activity.[5,6]
Guanylatecyclase enzyme has been proposed as a mediator in estrogen-induced vasodilation. However, their exact role and mechanism is highly controversial.[7,8]
A number of reports indicate that nitric oxide (NO) may play a pivotal role in mediating the effects of estrogens on the vasculature. This potent vasodilator is produced in the vascular endothelial cells.[9-12]
A direct action on the vascular smooth muscles has been also reported as another underlying mechanism of vasorelaxation incited by estrogens. In a previous study, the authors demonstrated that the relaxant effect of 17β-estradiol on human saphenous vein was elicited by calcium-dependent and -independent pathways.[13] The role of K^+ channels was also underlined in another study.[14]
It has been reported that estrogens could also modulate peripheral vascular synthesis of vasodilatory hormones. Prostacyclin is one of these hormones, which its production has been proposed as a pathway in estrogen-mediated vasorelaxation.[15,16]
Altogether, estrogens appear to reduce the risk of cardiovascular disease through a combination of mechanisms including changes in lipid profile, endothelial NO synthesis, cell proliferation and angiogenesis, and the regulation of vascular muscle cell (VSMC) Ca^{2+} and K^+ channels. These effects may be mediated through genomic and/or nongenomic pathways.[17]
Naderali et al.[1] showed that 17α-estradiol lacks any effect on classic estrogen receptors. Accordingly, they

***Corresponding author:** Hossein Babaei, Email: babaeih@tbzmed.ac.ir concluded that the known complications of estrogen-contained oral contraceptive pills, such as endometrial carcinoma and thrombosis, might not be seen with 17α-estradiol.

The mechanisms involved in the rapid vasorelaxant effects of 17α-Ethynylestradiol (17α-EE) are not well understood and are drastically controversial. In addition, there is lack of data in terms of the effects of 17α-EE on veins.

Since it is usually used in coronary artery bypass graft (CABG) surgery, the saphenous vein is of great important to physicians.[18] Furthermore, the incidence of acute closure and accelerated atherosclerosis has been reported high for this vein.[19]

The present study aims to examine, for the first time, the possible relaxant effects of 17α-EE on human saphenous vein in vitro and its possible mechanism(s).

Materials and Methods

Tissue preparation and isometric change recording

After being approved by the Ethics Committee of Tabriz University of Medical Sciences and in conformity with the principles outlined in the Declaration of Helsinki, vein segments were taken from excessive portions of saphenous veins from patients undergoing CABG surgery (n=71), including 58 males (mean age: 57.50±10.32, range: 36-74) and 13 females (mean age: 58.80±2.47, range: 44-71) at Madani Educational Heart Centre, Tabriz University of Medical Sciences, Tabriz, Iran.

Our preliminary experiments showed that there is no significant difference between the contractile or relaxant responses of the saphenous vein rings obtained from male patients and those obtained from female patients. However, to avoid any interference of confounding variables (cardiovascular health, smoking, medications, etc.) in each set of experiments control rings employed from the same male or female patients.

The acquired segments were immediately transferred from operating room to laboratory in ice-cold Krebs solution, trimmed of adjacent tissues and cut into 3-5 mm rings.

The presence and functionality of the endothelium was proven routinely at the beginning of the experiment when there was significant relaxation (more than %50) to acetylcholine (6 μM) in veins precontracted by phenylephrine (0.1μM).[20]

To investigate the role of endothelium in 17α-EE-induced relaxation, the luminal surface of some vein rings was thoroughly scraped off by using cotton thread. The lack of endothelium was confirmed when there was no relaxation in response to acetylcholine (6μM) in the rings precontracted with phenylephrine (0.1μM).[21]

For isometric change recording, two stainless steel triangle hooks introduced through the lumen of the vein rings, one fixed to the bottom of organ bath, while the other connected to a force-displacement transducer (LETICA, Spain). A computer-assisted data acquisition system (ADInstruments, Power Lab/4SP) recorded the changes in isometric tension during the experiments.[13,22]

The employed organ bath (10 ml) consisted of modified Krebs-Ringer bicarbonate solution (NaCl: 118mM, KCl: 4.7mM, KH_2PO_4: 1.2mM, $NaHCO_3$: 25mM, $MgSO_4.7H_2O$: 2.1mM, $CaCl_2$: 2.5mM, glucose: 11.1mM). The solution was aerated with a mixture of 95% O_2 and 5% CO_2, maintaining a pH of 7.3-7.4. The temperature was held constant at 37°C. The optimal tension was adjusted at 3g in all primary tests and throughout the experiments as previously established.[23,24] Each preparation was allowed to equilibrate for at least 60 min prior to initiation of experimental procedures, during which the bath solution was refreshed every 15 min and the tension was adjusted.

Effect of 17α-EE on isolated human saphenous vein rings

Since KCl and $PGF_{2\alpha}$ were shown to produce a stable and long-lasting contraction in human saphenous vein,[22] they were chosen as contractile agents in the present study. In order to obtain the submaximal concentration of these contractile agents, a concentration-response curve to each of them was constructed.

After achieving stable contraction by using either KCl or $PGF_{2\alpha}$, different concentrations of 17α-EE (2, 5, 10, 20 and 40 μM) were added for 40 min as a standard cutoff time in a non-cumulative manner. Each preparation was exposed to only one concentration of 17α-EE. From 17α-EE concentration response curve, 20 μM was chosen as an optimal submaximal concentration and used in all mechanistic experiments. The vehicle (ethanol, at final bath concentration no greater than 0.1%, v/v) alone had no significant relaxant effect on the contractile responses of the vein rings.

Effect of endothelium-removal on 17α-EE -induced vasodilatation

To assess the effect of endothelium, 17α-EE (20μM) was added to both intact and endothelium-denuded vein rings at the plateau of contraction produced by $PGF_{2\alpha}$ (0.8μM). Forty minutes later, the amount of relaxation was assessed and compared with control group.

Effect of guanylatecyclase (GC) inhibition on 17α-EE -induced vasodilatation

Methylene blue inhibits GC by oxidizing its hem iron, and reduces the relaxation elicited by sodium nitroprusside and NO. The effect of methylene blue on 17α-EE-induced relaxation was examined to determine a possible role of soluble GC. For this purpose, vein rings with intact endothelium were incubated with methylene blue (10 μM) for 20 min before induction of contraction with $PGF_{2\alpha}$ (0.8μM). Afterward, the relaxant responses to 17α-EE were documented.

Effect of NO synthesis inhibition on 17α-EE -induced vasodilatation

To assess the role of NO synthesis in 17α-EE-induced relaxation, vein rings with intact endothelium were challenged with N-nitro-L-arginine methyl ester

(L-NAME, 200µM) for 20 min prior to inducing contraction with $PGF_{2\alpha}$ (0.8µM).[25,26] The relaxant responses to 17α-EE were evaluated thereafter.

Effect of cyclooxygenase inhibition on 17α-EE-induced vasodilatation

Indomethacin, an inhibitor of cyclooxygenase, was used for 20 min at a dose of 10µM in some vein rings with intact endothelium.[27,28] After using contractile agents, 17α-EE (20µM) was added for 40 min in these tissues. As indomethacin was dissolved in pure ethanol, a group of vein rings using only pure ethanol (10µL) served as the control.

Effect of potassium channel inhibition on 17α-EE - induced vasodilatation

Tetraethyl ammonium (TEA) is a potassium channel blocker, with nonselective effect at high concentration.[29] In order to examine the effect of potassium channel blockade on 17α-EE-induced relaxation, a group of vein rings with intact endothelium were incubated with TEA (5mM) for 20 min before contraction with $PGF_{2\alpha}$ (0.8µM). Subsequently, the relaxant responses to 17α-EE were investigated.

Chemical Reagents and Drugs

Acetylcholine, 17α-EE, indomethacin, N-nitro-L-arginine methyl ester, methylene blue and tetraethyl ammonium all were purchased from Sigma. Phenylephrine was obtained from SinaDaru Co (Iran) and $PGF_{2\alpha}$ from Abureyhan Co. (Iran). Indomethacin and 17α-EE were dissolved in pure ethanol and the rest in distilled water. Ingredients of Krebs solution obtained from Merck.

Statistical analysis

The SPSS software version 12 (SPSS, USA) was used for statistical comparisons. Data are presented as mean ± standard error of the mean (SEM). The relaxant responses induced by 17α-EE were expressed as percentage of the initial contraction produced by either KCl or $PGF_{2\alpha}$. Linear regressions were performed by least square method for calculation of EC_{50}. The Student's t-test (Independent samples) was used to compare the data and p value less than 0.05 was considered as statistically significant.

Results

Effect of KCl and $PGF_{2\alpha}$ on isolated human saphenous vein rings

Both KCl (2-120 mM) and $PGF_{2\alpha}$ (0.05-2 µM) induced contraction in human saphenous vein tissues in a concentration-dependent manner. These responses reached a plateau after about 15-20 min, remaining stable for 60-70 min. Concentration-response curves to KCl and $PGF_{2\alpha}$ are depicted in Figure 1A and Figure 1B, respectively. Submaximal concentrations of $PGF_{2\alpha}$ and KCl(~ EC_{80}) were chosen for further experiments (0.8 µM and 60 mM, respectively).

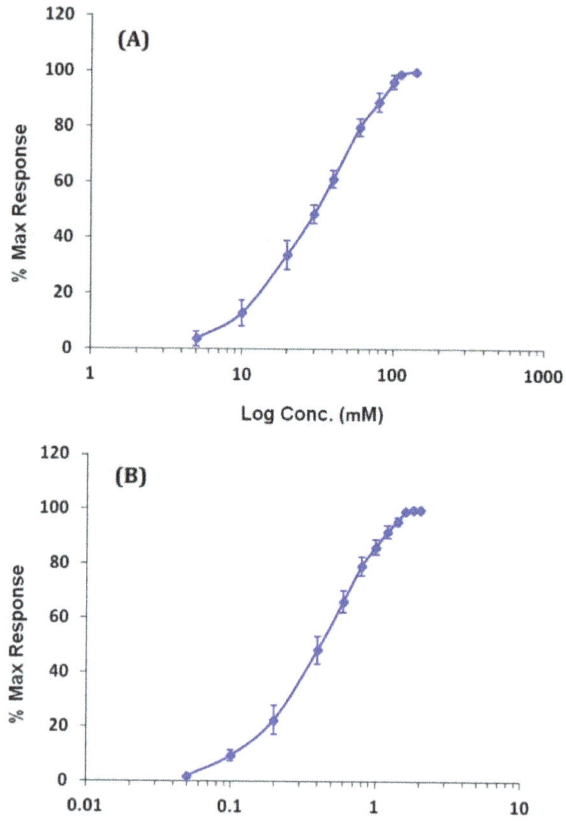

Figure 1. Concentration-response curves to KCl (A) and $PGF_{2\alpha}$ (B) in human saphenous vein.

Effect of 17α-EE on isolated human saphenous vein rings

The relaxant effects of increasing concentrations of 17α-EE (2, 5, 10, 20 and 40 µM) on the employed saphenous vein rings after 40 min are shown in Figure 2. The EC_{50} value for 17α-EE-induced relaxant effect in the specimens contracted by $PGF_{2\alpha}$ was about 20 µM. The relaxant response to 17α-EE was both repeatable and reversible (Figure 3).

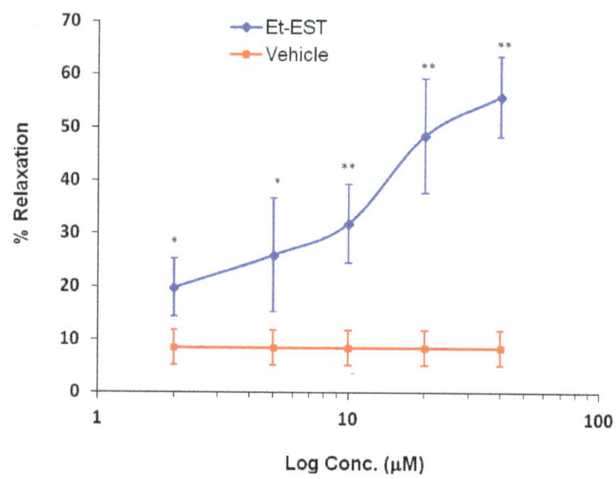

Figure 2. Relaxant effect of different concentrations of 17α-Ethynylestradiol (Et-EST) on human saphenous vein rings precontracted with $PGF_{2\alpha}$ (0.8 µM).
The relaxant responses (mean±SEM) are expressed as the percentage of the initial contraction produced by $PGF_{2\alpha}$. The vehicle volume remained fixed (10 µl) in all experiments (n=8) *:$p<0.05$, **: $p<0.01$.

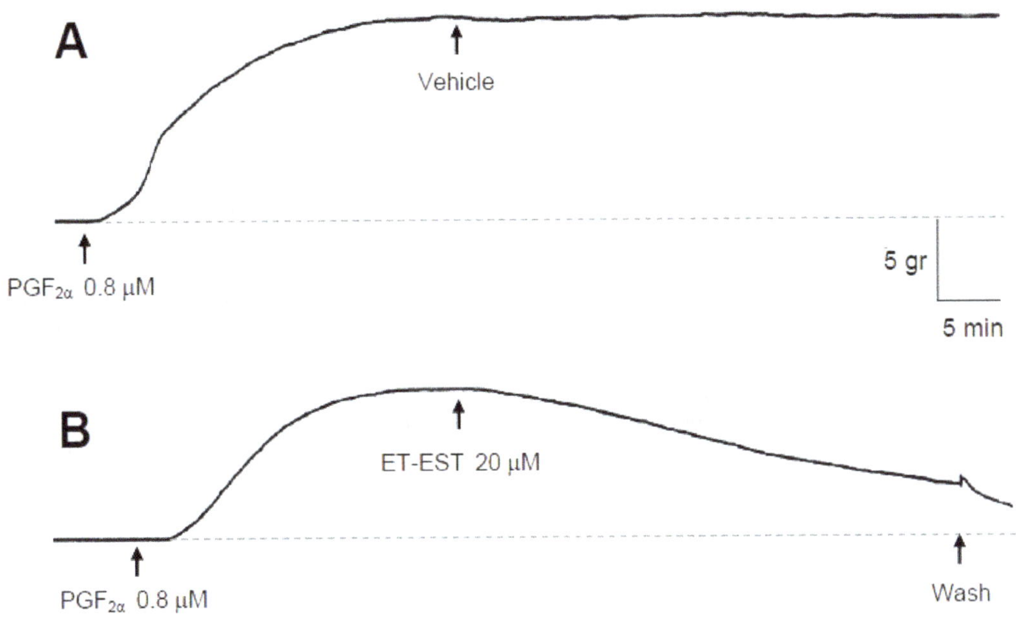

Figure 3. Representative trace showing stable contractile response to $PGF_{2α}$ (0.8 μM) (A) and acute relaxant response to 17α-Ethynylestradiol (ET-EST) (B) in human saphenous vein rings precontracted by $PGF_{2α}$

Effect of endothelium on 17α-EE -induced vasodilatation

The mean percent decrease in contractile response after adding 17α-EE was comparable between the two groups containing endothelium-free and endothelium-intact saphenous veins (60.4±9.6% vs. 48.6±10.8%, respectively (Figure 4). Therefore, denuding endothelium from the human saphenous vein rings did not change the vasorelaxant effect of 17α-EE significantly (p=0.21).

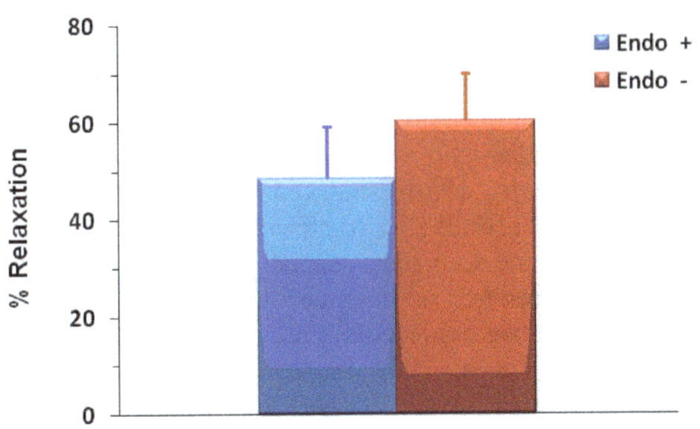

Figure 4. Effect of endothelium denudation on 17α-Ethynylestradiol (17α-EE)-induced vasodilatation in human saphenous vein rings precontracted with $PGF_{2α}$ (0.8μM).
Number of experiments=8. The difference was not statistically significant (p =0.21).

Effect of GC inhibition on 17α-EE -induced vasodilatation

The mean 17α-EE -induced relaxation was not significantly different between the samples incubated with methylene blue (GC-inhibitor) comparing with that in the controls (33.7±8.0% vs. 48.6±10.8%; respectively, p=0.14) (Figure 5).

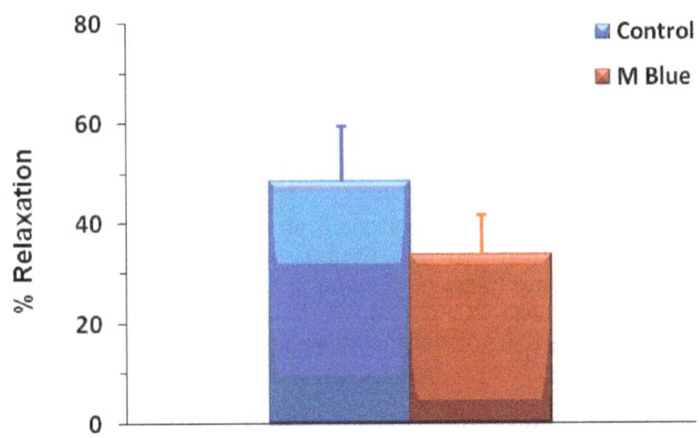

Figure 5. Effect of the inhibition of guanylatecyclase enzyme by using methylene blue (M Blue, 10μM) on 17α-Ethynylestradiol-induced vasodilatation in human saphenous vein rings precontracted with $PGF_{2α}$ (0.8μM). Number of experiments=8. The difference was not statistically significant (p=0.14).

Effect of NO synthesis inhibition on 17α-EE -induced vasodilatation

The mean 17α-EE-induced relaxation was 38.0±9.4% in the tissues incubated with L-NAME (NO synthase inhibitor), and 45.0±8.7% in the cases without L-NAME. There was not a significant difference between the two groups in this regard (p=0.23) (Figure 6).

Effect of cyclooxygenase inhibition on 17α-EE -induced vasodilatation

There was no significant difference between the veins incubated with indomethacin (cyclooxygenase inhibitor) and the control veins in terms of 17α-EE-induced relaxation (38.2±9.3% vs. 32.9±11.0%; p=0.33) (Figure 7).

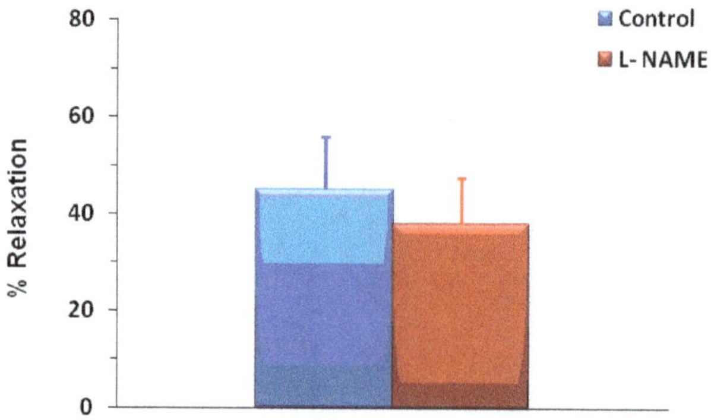

Figure 6. Effect of the inhibition of nitric oxide synthesis by using N-nitro-L-arginine methyl ester (L-NAME, 200µM) on 17α-Ethynylestradiol-induced vasodilatation in human saphenous vein rings precontracted with $PGF_{2\alpha}$ (0.8µM). Number of experiments=8. The difference was not statistically significant (p=0.23).

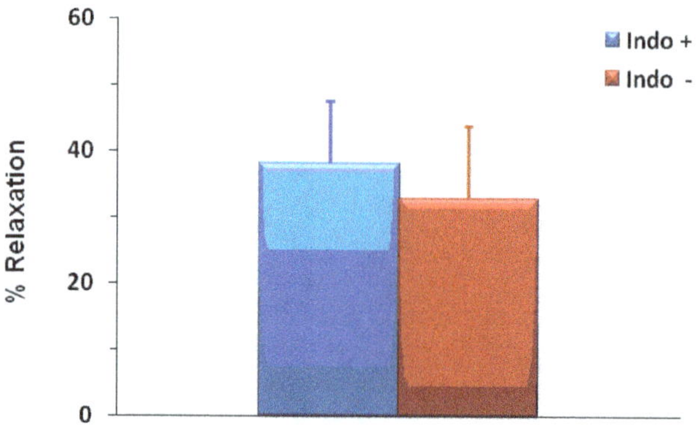

Figure 7. Effect of the inhibition of prostaglandin synthesis by using indomethacin (Indo, 10 µM) on 17α-Ethynylestradiol-induced vasodilatation in human saphenous vein rings precontracted with $PGF_{2\alpha}$ (0.8µM). Number of experiments=8. The difference was not statistically significant (p=0.33).

Effect of potassium channel inhibition on 17α-EE-induced vasodilatation

The mean 17α-EE-induced relaxation did not differ significantly between the veins incubated with TEA (potassium channel-inhibitor) and the control veins (38.6±6.1% vs. 45.2±10.7%, respectively; p=0.22) (Figure 8).

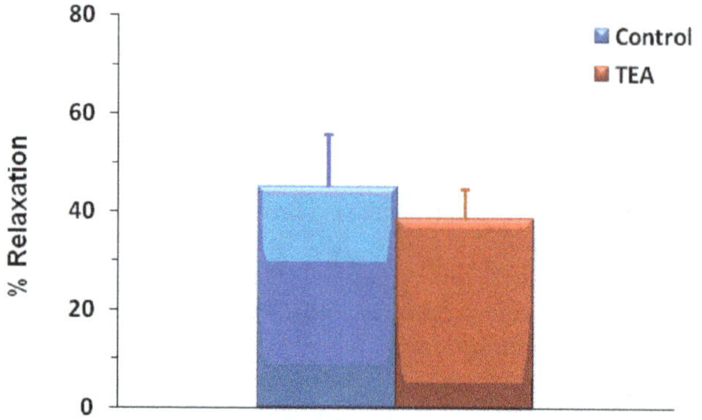

Figure 8. Effect of the inhibition of potassium channels by using tetraethyl ammonium (TEA, 5mM) on 17α-Ethynylestradiol-induced vasodilatation in human saphenous vein rings precontracted with $PGF_{2\alpha}$ (0.8µM). Number of experiments=8. The difference was not statistically significant (p=0.22).

Discussion

Estrogen-induced vasorelaxation is believed to be rendered through interacting with vascular smooth muscle, endothelial cells, and vessel wall.[30-32] Despite extensive research, however, the exact mechanisms underlying estrogen-induced vasorelaxation are unclear.[1] In addition, the underlying mechanism of vasorelaxation by estrogens varies from type to type.[2-4]

In the present study, the acute vasorelaxant effect of 17α-EE on isolated human saphenous vein rings precontracted with KCl or $PGF_{2\alpha}$ was investigated.

A direct effect of estrogens on the endothelium has been proposed as a possible mechanism of vasorelaxation.[33] In the present work, however, there was no significant difference between endothelium-denuded and endothelium-intact vein rings in terms of the mean percent decrease in contractile response after adding 17α-EE. It should be taken into consideration that estrogen-induced vasodilation can be either endothelium-dependent or –independent.[34,35] Likewise, other factors such as gender and hormonal status may play a role in this regard. For example, Martínez et al[36] showed that while gender and hormonal environment had no effect on the estrogen-induced, endothelium-independent component of the relaxation, both of them significantly modulated the estrogen-induced, endothelium-dependent component of the relaxation in rat aorta strips. The role of these possible confounding factors needs to be examined in further studies.

The other factor, which is proposed to have an effect on the vasorelaxation mediated by estrogens, is guanylatecyclase enzyme. In an attempt to clarify the role of this enzyme, methylene blue, an inhibitor of guanylatecyclase, was used.[37,38] In line with some previous reports, adding methylene blue did not modify estrogen-induced relaxation.[8]

Nitric oxide production is another mechanism that has been proposed in estrogen-induced vasorelaxation.[39,40] Thus, in another part of the present work the role of nitric oxide in 17α-EE-induced vasorelaxation was examined. Accordingly, there was no significant difference in the vein rings relaxation produced by 17α-EE in the presence or absence of L-NAME, a potent inhibitor of nitric oxide synthase.[25,26] In conformity with this finding, in a study on human omental artery, Vedernikov et al[41] concluded that the vasorelaxant effect of estrogen (17beta-estradiol) does not involve the products of endothelial nitric oxide. Shaw et al.[42] examined the vasorelaxing effects of 17-beta-estradiol on pre-contracted pressurized (50 mmHg) isolated rat mesenteric and coronary arteries. The vasodilatory responses in both types of artery were unaffected by L-NAME. Similar finding was also reported in another study in rabbit carotid artery.[43]

It is believed that estrogen stimulates nitric oxide production through both endothelium-dependent and independent pathways.[44] Since L-NAME exhibits some selectivity for the inhibition of particular isoforms of nitric oxide synthase,[45] it is possible that other ways of nitric oxide release remain unblocked even in the presence of L-NAME. To reach a definite conclusion in this regard, however, further clarifying studies are mandatory.

Some studies have suggested that the cardiovascular protection by estrogens may be exerted through the stimulation of prostaglandin synthesis in vessel wall. It has been demonstrated that chronic treatment by estrogen increases in vivo production of prostacyclin and attenuates the level of blood thromboxane in rabbits fed with highly atherogenic diet in comparison with placebo-treated animals.[46] To determine the possible role of prostaglandins in 17α-EE-induced vasorelaxation, we compared indomethacin-incubated tissues with control group. Again, and in conformity with a previous report,[43] no significant difference was detected between the two groups.

A widely discussed probable mechanism by which estrogen may exert its vasorelaxant effect is the alteration in potassium (K^+) channels. To assess this function in the present work, we assessed the 17α-EE-induced relaxation in the presence of TEA, an inhibitor of potassium channels.[47] There was not a significant difference between the two groups in this regard.

As discussed earlier, the results of various studies are widely heterogeneous, and sometimes inconclusive. The type of estrogen and contracturant, the presence or absence of endothelium, and the employed methodology to examine the acute effects may contribute to the variability in the response.[8,48,49] In addition, the vasodilatory effects of different estrogens could widely vary between specific species and/or vascular beds in systemic circulation.[50,51]

Conclusion

This is the first study, which examines the vasorelaxant effect of 17α-EE in human saphenous vein. This concentration-dependent relaxant effect occurs acutely (non-genomic), independent of the mechanisms associated with guanylatecyclase, cyclooxygenase, endothelium, NO and potassium channels.

Acknowledgments

We gratefully acknowledge funding from Drug Applied Research Center, Tabriz University of Medical Sciences and kind cooperation of operation rooms staff, Madani Educational Heart Centre, Tabriz University of Medical Sciences Tabriz, Iran.Results presented are from S. Fallh's Pharm D. thesis that was approved by students' research committee of Tabriz University of Medical Sciences.

Conflict of Interest

The authors report no conflicts of interest.

References

1. Naderali EK, Smith SL, Doyle PJ, Williams G. Vasorelaxant effects of oestradiols on guinea pigs: a role for gender differences. *Eur J Clin Invest* 2001;31(3):215-20.
2. Freay AD, Curtis SW, Korach KS, Rubanyi GM. Mechanism of vascular smooth muscle relaxation by estrogen in depolarized rat and mouse aorta. Role of nuclear estrogen receptor and Ca2+ uptake. *Circ Res* 1997;81(2):242-8.
3. Reis SE, Gloth ST, Blumenthal RS, Resar JR, Zacur HA, Gerstenblith G, et al. Ethinyl estradiol acutely attenuates abnormal coronary vasomotor responses to acetylcholine in postmenopausal women. *Circulation* 1994;89(1):52-60.
4. Bhalla HL, Arora MK, Saxena KK, Surin WR. Chronic use of 17β-Ethinyl estradiol on cardiovascular hemodynamic profile: "Friend or foe"? *J Pharm Negative Results* 2013;4:54-9.
5. Liu PY, Death AK, Handelsman DJ. Androgens and cardiovascular disease. *Endocr Rev* 2003;24(3):313-40.
6. Tostes RC, Nigro D, Fortes ZB, Carvalho MH. Effects of estrogen on the vascular system. *Braz J Med Biol Res* 2003;36(9):1143-58.
7. Gruetter CA, Gruetter DY, Lyon JE, Kadowitz PJ, Ignarro LJ. Relationship between cyclic guanosine 3':5'-monophosphate formation and relaxation of coronary arterial smooth muscle by glyceryl trinitrate, nitroprusside, nitrite and nitric oxide: effects of methylene blue and methemoglobin. *J Pharmacol Exp Ther* 1981;219(1):181-6.
8. Martinez C, Sanchez M, Hidalgo A, De Boto MJ. Mechanisms of diethylstilbestrol-induced relaxation in rat aorta smooth muscle. *Vascul Pharmacol* 2003;40(4):197-204.
9. Furchgott RF, Zawadzki JV. The obligatory role of endothelial cells in the relaxation of arterial smooth muscle by acetylcholine. *Nature* 1980;288(5789):373-6.
10. Ignarro LJ, Buga GM, Wood KS, Byrns RE, Chaudhuri G. Endothelium-derived relaxing factor produced and released from artery and vein is nitric oxide. *Proc Natl Acad Sci U S A* 1987;84(24):9265-9.
11. Palmer RM, Ashton DS, Moncada S. Vascular endothelial cells synthesize nitric oxide from L-arginine. *Nature* 1988;333(6174):664-6.
12. Palmer RM, Ferrige AG, Moncada S. Nitric oxide release accounts for the biological activity of endothelium-derived relaxing factor. *Nature* 1987;327(6122):524-6.
13. Babaei H, Azarmi Y. 17beta-estradiol inhibits calcium-dependent and -independent contractions in isolated human saphenous vein. *Steroids* 2008;73(8):844-50.
14. Babaei H, Azarmi Y. Effect of potassium channels and endothelium derived hyperpolarizing factor on vasorelaxant effect of 17β-estradiol in human saphenous vein. *Pharma Sci* 2008;4:55-66

15. Sherman TS, Chambliss KL, Gibson LL, Pace MC, Mendelsohn ME, Pfister SL, et al. Estrogen acutely activates prostacyclin synthesis in ovine fetal pulmonary artery endothelium. *Am J Respir Cell Mol Biol* 2002;26(5):610-6.
16. Ospina JA, Krause DN, Duckles SP. 17beta-estradiol increases rat cerebrovascular prostacyclin synthesis by elevating cyclooxygenase-1 and prostacyclin synthase. *Stroke* 2002;33(2):600-5.
17. Falkenstein E, Tillmann HC, Christ M, Feuring M, Wehling M. Multiple actions of steroid hormones--a focus on rapid, nongenomic effects. *Pharmacol Rev* 2000;52(4):513-56.
18. Tarzamni MK, Eshraghi N, Fouladi RF, Afrasiabi A, Halimi M, Azarvan A. Atherosclerotic changes in common carotid artery, common femoral artery, and ascending aorta/aortic arch in candidates for coronary artery bypass graft surgery. *Angiology* 2012;63(8):622-9.
19. Ouyang P, Tardif JC, Herrington DM, Stewart KJ, Thompson PD, Walsh MN, et al. Randomized trial of hormone therapy in women after coronary bypass surgery. Evidence of differential effect of hormone therapy on angiographic progression of disease in saphenous vein grafts and native coronary arteries. *Atherosclerosis* 2006;189(2):375-86.
20. Azarmi Y, Babaei H, Alizadeh F, Gharebageri A, Fouladi DF, Nikkhah E. Allopurinol Prevents Nitroglycerin-induced Tolerance in Rat Thoracic Aorta. *J Cardiovasc Pharmacol* 2014;63(2):113-9.
21. Babaei H, Gharehbagheri A, Eteraf Oskouei T, Delazar A, Asnaashari S, Bamdad Mogadam S. Role of endothelium on Vasorelaxant effect of Ribes biebersteinii fruit total extract on rat aorta. *Pharm Sci* 2009;15(2):159- 68.
22. Babaei H, Ebrahimi F, Shahbazi Mojarrad J, Azarmi Y, Gharehbagheri A. Vasorelaxant effect of a newly synthesized dihydropyridine ethyl ester (DHPEE) on rat thoracic aorta: Dual Mechanism of action. *Adv Pharm Bull* 2011;1(1):10-7.
23. Azarmi Y, Babaei H. Effect of endothelium and cGMP on vasorelaxant effect of 17b estradiol on human saphenous vein. *Pharm Sci* 2006;11(4):79-85.
24. Babaei H, Azarmi Y. Comparative effect of genistein and 17b-estradiol on human saphenous vein and rat aorta. *Pharm Sci* 2005;10(2):101-10.
25. Bilfinger TV, Vosswinkel JA, Cadet P, Rialas CM, Magazine HI, Stefano GB. Direct assessment and diminished production of morphine stimulated NO by diabetic endothelium from saphenous vein. *Acta Pharmacol Sin* 2002;23(2):97-102.
26. Sahin AS, Atalik KE, Sahin TK, Dogan N. Cooling and response to hydrogen peroxide in human saphenous vein: role of the endothelium. *Fundam Clin Pharmacol* 2005;19(3):341-6.
27. Leung FP, Yao X, Lau CW, Ko WH, Lu L, Huang Y. Raloxifene relaxes rat intrarenal arteries by inhibiting Ca2+ influx. *Am J Physiol Renal Physiol* 2005;289(1):F137-44.
28. Torregrosa G, Burguete MC, Perez-Asensio FJ, Salom JB, Gil JV, Alborch E. Pharmacological profile of phytoestrogens in cerebral vessels: in vitro study with rabbit basilar artery. *Eur J Pharmacol* 2003;482(1-3):227-34.
29. Omae T, Nagaoka T, Tanano I, Yoshida A. Pioglitazone, a peroxisome proliferator-activated receptor-gamma agonist, induces dilation of isolated porcine retinal arterioles: role of nitric oxide and potassium channels. *Invest Ophthalmol Vis Sci* 2011;52(9):6749-56.
30. Diaz M, Ramirez CM, Marin R, Marrero-Alonso J, Gomez T, Alonso R. Acute relaxation of mouse duodenum [correction of duodenun] by estrogens. Evidence for an estrogen receptor-independent modulation of muscle excitability. *Eur J Pharmacol* 2004;501(1-3):161-78.
31. Nakajima T, Kitazawa T, Hamada E, Hazama H, Omata M, Kurachi Y. 17beta-Estradiol inhibits the voltage-dependent L-type Ca2+ currents in aortic smooth muscle cells. *Eur J Pharmacol* 1995;294(2-3):625-35.
32. Grady D, Rubin SM, Petitti DB, Fox CS, Black D, Ettinger B, et al. Hormone therapy to prevent disease and prolong life in postmenopausal women. *Ann Intern Med* 1992;117(12):1016-37.
33. Rodriguez J, Garcia De Boto MJ, Hidalgo A. Mechanisms involved in the relaxant effect of estrogens on rat aorta strips. *Life Sci* 1996;58(7):607-15.
34. Andersen HL, Weis JU, Fjalland B, Korsgaard N. Effect of acute and long-term treatment with 17-beta-estradiol on the vasomotor responses in the rat aorta. *Br J Pharmacol* 1999;126(1):159-68.
35. Raddino R, Pela G, Uberti D, Portera C, Ferrari R, Scarabelli TM, et al. Estrogen derivative relaxes rabbit aorta via the endothelial receptor system. *Ital Heart J* 2001;2(1):49-54.
36. Martinez C, Lopez C, Hidalgo A, Sanchez M, Garcia De Boto MJ. Gonadectomy eliminates endothelium-dependent diethylstilbestrol-induced relaxant effect in rat aorta. *Pharmacology* 2003;67(3):136-42.
37. Friebe A, Koesling D. Regulation of nitric oxide-sensitive guanylyl cyclase. *Circ Res* 2003;93(2):96-105.
38. Mayer B, Brunner F, Schmidt K. Inhibition of nitric oxide synthesis by methylene blue. *Biochem Pharmacol* 1993;45(2):367-74.
39. Hekimoglu A, Celik F, Tas T, Ece A, Kavak V. The contribution of nitric oxide on the relaxation effects of diethylstilbestrol. *Saudi Med J* 2008;29(5):662-7.
40. Momoi H, Ikomi F, Ohhashi T. Estrogen-induced augmentation of endothelium-dependent nitric oxide-mediated vasodilation in isolated rat cerebral small arteries. *Jpn J Physiol* 2003;53(3):193-203.
41. Vedernikov YP, Belfort MA, Saade GR, Garfield RE. Inhibition of cyclooxygenase but not nitric oxide synthase influences effects on the human omental artery of the thromboxane A2 mimetic U46619 and

17beta-estradiol. *Am J Obstet Gynecol* 2001;185(1):182-9.
42. Shaw L, Taggart MJ, Austin C. Mechanisms of 17 beta-oestradiol induced vasodilatation in isolated pressurized rat small arteries. *Br J Pharmacol* 2000;129(3):555-65.
43. Salom JB, Burguete MC, Perez-Asensio FJ, Centeno JM, Torregrosa G, Alborch E. Acute relaxant effects of 17-beta-estradiol through non-genomic mechanisms in rabbit carotid artery. *Steroids* 2002;67(5):339-46.
44. White RE. Estrogen and vascular function. *Vascul Pharmacol* 2002;38(2):73-80.
45. Furfine ES, Harmon MF, Paith JE, Garvey EP. Selective inhibition of constitutive nitric oxide synthase by L-NG-nitroarginine. *Biochemistry* 1993;32(33):8512-7.
46. Fogelberg M, Vesterqvist O, Diczfalusy U, Henriksson P. Experimental atherosclerosis: effects of oestrogen and atherosclerosis on thromboxane and prostacyclin formation. *Eur J Clin Invest* 1990;20(1):105-10.
47. Chan W, Yao X, Ko W, Huang Y. Nitric oxide mediated endothelium-dependent relaxation induced by glibenclamide in rat isolated aorta. *Cardiovasc Res* 2000;46(1):180-7.
48. Teoh H, Quan A, Leung SW, Man RY. Vascular effects of estrone and diethylstilbestrol in porcine coronary arteries. *Menopause* 2009;16(1):104-9.
49. Martinez C, Sanchez M, Hidalgo A, Garcia De Boto MJ. Involvement of K(ATP) channels in diethylstilbestrol-induced relaxation in rat aorta. *Eur J Pharmacol* 2001;413(1):109-16.
50. Hilgers RH, Oparil S, Wouters W, Coelingh Bennink HJ. Vasorelaxing effects of estetrol in rat arteries. *J Endocrinol* 2012;215(1):97-106.
51. Reslan OM, Yin Z, Do Nascimento GR, Khalil RA. Subtype-specific Estrogen Receptor-mediated Vasodilator Activity in the Cephalic, Thoracic, and Abdominal Vasculature of Female Rat. *J Cardiovasc Pharmacol* 2013;62(1):26-40.

Anti-Inflammatory Effect of Taurine in Burned Patients

Sima Lak[1], Alireza Ostadrahimi[2]*, Behrooz Nagili[1], Mohammad Asghari-Jafarabadi[3], Sanaz Beigzali[4], Feridoon Salehi[5], Roxana Djafarzadeh[6]

[1] *Infectious and Tropical Disease Research Centre, Tabriz University of Medical Sciences, Tabriz, Iran.*
[2] *Nutrition Research Center, Faculty of Health and Nutrition, Tabriz University of Medical Sciences, Tabriz, Iran.*
[3] *Road Traffic Injury Prevention Centre, Tabriz University of Medical Sciences, Tabriz, Iran.*
[4] *Student Research Committee, Faculty of Medicine, Tabriz University of Medical Sciences, Tabriz, Iran.*
[5] *Burn Center, Sina Hospital, Tabriz University of Medical Sciences, Tabriz, Iran.*
[6] *Scientific Associate, Global eLearning Academy, Geneva, Switzerland.*

Article info

Keywords:
- Burns
- Nutrition
- Taurine
- Systematic Inflammatory Response Syndrome

Abstract

Purpose: Burn induced inflammatory response can be mediated by reactive oxygen metabolites and accompanied by multiple organ dysfunction. Taurine has protective effects against various inflammatory conditions. The aim of this study was to determine the effect of Taurine supplement in thermal burn victims.

Methods: Thirty patients with severe thermal burns were enrolled in this randomized double-blinded clinical trial. These patients were randomly divided into two equal groups (namely Control and Taurine groups), where both received isocaloric and isonitrogenous formula. One group was supplemented with 50 mg/kg of Taurine per day for a duration of 10 days. Blood samples were obtained to measure Interleukin-10 (IL-10), high-sensitivity C-reactive protein (hs-CRP), and Tumor Necrosis Factor alpha (TNF-α) levels at the beginning and the end of the study.

Results: Change in serum level of IL-10 in Taurine group was more than Control group [-13.60(-31.40, -10.40) compared to -4.00(-20.00, -0.20) respectively; $P = 0.030$]. This change was significant in patients with more than 30% TBSA of burn [-14.20(-31.40, -10.40) compared to -2.40(-9.60, 0.40) respectively; $P = 0.013$]. As for the hs-CRP and TNF-α levels, the difference between the two groups were not significant.

Conclusion: Based on the results obtained, Taurine supplement showed a positive outcome on anti-inflammatory cytokine IL-10 in all burn patients. This effect was even more significant in patients with higher percentage of burn area. Taurine had no significant effect on the inflammatory marker hs-CRP and the pro-inflammatory cytokine TNF-α level. For a more thorough verification, measurement of a wider range of inflammatory cytokines in more frequent time intervals are suggested.

Introduction

Extensive tissue destruction are the major causes of mortality and morbidity. Following the initial resuscitation period, patients develop systemic inflammatory response syndrome (SIRS).[1] The activation of a pro-inflammatory cascade after burn injury appears to be important in the development of subsequent immune dysfunction, susceptibility to sepsis, and development of SIRS and multiple organ dysfunction syndrome (MODS), which primarily contribute to morbidity and mortality in severe burn injuries.[2] Following the initial pro-inflammatory phase, anti-inflammatory response follows primarily as a release of IL-10, IL-4, prostaglandin E2, soluble TNF receptors and IL-1 receptor antagonists.[3] The temporal relationship between a pro-inflammatory and anti-inflammatory cytokine response is not fully understood but anti-inflammatory mediators are known to suppress the cellular immune response. The anti-inflammatory response overcome the pro-inflammatory state, leading to a functional state of depressed immune response. This state causes, impaired antibody production and diminished phagocytosis, which puts patients in an increased risk for additional infectious state.[4,5] IL-10 is an important anti-inflammatory cytokine. It is classified as a Th2-type cytokine and known to be an important factor in maintaining homeostasis of overall immune responses.[6,7] With its immunosuppressive properties, IL-10 is produced by monocytes and T helper cells, including activated T cells and B cells.[8] In addition, it has been shown to suppress a wide range of inflammatory responses.

Taurine (2-aminoethylsulphonic acid) is derived from the methionine and cysteine metabolism. As a semi-essential amino acid with high concentration in mammalian cells and plasma, Taurine plays an important role in various essential biological processes.[9,10] Taurine is presented in neutrophilic granulocytes, lymphocytes and monocytes.[11,12] It is an antioxidant and has tissue

***Corresponding author:** Alireza Ostadrahimi, Email: ostadrahimi@tbzmed.ac.ir

protective effects in oxidant induced injuries. It can reduce cell injuries followed by ischemia and reperfusion phenomena.[13-15] It is effective in the maintenance of vascular tone and exerts a vasodilator,[16] osmoregulator, intracellular calcium canal regulator effects. As part of an anti-inflammatory process, Taurine (within monocytes and neutrophils) reacts with hypochlorous acid (HOCL) to produce Taurine chloramines (TauCL). TauCL is less toxic than HOCL and is a powerful regulator of inflammation. It regulates the pro-inflammatory mediators in inflammatory cells.[17,18]

In this study, we aimed to investigate the levels of pro-inflammatory and anti-inflammatory cytokines over a time interval (days 1 and 9), in order to determine the relationship between the effects of Taurine and the levels of these cytokines (IL-10, hs-CRP, and TNF-α) on burned patients.

Materials and Methods

This was an interventional study, single-centre, double-blind, and block Randomised Clinical Trial. It was conducted on 30 patients with severe burns, admitted to the Burns Ward of Sina Hospital (Tabriz, Iran).

Eligibility Criteria

Inclusion Criteria – Patients in this study were admitted within the first day of obtaining a burn injury, with a Total Body Surface Area (TBSA) of burn with greater than 20%. The age range was between 18-85 years with an expected hospital stay of 10 days. These patients were likely to have at least 48 hours of enteral nutrition.

Exclusion Criteria – Pregnant women, patients with cardiogenic shock, severe inhalation injury, hepatic failure, renal failure, congenital amino acid metabolism impairment, and enteral feeding contraindication were excluded from this study.

Age Limits – The age limit was above 18 years of age.

Experimental Design

The patients were divided into two groups of 15 by a random allocation software. One group was defined as the Control group and consisted of 10 males and 5 females aged between 18 to 60 years of age (Group C: n = 15, Age Range 18-60, Average 36.27 ± 14.35). The second group, defined as Taurine group, also consisted of 10 males and 5 females with an age range between 21 to 72 years (Group T: n = 15, Age Range 21-72, Average 37.38 ± 14.08). Both groups received the routine therapy for management of burns after admission.

Nutrition

All the subjects received hourly enteral feeding of commercially prepared meal (EnteraMeal Standard Karen Pharma and Food supplement Co., Iran), 1kcal.ml^{-1}: 14% Protein, 54% Carbohydrate, and 32% Fat) within the first hour of admission. Protein was also added to patients with burns more than 30% TBSA starting day 3. This was to maintain their protein levels at about 1.5-2 mg.kg^{-1}. The composition of the diet was identical for each group. The calorie requirement was calculated according to the Harris-Benedict equation which gives an estimate of Resting Energy Expenditure (REE) x 1.5.Taurine group received an additional daily intake of Taurine supplement (Euro OTC Pharma GmbH, Germany) of 50 mg.kg^{-1} (with a maximum dose of 4g per day). This intervention lasted for about 10 days from the admission day used as the baseline and the second blood sample measurement on day 9.

Biochemical Assessment

Blood samples were obtained on days 1 and 9 after injury in order to measure IL-10, hs-CRP and TNF-α levels. Serum were separated immediately after centrifugation and frozen at -70°C until it was assayed. Serum levels of IL-10, TNF-α, and hs-CRP were measured using commercially available Enzyme-Linked ImmunoSorbant Assay (ELISA) kits (eBioscience, Austria).

Statistical Analysis

Data were analysed using SPSS (Version 21). Data distribution was assessed using Kolmogorov-Smirnov test. Normally distributed variables were presented as Mean ± Standard Deviation (M ± SD). Comparison of time points (Day 1 and Day 9) within each group was assessed by Dependent (Paired) Samples t-test. Comparisons between groups were made with Independent (Unpaired) Samples t-test. Non-normally distributed variables were presented as the Median and Interquartile Range (IQR) (standard 25th-75th percentile). Comparisons of non-normally distributed samples were performed using Wilcoxon Signed-Ranks test within each group, and Mann-Whitney U test to compare differences between the two groups. The probability less than 0.05 ($P < 0.05$) were considered significant.[19]

Results

General characteristics of the patients are shown in Table 1. The majority of the patients were male (66.7%). The age range was between 18-72 years (n=30; age average of 36.27 ± 14.86 in Group C and 37.73 ± 14.57 in Group T; Table 1). The Extent of Total Body Surface Area (TBSA) in all the burn patients ranged between 20% and 60% (TBSA%: 31.07 ± 12.40 in Group C and 32.33 ± 12.25 in Group T; Table 1).

Table 1. Characteristics of Study Subjects

Characteristics	Group C (n=15)	Group T (n=15)
Age[1] (yr)	36.27 ± 14.86	37.73 ± 14.57
Age Range (yr)	18-60	21-72
Sex[2] (M:F)	10:5	10:5
Weight[1] (kg)	72.67 ± 17.99	68.33 ± 14.68
Height[1] (cm)	167.13 ± 12.30	167.27 ± 7.03
TBSA[1] (%)	31.07 ± 12.40	32.33 ± 12.25
TBSA < 30%	22.25 ± 2.76	23.13 ± 2.80
TBSA ≥ 30%	41.14 ± 11.29	42.86 ± 9.94
Sepsis[3] (n, %)	2, 13.33	1, 6.67
Mortality[3] (n, %)	1, 6.67	1, 6.67

[1] Data for *Age*, *Weight*, *Height*, and *TBSA* are presented as Means ± Standard Deviation (M ± SD)
[2] Data for *Sex* are presented as frequency ratio (Male:Female)
[3] Data for *Sepsis* and *Mortality* are presented as Frequency and Percentage (Frequency, Percentage)

Patients in T group had a more significant decreased levels of IL-10 compared with C group subjects (-13.60[-31.40, -10.40] compared with -4.00[-20.00, -0.20] respectively; $P = 0.030$; Table 2). In particular, patients with severe burn (TBSA $\geq$ 30%) showed a more significant change (-14.20[-31.40, -10.40] compared with -2.40[-9.60, 0.40] respectively; $P = 0.013$; Table 2).
Hs-CRP levels were increased in group C (0.83 ± 1.54; $P = 0.056$, Table 2) while group T showed a non-significant decrease (-0.46 ± 2.33; $P > 0.05$, Table 2). The difference between the two groups was not significant ($P = 0.087$; Table 2). There was no significant difference between the two groups based on severity.
Plasma TNF-α levels increased significantly in Control group (0.71 ± 1.42; $P = 0.038$, Table 2). There was a non-significant increase in TNF-α levels of group T (0.08 ± 1.57; $P > 0.05$, Table 2). The difference between the two groups was not significant ($P = 0.131$; Table 2). Comparing the two groups based on severity of burn did not show any significance neither.

Table 2. Effect of Taurine Supplement on Inflammatory Markers

Variable	Group C			Group T			P**
	Day 1	Day 9	P*	Day 1	Day 9	P*	
IL-10[1]	**19.20 (6.40,26.80)**	**6.60 (5.40,10.40)**	**0.004**	**25.60 (15.00,44.60)**	**7.20 (5.40,13.20)**	**0.001**	**0.030**
IL-10[1] < 30%	24.10 (7.15,29.05)	5.80 (5.10, 9.40)	0.013	23.70 (15.75,74.78)	6.90 (4.65, 8.60)	0.006	0.377
IL-10[1] ≥ 30%	9.00 (6.40, 26.80)	9.60 (6.60,17.80)	0.102	29.40 (13.00,44.60)	7.20 (5.60,13.20)	0.009	0.013
hs-CRP[2]	**7.99 ± 1.77**	**8.82 ± 1.09**	**0.056**	**8.89 ± 1.56**	**8.43 ± 1.52**	**0.458**	**0.087**
hs-CRP[2]<30%	6.99 ± 1.37	8.46 ± 0.82	0.025	8.24 ± 1.86	7.85 ± 1.85	0.745	0.168
hs-CRP[2]≥30%	9.15 ± 1.48	9.24 ± 1.28	0.434	9.63 ± 3.38	9.09 ± 3.18	0.060	0.156
TNF-α[2]	**10.76 ± 0.81**	**11.11 ± 0.90**	**0.038**	**11.11 ± 1.12**	**11.19 ± 1.41**	**0.423**	**0.131**
TNF-α[2]<30%	10.45 ± 0.65	11.63 ± 1.17	0.043	10.90 ± 0.95	11.68 ± 1.03	0.088	0.309
TNF-α[2]≥30%	11.11 ± 0.88	11.29 ± 0.49	0.322	11.36 ± 4.20	10.64 ± 3.72	0.108	0.093

[1] Data for IL-10 is presented as Median (IQR)
[2] Data for hs-CRP and TNF-α are presented as Means ± Standard Deviation (M ± SD)
* Indicates the P value comparing time points within a single group using Paired t-test or Wilcoxon Signed-Rank test
** Indicates the P value comparing the mean difference between two groups using Unpaired t-test or Mann-Whitney test

Discussion

The aim of this study was to assess the administration of a Taurine supplement and its effect on the inflammatory response in severely burned patients.
The survival rates for burn patients have improved significantly over the last few decades due to advances in intensive care and burn centers. Burn wound infection is caused by impaired systematic and local immune responses. The functional integrity of immune responses after injury is very important. Several studies have reported an elevated levels of macrophage derived mediators in tissues of burned animals and patients, including TNF-α, which in turn influence lymphocyte responses. This dysregulation of macrophage activity leads to increased pro-inflammatory factors and increased susceptibility to sepsis.[20]
Usually, the exceeding release of pro-inflammatory cytokines is only short lived, whereas the suppression of the cellular defence function mediated by anti-inflammatory cytokines and other mediators lasts longer. This suppression may prompt a new episode of infection and subsequently may trigger a new peak of the systemic inflammatory response.[21]
Septic patients are characterized by their inability to eliminate invading pathogens and susceptibility to secondary nosocomial infections. In injured patients, an increased production of IL-10 is correlated with subsequent sepsis.[22] This increase which occurs in burn injuries, results in a deficient immune response to infection and an increase in sepsis-related mortality.[23] Lyons et al. showed that in a burned mouse, this cytokine decreases resistance to infection.[22]
Taurine can provide a range of benefits through its antioxidant and anti-inflammatory effects. It also has been shown to be tissue- protective in variety of models which result in inflammation.[17] Taurine can act as a trap for HOCl forming the long-lived oxidant Tau-NHCl, which is more stable and less toxic than HOCl. Moreover, Tau-NHCl down-regulates the generation of pro-inflammatory mediators by phagocytic cells, such as TNF-α and IL-1β.[17,18] This process suppresses the inflammatory reaction and protects cells from the cytotoxic and cytolytic actions of HOCl.[24] Vermeulen et al reported a longer duration of mechanical ventilation and ICU support in critically ill patients with low plasma Taurine.[25] Low level of plasma Taurine was also reported in in critically ill septic[26] patients, and after trauma.[27,28] In this study, serum levels of IL-10 were measured on days 1 and 9 of admission. The first measurement showed higher values of cytokine, whereas the second measurement revealed a decrease. This was more noticeable in the Taurine supplemented group and demonstrates that this supplement can meliorates IL-10 level compared with the control group. Strongly decreased IL-10 levels by Taurine supplementation in brain injured rats was also shown by Su et al.[29] Furthermore, as a commonly used marker of acute inflammation,[30] the hs-CRP level reduction in the Taurine group shows faster control of the burn induced inflammation.

Patients in group T showed IL-10 levels that were significantly lower than of patients in control group (P<0.05). Furthermore, IL-10 level drop were significantly lower than the control group (P<<0.05).

Next we compared the hs-CRP and TNF-α profile in two groups (Table 2). There were no significant changes in serum concentrations of hs-CRP and TNF-α throughout the study period. Serum concentration did increase slightly although this change did not show statistical significance. Serum concentrations of these inflammatory markers are shown in Table 2.

Taurine is also suggested to be more effective in patients with a greater TBSA percentage, the stronger effect of the supplementation on patients with severe burns may be due to the presence of more inflammation and oxidative stress, and the subsequent need for more anti-oxidants and anti-inflammatory effects (Figure1). As more usage and decrease of antioxidants can be seen in injuries of greater severity or systemic inflammatory response syndrome.[31,32]

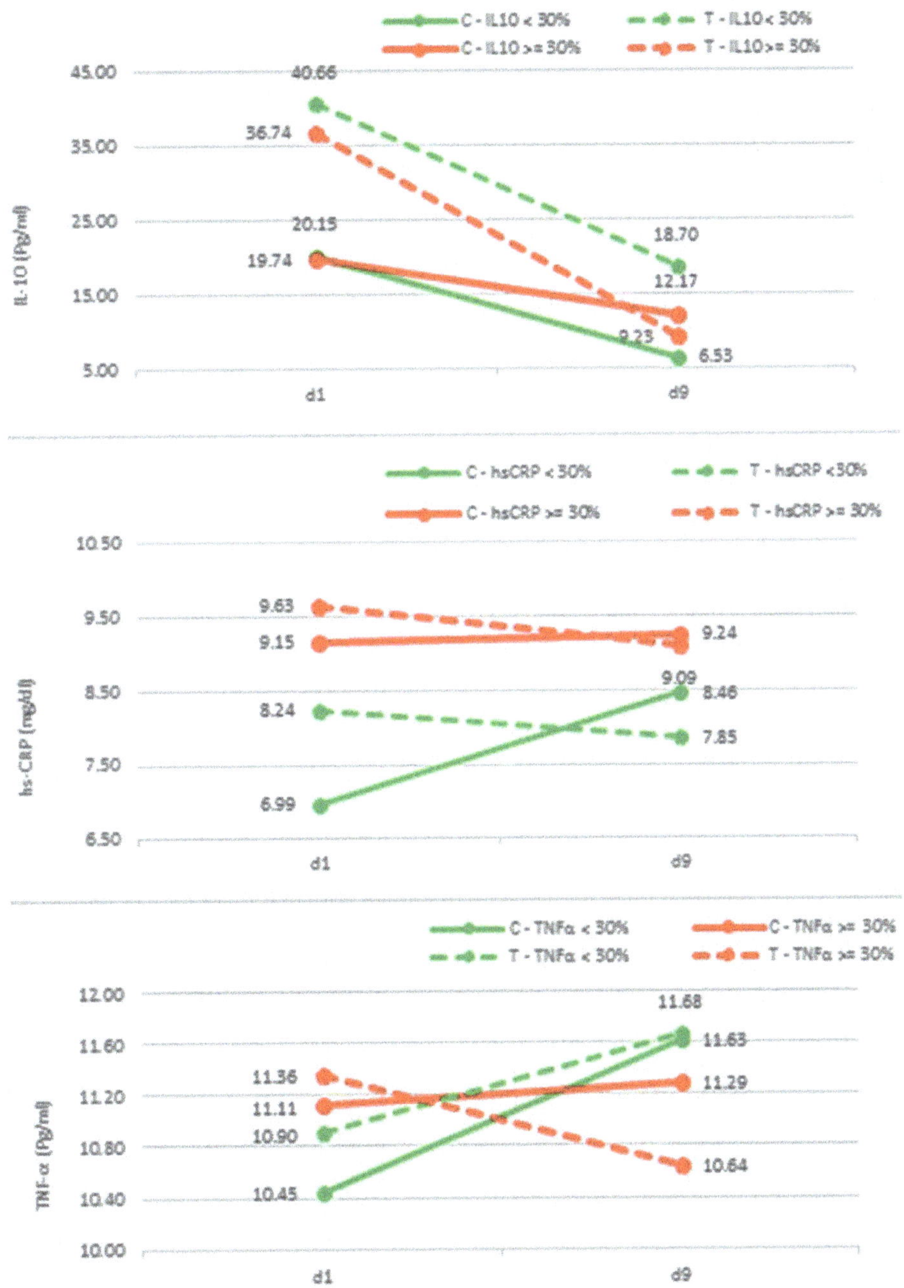

Figure 1. The Mean Difference of IL-10, hs-CRP, and TNF-α serum Level[1]

[1]The mean difference of IL-10, hs-CRP and TNF-α serum levels are shown in days 1 and 9 of admission to hospital in both C (Control) and T (Taurine) groups. *Group C* is shown with a solid line whereas *group T* is shown with a dashed line. Mean average of measurements for *TBSA* percentage of <30% in each group are indicated with green color while the *TBSA* percentage ≥30% are indicated with color red.

Taurine is also suggested to be more effective in patients with a greater TBSA percentage, the stronger effect of the supplementation on patients with severe burns may be due to the presence of more inflammation and oxidative stress, and the subsequent need for more anti-oxidants and anti-inflammatory effects. As more usage and decrease of antioxidants can be seen in injuries of greater severity or systemic inflammatory response syndrome.[27,28]

After the first week of our study, there was less sepsis in the Taurine group than in the control group. However, the difference was not significant. All of our findings suggest that, Taurine supplement lowers inflammation.

On the basis of our present results, it is tempting to hypothesize that decreased levels of IL-10 may favor a benefit from a therapy with Taurine supplement. However, these preliminary data need to be confirmed with larger number of patient studies. The main limitations of this study were the low sample of patients followed by a short term of study. In order to obtain more accurate results, larger samples, more groups administered different doses of the supplement, and more frequent time interval measurements would help us to reach stronger conclusions.

Conclusion

Despite improvements in the early care of burn, SIRS, MODS and severe sepsis remain major causes of mortality in burn patients. Most often, an inadequate nutrition leads to increased mortality. This study, regardless of the mechanism behind, clearly shows the benefit of Taurine supplement in burn injury patients especially the more severe ones by modifying the serum inflammatory cytokine levels. Further studies are required in order to identify the exact mechanism responsible for the efficacy of this nutritional supplement and the appropriate timing in order to determine if it should be administered to burn injury patients as a routine.

Acknowledgments

This is a report of a database from PhD thesis of Dr. Sima Lak entitled *'Effect of Taurine Supplementation and types of Nutrition on Inflammatory Factors and Clinical Outcome in Severely Burned Patients with SIRS Receiving Enteral Nutrition'* registered in Infectious and Topical Diseases Research Centre, Tabriz University of Medical Sciences, Tabriz, Iran. This work was fully supported by Infectious and Topical Diseases Research Centre (Grant No. 10701), Tabriz University of Medical Sciences, Tabriz, Iran. We wish to thank all participated patients and colleagues in Burn Centre of SINA hospital for their assistance.

Conflict of Interest

The authors report no conflicts of interest.

References

1. Fazal N. T Cell Suppression in Burn and Septic Injuries. In: Kapur S, editor. Immunosuppression Role in Health and Diseases. USA: In Tech; 2012.
2. Dahiya P. Burns as a model of SIRS. *Front Biosci* 2009;14:4962-7. doi: 10.2741/3580
3. Bone RC. Sir Isaac Newton, sepsis, SIRS, and CARS. *Crit Care Med* 1996; 24(7):1125-8. doi: 10.1097/00003246-199607000-00010.
4. Astiz ME, Rackow EC. Septic shock. *Lancet* 1998;351(9114):1501-5. doi: 10.1016/S0140-6736(98)01134-9
5. Kim HS, Kim JH, Yim H, Kim D. Changes in the levels of interleukins 6, 8, and 10, tumor necrosis factor alpha, and granulocyte-colony stimulating factor in korean burn patients: Relation to burn size and postburn time. *Ann Lab Med* 2012;32(5):339-44. doi: 10.3343/alm.2012.32.5.339
6. Klamt F, Shacter E. Taurine chloramine, an oxidant derived from neutrophils, induces apoptosis in human b lymphoma cells through mitochondrial damage. *J Biol Chem* 2005;280(22):21346-52. doi: 10.1074/jbc.M501170200
7. Piao S, Cha YN, Kim C. Taurine chloramine protects raw 264.7 macrophages against hydrogen peroxide-induced apoptosis by increasing antioxidants. *J Clin Biochem Nutr* 2011;49(1):50-6. doi: 10.3164/jcbn.10-120
8. Stober CB, Lange UG, Roberts MT, Alcami A, Blackwell JM. Il-10 from regulatory t cells determines vaccine efficacy in murine leishmania major infection. *J Immunol* 2005;175(4):2517-24.
9. Huang Y, Li Z, Yang Z. Roles of ischemia and hypoxia and the molecular pathogenesis of post-burn cardiac shock. *Burns* 2003;29(8):828-33.
10. Youn YK, Suh GJ, Jung SE, Oh SK, Demling R. Recombinant human growth hormone decreases lung and liver tissue lipid peroxidation and increases antioxidant activity after thermal injury in rats. *J Burn Care Rehabil* 1998;19(6):542-8.
11. Eschwege P, Paradis V, Conti M, Holstege A, Richet F, Deteve J, et al. In situ detection of lipid peroxidation by-products as markers of renal ischemia injuries in rat kidneys. *J Urol* 1999;162(2):553-7.
12. Demling RH, Lalonde C. Systemic lipid peroxidation and inflammation induced by thermal injury persists into the post-resuscitation period. *J Trauma* 1990;30(1):69-74.
13. Motoyama T, Okamoto K, Kukita I, Hamaguchi M, Kinoshita Y, Ogawa H. Possible role of increased oxidant stress in multiple organ failure after systemic inflammatory response syndrome. *Crit Care Med* 2003;31(4):1048-52. doi: 10.1097/01.CCM.0000055371.27268.36
14. Huxtable RJ. Physiological actions of taurine. *Physiol Rev* 1992;72(1):101-63.

15. Sturman JA. Taurine in development. *Physiol Rev* 1993;73(1):119-47.
16. Maher SG, Condron CE, Bouchier-Hayes DJ, Toomey DM. Taurine attenuates cd3/interleukin-2-induced t cell apoptosis in an in vitro model of activation-induced cell death (aicd). *Clin Exp Immunol* 2005;139(2):279-86. doi: 10.1111/j.1365-2249.2005.02694.x
17. Schuller-Levis GB, Park E. Taurine and its chloramine: Modulators of immunity. *Neurochem Res* 2004;29(1):117-26.
18. Kingston R, Kelly CJ, Murray P. The therapeutic role of taurine in ischaemia-reperfusion injury. *Curr Pharm Des* 2004;10(19):2401-10.
19. Asghari-Jafarabadi M, Soltani A, Mohammadi SM. Statistical Series: Tests for Comparing of Means. *J Diabetes Lipid Disord* 2013; 12(4): 265-91.
20. O'Riordain MG, Collins KH, Pilz M, Saporoschetz IB, Mannick JA, Rodrick ML. Modulation of macrophage hyperactivity improves survival in a burn-sepsis model. *Arch Surg* 1992;127(2):152-7; discussion 7-8.
21. Heyland DK, Dhaliwal R, Day AG, Muscedere J, Drover J, Suchner U, et al. Reducing deaths due to oxidative stress (the redoxs study): Rationale and study design for a randomized trial of glutamine and antioxidant supplementation in critically-ill patients. *Proc Nutr Soc* 2006;65(3):250-63.
22. Lyons A, Kelly JL, Rodrick ML, Mannick JA, Lederer JA. Major injury induces increased production of interleukin-10 by cells of the immune system with a negative impact on resistance to infection. *Ann Surg* 1997;226(4):450-8; discussion 8-60.
23. Sherry RM, Cue JI, Goddard JK, Parramore JB, DiPiro JT. Interleukin-10 is associated with the development of sepsis in trauma patients. *J Trauma* 1996;40(4):613-6; discussion 6-7.
24. Sun M, Zhao YM, Gu Y, Xu C. Therapeutic window of taurine against experimental stroke in rats. *Transl Res* 2012;160(3):223-9. doi: 10.1016/j.trsl.2012.02.007
25. Chiarla C, Giovannini I, Siegel JH, Boldrini G, Castagneto M. The relationship between plasma taurine and other amino acid levels in human sepsis. *J Nutr* 2000;130(9):2222-7.
26. Paauw JD, Davis AT. Taurine concentrations in serum of critically injured patients and age- and sex-matched healthy control subjects. *Am J Clin Nutr* 1990;52(4):657-60.
27. Boelens PG, Houdijk AP, de Thouars HN, Teerlink T, van Engeland MI, Haarman HJ, et al. Plasma taurine concentrations increase after enteral glutamine supplementation in trauma patients and stressed rats. *Am J Clin Nutr* 2003;77(1):250-6.
28. Vermeulen MA, van Stijn MF, Visser M, Lemmens SM, Houdijk AP, van Leeuwen PA, et al. Taurine concentrations decrease in critically ill patients with shock given enteral nutrition. *JPEN J Parenter Enteral Nutr* 2015. doi: 10.1177/0148607114567199
29. Su Y, Fan W, Ma Z, Wen X, Wang W, Wu Q, et al. Taurine improves functional and histological outcomes and reduces inflammation in traumatic brain injury. *Neuroscience* 2014;266:56-65. doi: 10.1016/j.neuroscience.2014.02.006
30. Povoa P. C-reactive protein: A valuable marker of sepsis. *Intensive Care Med* 2002;28(3):235-43. doi: 10.1007/s00134-002-1209-6
31. Alonso de Vega JM, Diaz J, Serrano E, Carbonell LF. Oxidative stress in critically ill patients with systemic inflammatory response syndrome. *Crit Care Med* 2002;30(8):1782-6.
32. Tsai K, Hsu T, Kong C, Lin K, Lu F. Is the endogenous peroxyl-radical scavenging capacity of plasma protective in systemic inflammatory disorders in humans? *Free Radic Biol Med* 2000;28(6):926-33.

Cytoprotective Effects of Melatonin Against Amitriptyline-Induced Toxicity in Isolated Rat Hepatocytes

Shohreh Taziki[1,2], Mohammad Reza Sattari[3,4], Siavoush Dastmalchi[5], Mohammad Ali Eghbal[6,3]*

[1] *Ischemic Disorders Research Center, Golestan University of Medical Sciences, Gorgan, Iran.*
[2] *Students' Research Committee, Faculty of Pharmacy, Tabriz University of Medical Science, Tabriz, Iran.*
[3] *Department of Pharmacology and Toxicology, Faculty of Pharmacy, Tabriz University of Medical Sciences, Tabriz, Iran.*
[4] *Neurosciences Research Centre, Tabriz University of Medical Sciences, Tabriz, Iran.*
[5] *Biotechnology Research Center, Tabriz University of Medical Sciences, Tabriz, Iran.*
[6] *Drug Applied Research Center, Tabriz University of Medical Sciences, Tabriz, Iran.*

Article info

Keywords:
- Amitriptyline
- Melatonin
- Oxidative stress
- Hepatocytes
- Mitochondrial membrane potential
- GSH

Abstract

Purpose: Amitriptyline, one of the commonly used tricyclic antidepressants, caused rare but severe hepatotoxicity in patients who received it continuously. Previous findings showed that the intermediate metabolites of amitriptyline produced by CYP450 are involved in hepatic injury. Melatonin is an antiaging and antioxidant hormone synthesized from pineal gland. The aim of present study was to evaluate the protective role of melatonin in an *in vitro* model of isolated rat hepatocytes.
Methods: Markers such as cell viability, reactive oxygen species formation, lipid peroxidation, mitochondrial membrane potential, and hepatocytes glutathione content were evaluated every 60 minutes for 180 minutes.
Results: Present results indicated that administration of 1mM of melatonin effectively reduced the cell death, ROS formation and lipid peroxidation, mitochondrial membrane potential collapse, and reduced cellular glutathione content caused by amitriptyline.
Conclusion: Our results indicated that melatonin is an effective antioxidant in preventing amitriptyline-induced hepatotoxicity. We recommend further *in vivo* animal and clinical trial studies on the hepatoprotective effects of melatonin in patients receiving amitriptyline.

Introduction

Melatonin is produced in the vertebrate pineal gland, the retina and possibly some other organs. This hormone plays several physiological roles such as regulation of sleep. Also there are many reports that melatonin's antioxidant action contributes to the protection of the organism from carcinogenesis and neurodegenerative disorders. It acts as a potent antioxidant by mechanisms such as stimulation of antioxidant enzymes, increasing the efficiency of mitochondrial oxidative phosphorylation and reducing free radical generation and direct free radical scavenging.[1-4] There are many reports on melatonin's protective effects against different chemicals-induced hepatotoxicity.[5,6]

It has been reported that amitriptyline increased liver enzymes in patients that received it continuously.[7] It is assumed that the accumulation of the aren oxide metabolites could be the responsible mechanism for the cellular damage caused by this drug.[8-10] It was previously reported that amitriptyline induced oxidative stress, it increased ROS formation and lipid peroxidation also amitriptyline increased GSH consumption in isolated rat hepatocytes.[9] In addition, a previous study showed that amitriptyline caused mitochondrial membrane potential reduction.[9] Based on our medical article data bases, there are few studies on the hepatoprotective role of antioxidants against amitriptyline-induced hepatotoxicity. In the present study, we investigated, for the first time, the protective roles of melatonin against cytotoxicity induced by amitriptyline towards freshly isolated rat hepatocytes.

Trypan blue exclusion test was used to measuring the percent of viable cells. The possibility of reactive oxygen species formation and lipid peroxidation was assessed and the effect of amitriptyline on intracellular glutathione was evaluated. In addition, the effect of amitriptylin on hepatocyte mitochondria was studied.

Materials and Methods

Chemicals

Amitriptyline, melatonin (N-Acetyl-5-methoxytryptamine) and Collagenase were obtained Sigma Aldrich chemical Co (St. Louis, USA). Other reagents were purchased from Merck chemical CO (Darmstadt, Germany).

Amitriptyline was dissolved in water and melatonin was dissolved in methanol. The amount of solvent in media was less than 20μl. The solvents had no effects on toxin or antioxidant effects. Male Sprague-Dawley rats (250–

***Corresponding author:** Mohammad Ali Eghbal , Email: m.a.eghbal@hotmail.com

300 g) were housed in ventilated plastic cages with 12h light photoperiod and an environmental temperature of 21-23°C with a 50-60% relative humidity. Animals were fed a normal chow diet and water ad libitum. The animals were handled and used according the animal handling protocol that approved by a local ethic committee in Tabriz University of medical sciences, Tabriz, Iran.

The rat liver was perfused with different buffer solutions through the portal vein. Hepatocytes were isolated from liver using collagenase perfusion technique which has been described in details before by Eghbal et al.[9] The collagenase enzyme in buffer solution destructed the liver tissue and lead to easily isolated of hepatocytes during the next steps.[9] Isolated hepatocytes (10 mL, 10^6 cells/mL) were suspended in the Krebs-Henseleit buffer (pH=7.4) in continuously rotating round bottom flasks, under an atmosphere of carbogen gas (95% O_2 and 5% CO_2) in a 37 °C water bath. Only the cells with viability of over the 85% were used.

Cell viability

Hepatocytes viability was measured by the trypan blue (0.1%, w/v) exclusion test microscopically.[11,12] Hepatocytes viability was determined every 60 minutes for 180 minutes to evaluate the effect of amitriptyline on cell viability, determining LC_{50} (lethal concentration 50%) dose of amitriptyline and testing the protective effects of melatonin against cell death induced by amitriptyline.[9,13-15]

Reactive oxygen species formation

To determine the extent of ROS generation by amitriptyline, 1.6 µl of 2.7- dichlorofluoresceine diacetate was added to hepatocytes flasks. DCFH-DA hydrolyzed to non-fluorescent DCFH in hepatocytes, DCFH reacted with ROS and became highly fluorescent. In 60,120,180 min 1 ml(10^6cell) of samples centrifuged at 3000g for 1 min, then the fluorescence of supernatant was detected fluorimetrically at excitation and emission wavelength of 490nm and 520nm respectively.[16-20]

Lipid peroxidation Measurement

Hepatocytes lipid peroxidation was detected by measuring of thiobarbituric acid reactive substance (TBARS) that formed during the decomposition of lipid hydro peroxides. 250µl of trichloroacetic acid (TCA, 70%w/v) was added to 1ml of hepatocytes suspension (10^6cell) and centrifuged at 3000g for 15 min, then 1 ml of thiobarbituric acid (0.8%w/v) added to supernatant and boiled for 20 min. The absorbance was measured at 532nm in an Ultrospec 2000 spectrophotometer.[21,22]

Mitochondrial membrane potential

Mitochondrial membrane potential was evaluated as a marker of toxicity induced by amitriptyline. To determining mitochondrial membrane potential Rhodamine 123 (the fluorescent dye) was used. This dye accumulates in intact mitochondria by facilitated diffusion. When the mitochondrial membrane potential is reduced by a toxin the amount of Rhodamine 123 in media is increased. One mL sample was taken from the cell suspension at programmed time points, and centrifuged at 1000 rpm for 1 minute. The cell was resuspensed in 2 ml of krebs-Henseleit buffer containing 1.5 µM Rhodamine 123 and incubated at 37°C water bath for 10 minutes. Hepatocytes were separated by centrifugation (3000 rpm for one minute) and the amount of rhodamine 123 appearing in the incubation medium were determined fluorimeterically at 490 nm excitation and 520 nm emission wavelengths using a Jasco® FP-750 spectrofluorometer.[1,23]

Determination of Hepatocytes GSH/GSSG content

To determine the hepatocyte glutathione (GSH) content the method of Ellman was used.[24] A 1 ml aliquot of the cell suspension (10^6 cells) was taken and 2 ml of 5% TCA was added and centrifuged. Then 0.5 ml of Ellman's reagent (0.0198% DTNB in 1% sodium citrate) and 3 ml of the phosphate buffer (pH 8.0) were added. The absorbance of the developed color was measured at 412 nm using a Biotech Pharmacia Ultrospec® 2000 spectro-photometer. Cell samples were reduced with potassium borohydride (KBH4) to prevent GSH oxidation during the experiment.[25] The enzymatic recycling method was used to assess the hepatocyte oxidized glutathione (GSSG) level.[26] Cellular GSH content was covalently bonded to 2-vinylpyridine at first. Then the excess 2-vinylpyridine was neutralized with thriethanolamine, and GSSG was reduced to GSH using the glutathione reductase enzyme and NADPH. The amount of GSH formed was measured as already described for GSH using the Ellman reagent (0.0198% DTNB in 1% sodium citrate).[2,27]

Statistical analysis

Results are given as the Mean±SEM for at least three independent experiments. Statistical analysis for the control and experimental groups was performed by a one-way ANOVA (analysis of variance) test followed by a Tukey's post hoc test. A $P < 0.05$ was considered as a significant difference.

Results

Trypan blue exclusion test was used to determine the ability of hepatocytes to maintain their viability with amitriptyline alone or in combination with melatonin.

Previous finding showed that amitriptyline caused cell death in a concentration dependent manner. The concentration in which amitriptyline caused 50 % cell death (LC_{50}) was found to be 40µM.[9] Our findings indicated that an effective dose of melatonin that provided suitable protection was 1mM (Table 1). Melatonin administration effectively prevented cell death induced by amitriptyline ($P<0.05$) (Table 1).

Markers such as ROS formation, lipid peroxidation, cellular glutathione content, and mitochondrial membrane potential were measured to study the mechanism by which melatonin protected hepatotoxicity induced by amitriptyline.

Table 1. Protective effect of melatonin against amitriptyline induced toxicity in isolated rat hepatocytes

Cytotoxicity (% Trypan blue uptake)			
Incubate	time(min):60	120	180
Control (only hepatocytes)	21±1	24±1	28±1
+Methanol 10µl	23±2	26±1	30±2
+Melatonine 1mM	20±3	22±2	24±3
+ Amitriptyline 40µm	41±3*	52±3*	59±2*
+ Melatonin 1mM	21±3 **	30±2**	37±2**
+Amitriptyline 200µM	100	100	100
+Amitriptyline 100µM	100	100	100
+Amitriptyline 20µM	32±3	40±5	50±2

Isolated rat hepatocytes (10^6 cells/mL) were incubated at 37°C in rotating round bottom flasks with 95 % O_2 and 5 % CO_2 in Krebs-Henseleit buffer (pH 7.4).
The results shown represent Mean±SE for three separate experiments.
*: Significantly different as compared to control group (P<0.05).
**: Significantly different from amitriptyline-treated group (P<0.05)

According to Figure 1, when hepatocytes were treted with melatonin (1 mM), the amount of ROS formed by amiytriptyline was suppressed drastically (P<0.05).

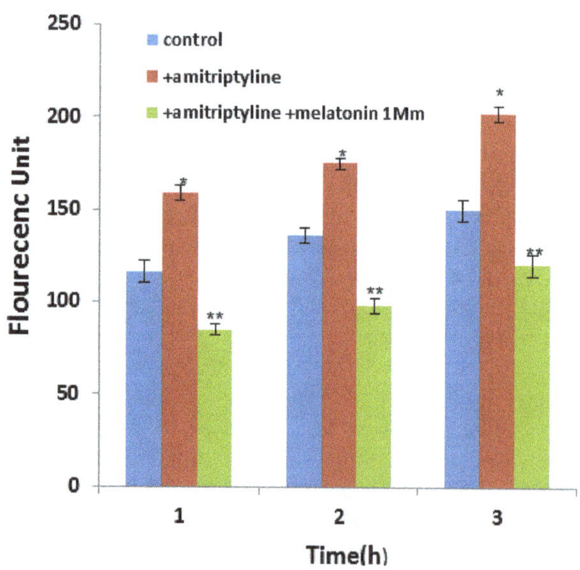

Figure 1. Protective effect of melatonin against amitriptyline induced ROS formation in isolated rat hepatocytes
Isolated rat hepatocytes (10^6 cells/mL) were incubated at 37 °C in rotating round bottom flasks with 95 % O_2 and 5 % CO_2 in Krebs-Henseleit buffer (pH 7.4).
The results shown represent Mean ± SE for three separate experiments.
*: Significantly different as compared to control group (P<0.05).
**: Significantly different from amitriptyline-treated group (P<0.05)

Previous findings showed that a notable amount of thiobarbituric acid reactive substances (TBARS) was formed in amitriptyline-treated rat hepatocytes as compared to the control group.[9] This indicates lipid peroxidation induced by cytotoxic concentrations of the drug. As shown in Figure 2 incubation of hepatocytes with 1mM of melatonin, prevented lipid peroxidation induced by amitriptyline (P<0.05).

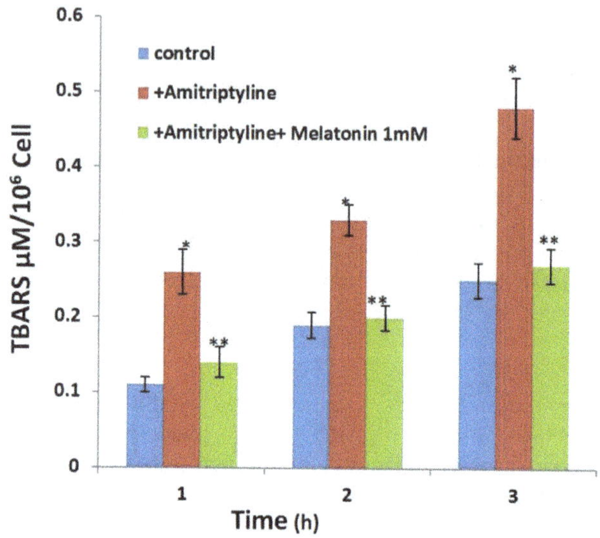

Figure 2. Protective effect of melatonin on lipid peroxidation induced by amitriptyline
Isolated rat hepatocytes (10^6 cells/mL) were incubated at 37 °C in rotating round bottom flasks with 95 % O_2 and 5 % CO_2 in Krebs-Henseleit buffer (pH 7.4).
The results shown represent Mean ± SE for three separate experiments.
*: Significantly different as compared to control group (P<0.05).
**: Significantly different from amitriptyline-treated group (P<0.05)

Previous findings showed that the LC_{50} dose of amitriptyline (40 µM) caused a reduction in mitochondrial membrane potential as measured by rhodamine 123 test.[9] This indicates that mitochondria could be a target for amitriptyline.[9] Melatonin was administered with amitriptyline to investigate if it could alleviate mitochondrial injury induced by amitriptyline. In comparison between the groups receiving amitriptyline alone and the group receiving amitriptyline in combination with 1mM melatonin, the degree of permeability of Rhodamine to the mitochondria was increased by melatonin significantly. It was found that melatonin effectively prevented mitochondrial depolarization caused by amitriptyline (Table 2).
Previous findings indicated that hepatocytes glutathione content was diminished notably when hepatocytes were treated with amitriptyline (40µm).[9] According to Table 3, comparing the group receiving only amitriptyline to the group receiving amitriptyline and 1mM melatonin, GSH content of cells was conspicuously increased in the melatonin-supplemented groups (P<0.05).

Table 2. protective effect of melatonin on mitochondrial toxicity induced by amitriptyline

% Control			
Incubation time (min): Incubate	60	120	180
Control (only hepatocytes)	100±0	94±2	85±3
+ Amitriptyline 40µm	60±3*	52±1*	43±3*
+ melatonin 1mM	80±3 **	68±4 **	60±3**

Isolated rat hepatocytes (10^6 cells/mL) were incubated at 37°C in rotating round bottom flasks with 95 % O_2 and 5 % CO_2 in Krebs-Henseleit buffer (pH 7.4).
The results shown represent Mean ± SE for three separate experiments.
*: Significantly different as compared to control group (P<0.05).
**: Significantly different from amitriptyline-treated group (P<0.05)

Table 3. Effect of melatonin on GSH consumption in presence of amitriptyline

% Control			
Incubation time (min): Incubate	60	120	180
Control (only hepatocytes)	100±0	84±3	75±3
+ Amitriptyline 40µm	65±2*	54±3*	45±3*
+ melatonin 1mM	90±1 **	76±2 **	65±3**

Isolated rat hepatocytes (10^6 cells/mL) were incubated at 37°C in rotating round bottom flasks with 95 % O_2 and 5 % CO_2 in Krebs-Henseleit buffer (pH 7.4). The results shown represent Mean±SE for three separate experiments.
*: Significantly different as compared to control group (P<0.05).
**: Significantly different from amitriptyline-treated group (P<0.05)

According to previous results, the amount of oxidized glutathione (GSSG) was increased in hepatocytes treated with 40µm amitriptyline.[9] According to Table 4, GSSG levels of amitriptyline-exposed cells were notably diminished in the melatonin-supplemented groups (P<0.05).

Table 4. Effect of melatonin on GSSG level in presence of amitriptyline

% Control			
Incubation time (min): Incubate	60	120	180
Control (only hepatocytes)	100±0	110±2	131±6
+ Amitriptyline 40µm	123±3*	143±2*	190±2*
+ melatonin 1mM	81±4**	115±6**	135±5**

Isolated rat hepatocytes (10^6 cells/mL) were incubated at 37°C in rotating round bottom flasks with 95 % O_2 and 5 % CO_2 in Krebs-Henseleit buffer (pH 7.4). GSSG level was measured as described by Irfan Rahman *et al* (2006)
The results shown represent Mean±SE for three separate experiments.
*: Significantly different as compared to control group (P<0.05).
**: Significantly different from amitriptyline-treated group (P<0.05)

Discussion

We have recently demonstrated that the cytotoxicity induced by amitriptyline was accompanied with ROS formation, lipid peroxidation, and mitochondrial depolarization. Moreover, reduction in cellular glutathione content was occurred. These results confirm the existence of the process of oxidative stress in hepatotoxicity due to amitriptyline.[9] Present results showed that hepatocytes supplementation with 1mM melatonin reduced cell death induced by amitriptyline and diminished the consequences of amitriptyline induced toxicity such as ROS generation, TBARS production and mitochondrial collapse. The protective effects of melatonin against amitriptyline could be due to its capability in scavenging reactive metabolites and conjugating with them. These findings are in line with the previous studies regarding the radical scavenger effects of melatonin.[3,4] Melatonin can rise the glutathione saving and decreases GSSG formation during amitriptyline toxicity notably (Table 3, 4). This might indicate the importance of melatonin in alleviating oxidative stress and scavenging reactive species to prevent the glutathione consumption as one of the main cellular defense mechanisms against toxic insults. This finding also supports the previous studies regarding the antioxidant effects of melatonin.[3,4] Mitochondrial depolarization can cause energy crisis and releasing of apoptotic signaling molecules, which could finally encounter cell death.[27] Administrations of 1mM melatonin provide protection against amitriptyline-induced mitochondrial collapse. There may be other functions of melatonin, yet undiscovered, which enhance its ability to protect against molecular damage by oxygen and toxic reactants. Protective effect of melatonin against amitriptyline-induced mitochondrial damage is through its activity in attenuating oxidative stress and scavenging reactive species.

Conclusion

According to our results, it could be concluded that melatonin is an effective protective agent in preventing amitriptyline-induced hepatotoxicity. We recommend further clinical trial studies on the antioxidant effects of melatonin in patients receiving amitriptyline. Also, the protective effect of melatonin against amitriptyline-induced toxicity proposes this agent as the subject of further studies for preventing different xenobiotics-induced liver damages, especially those accompanied by oxidative stress.

Acknowledgments

The authors are indebted to "Drug Applied Research Center" of Tabriz University of Medical Sciences for financial support of this study and providing technical facilities. The authors are thankful to the "students' research committee "of Tabriz University of Medical Sciences, Tabriz-Iran, for providing technical supports to the study. This article is written based on the results of thesis No.66, submitted to Tabriz University of Medical Sciences, Tabriz-Iran in fulfillment of the requirements of PhD Degree, of Shohreh Taziki.

Conflict of Interest
The authors report no conflicts of interest.

Abbreviation
ROS, reactive oxygen species; MMP, mitochondrial membrane potential; TBARS, Thiobarbituric acid reactive substance

References

1. Abdoli N, Azarmi Y, Eghbal MA. Protective Effects of N-acetylcysteine Against the Statins Cytotoxicity in Freshly Isolated Rat Hepatocytes. *Adv Pharm Bull* 2014;4(3):249-54. doi: 10.5681/apb.2014.036
2. Heidari R, Babaei H, Roshangar L, Eghbal MA. Effects of Enzyme Induction and/or Glutathione Depletion on Methimazole-Induced Hepatotoxicity in Mice and the Protective Role of N-Acetylcysteine. *Adv Pharm Bull* 2014;4(1):21-8. doi: 10.5681/apb.2014.004
3. Reiter RJ, Tan DX, Mayo JC, Sainz RM, Leon J, Czarnocki Z. Melatonin as an antioxidant: biochemical mechanisms and pathophysiological implications in humans. *Acta Biochim Pol* 2003;50(4):1129-46.
4. Kostoglou-Athanassiou I. Therapeutic applications of melatonin. *Ther Adv Endocrinol Metab* 2013;4(1):13-24. doi: 10.1177/2042018813476084
5. Garcia-Rubio L, Matas P, Miguez MP. Protective effect of melatonin on paraquat-induced cytotoxicity in isolated rat hepatocytes. *Hum Exp Toxicol* 2005;24(9):475-80. doi: 10.1191/0960327105ht548oa
6. Pan M, Song YL, Xu JM, Gan HZ. Melatonin ameliorates nonalcoholic fatty liver induced by high-fat diet in rats. *J Pineal Res* 2006;41(1):79-84. doi: 10.1111/j.1600-079x.2006.00346.x
7. Selim K, Kaplowitz N. Hepatotoxicity of psychotropic drugs. *Hepatology* 1999;29(5):1347-51. doi: 10.1002/hep.510290535
8. Abernathy CO, Lukacs L, Zimmerman HJ. Toxicity of tricyclic antidepressants to isolated rat hepatocytes. *Biochem Pharmacol* 1975;24(3):347-50. doi: 10.1016/0006-2952(75)90216-6
9. Taziki S, Sattari MR, Egbal MA. Evaluation of amitriptyline-induced toxicity in freshly isolated rat hepatocytes and the protective role of taurine. *Life Sci J* 2013;10(8s): 314-20.
10. Mostafalou S, Eghbal MA, Nili-Ahmadabadi A, Baeeri M, Abdollahi M. Biochemical evidence on the potential role of organophosphates in hepatic glucose metabolism toward insulin resistance through inflammatory signaling and free radical pathways. *Toxicol Ind Health* 2012;28(9):840-51. doi: 10.1177/0748233711425073
11. Moldéus P, Högberg J, Orrenius S. Isolation and use of liver cells. *Method Enzymol* 1978;52:60-71. doi: 10.1016/s0076-6879(78)52006-5
12. Heidari R, Babaei H, Eghbal MA. Ameliorative effects of taurine against methimazole-induced cytotoxicity in isolated rat hepatocytes. *Sci Pharm* 2012;80(4):987-99. doi: 10.3797/scipharm.1205-16
13. Heidari R, Babaei H, Eghbal MA. Cytoprotective Effects of Organosulfur Compounds against Methimazole Induced Toxicity in Isolated Rat Hepatocytes. *Adv Pharm Bull* 2013;3(1):135-42. doi: 10.5681/apb.2013.023
14. Eghbal MA, Abdoli N, Azarmi Y. Efficiency of hepatocyte pretreatment with coenzyme Q10 against statin toxicity. *Arh Hig Rada Toksikol* 2014;65(1):101-8. doi: 10.2478/10004-1254-65-2014-2398
15. Nafisi S, Heidari R, Ghaffarzadeh M, Ziaee M, Hamzeiy H, Garjani A, et al. Cytoprotective effects of silafibrate, a newly-synthesised siliconated derivative of clofibrate, against acetaminophen-induced toxicity in isolated rat hepatocytes. *Arh Hig Rada Toksikol* 2014;65(2):169-78. doi: 10.2478/10004-1254-65-2014-2434
16. Anoush M, Eghbal MA, Fathiazad F, Hamzeiy H, Kouzehkonani NS. The protective effects of garlic extract against acetaminophen-induced oxidative stress and glutathione depletion. *Pak J Biol Sci* 2009;12(10):765-71. doi: 10.3923/pjbs.2009.765.771
17. Chan TS, Moridani M, Siraki A, Scobie H, Beard K, Eghbal MA, et al. Hydrogen peroxide supports hepatocyte P450 catalysed xenobiotic/drug metabolic activation to form cytotoxic reactive intermediates. *Adv Exp Med Biol* 2001;500:233-6. doi: 10.1007/978-1-4615-0667-6_34
18. Heidari R, Babaei H, Eghbal MA. Cytoprotective effects of taurine against toxicity induced by isoniazid and hydrazine in isolated rat hepatocytes. *Arh Hig Rada Toksikol* 2013;64(2):15-24. doi: 10.2478/10004-1254-64-2013-2297
19. Eghbal MA, Taziki S, Sattari MR. Mechanisms of phenytoin-induced toxicity in freshly isolated rat hepatocytes and the protective effects of taurine and/or melatonin. *J Biochem Mol Toxicol* 2014;28(3):111-8. doi: 10.1002/jbt.21542
20. Mostafalou S, Abdollahi M, Eghbal MA, Saeedi Kouzehkonani N. Protective effect of NAC against malathion-induced oxidative stress in freshly isolated rat hepatocytes. *Adv Pharm Bull* 2012;2(1):79-88. doi: 10.5681/apb.2012.011
21. Smith MT, Thor H, Hartzell P, Orrenius S. The measurment of lipid peroxidation in isolated hepatocytes. *Biochem Pharmacol* 1982;31(1):19-26. doi: 10.1016/0006-2952(82)90230-1
22. Abdoli N, Heidari R, Azarmi Y, Eghbal MA. Mechanisms of the statins cytotoxicity in freshly isolated rat hepatocytes. *J Biochem Mol Toxicol* 2013;27(6):287-94. doi: 10.1002/jbt.21485

23. Eghbal MA, Pennefather PS, O'brien PJ. H2S cytotoxicity mechanism involves reactive oxygen species formation and mitochondrial depolarisation. *Toxicology* 2004;203(1-3):69-76. doi: 10.1016/j.tox.2004.05.020
24. Reiner CK, Kada G, Gruber HJ. Quick measurement of protein sulphydryls with Ellman'sreagent and with 4,4′-dithiodipyridine. *Anal Bioanal Chem* 2002;373(4-5):266-76. doi: 10.1007/s00216-002-1347-2
25. Kleinman WA, Richie JP, Jr. Status of glutathione and other thiols and disulfides in human plasma. *Biochem Pharmacol* 2000;60(1):19-29. doi: 10.1016/s0006-2952(00)00293-8
26. Rahman I, Kode A, Biswas SK. Assay for quantitative determination of glutathione and glutathione disulfide levels using enzymatic recycling method. *Nat Protoc* 2006;1(6):3159-65. doi: 10.1038/nprot.2006.378
27. Taziki S, Sattari MR, Eghbal MA. Mechanisms of trazodone-induced cytotoxicity and the protective effects of melatonin and/or taurine toward freshly isolated rat hepatocytes. *J Biochem Mol Toxicol* 2013;27(10):457-62. doi: 10.1002/jbt.21509

Comparative Study on the Effects of Ceftriaxone and Monocytes on Recovery after Spinal Cord Injury in Rat

Javad Tajkey[1], Alireza Biglari[2]*, Bohlol Habibi Asl[1]*, Ali Ramazani[3], Saeideh Mazloomzadeh[4]

[1] *Department of Pharmacology, School of Pharmacy, Tabriz University of Medical Sciences, Tabriz, Iran.*
[2] *Department of Genetics and Molecular Medicine, School of Medicine, Zanjan University of Medical Sciences, Zanjan, Iran.*
[3] *Zanjan Pharmaceutical Biotechnology Research Center, Zanjan University of Medical Sciences, Zanjan, Iran.*
[4] *Department of Epidemiology, School of Medicine, Zanjan University of Medical Sciences, Zanjan, Iran.*

Article info

Keywords:
· Spinal cord injury
· Ceftriaxone
· Monocyte
· Rat model

Abstract
Purpose: Comparison between the efficacy of ceftriaxone and monocytes on improvement neuron protection and functional recovery after spinal cord injury (SCI) in rat.
Methods: Rats were randomly divided into three groups of ten. Spinal cord injury w performed on rats under general anesthesia using the weight dropping method. Ceftriaxone w injected intraperitoneally 200 mg/kg/day for seven days after SCI. Monocytes were injected 2 10^5 cells 4 days after SCI. Hind limb motor function was assessed using the Basso, Beattie a Bresnahan (BBB) scale. Corticospinal tract (CST) axons were traced by injection of biot dextran amine (BDA) into the sensorimotor cortex.
Results: There were statistically significant differences in BBB scores in ceftriaxone comparison to both monocytes receiving and control groups. On the other hand there we statistically significant differences in axon counting in both ceftriaxone and monocyt receiving groups in comparison to control group.
Conclusion: Our findings suggest that ceftriaxone improves functional recovery more effecti than monocytes in rats after SCI. These results are from an experimental model and validation required for further investigation.

Introduction

As many as 500,000 people suffer a spinal cord injury (SCI) each year. Up to 90% of SCI cases are due to traumatic causes such as road traffic crashes, falls and violence.[1,2] However, early interventions can likely spare most tissues and cells, producing a minimum degree of deficit and lead to maximum functional recovery. Monocytes exert anti-inflammatory effects on damaged tissues and overlay the way for the extension of axons. But at the time of SCI, monocyte responses at the site of injury become inefficient, which may be due to reduced numbers of monocytes entering the site of injury from the blood stream. Previous studies have primarily focused on artificial infiltration of monocytes into the site of nerve injury. In recent years, extensive use of anti-inflammatory agents such as methylprednisolone has been implicated in SCI.[3,4] However, despite the initial hopefulness, methylprednisolone has not demonstrated a significant clinical efficacy.[5-7] Nevertheless, secondary injury after SCI can make post-traumatic inflammatory reactions. As a result, certain inflammatory mediators, namely cytokines, proteases and reactive oxygen species, can trigger the activation of apoptosis executioners like caspases, which will eventually result in neuronal loss and permanent neurological deficit.[8-10] Recently, a number of novel important concepts of secondary injury have been proposed. Toxic chemicals released by axons, damaged cells and blood vessels attack to intact neighbor cells. Glutamate as a neurotransmitter plays a critical role excessively disruptive process which has been called excitotoxicity.[11] Moreover, one of the glutamate receptors (AMPA: α-amino-3-hydroxy-5-methyl-4-isoxazole propionic acid) plays a significant role in oligodendrocyte injury. Glutamate transport is the only known mechanism of extracellular glutamate clearance and glutamate transporter 1 (GLT-1) is the major glutamate transporter of the mammalian brain. Ceftriaxone has recently been discovered to up-regulate GLT-1 expression in the CNS through increasing *GLT-1* transcription.[12,13] Moreover, ceftriaxone improves neuron protection and functional recovery in rat spinal cord injury models[14] and recent studies have extensively focused on molecular and cellular therapeutic interventions. Therefore, the present study has designed to compare the effects of monocytes and ceftriaxone on spinal cord injury in the rats.

Materials and Methods

Animal model

This study was conducted on female Sprague-Dawley rats (10 weeks, 200–245 g) that were obtained from the animal colony at the local institute. Animal experiments conformed to institutional standards. The animals were

***Corresponding authors:** Bohlol Habibi Asl and Alireza Biglari, Emails: habibib@tbzmed.ac.ir, biglari@zums.ac.ir randomly divided into three groups of ten. SCI was performed under general anesthesia, using intraperitoneal ketamine (80 mg/kg) and xylazine (10 mg/kg) injection, by the weight dropping method in which a 10 g metal rod was dropped on the laminectomized area from a height of 5 cm.

Animal grouping

Group one received normal saline for seven days post SCI, group two received 2×10^5 monocytes injected in site of injury on forth day post SCI and group three received ceftriaxone, injected intraperitoneally 200 mg/kg/day.

A Basso, Beattie and Bresnahan (BBB) score test[15] was performed for six weeks. Two weeks before the end of the BBB test, biotin dextran amine (BDA) was injected intracerebrally and tissue staining was performed at the end of the six weeks.

Extraction and Cell Culture

In order to monocytes extraction, blood samples were taken from the hearts of several rats and kept on ice in tubes containing EDTA. Equal in volume to the blood sample, ficoll was added to falcon tubes and the blood samples were diluted with Phosphate buffer saline (PBS) and gently added to the falcon tubes so that the samples did not mix with the ficoll. The tubes containing the samples were centrifuged at 400×*g* for 30 min at 18-20°C. In the next stage, the intended layer that contained monocytes was transferred to another tube and 6 ml of PBS was added. These samples were then centrifuged at 100×*g* for 10 min at 18–20°C. The upper layer was discarded and the remaining deposit was suspended with RPMI-1640 medium in 5% fetal bovine serum (FBS). This suspension was incubated at 37°C with 5% CO_2 and then incubated for 2 h. Then the upper mixture was removed and a new cell culture containing 100 ng of monocyte colony-stimulating factor (MCSF) in 1 ml was added to the flask. It can be concluded that most of the attached cells are monocytes because monocytes are able to attach to the bottom of the flask but the other blood cells are unable to attach to the bottom of the flask within 2 h.

Locomotor Assessment

Following SCI, hind limb motor function was assessed weekly based on the BBB scale, as previously described.[14]

Biotin Dextran Amine Detection

Biotin dextran amine (BDA) was injected intracerebrally two weeks prior to end of BBB by creating a hole situated 2 mm posterior and 2 mm right of Bregma, according to previous methods.[14] Tissue section preparation and staining was performed at the end of the six weeks. Sections were washed in PBS containing 0.1% Triton X-100, incubated for 1 h with avidin and biotinylated horseradish peroxidase (HRP) (NeuroTrace™ BDA-10,000 Neuronal Tracer Kit, N-7167), washed in PBS and then reacted with 3,3'-diaminobenzidine (DAB) in 50 mM Tris buffer, pH 7.6, 0.024% hydrogen peroxide and 0.5% nickel chloride. Following BDA administration and subsequent staining with DAB, which leads to black deposit formation[16,17] then ten sequential cross sections, 5 micrometers apart, were randomly prepared. Cross-sections from the rostral-most block were used to determine the extent of corticospinal tract (CST) labeling above the lesion, the number of BDA-labeled axon arbors that entered the gray matter of the thoracic spinal cord at the thoracic vertebrae (T_{10}) and the number of BDA-labeled axon arbors that entered the gray matter of the thoracic spinal cord above the lesion.[16,17] The axons were counted using software (imaging software for life science microscopy) attached to a microscope (Olympus Bx52, Japan).

Drug

Ceftriaxone was dissolved in sterile endotoxin-free 0.9% normal saline at 60 mg/ml and stored at 4°C. This solution was injected intraperitoneally into group three. For intraperitoneal injections, the 60-µg/µl ceftriaxone stock was diluted with normal saline to obtain 30 µg/µl of the drug then 5 µl of the diluted ceftriaxone was injected (227 nmol).

Cell injection

Monocytes numbering 2×10^5 were suspended in 2 µl PBS and stereotaxically injected into the caudal border of the lesion through a Hamilton syringe with a 30 G needle.

Data evaluation and statistical analysis

Values were expressed as means ± standard deviations. Sample size (n) for each group was 10 rats. Comparisons were performed using analysis of variance (ANOVA) followed by post-hoc Scheffe tests. P values less than 0.05 were considered significant. All statistical analyses were performed using SPSS version 10.0 computer software program for Windows (SPSS Inc, Chicago, IL, USA).

Results

Comparison of the effect of ceftriaxone and monocytes injection on hindlimb motor function after SCI

Following SCI and ceftriaxone administration, there was significant recovery of locomotion over the first week. There were significant differences for BBB scores between experimental groups in the second ($P<0.005$), third ($P<0.001$), fourth ($P<0.001$), fifth ($P<0.004$), and sixth ($P<0.001$) weeks (Figure 1). Pair wise comparisons showed no significant differences between groups in the first week ($P = 0.058$).

Following SCI and administration of monocytes, there was no correlation with the control group (normal saline) but in contrast to the above finding, there was a correlation with the first group (ceftriaxone) (Figure 1).

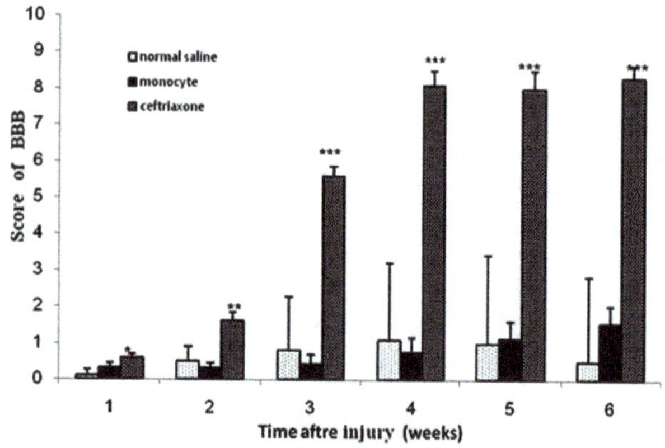

Figure 1. Effect of Ceftriaxone (200 mg/kg/day/ip) and Monocytes injection on hindlimb motor function after the spinal cord injury. Each bar represents mean ±SEM (n = 10) per group). $^*p<0.05$, $^{**}p<0.01$, $^{***}p<0.001$ significantly different from the normal sline group. (BBB):Beattie and Bresnahan score

Effect of ceftriaxone and monocytes injection on axonal regeneration

Following SCI and either ceftriaxone or monocytes injection, there was a significant increase in axon number in both groups compared to the control group ($P<0.001$). The mean score of BBB in the ceftriaxone group was different from the other groups in the second, third, fourth, and sixth weeks. At the same time, there was a significant increase in axon number in the ceftriaxone and monocytes groups compared to the control group ($P<0.001$), whereas this difference was not significant between the ceftriaxone and monocytes groups (Figure 2).

Discussion

Molecular therapies after SCI serve several goals, including protection of neurons from secondary cell death, promotion of axonal growth, and improving nerve conduction.[18,19] Several goals are achieved by cellular transplantation after SCI, including the filling of cavities or cysts, the generation of new neurons or myelinating cells, and to provide an appropriate environment for regeneration of axons.[20-22] The nature of the macrophage response has been proposed as the likely cause of the failure of the spinal cord to recover. This is different from the situation observed in the regenerative peripheral nervous system (PNS).[23-26] After transection and transplantation of activated macrophages incubated with PNS or skin tissue in rats, recovery of hind limb function occurs. Fibers extend across the lesion, and recovered functions were terminated by re-transection of the spinal cord.[27] However, the extent of recovery was similar to the results obtained from the transplant of other cell types and succeeded only in a rat subgroup.[22,28,29] On the contrary, tissue survival and hind limb recovery are hindered by the activation of intrinsic macrophages at the lesion site with microinjections of a pro-inflammatory agent.[30] Improvement of Hind limb usage during locomotion, increased white matter sparing, and functional recovery have been the result of macrophage depletion after SCI.[28,31] Thus, our study investigated whether treatment with monocytes improved ambulatory ability and prevention of paralysis in rat models of SCI.

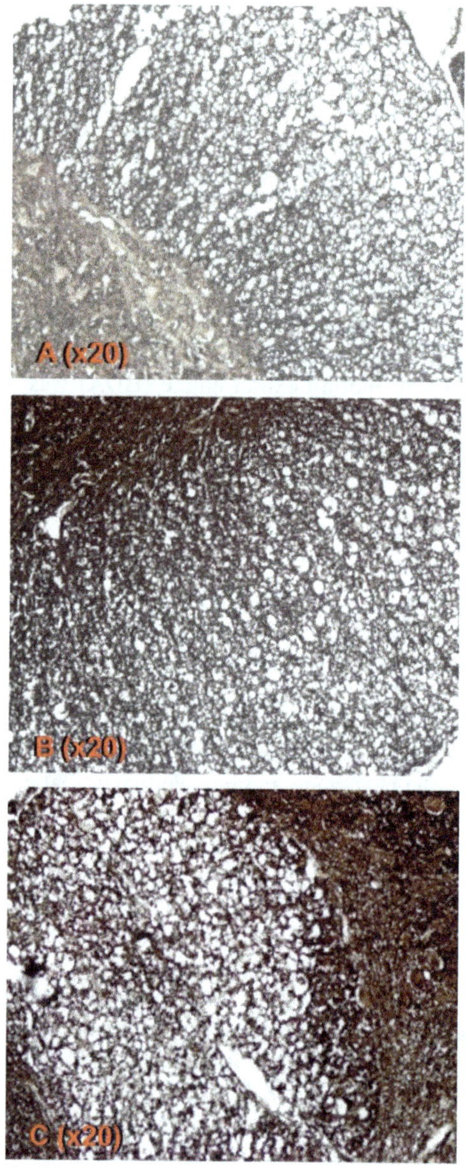

Figure 2. Distribution and density of CST axons in a PBS injected normal saline (A) ,Monocyte treated (B), Ceftriaxone (C).

Our findings show that monocytes alone cannot improve locomotor function, which is consistent with previous findings. Activated monocytes have been used *in vitro* to restore spinal lesions in most studies,[30] and identifying the phenotype of monocytes, factors, and cytokines secreted from monocytes prior to injection is most significant. In 1998, Rapalino et al. injected macrophages produced through the concurrent culture with peripheral nerve pieces into spinal lesions in rat, and concluded that the injection of activated macrophages results in motor improvement.[23] In 2003, Boumstein et al. injected skin-coincubated macrophages into spinal lesion sites in rat that resulted in improved motor recovery.[32] Previous studies also suggest a longer period of at least eight weeks to show effects of monocytes on locomotor improvement.[23,32-34]

Following treatment with ceftriaxone, there is a significant recovery rate in treated animals in subsequent weeks ($p<0.001$).

Ceftriaxone administration significantly promoted axonal regeneration in experimental and control groups ($P<0.001$, Figure 3), showing an important role of ceftriaxone in the regulation of axonal growth.

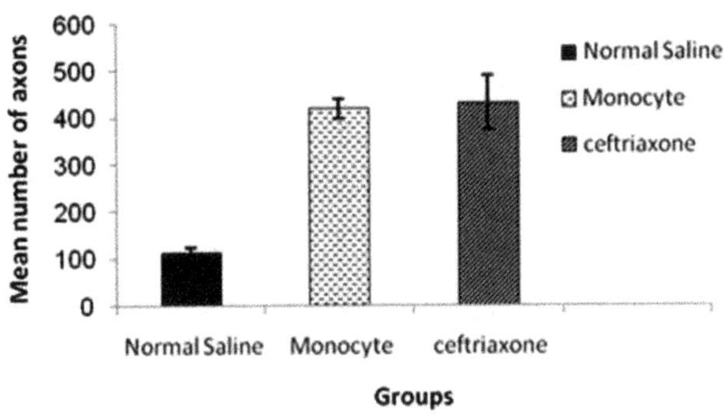

Figure 3. Comparative effect of Ceftriaxone (200 mg/kg/day/ip) and Monocytes injection on Number of axons in different experimental groups. Each bar represents mean ±SEM (n = 10 per group).

The secondary injury phase of SCI involves auto-destructive events like reactive oxygen species-induced lipid peroxidation,[35] caspase-3 activation,[36,37] and glutamate production. These findings suggest that compounds that can protect cells from excess glutamate can limit spinal cord destruction.[38] It is also believed that the injury cascade of neurodestructive events will extend when secondary injury increases because of delayed treatment.[4] The first scientifically grounded pharmacological treatment for SCI dates back to the 1990s. Although a clinical study showed that a high dose of the steroid methylprednisolone decreased disability when administered within 8 h of trauma,[39] treatment with a high dose of methylprednisolone was later reported to be associated with complications, including wound infection and increased frequency of gastric bleeding; methylprednisolone treatment remains controversial in many countries.[40-42] Furthermore, although treatment with this drug might result in the reduction of swelling, inflammation, glutamate release, and free-radical accumulation, the specific mechanism of action remains unclear.[41] In a similar study, experimental drugs including monosialoganglioside sodium (GM-1 ganglioside), naloxone, and tirilazad were tested in multicenter clinical trials, but the desired results were not achieved.[43] However, significant improvement in functional recovery (BBB) after SCI was reported in another study in which minocycline was administered early (0.5–24 h).[44] The results of another similar study suggested that drugs that impede AMPA-type glutamate receptors turn out to be efficacious in keeping lesions and disability to a minimum.[45] Specific AMPA-receptor antagonists have also been tested in patients with SCI in recent years.[38] A large number of studies assert that glutamate and its structural analogues could have both short and long-term poisonous impacts on cortical and motor neurons.[46-48] The exposure of neurons to abnormally high concentrations of glutamate results from the defective clearance of glutamate from the extracellular space.[38] Glutamate neurotransmission is greatly regulated, mainly via glutamate transporters. The glutamate transporter GLT-1 is principally responsible for glutamate clearance in the spinal cord.[49] Down-regulation of GLT-1 can happen in activated astrocytes, and is associated with increased extracellular glutamate and neuroexcitation.[12] During other conditions, astrocyte activation occurs subsequent to spinal cord destruction. Recently, glutamate transporters have emerged as a potential therapeutic target in a wide range of acute and chronic neurological disorders, owing to their novel mode of action. The modulation of GLT-1, a primary glutamate transporter, provides neuroprotection in different models of ischemic injury and motoneuron degeneration.[50] Therefore, an attempt was made to explore the neuroprotective potential in spinal cord injury using ceftriaxone, a GLT-1 modulator. In the present study, treatment with ceftriaxone resulted in significant differences in BBB scores compared to the control group. Furthermore, ceftriaxone also promoted axon regeneration and impeded neuronal damage and eventual cell death, and improved motor function.

In spite of a lack of difference in axon counting following monocytes administration, further study is needed to investigate the reasons for increasing cell count and low locomotor improvement, in contrast to what is seen by ceftriaxone administration.

Conclusion

In conclusion, our study shows that ceftriaxone improved the functional recovery in the injured rats following SCI more effective than monocytes administration. Further investigations with new procedures such as co-administration of ceftriaxone with monocytes or gene therapies approaches to improve spinal cord injury are required.

Acknowledgments

We thank the research deputy of Tabriz and Zanjan University of Medical Sciences (ZUMS) for financial support of this project (Ph.D. thesis).

Conflict of Interest

Authors declare no conflict of interest.

References

1. Price C, Makintubee S, Herndon W, Istre GR. Epidemiology of traumatic spinal cord injury and acute hospitalization and rehabilitation charges for

spinal cord injuries in Oklahoma, 1988-1990. *Am J Epidemiol* 1994;139(1):37-47.

2. French DD, Campbell RR, Sabharwal S, Nelson AL, Palacios PA, Gavin-Dreschnack D. Health care costs for patients with chronic spinal cord injury in the Veterans Health Administration. *J Spinal Cord Med* 2007;30(5):477-81.
3. Miekisiak G, Kloc W, Janusz W, Kaczmarczyk J, Latka D, Zarzycki D. Current use of methylprednisolone for acute spinal cord injury in Poland: survey study. *Eur J Orthop Surg Traumatol* 2014;24 Suppl 1:269-73. doi: 10.1007/s00590-014-1422-3
4. Bracken MB, Shepard MJ, Holford TR, Leo-Summers L, Aldrich EF, Fazl M, et al. Methylprednisolone or tirilazad mesylate administration after acute spinal cord injury: 1-year follow up. Results of the third National Acute Spinal Cord Injury randomized controlled trial. *J Neurosurg* 1998;89(5):699-706. doi: 10.3171/jns.1998.89.5.0699
5. Hurlbert RJ. Methylprednisolone for acute spinal cord injury: an inappropriate standard of care. *J Neurosurg* 2000;93(1 Suppl):1-7. doi: 10.3171/spi.2000.93.1.0001
6. Sayer FT, Kronvall E, Nilsson OG. Methylprednisolone treatment in acute spinal cord injury: the myth challenged through a structured analysis of published literature. *Spine J* 2006;6(3):335-43. doi: 10.1016/j.spinee.2005.11.001
7. Short DJ, El Masry WS, Jones PW. High dose methylprednisolone in the management of acute spinal cord injury - a systematic review from a clinical perspective. *Spinal Cord* 2000;38(5):273-86. doi: 10.1038/sj.sc.3100986
8. Chong ZZ, Li F, Maiese K. Oxidative stress in the brain: novel cellular targets that govern survival during neurodegenerative disease. *Prog Neurobiol* 2005;75(3):207-46. doi: 10.1016/j.pneurobio.2005.02.004
9. Young W, Kume-Kick J, Constantini S. Glucocorticoid therapy of spinal cord injury. *Ann N Y Acad Sci* 1994;743:241-63; discussion 63-5. doi: 10.1111/j.1749-6632.1994.tb55796.x
10. Cavallucci V, D'amelio M. Matter of life and death: the pharmacological approaches targeting apoptosis in brain diseases. *Curr Pharm Des* 2011;17(3):215-29. doi: 10.2174/138161211795049705
11. Azbill RD, Mu X, Springer JE. Riluzole increases high-affinity glutamate uptake in rat spinal cord synaptosomes. *Brain Res* 2000;871(2):175-80. doi: 10.1016/s0006-8993(00)02430-6
12. Ramos KM, Lewis MT, Morgan KN, Crysdale NY, Kroll JL, Taylor FR, et al. Spinal upregulation of glutamate transporter GLT-1 by ceftriaxone: therapeutic efficacy in a range of experimental nervous system disorders. *Neuroscience* 2010;169(4):1888-900. doi: 10.1016/j.neuroscience.2010.06.014
13. Rothstein JD, Patel S, Regan MR, Haenggeli C, Huang YH, Bergles DE, et al. Beta-lactam antibiotics offer neuroprotection by increasing glutamate transporter expression. *Nature* 2005;433(7021):73-7. doi: 10.1038/nature03180
14. Tajkey J, Ramazani A, Biglari A, Mazlomzadeh S, Habibi Asl B. Ceftriaxone Improves Neuron Protection and Functional Recovery in Rat Model of Spinal Cord Injury. *Ann Res Rev Biol* 2014;4(12):1958-67. doi: 10.9734/arrb/2014/8308
15. Basso DM, Beattie MS, Bresnahan JC. A sensitive and reliable locomotor rating scale for open field testing in rats. *J Neurotrauma* 1995;12(1):1-21. doi: 10.1089/neu.1995.12.1
16. Innocenti GM, Clarke S, Kraftsik R. Interchange of callosal and association projections in the developing visual cortex. *J Neurosci* 1986;6(5):1384-409.
17. Vercelli A, Repici M, Garbossa D, Grimaldi A. Recent techniques for tracing pathways in the central nervous system of developing and adult mammals. *Brain Res Bull* 2000;51(1):11-28. doi: 10.1016/s0361-9230(99)00229-4
18. Anderson KD. Targeting recovery: priorities of the spinal cord-injured population. *J Neurotrauma* 2004;21(10):1371-83. doi: 10.1089/neu.2004.21.1371
19. Eaton MJ. Cell and molecular approaches to the attenuation of pain after spinal cord injury. *J Neurotrauma* 2006;23(3-4):549-59. doi: 10.1089/neu.2006.23.549
20. Li J, Lepski G. Cell transplantation for spinal cord injury: a systematic review. *Biomed Res Int* 2013;2013:786475. doi: 10.1155/2013/786475
21. Liu S, Li C, Xing Y, Tao F. Role of Stem Cell Transplantation in Remyelination and Pain Relief after Spinal Cord Injury. *J Stem Cell Res Ther* 2014;4(1):158-9. doi: 10.4172/2157-7633.1000158
22. Peterson ME. Effects of megestrol acetate on glucose tolerance and growth hormone secretion in the cat. *Res Vet Sci* 1987;42(3):354-7.
23. Rapalino O, Lazarov-Spiegler O, Agranov E, Velan GJ, Yoles E, Fraidakis M, et al. Implantation of stimulated homologous macrophages results in partial recovery of paraplegic rats. *Nat Med* 1998;4(7):814-21. doi: 10.1038/nm0798-814
24. Geissmann F, Jung S, Littman DR. Blood monocytes consist of two principal subsets with distinct migratory properties. *Immunity* 2003;19(1):71-82. doi: 10.1016/s1074-7613(03)00174-2
25. Piltti KM, Salazar DL, Uchida N, Cummings BJ, Anderson AJ. Safety of human neural stem cell transplantation in chronic spinal cord injury. *Stem Cells Transl Med* 2013;2(12):961-74. doi: 10.5966/sctm.2013-0064
26. Hirschberg DL, Schwartz M. Macrophage recruitment to acutely injured central nervous system is inhibited by a resident factor: a basis for an immune-brain barrier. *J Neuroimmunol* 1995;61(1):89-96. doi: 10.1016/0165-5728(95)00087-i

27. Reier PJ. Cellular transplantation strategies for spinal cord injury and translational neurobiology. *NeuroRx* 2004;1(4):424-51. doi: 10.1602/neurorx.1.4.424
28. Konieczny L. The formation of cold immunoglobulin complexes. *Bull Acad Pol Sci Biol* 1979;27(1):1-6.
29. Moon L, Bunge MB. From animal models to humans: strategies for promoting CNS axon regeneration and recovery of limb function after spinal cord injury. *J Neurol Phys Ther* 2005;29(2):55-69. doi: 10.1097/01.npt.0000282512.16964.94
30. Popovich PG, Guan Z, Mcgaughy V, Fisher L, Hickey WF, Basso DM. The neuropathological and behavioral consequences of intraspinal microglial/macrophage activation. *J Neuropathol Exp Neurol* 2002;61(7):623-33.
31. Popovich PG, Guan Z, Wei P, Huitinga I, Van Rooijen N, Stokes BT. Depletion of hematogenous macrophages promotes partial hindlimb recovery and neuroanatomical repair after experimental spinal cord injury. *Exp Neurol* 1999;158(2):351-65. doi: 10.1006/exnr.1999.7118
32. Bomstein Y, Marder JB, Vitner K, Smirnov I, Lisaey G, Butovsky O, et al. Features of skin-coincubated macrophages that promote recovery from spinal cord injury. *J Neuroimmunol* 2003;142(1-2):10-6. doi: 10.1016/s0165-5728(03)00260-1
33. Schwartz M, Yoles E. Macrophages and dendritic cells treatment of spinal cord injury: from the bench to the clinic. *Acta Neurochir Suppl* 2005;93:147-50. doi: 10.1007/3-211-27577-0_25
34. Lin LF, Doherty DH, Lile JD, Bektesh S, Collins F. GDNF: a glial cell line-derived neurotrophic factor for midbrain dopaminergic neurons. *Science* 1993;260(5111):1130-2. doi: 10.1126/science.8493557
35. Iwasa K, Ikata T, Fukuzawa K. Protective effect of vitamin E on spinal cord injury by compression and concurrent lipid peroxidation. *Free Radic Biol Med* 1989;6(6):599-606. doi: 10.1016/0891-5849(89)90067-1
36. Citron BA, Arnold PM, Sebastian C, Qin F, Malladi S, Ameenuddin S, et al. Rapid upregulation of caspase-3 in rat spinal cord after injury: mRNA, protein, and cellular localization correlates with apoptotic cell death. *Exp Neurol* 2000;166(2):213-26. doi: 10.1006/exnr.2000.7523
37. Springer JE, Azbill RD, Knapp PE. Activation of the caspase-3 apoptotic cascade in traumatic spinal cord injury. *Nat Med* 1999;5(8):943-6. doi: 10.1038/11387
38. Rothstein JD, Martin LJ, Kuncl RW. Decreased glutamate transport by the brain and spinal cord in amyotrophic lateral sclerosis. *N Engl J Med* 1992;326(22):1464-8. doi: 10.1056/nejm199205283262204
39. Bracken MB, Shepard MJ, Collins WF, Holford TR, Young W, Baskin DS, et al. A randomized, controlled trial of methylprednisolone or naloxone in the treatment of acute spinal-cord injury. Results of the Second National Acute Spinal Cord Injury Study. *N Engl J Med* 1990;322(20):1405-11. doi: 10.1056/NEJM199005173222001
40. Ducker TB, Zeidman SM. Spinal cord injury. Role of steroid therapy. *Spine (Phila Pa 1976)* 1994; 19(20):2281-7. doi: 10.1097/00007632-199410150-00006
41. Bracken MB, Shepard MJ, Holford TR, Leo-Summers L, Aldrich EF, Fazl M, et al. Administration of methylprednisolone for 24 or 48 hours or tirilazad mesylate for 48 hours in the treatment of acute spinal cord injury. Results of the Third National Acute Spinal Cord Injury Randomized Controlled Trial. National Acute Spinal Cord Injury Study. *JAMA* 1997;277(20):1597-604. doi: 10.1001/jama.277.20.1597
42. Young W. Methylprednisolone treatment of acute spinal cord injury: an introduction. *J Neurotrauma* 1991;8 Suppl 1:S43-6.
43. Geisler FH. Clinical trials of pharmacotherapy for spinal cord injury. *Ann N Y Acad Sci* 1998;845(1):374-81. doi: 10.1111/j.1749-6632.1998.tb09689.x
44. Festoff BW, Ameenuddin S, Arnold PM, Wong A, Santacruz KS, Citron BA. Minocycline neuroprotects, reduces microgliosis, and inhibits caspase protease expression early after spinal cord injury. *J Neurochem* 2006;97(5):1314-26. doi: 10.1111/j.1471-4159.2006.03799.x
45. Wrathall JR, Teng YD, Choiniere D. Amelioration of functional deficits from spinal cord trauma with systemically administered NBQX, an antagonist of non-N-methyl-D-aspartate receptors. *Exp Neurol* 1996;137(1):119-26. doi: 10.1006/exnr.1996.0012
46. Weiss JH, Koh JY, Choi DW. Neurotoxicity of beta-N-methylamino-L-alanine (BMAA) and beta-N-oxalylamino-L-alanine (BOAA) on cultured cortical neurons. *Brain Res* 1989;497(1):64-71. doi: 10.1016/0006-8993(89)90970-0
47. Choi DW, Rothman SM. The role of glutamate neurotoxicity in hypoxic-ischemic neuronal death. *Annu Rev Neurosci* 1990;13:171-82. doi: 10.1146/annurev.ne.13.030190.001131
48. Urca G, Urca R. Neurotoxic effects of excitatory amino acids in the mouse spinal cord: quisqualate and kainate but not N-methyl-D-aspartate induce permanent neural damage. *Brain Res* 1990;529(1-2):7-15. doi: 10.1016/0006-8993(90)90805-l
49. Yamada K, Watanabe M, Shibata T, Nagashima M, Tanaka K, Inoue Y. Glutamate transporter GLT-1 is transiently localized on growing axons of the mouse spinal cord before establishing astrocytic expression. *J Neurosci* 1998;18(15):5706-13.
50. Verma R, Mishra V, Sasmal D, Raghubir R. Pharmacological evaluation of glutamate transporter 1 (GLT-1) mediated neuroprotection following cerebral ischemia/reperfusion injury. *Eur J Pharmacol* 2010;638(1-3):65-71. doi: 10.1016/j.ejphar.2010.04.021

Short-Term Treatment with Silymarin Improved 6-OHDA-Induced Catalepsy and Motor Imbalance in Hemi-Parkisonian Rats

Rasool Haddadi[1], Shahla Eyvari Brooshghalan[2], Safar Farajniya[2], Alireza Mohajjel Nayebi[2,3]*, Hamdolah Sharifi[4]

[1] *Department of Pharmacology and Toxicology, Faculty of Pharmacy, Hamadan University of Medical Science, Hamadan, Iran.*
[2] *Drug Applied Research Center, Tabriz University of Medical Sciences, Tabriz, Iran.*
[3] *Clinical Psychiatry Research Center, Tabriz University of Medical Sciences, Tabriz, Iran.*
[4] *Department of Pharmacology, Faculty of Pharmacy, Urmia University of Medical Science, Urmia, Iran.*

Article info

Keywords:
· Silymarin
· 6-OHDA
· Catalepsy
· Motor disturbance
· Rat

Abstract
Purpose: Parkinson's disease (PD) is a common neurodegenerative disorder characterized by disabling motor abnormalities, which include tremor, muscle stiffness, paucity of voluntary movements, and postural instability. Silymarin (SM) or milk thistle extract, is known to own antioxidative, anti-apoptotic, anti-inflammatory and neuroprotective effects. In the present study, we investigated the effect of intraperitoneal (i.p) administration of SM, on 6-OHDA-induced motor-impairments (catalepsy and imbalance) in the rats.
Methods: Experimental model of PD was induced by unilateral infusion of 6-hydroxydopamine (6-OHDA; 8 µg/2 µl/rat) into the central region of the substantia nigra pars compacta (SNc). Catalepsy and motor coordination were assessed by using of bar test and rotarod respectively.
Results: The results showed a significant ($p<0.001$) increase in catalepsy of 6-OHDA-lesioned rats whereas; in SM (100, 200 and 300 mg/kg, i.p for 5 days) treated hemi-parkinsonian rats catalepsy was decreased markedly ($p<0.001$). Furthermore, there was a significant ($p<0.001$) increase in motor-imbalance of 6-OHDA-lesioned rats. SM improved motor coordination significantly ($p<0.001$) in a dose dependent manner and increased motor balance.
Conclusion: In conclusion, we found that short-term treatment with SM could improve 6-OHDA-induced catalepsy and motor imbalance in rats. We suggest that SM can be used as adjunctive therapy along with commonly used anti-parkinsonian drugs. However, further clinical trial studies should be carried out to prove this hypothesis.

Introduction

Parkinson's disease (PD) is a progressive neurodegenerative disorder of the central nervous system which affects more than 4 million people over age 60 worldwide.[1] The disorder affects different areas of the brain, specially a region called the substantia nigra pars compacta (SNc) that controls balance and movement.[2] Often the first manifestation of PD is tremor of a limb, particularly when the body is at rest. Typically, the tremor begins on one side of the body, usually in one hand. Other characteristic symptoms include rigidity or stiffness of the limbs and trunk, slow movement (bradykinesia) or the inability to move (akinesia), and impaired balance and coordination (postural instability).[3] These features occur when dopaminergic neurons in the SNc die or become impaired.[2,3] Normally, dopaminergic cells produce dopamine, which transmits signals within the brain to produce smooth physical movements. When these dopamine-producing neurons die or become impaired, communication between the brain and muscles weakens, and eventually, the brain is unable to control muscle movement. The primary cause of PD is still unknown although aging appears to be a major risk factor. Indeed, mitochondrial impairment and elevated oxidative stress have been linked to the PD pathogenesis.[4] It is well agreed that chronic neuro-inflammation has part in the pathogenesis of the disease.[5,6]

Milk thistle (*Silybum marianum*) extract, silymarin (SM), is a polyphenolic flavonoid which has become so popular among herbalists throughout the world to maintaining liver health. SM is commonly used to treat liver diseases and has antioxidative,[7] anti-apoptotic,[8] anti-inflammatory,[9,10] neuroprotective properties against neuronal damages and brain aging.[11,12]

SM effect against oxidative stress is due to the scavenging of free radicals, activation of superoxide dismutase[13,14] and increase in reduced glutathione.[14] Furthermore, previous studies showed protective effects of SM in several experimental models of neuronal injury, especially in focal cerebral ischemia and cerebral ischemia–reperfusion-induced brain injury in rats.[15,16] Because of less information about its effect on PD, in this study we

***Corresponding author:** Alireza Mohajjel Nayebi, Email: nayebia@tbzmed.ac.ir

investigated the effect of SM on 6-OHDA-induced motor disturbance in hemi-parkinsonian rats.

Materials and Methods

Chemicals

All chemicals were purchased from Sigma Chemical Co. (USA). Solutions were made freshly on the days of experiment by dissolving drugs in physiological saline (0.9% NaCl) except for SM which was dissolved in 50% polyethylene glycol (PEG). The drugs were injected intraperitoneally (i.p) except for 6-OHDA which was injected into SNc.

Animals

Male Wistar rats (240±20 g) were used in this study. The animals were given food and water at liberty and were housed in standard polypropylene cages, four per cage at an ambient temperature of 25±2 °C under a 12-h light/12-h dark cycle. Animals were habituated to the testing conditions including being transferred to the experimental environment, handled, weighed, and restrained on the test platform for 10 min; 2 days before the behavioral investigations were conducted. The present study was carried out in accordance with the ethical guidelines for the Care and Use of Laboratory Animals of Tabriz University of Medical Sciences, Tabriz, Iran (National Institutes of Health Publication No. 85-23, revised 1985).

Experimental protocol

In the beginning of study only the rats that showed normal immobilization in bare test were subjected to further experimentation. The healthy animals were allocated randomly into 8 groups each consisting of eight rats by using simple random sampling method. Rats in group 1 (control group) received no injection and were left untreated for the entire period of the experiment as intact animals. Rats in group 2 (sham-operated) were injected with saline into SNc and were left untreated for the entire period of the experiment. Rats in group 3 (Lesioned (L) group) received only administration of 6-OHDA into SNc. Rats in group 4 (L + vehicle) were received intra-nigral administration of 6-OHDA in the same way as group 3 and then, after recovery period, treated with PEG for 5 consecutive days (days 22 to day 26). Rats in groups 5, 6 and 7 (L + SM) were received intra-SNc administration of 6-OHDA in the same way as group 3 and then, after recovery period, all animals that showed parkinsonian features were treated with i.p injection of SM 100, 200, 300 mg/kg, once daily for 5 consecutive days. Rats in group 8 (SM treated healthy animals) were treated with i.p injection of SM 200mg/kg once daily (9 a.m.) for 5 days.

Surgical procedures

The animals were anesthetized by i.p injection of ketamine (80 mg/kg) and xylazine (10 mg/kg). After the rats were deeply anaesthetized (loss of corneal and toe pad reflexes), they were fixed in a stereotaxic frame (Stoelting, Wood Lane, IL, USA) in the flat position and stereotaxicaly injected with 6-OHDA into SNc through a 23 gauge sterile stainless steel guide cannula. The coordinates for this position were based on the rat brain atlas:[17] anteroposterior from bregma (AP) = -5.0 mm, mediolateral from the midline (ML) = 2.1 mm and dorsoventral from the skull (DV) = -7.7mm. Desipramine (25 mg/kg, i.p) was injected 30 min before intra-SNc injection of 6-OHDA to avoid degeneration of noradrenergic neurons. Then 6-OHDA (8 μg/ per rat in 2 μl saline with 0.2 % ascorbic acid) was infused by infusion pump at the flow rate of 0.2 μl/min into the right SNc. At the end of injection, guide cannula was kept for an additional 5 min and then was withdrawn slowly. All of these procedures were repeated in Sham-operated animals but they were received only 2 μl vehicle of 6-OHDA.

Cannula verification

For confirmation of placement of the cannula in the SNc, at the end of experiments all rats with guide cannula were euthanized by a high dose of ether. The brains with the injecting tube in situ were removed and placed in a formaldehyde (10%) solution. After 1 week, the tissues were embedded in paraffin. Then serial sections (3 μm) were cut with a microtome (Leitz, Germany), and the placement of the tip of the cannula in the SNc was microscopically controlled. Data from rats with an incorrect placement of the cannula were excluded from the analysis.

Behavioral analysis

All tests were carried out between 9.0 a.m. and 3.0 p.m. Animals were transferred to the experimental room at least 1 h before the test in order to let them acclimatize to the test environment. All experiments were carried out by an observer who was blind to the identity of treatments.

Catalepsy assay test

Catalepsy was assessed by using a standard wooden bar test in the days of 21, 22 and 26 after 6-OHDA injection (Figure 1). Anterior limbs of rat gently extended on 9 cm high bar (0.9 cm in diameter) and the duration of retention of rats in this imposed posture was considered as the bar test elapsed time. The end point of catalepsy was designated to occur when both front paws were removed from the bar or if the animal moved its head in an exploratory manner. The cut-off time of the test was 600 sec. The animals were pre-trained to maintain their anterior limb on the bar for 2 consecutive days before main test. Catalepsy was assessed three weeks after neurotoxin injection and 1 and 5 days after intra-peritoneal (i.p) injection of SM in four consecutive times with one hour interval (time 5, 60, 120 & 180 minute).

Rotarod assay test

Assessment of motor coordination was done by using rotarod test.[18] This test was performed on the day 21 after 6-OHDA injection, 1 and 5 days after i.p injection of SM (Figure 1) in four consecutive times, each lasting 720 s, with one hour inter-trial period. Rats were mounted on the rotarod (18 RPM) and the time latency to fall from the rod was automatically recorded. All rats were pre-trained for 2 days in order to reach a stable performance. Animals staying during 720 s were taken from the rotarod and their retention time on rotarod considered 720 s. Values were expressed as retention time on the rotarod in the four test trails (5, 60, 120 & 180 minute).

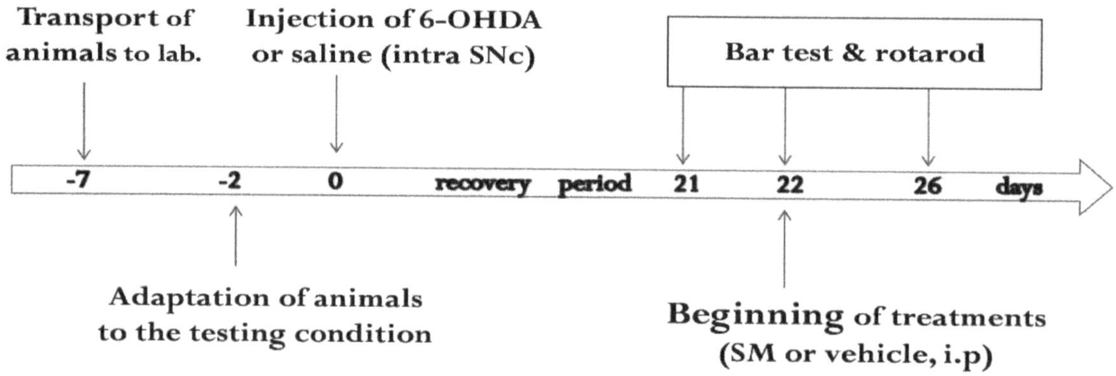

Figure 1. Schematic representation of the experimental procedure; see text for details.

Statistical analysis

Statistical analysis of each data set was performed by use of SPSS software (version 16.0). Data were expressed as the mean±SEM, and were analyzed by one-way ANOVA in each experiment. In the case of significant variation ($p<0.05$), the values were compared by Tukey test.

Results

Effect of intra-SNc injection of 6-OHDA on Catalepsy

Rats were divided into three groups: normal, sham operated and 6-OHDA (8 µg/2µl/rat)-injected group. Drugs or vehicle were injected into the SNc through the implanted guide cannula. As it has been shown in Figure 2, 6-OHDA was able to induce significant ($p<0.001$) catalepsy in comparison with both normal and sham-operated rats.

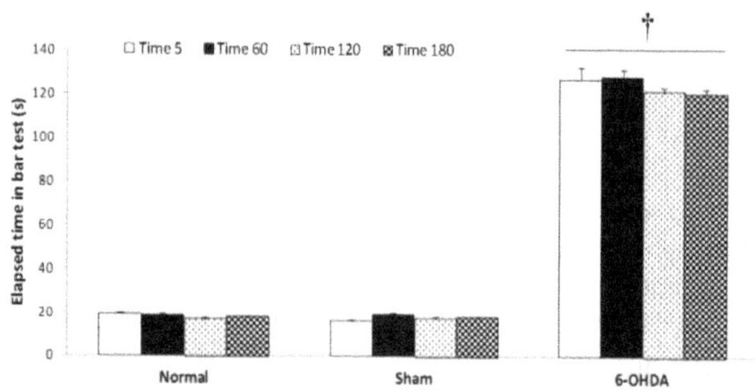

Figure 2. The results of bar test in normal, sham-operated and 6-OHDA-lesioned (8 µg/2 µl/rat) rats. Each bar represents the mean±SEM of elapsed time (s); n=8 rats for each group; †p<0.001 as compared with normal and sham-operated groups.

Effect of short-term administration of SM on 6-OHDA induced catalepsy

The effect of short-term treatment with SM (100, 200 and 300mg/kg, *i.p*) and its vehicle on catalepsy was investigated in 6-OHDA-lesioned rats for 5 consecutive days (Figure 3). In these groups catalepsy was assessed on day 21 after surgery for 4 repeated times (5, 60, 120 and 180 min). Rats that showed catalepsy were treated with SM and then catalepsy was assessed by bar test at 1 and 5 days after beginning of treatment. The results indicated that treatment with SM for 5 days (in all 3 doses) significantly ($p<0.001$) attenuated the severity of 6-OHDA induced catalepsy, but in the first day of treatment, only SM 300 mg/kg ($p<0.05$) decreased 6-OHDA-induced catalepsy (Figure 3A). No alteration was observed on bar test elapsed time in vehicle-treated rats (Figure 3B).

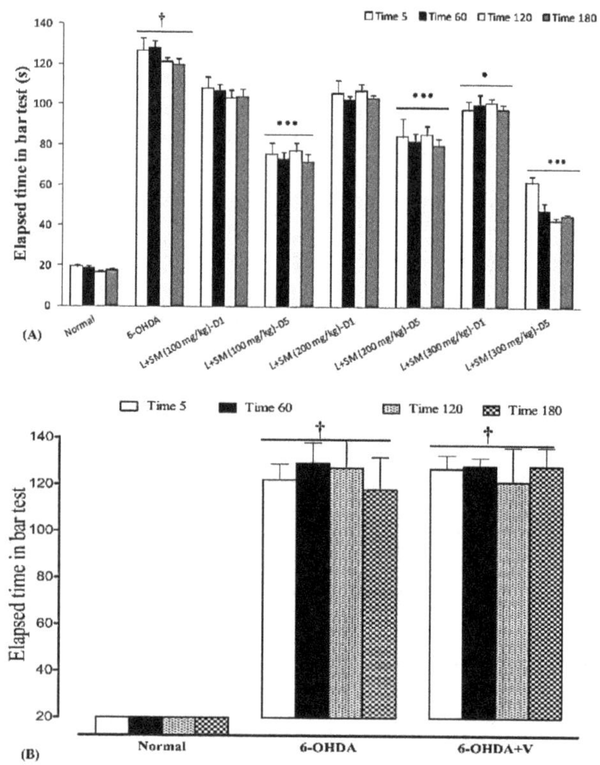

Figure 3. The results of bar test in 6-OHDA (8 µg/2 µl/rat)-lesioned rats which were treated with silymarin (100, 200 and 300mg/kg, i.p for 15 days) (Figure 3A) and silymarin vehicle (Figure 3B). Each bar represents the mean±SEM of catalepsy time (s); n=8 rats for each group; *p<0.05; ***p<0.001 as compared with 6-OHDA Lesioned group; †p<0.001 when compared with normal rats. (SM=Silymarin); (V=Vehicle of Silymarin); (D = Day).

Effect of intra-SNc injection of 6-OHDA on motor-balance

The effect of intra-SNc injection of 6-OHDA on motor coordination was evaluated by rotarod test. The time duration to fall from rotating rod was evaluated in three groups of rats: normal, sham operated and 6-OHDA (8 µg/2µl/rat)-lesioned rats. Drugs and vehicle were injected into the SNc through the implanted guide cannula. As it has been shown in Figure 4, 6-OHDA was able to induce significant ($p<0.001$) motor imbalance in comparison with both normal and sham-operated.

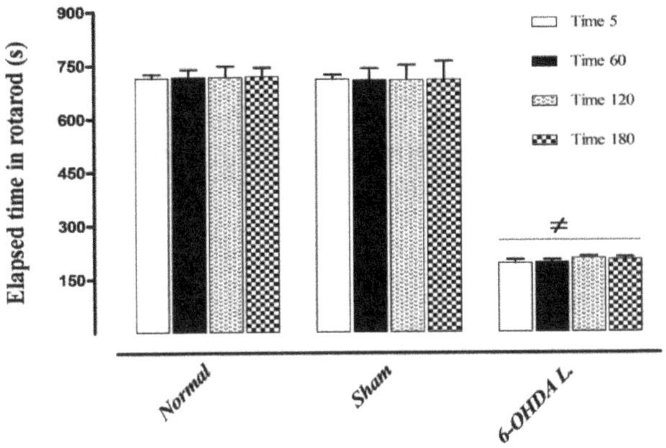

Figure 4. The rotarod test results of normal, sham-operated and 6-OHDA-lesioned (8 µg/2 µl/rat) rats. Each bar represents the mean±SEM of elapsed time on the rod (s); n=8 rats for each group; ≠p<0.001 as compared with normal and sham-operated groups (L=Lesioned).

Effect of SM on 6-OHDA induced motor incoordination

The effect of SM (100, 200 and 300mg/kg, i.p) and its vehicle on 6-OHDA-induced motor incoordination was assessed by rotarod. In these groups motor balance was tested 3 weeks after surgery for 4 repeated times (5, 60, 120 and 180 min). Rats that showed motor imbalance were treated with SM and then motor-balance was assessed 1 and 5 days after beginning of treatment. The results indicated that SM (100, 200 and 300mg/kg) after 5 days significantly ($p<0.05$, 0.01 and 0.001) improved motor balance in 6-OHDA-lesioned rats in a dose and time dependent manner. However, SM (300mg/kg) increased ($p<0.001$) motor balance in 6-OHDA-lesioned rats in the first day of treatment (Figure 5A). In vehicle treated rats, there was not any alteration on rotarod elapsed time (Figure 5B).

Discussion

We have recently reported that pre-treatment with SM amends the 6-OHDA-induced motor impairments by inhibition of inflammatory pathways and oxidative stress.[11,19] In this study we tried to investigate the effect of SM on 6-OHDA-induced catalepsy and motor imbalance which were assessed by bar test and rotarod respectively. Catalepsy which is commonly assessed by bar test is a valid marker of the nigrostriatal neurodegeneration.[11,20] In rodents, this is a standard test for evaluation of 6-OHDA and neuroleptic drugs-induced akinesia.[21-24] In the present study we observed that intra-SNc injection of 6-OHDA resulted in motor impairments (increased catalepsy and decreased motor-balance) in rats which were attenuated by short term treatment with SM. This is in accordance to findings of other researchers[21,24,25] who reported that 6-OHDA (8-12µg) caused catalepsy and motor-impairment through induction of progressive neurodegeneration of SNc neurons.[22] It is well established that 6-OHDA induced hemi-parkinsonian rats are a standard experimental model of PD and can be used in investigating of potential neuroprotective effect of drugs.[26-29] 6-OHDA is a neurotoxin which structurally is similar to dopamine and norepinephrine. After its injection, 6-OHDA is up taken by dopaminergic neurons and then readily oxidized to hydrogen peroxide and paraquinone.[30] It does not cross the blood–brain barrier. Thus, it is widely used to induce experimental models of PD by stereotaxic injection directly into the nigro-striatal region. It has been reported that 6-OHDA increases TNF-α levels in SNc, striatum and cerebrospinal fluid.[25,31] Furthermore, 6-OHDA causes to neurodegeneration through inhibition of mitochondrial respiratory enzymes and induction of oxidative stress.[32] It seems that also toxic effects of 6-OHDA are partly mediated through activation of microglia.[33]

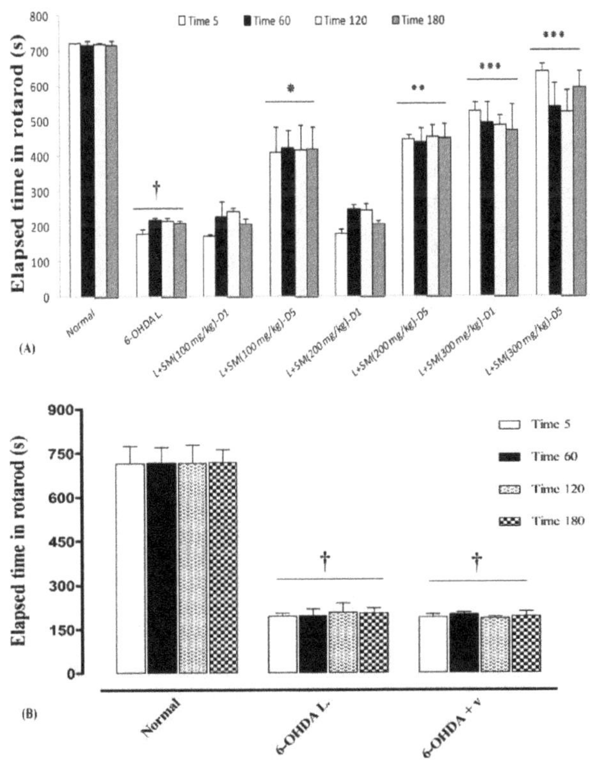

Figure 5. The rotarod test results of 6-OHDA (8 µg/2 µl/rat)-lesioned rats that short-term treated with silymarin (100, 200 and 300mg/kg, i.p for 15 days) (Figure 5A) and silymarin vehicle (Figure 5B). Each bar represents the mean±SEM of elapsed time (s) on the rod; n = 8 rats for each group; †p<0.001 between normal and 6-OHDA groups; *p<0.05; **p<0.01; ***p<0.001 when compared with 6-OHDA-lesioned rats. (SM=Silymarin); (V=Vehicle of silymarin); (L=Lesioned); (D=Day).

Several useful effects have been reported for SM in different cultured neuronal cell lines and animal studies.[12,34] However, less information is available about its effects on motor disturbances in experimental models of PD. In this study we observed that short-term (5 days) treatment with SM could improve 6-OHDA-induced catalepsy. An important finding of this study is that single high dose of SM (300mg/kg) in the first day could decrease catalepsy in bar test. This is in accordance with previous studies showing that pre-treatment with SM and its acute administration decreased catalepsy and rotational behavior in hemi-parkinsonian rats by protecting nigrostriatal neurons against neurodegenerative process.[11,34,35] According to the results, intra-nigral injection of 6-OHDA impaired motor coordination so that rats fail to maintain their balances on rotarod and the duration of walking on the rotating drum significantly decreased in lesioned rats when compared with sham-operated group. On the other hand, our results showed a significant decrease in the 6-OHDA induced motor imbalance in lesioned rats which were treated by different doses of SM for five days. Furthermore, SM (300mg/kg) could improve motor-balance in the first day of treatment and increased retention time on rotarod. In rotarod, which is considered as a standard test for evaluation of motor-balance, performance is measured by the period of time that an animal stays up and walks on the rod and the latency to fall off the drum was recorded.[20,25,36] In 6-OHDA-lesioned rats loss of dopaminergic neurons and reduction of striatal dopamine levels is an essential cause of motor incoordination. In fact, unilateral lesion of SNc obliges animal to change its weight irregularly for movement and balance; therefore this lead to motor disturbance and asymmetry.[3,21,22]

Because of high density of microglia in the SNc, the neurons of this area are over sensitized to inflammatory affront as a major exciter of neurodegenerative disease[37] and activation of this microglia lead to release of pro-inflammatory cytokines, which have an important role in neurotoxicity.[38] Previous studies revealed that SM down-regulates nuclear factor kappa B (NF-kB) activation in DA neurons,[16,34] reduces brain myeloperoxidase activity[11] and inhibits cerebral cyclooxygenase-2(COX-2),[16] and subsequently decreases release of pro-inflammatory cytokines[11,18]. These properties may explain the observed motor improving effects of SM in hemi-parkinsonian rats. Additionally, SM decreases brain lipids peroxidation and Malondialdehyde as an index of the oxidative stress severity[19,35] and increases the level of brain superoxide dismutase (SOD) and glutathione reductase (GR) as antioxidant enzymes[35] in experimental models of PD. It can be postulated that reported neuroprotective effects of SM are mediated at least in part through its anti-oxidant activity.

Conclusion

The short-term administration of SM attenuated 6-OHDA induced catalepsy and motor imbalance. According to the obtained results, we suggest that SM may be used as a potential adjunctive therapy together with routinely used antiparkinsonian drugs. However, further clinical investigations should be carried out to prove it.

Acknowledgments

We wish to thank the Director of Drug Applied Research Center, Tabriz University of Medical Sciences for supporting this study.

Furthermore, we appreciate manager of Goldaru Herbal Pharmaceutical Laboratories for donating pure silymarin powder.

Conflict of Interest

The authors declare that they have no competing interest.

References

1. Warner TT, Schapira AH. Genetic and environmental factors in the cause of parkinson's disease. *Ann Neurol* 2003;53 Suppl 3:S16-23; discussion S-5. doi: 10.1002/ana.10487
2. Jenner P, Olanow CW. The pathogenesis of cell death in parkinson's disease. *Neurology* 2006;66(10 Suppl 4):S24-36.
3. Dauer W, Przedborski S. Parkinson's disease: Mechanisms and models. *Neuron* 2003;39(6):889-909.
4. Obeso JA, Rodriguez-Oroz MC, Goetz CG, Marin C, Kordower JH, Rodriguez M, et al. Missing pieces in the parkinson's disease puzzle. *Nat Med* 2010;16(6):653-61. doi: 10.1038/nm.2165
5. Hirsch EC, Hunot S. Neuroinflammation in parkinson's disease: A target for neuroprotection? *Lancet Neurol* 2009;8(4):382-97. doi: 10.1016/S1474-4422(09)70062-6
6. Lee JK, Tran T, Tansey MG. Neuroinflammation in parkinson's disease. *J Neuroimmune Pharmacol* 2009;4(4):419-29. doi: 10.1007/s11481-009-9176-0
7. Mandegary A, Saeedi A, Eftekhari A, Montazeri V, Sharif E. Hepatoprotective effect of silyamarin in individuals chronically exposed to hydrogen sulfide; modulating influence of tnf-alpha cytokine genetic polymorphism. *Daru* 2013;21(1):28. doi: 10.1186/2008-2231-21-28
8. Manna SK, Mukhopadhyay A, Van NT, Aggarwal BB. Silymarin suppresses tnf-induced activation of nf-kappa b, c-jun n-terminal kinase, and apoptosis. *J Immunol* 1999;163(12):6800-9.
9. Gupta OP, Sing S, Bani S, Sharma N, Malhotra S, Gupta BD, et al. Anti-inflammatory and anti-arthritic activities of silymarin acting through inhibition of 5-lipoxygenase. *Phytomedicine* 2000;7(1):21-4. doi: 10.1016/S0944-7113(00)80017-3
10. Esmaily H, Vaziri-Bami A, Miroliaee AE, Baeeri M, Abdollahi M. The correlation between nf-kappab inhibition and disease activity by coadministration of

silibinin and ursodeoxycholic acid in experimental colitis. *Fundam Clin Pharmacol* 2011;25(6):723-33. doi: 10.1111/j.1472-8206.2010.00893.x

11. Haddadi R, Mohajjel Nayebi A, Brooshghalan SE. Pre-treatment with silymarin reduces brain myeloperoxidase activity and inflammatory cytokines in 6-ohda hemi-parkinsonian rats. *Neurosci Lett* 2013;555:106-11. doi: 10.1016/j.neulet.2013.09.022
12. Galhardi F, Mesquita K, Monserrat JM, Barros DM. Effect of silymarin on biochemical parameters of oxidative stress in aged and young rat brain. *Food Chem Toxicol* 2009;47(10):2655-60. doi: 10.1016/j.fct.2009.07.030
13. Muzes G, Deak G, Lang I, Nekam K, Gergely P, Feher J. Effect of the bioflavonoid silymarin on the in vitro activity and expression of superoxide dismutase (sod) enzyme. *Acta Physiol Hung* 1991;78(1):3-9.
14. Nencini C, Giorgi G, Micheli L. Protective effect of silymarin on oxidative stress in rat brain. *Phytomedicine* 2007;14(2-3):129-35. doi: 10.1016/j.phymed.2006.02.005
15. Raza SS, Khan MM, Ashafaq M, Ahmad A, Khuwaja G, Khan A, et al. Silymarin protects neurons from oxidative stress associated damages in focal cerebral ischemia: A behavioral, biochemical and immunohistological study in wistar rats. *J Neurol Sci* 2011;309(1-2):45-54. doi: 10.1016/j.jns.2011.07.035
16. Hou YC, Liou KT, Chern CM, Wang YH, Liao JF, Chang S, et al. Preventive effect of silymarin in cerebral ischemia-reperfusion-induced brain injury in rats possibly through impairing nf-kappab and stat-1 activation. *Phytomedicine* 2010;17(12):963-73. doi: 10.1016/j.phymed.2010.03.012
17. Paxinos G, Watson C. The rat brain in stereotaxic coordinates. San Diego: Elsevier Academic Press; 2007.
18. Mohajjel Nayebi A, Nazemiyeh H, Omidbakhsh R, Çobanoglu S. Analgesic effect of the methanol extract of Erica arborea (L.) in mice using formalin test. *Daru* 2008;16(4): 229-32.
19. Haddadi R, Nayebi AM, Farajniya S, Brooshghalan SE, Sharifi H. Silymarin improved 6-ohda-induced motor impairment in hemi-parkisonian rats: Behavioral and molecular study. *Daru* 2014;22:38. doi: 10.1186/2008-2231-22-38
20. Carvalho MM, Campos FL, Coimbra B, Pego JM, Rodrigues C, Lima R, et al. Behavioral characterization of the 6-hydroxidopamine model of parkinson's disease and pharmacological rescuing of non-motor deficits. *Mol Neurodegener* 2013;8:14. doi: 10.1186/1750-1326-8-14
21. Schwarting RK, Huston JP. The unilateral 6-hydroxydopamine lesion model in behavioral brain research. Analysis of functional deficits, recovery and treatments. *Prog Neurobiol* 1996;50(2-3):275-331.
22. Deumens R, Blokland A, Prickaerts J. Modeling parkinson's disease in rats: An evaluation of 6-ohda lesions of the nigrostriatal pathway. *Exp Neurol* 2002;175(2):303-17. doi: 10.1006/exnr.2002.7891
23. Sharifi H, Mohajjel Nayebia A, Farajnia S. The effect of chronic administration of buspirone on 6-hydroxydopamine-induced catalepsy in rats. *Adv Pharm Bull* 2012;2(1):127-31. doi: 10.5681/apb.2012.019
24. Sharifi H, Mohajjel Nayebia A, Farajnia S. Dose-dependent effect of flouxetine on 6-ohda-induced catalepsy in male rats: A possible involvement of 5-ht1a receptors. *Adv Pharm Bull* 2013;3(1):203-6. doi: 10.5681/apb.2013.033
25. Sharifi H, Nayebi AM, Farajnia S, Haddadi R. Effect of chronic administration of buspirone and fluoxetine on inflammatory cytokines in 6-hydroxydopamine-lesioned rats. *Drug Res (Stuttg)* 2014. doi: 10.1055/s-0034-1374615
26. Sharifi H, Mohajjel Nayebi A, Farajnia S. 8-oh-dpat (5-ht1a agonist) attenuates 6-hydroxy- dopamine-induced catalepsy and modulates inflammatory cytokines in rats. *Iran J Basic Med Sci* 2013;16(12):1270-5.
27. Mahmoudi J, Nayebi AM, Samini M, Reyhani-Rad S, Babapour V. Buspirone improves the anti-cataleptic effect of levodopa in 6-hydroxydopamine-lesioned rats. *Pharmacol Rep* 2011;63(4):908-14.
28. Mahmoudi J, Mohajjel Nayebi A, Samini M, Reyhani-Rad S, Babapour V. 5-ht(1a) receptor activation improves anti-cataleptic effects of levodopa in 6-hydroxydopamine-lesioned rats. *Daru* 2011;19(5):338-43.
29. Nayebi AM. Hypothesis: A promising effect of 5-HT1A receptor agonists in alleviating motor symptoms of Parkinson's disease. *Afr J Pharm Pharmaco* 2010; 4(6):289-290.
30. Heikkila R, Cohen G. Inhibition of biogenic amine uptake by hydrogen peroxide: A mechanism for toxic effects of 6-hydroxydopamine. *Science* 1971;172(3989):1257-8.
31. Mogi M, Togari A, Tanaka K, Ogawa N, Ichinose H, Nagatsu T. Increase in level of tumor necrosis factor (tnf)-alpha in 6-hydroxydopamine-lesioned striatum in rats without influence of systemic l-dopa on the tnf-alpha induction. *Neurosci Lett* 1999;268(2):101-4.
32. Glinka Y, Gassen M, Youdim MB. Mechanism of 6-hydroxydopamine neurotoxicity. *J Neural Transm Suppl* 1997;50:55-66.
33. Whitton PS. Inflammation as a causative factor in the aetiology of parkinson's disease. *Br J Pharmacol* 2007;150(8):963-76. doi: 10.1038/sj.bjp.0707167
34. Wang MJ, Lin WW, Chen HL, Chang YH, Ou HC, Kuo JS, et al. Silymarin protects dopaminergic neurons against lipopolysaccharide-induced neurotoxicity by inhibiting microglia activation. *Eur J Neurosci* 2002;16(11):2103-12.

Therapeutic Efficacy of Orally Delivered Doxorubicin Nanoparticles in Rat Tongue Cancer Induced by 4-Nitroquinoline 1-Oxide

Monir Moradzadeh Khiavi[1], Ahamd Rostami[2], Hamed Hamishekar[3], Mehran Mesgari Abassi[3], Amirala Aghbali[2], Roya Salehi[3], Bita Abdollahi[3], Soheila Fotoohi[3], Mahmud Sina[2]*

[1] *Department of Oral and Maxillofacial Pathology, School of Dentistry, Tehran University of Medical Sciences, International campus, Tehran, Iran.*
[2] *Department of Oral and Maxillofacial Pathology, School of Dentistry, Tabriz University of Medical Sciences, Tabriz, Iran.*
[3] *Drug Applied Research Center, Tabriz University of Medical Sciences, Tabriz, Iran.*

Article info

Keywords:
· Doxorubicin
· Squamous cell carcinoma
· Oral
· 4-NQO
· Rats
· Nanoparticles

Abstract
Purpose: Oral cancer is one of the most significant cancers in the world, and squamous cell carcinoma makes up about 94% of oral malignancies. The aim of the present study was to compare the efficacy of doxorubicin plus methotrexate - loaded nanoparticles on tongue squamous cell carcinoma induced by 4NQO and compare it with the commercial doxorubicin and methotrexate delivered orally on seventy SD male rats.
Methods: 70 rats were divided into five groups. During the study, the animals were weighed by a digital scale once a week. Number of mortalities was recorded in the data collection forms. At the end of the treatment, biopsy samples were taken from rat tongues in order to evaluate the severity of dysplasia and the extent of cell proliferation. The results were analyzed using ANOVA, descriptive statistics and chi-square test.
Results: No statistically significant difference was found in the mean weight of five groups ($p>0.05$). No significant relationship was found between groups and mortality rate ($P = 0.39$). In addition, there was a significant relationship between groups and the degree of dysplasia ($P <0.001$). The statistical analysis showed a significant relationship between groups and the rate of cell proliferation ($p <0.001$).
Conclusion: The results of the present study showed that the use of doxorubicin plus methotrexate - loaded nanoparticles orally had more therapeutic effects than commercial doxorubicin plus methotrexate.

Introduction

Head and neck tumors include a major group of neoplasms in worldwide, and are on the rise in many parts of the world. The most common of this disease, is cancer of the mouth approximately 90% are squamous cell carcinoma (SCC).[1] Based on the reports of the World Health Organization, oral cavity carcinoma is the sixth most common cancer after lung, prostate, colorectal, stomach and bladder cancers in men and is the tenth most common, colorectal, cancer in women.[1] Most of the invasive oral carcinomas originate from altered oral pre-cancerous lesions and have a likelihood of progressing to SCC. Tumor progression in epithelial cells is classified into normal epithelium, hyperplasic (non-dysplastic), carcinoma in situ and invasive carcinomas.[1]

Squamous cell carcinoma is a multi-factorial disease. These factors are divided into two groups of internal and external factors. External factors, which include; smoking, alcoholism, syphilis and solar radiation (Vermilion lip cancer), and the internal factors, include systemic or the generalized conditions such as general malnutrition or iron deficiency anemia.[2,3] Developing this type of cancer results in changes of the patient's appearance, decreased quality of life, and most importantly decreased eating ability.[4]

Various treatments have been carried out on squamous cell carcinoma. The standard treatments for this disease include surgery, chemotherapy and radiation, each of which has its own complications. The side effects of chemotherapy include soreness of the mouth, throat, weight loss, thrombocytopenia, vomiting, anorexia, diarrhea, and constipation. The surgical patients in the more advanced stages of this disease may face dysphagia and dysphonia, and most likely deformity of the face. The side effects of radiation therapy include, dry mouth, sensitive teeth/ mucosa with extensive dental caries and dysphagia.[6]

Doxorubicin is one of the most effective anti-cancer drugs. It is prescribed often in combination with other anti-cancer drugs for the treatment of the various cancers. Doxorubicin is a subgroup of anthracycline, which is a branch of antibiotics produced by Streptomyces Peucetius and a variety Cassius.[7]

***Corresponding author:** Mahmud Sina, Email: sinam@tbzmed.ac.ir

Anthracycline, doxorubicin, daunorubicin, adriamycin and epirubicin are antineoplastic antibiotics with a wide range of clinical applications, doxorubicin acts against a number of tumors, such as sarcomas and carcinomas. This drug is also used in hematological malignancies (leukemia, lymphoma and multiple myeloma).[7] However, the commercial form of this drug has severe side effects, one of which is cardiac toxicity. Hence, the use of doxorubicin for treatment of cancer patients has some limitations.[8,9] Much efforts has been taken to solve this problem and reduce the adverse effects, among which is its confinement within the nanoparticle systems. One of the goals of nanotechnology is (DNA-based nanobots) to target cancer cells, this is accomplished by the molecular delivery of drugs that trigger cell suicide in leukemia and lymphoma cells.[10] Nanoparticles include different types of colloidal systems with a submicron scale (smaller than one micrometer). They may be inorganic, liposomal or polymeric. One of the main advantages of nanoparticles is their dwarfed size, which makes it easy to bypass the biological membranes and deliver the drugs directly to the nuclei of cancer cells. Another advantage is the high density of the pharmaceutical agent that can be used to achieve different drug release characteristics.[11]

Because of the high level of nanoparticles, these particles are capable of carrying a payload of multiple drug particles directly to the nuclei of the cancerous cell. The nanoparticles are also capable of penetrating deep into the tumor tissue, thus delaying the detection by the immune cells, and reaching the targeted cells. The particles enter into cancerous tumors in large numbers, and form a homogenous fluid with low viscosity and remain in the tumor tissue for an extended period. In view of the fact that the cancerous cell mediums have an acidic pH of 4-5.8, the controlled delivery systems for the treatment of cancer should be designed in such a way that prevents drug release at a physiologic pH, and/or minimizes the release, with the maximum delivery of the drug released in the acidic environment. Since the ideal controlled delivery systems for the treatment of cancer contain a maximum release in acidic environments, the delivery system used is injection or implants depending on the type of medication prescribed; moreover, this delivery system is necessary to prevent the toxic effects of these drugs in an oral form.[12]

The aim of this study was to assess the efficacy of doxorubicin plus methotrexate - loaded nanoparticles (in a soluble form and loaded on polymeric nanoparticles) on the tongue squamous cell carcinoma. The SCC was induced by 4-Nitroquinoline 1-Oxide(4NQO) and compare with the commercial doxorubicin and methotrexate delivered orally on seventy Sprague Dawley (SD) male rats in the laboratory animals section of Drug Applied Research Center and School of Dentistry, Tabriz University of MedicalSciences.

Materials and Methods

Studied Animals

In this experimental study, 70 (5 groups of 14 each) SD male rats were selected with the following features: Age range of 2.5- 3 months, an approximate weight of 150± 50g. The rats were kept at 22 ±2 °C and12 hours light cycle, 60 ± 0.5 percent ambient humidity and available food conditions.

Chemicals

The powder 4-nitroquinoline1-oxide (4NQO) was purchased from Sigma (Poole, UK) to induce carcinoma of tongue.[13-15] The 500 ml of 4NQO solution 30 ppm was regularly prepared for each cage three times per-week (every other day for 14 weeks). The solution preparation was 15 mg of 4NQO weighed by a digital scale, and dissolved in 498.5ml of water, bottled and covered with foil to protect it from light exposure.[13-15]

Anticancer drug loaded nanoparticles

Nanoparticle synthesis was studied and discussed by Salehi et al, briefly, an appropriate amount of synthesized nanoparticles was stirred in a solution of methotrexate by ultrasonic device for 5 minutes. After stirring the mixture (methotrexate-loaded nanoparticles), it was placed in a dark condition, next doxorubicin hydrochloride was added to the mixture of methotrexate and loaded with nanoparticles by ultrasonic device for 3 minutes (Sonics Vibra cell, Model: VCX 130PB, Newton, CT). The final ratio of carrier/drug was 5 to 1 for both drugs. This mixture was kept in a magnetic stirrer at room temperature for 24 hours in a dark condition; until the Methotrexate-doxorubicin was loaded nanoparticles remained for 2 hours to allow the deposition. The methotrexate-doxorubicin loaded nanoparticles were centrifuged at 14,000 rpm for 15 minutes. Subsequently, it was dried for 24 hours at room temperature and stored in the container until further use by the study.[16]

The doxorubicin were loaded with anti-cancer drugs were diluted with a physiologic saline solution to the appropriate concentration before use on the animals.

Experimental design

The seventy rats were divided into 5 groups of 14. The Table 1 shows the studied groups briefly.

Group N: the control-group, were fed a normal diet and no intervention was performed.

Group K: the carcinoma control group, received 4-NQO at the concentration of 30 ppm in their drinking water for 14 weeks without any treatment.

Group F: the nanodrug control group, received 6mg the doxorubicin plus methotrexate-loaded nanoparticles once a day on days of 2, 5 and 8 of the study in order to evaluate the probable side effects of the drug.

Groups E and D were the treatment groups and received 4-NQO at the concentration of 30 ppm in their drinking water for 14 weeks and then they also orally received commercial doxorubicin (made by a pharmaceutical company, Italy) and the DOX-MTX-loaded nanoparticles respectively once a day on days of 2, 5 and 8 of the study.

Accordingly, groups D and E were divided into two groups of 7 rats:

Group D1 and D2: Received 1.5 and 6 mg doxorubicin plus methotrexate-loaded nanoparticles, respectively.

Group E1 and E2: Received 1.5 and 6 mg commercial doxorubicin plus methotrexate, respectively.

During the study, the animals were weighed by digital scale within an accuracy of 1g once a week, and recorded in grams on the data collection form.

The rats in each group were counted and the number of mortalities was recorded in the data collection forms daily, and evaluated with consideration of their relationship to their groups and the other groups.

Table 1. The studied groups

Groups	4NQO	Drug
N	-	-
K	×	-
F	-	×(Nanodrug)
D	×	×(Nanodrug)
E	×	×(commercial drug)

-: The groups that didn't receive 4NQO or any drugs
×: The groups that received 4NQO or any drugs

Histopathologiocal evaluation

Following treatment for three month with the doxorubicin plus methotrexate, the rats were anesthetized with ether by use of the anesthetic chamber and tongue biopsies were taken from the groups-N, K, D and E.[17] The samples were fixed in 10% formalin for 24 hours, and paraffin blocks were prepared from the samples. Next, sections of 5-micron thickness were prepared for staining with hematoxylin and eosin, the prepared samples were studied by both pathologists using light microscope, Olympus BX50F4 with a magnification of ×400. Every morphological changes of the epithelium including enlarged nuclei and cells, increased nuclear to cytoplasmic ratio, pleomorphic nuclei and cells, dyskeratosis and increased mitotic activity were scaled.

For evaluation of the malignant changes in each sample, the changes of the epithelium were classified as follows: no lesion, mild dysplasia, moderate dysplasia, severe dysplasia and squamous cell carcinoma. Ki-67 was used as an immunohistochemistry marker to study the cellular proliferation. The 4-micron sections were prepared from paraffin blocks using the specific assay kit for staining, Ki67 (monoclonal antibody Ki-67 protein; DO-7 Novocastra, Anti-mouse) in groups N, K, D and E. Immunostaining for Ki-67 was performed according to the manufacturer's instructions (Dako, Denmark). Ki-67 precipitate on the cellular nuclei renders them a brown color. Therefore, the sections were studied by both pathologists using a light microscope, OlymposBX50 F4, made in Japan, with a magnification of ×400. It should be noted that assessing and evaluating Ki-67 marker begin with counting the total number of cells in the microscopic field with a magnification of × 400 and the number of cells, which had stained nuclei, were counted and was expressed as a percentage of the total cells in the field. Cells that were associated with the expression of Ki-67 create brown insoluble sediments; Ki-67 transforms the nuclei brown. Therefore, they were separately counted in10 fields, thus, the end the mean percentage was expressed as a total of10 fields. Therefore, the percentage data obtained was placed in one of the subgroups. Based on these studies, these sections were divided into four categories (negative, weak, moderate, severe). If less than 10 percent of the section was stained, it was considered negative, 10-25%, weak(+), 26-50%, moderate(++), more than 50%, severe(+++).[18,19]

Statistical analysis

The obtained data was analyzed using analysis of variance (ANOVA) statistical methods, SPSS.15 and descriptive statistic methods (frequency and percentage) and Chi square test were used to study the mortality rate. The data was also analyzed by the nonparametric ANOVA test (Kruskal-Wallis) to compare the mean weight loss in the different groups, the significance level of tests was at 0.05.

Ethical considerations

All ethical considerations were met based on Helsinki Protocol and the University Research Ethics Committee approvals. Since this article is the result of a research project approved by the Research Committee, Tabriz University of Medical Sciences, the ethical considerations have been approved by the its ethics committee.

Results

Weight changes

In total, no weight loss was observed in any of the study groups at their first and last weight measurement. The maximum amount of weight gain was observed in-group D (Figure 1). One-way ANOVA test with repeated measurements were used to investigate the statistical significant differences between the mean weights. The results are shown in Table 2, No statistically significant difference was shown in mean weight in the five groups ($p>0.05$).The mean weight in Groups D1 and E1 were greater than D2 and E2 respectively, the difference was significant ($p<0.05$), the results are illustrated in Table 3.

Mortality

Statistical analysis indicated a lack of relationship between the groups and the rate of mortality ($p= 0.39$). The results of mortality rates of study the groups are illustrated in Table 2.

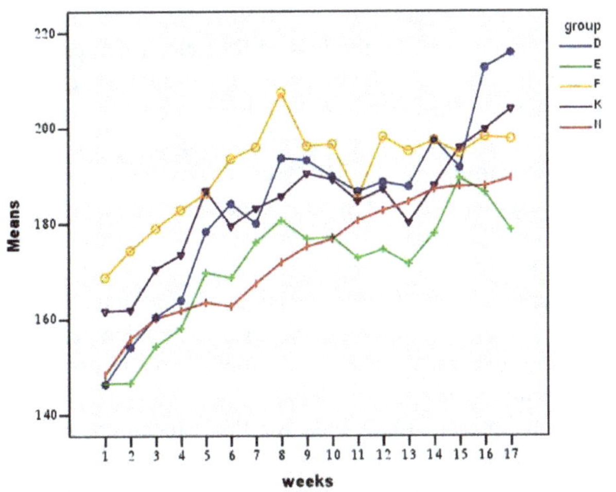

Figure 1. Mean weight of the studied groups in the seventeen –week length

Table 2. Weight gain and death rate of treated and nontreated rats in groups

Groups	N	K	F	D	E
Weight gain Mean (grams) (SD)	173.2 (±32.23)	170.9 (±20.4)	178.1 (±29.52)	170.98 (±36.67)	183.87 (±43.99)
Death rate n (%)	0	7%	0	0	0

Table 3. Mean weight in two doses

Variables	D		E	
	D1	D2	E1	E2
Weight(SD)	206.6(±9)	161.1(±9)	199.4(±4.1)	142.6(±4.1)

Dysplasia

In Group-D, the most common lesion was mild dysplasia (Figure 2), in Group-E moderate dysplasia and in Group-K, SCC (Figure 3). The results of the evaluation of the lesions in the study groups are given in Table 4.The statistical results demonstrated a relationship between the study groups and the dysplasia rate ($p<0.001$). There was no relationship between drug dose and dysplasia rate within each group ($p>0.05$). The results of the evaluation of the lesions in the study groups and the drug doses are shown in Table 5.

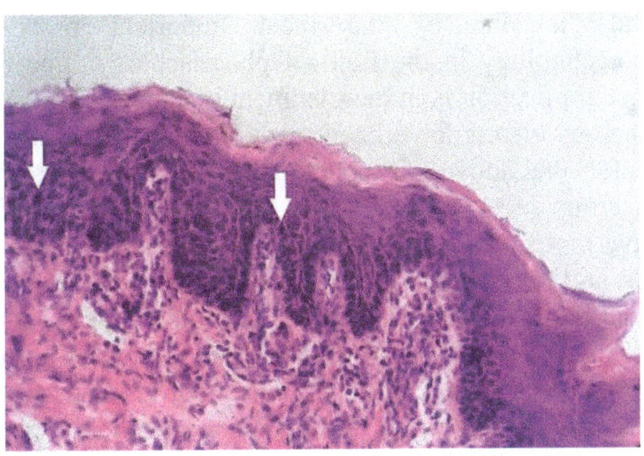

Figure 2. Mild epithelial dysplasia (H&E ×200), shows nuclear hyperchromatism and plomorphism (arrows) in the basal and parabasal layers.

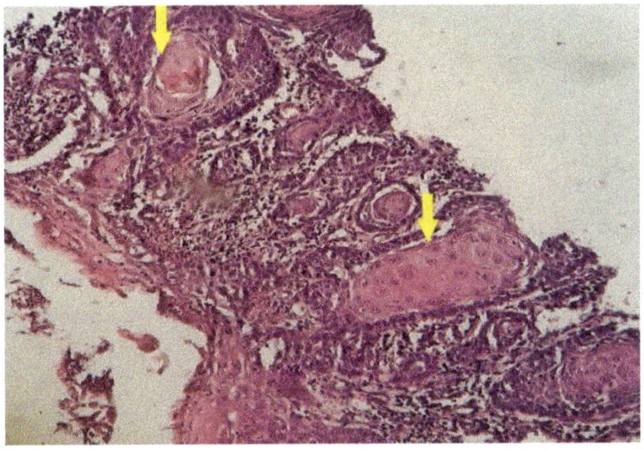

Figure 3. Squamous cell carcinoma shows invasive islands of dysplastic epithelial cells (arrows) (H&E, ×400)

Table 4. Frequency and percentage of the generated lesions in the studied group

groups	Without Dysplasia	Mild epithelial dysplasia	Moderate epithelial dysplasia	Severe epithelial dysplasia	SCC
D	2(14.3)	10(71.4)	2(14.3)	0	0
E	0	0	8(517)	6(42.9)	0
K	0	0	0	2(14.3)	12(85.7)

Table 5. Frequency and percentage of lesions in the study group based on drug dose

groups	Without Dysplasia	Mild epithelial dysplasia	Moderate epithelial dysplasia	Severe epithelial dysplasia	SCC
D1	0	5(53.7)	2(14.3)	0	0
D2	2(14.3)	5(53.7)	0	0	0
E1	0	0	3(21.4)	4(28.6)	0
E2	0	0	5(53.7)	2(14.3)	0

Ki- 67 expression

The results revealed that the level of Ki-67 expression in Group-N, which was the control-group, was entirely negative(-), and Group-D was a typically weak expression (+),while the expression of this marker in group-E was moderate (+ +), and in Group K, severe (+++) (Figure 4). Figure 5 displayed a mild Ki-67 expression (+) in group-D (which received the nano drug).

Results of the evaluation of Ki - 67 expressions in the study groups are illustrated in Table 6. The Chi-square test was used to evaluate the relationship between the study groups and rate of Ki-67 expression. In each group, the results demonstrated a significant relationship between the study groups and the rate of Ki-67 expression ($P<0.001$). In addition, there was no relationship between the drug dose and Ki-67 expression within each group ($p>0.05$). Ki-67expression results based on the drug doses in the study groups are given in Table 7.

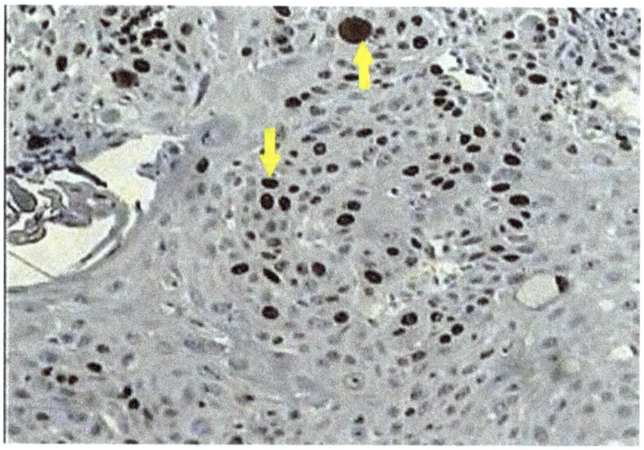

Figure 4. Severe expression of ki-67 in epithelial cells with nuclear staining (arrows) (IHC, ×400)

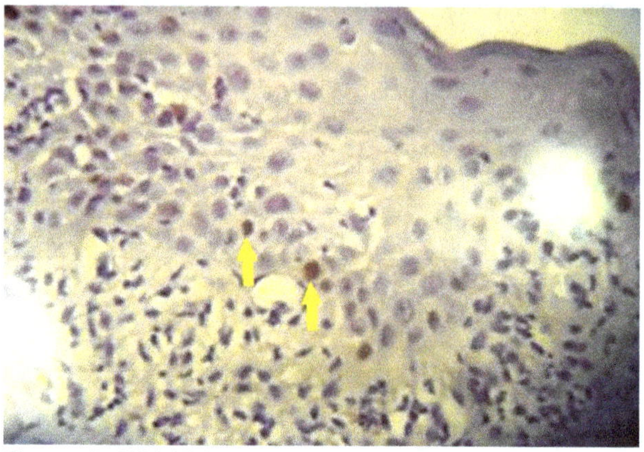

Figure 5. Mild Ki-67 expression in group D which received nanoparticle-based doxorubicin. A few nucleus have been stained in this figure (arrows)(IHC,× 400)

Table 6. Frequency and percentage of Ki-67 expression in the studied group

groups	Negetive(-)	Weak(+)	Moderate(++)	Severe(+++)
N	14(100)	0	0	0
D	3(21.4)	9(64.3)	2(14.3)	0
E	0	6(42.9)	6(42.9)	2(14.3)
K	0	0	0	14(100)

Table 7. Frequency and percentage of proliferation in the studied groups based on the drug dose.

groups	Negative(-)	Weak(+)	Moderate(++)	Severe(+++)
D1	1(7.1)	4(28.6)	2(14.3)	0
D2	2(14.3)	5(35.7)	0	0
E1	0	2(14.3)	3.(21.4)	2(14.3)
E2	0	4(28.6)	3.(21.4)	0

Discussion

In this study, 4NQO was used to induce cancer, 4-Nitroquinoline 1-oxide (4NQO) is a potent chemical carcinogens and its carcinogenic activity is due to its enzymatic activity and reduction of nitro groups. The carcinogenic metabolite of 4-Nitroquinoline 1-oxide (4NQO) is created by the loss of four electrons resulting in the production 4-hydroxy amino quinoline 1-oxide (4HAQO).[20] This material has been used in previous studies to induce oral cancer in rat tongues.[13,14] Clinical and histopathologic studies have shown that squamous cell carcinoma due to 4NQO is considered the equivalent to human squamous cell carcinoma.[20,21,22] Squamous cell carcinoma(SCC)makes-up approximately 95% of all the oral malignancies. It is associated with various factors such as smoking, alcohol, nutritional deficiencies, and radiation exposure, also to a number of viruses and suppression of immune system.[2]

The conventional treatments for this cancer are radical surgery, radiation and chemotherapy. Despite the recent advances in cancer treatments today, the survival rate in patients with squamous cell carcinoma remains at a 50 to 59%.[2] Chemotherapy is a systemic treatment which controls the metastatic spread of tumors by destroying the cancerous cells. Using the appropriate dose of anti-cancer agents, and chemotherapy can destroy a large percentage of the cancerous cells. There are a number of various chemotherapy drugs available in the market today, some of which are used separately, however, in most cases, a combination of medications are used adjunctly.[23]

A range of drugs have been used for the purpose of chemotherapy such as cisplatin and doxorubicin, of which each can have severe side effects.[10,23]

The creation of nanotechnology has given medicine a new option and tool for the delivery and accurate transfer of the medications necessary for treating cancer.[24]

The main purpose of nanotechnology in the field of pharmacology is providing an efficient and accurate transfer of the drug to the desired target with minimal side effects and toxicity. Nanocarrier may have the following functions:

- protect a drug from destruction;
- increase drug absorption through facilitating its distribution across the intestinal membrane;
- result in the balanced effect of the drug on the body and alter the tissue distribution.[7,8]

Thus it can lead to the protection of large amounts of prescribed medication, which could be destroyed by the liver and spleen.Without a doubt, the use of colloidal metals is one of the most important parts of nanotechnology in the field of pharmacology. The first direct application is in the treatment of cancer.[7,8] To date, numerous efforts have been made and are being carried out for the active controlled transfer of drugs to the cancerous cells, most of which have focused on loading active molecules, such as antibodies that bind to cancer cells on the liposome's containing the anti-cancer drug.[9] Because of the ability of the chemotherapy nanodrug with its different coatings to penetrate the tumor tissues, Peer and Valetti revealed that the nanodrugs made with a liposomal coating were one of the most reliable carrier systems designed to receive moreover, deliver the chemotherapy nanodrugs.[25,26]

In this study, doxorubicin plus methotrexate-loaded stimuli responsive silica based nanoparticles was used. The results established that the above-mentioned system had a greater efficacy. Doxorubicin is a drug that is used to treat a variety of tumors such as sarcomas and carcinomas. Additionally, these drugs are used in hematologic malignancies (leukemia, lymphoma and multiple myeloma).[10]

Multiple studies have been carried out on the efficacy of doxorubicin in animal models.

Wang et al carried out a study targeting the therapy of hepatocellular carcinoma using pro-drugs (an inactive form) of doxorubicin. In the above-mentioned study, an increased anti-metastatic activity and decreased toxicity was observed.[27]

In a previous study by Siegal et al, they compared the efficacy of free doxorubicin with its liposomal form in animal models that had brain tumors as a secondary cancer and revealed that the use of liposome's as a carrier of cytotoxic drugs improved the treatment efficacy of the drug in brain tumors.[28]

Lingha evaluated the amount of drug released after treatment with free doxorubicin as compared to the injectable nanocarrier doxorubicin in mice implanted with breast cancers, and concluded that the application of liposomal nanodrugs increased the bioavailability of the drug and consequently, its effectiveness.[29]

Steiniger studied the effects of the nanodrugs in vivo in the treatment of glioblastoma and concluded that doxorubicin bound to nanoparticles provided greater therapeutic potential in the treatment of human glioblastoma.[30] However, to the knowledge of this study, no research has been published on the effects of nanodrugs on squamous cellcarcinoma, which was the investigative work of this study.

This investigative research on the histopathologic evaluation of the study groups revealed a significant decrease in the malignancy grade of the groups receiving doxorubicin plus methotrexate-loaded stimuli responsive silica based nanoparticles compared with its commercial form ($P < 0.001$),which demonstrated the efficacy of the nanodrug as compared to that of commercial formulary. The results of previous studies regarding various tumors are consistent with those of the present study.[27-30]

In this study, Ki-67 marker were used to evaluate the efficacy of doxorubicin plus methotrexate-loaded nanoparticles in the treatment of squamous cell carcinoma. Ki-67 is one of the most well known cell cycle-related proteins that are used in the diagnostic histopathology. This marker is a protein that is expressed on proliferated,malignant cells, and used as a marker of cell proliferation.[18,19] The efficacies of nanodrugs were evaluated using other immunohistochemical markers in various studies.[18,19]

The results of Stefani's study on glioblastoma tumor demonstrated a decrease in the expression of GFAP and VEGF markers in the groups treated by doxorubicin plus methotrexate-loaded stimuli responsive silica based nanoparticles. Since the decrease in the expression of these markers is effective in the improvement of patient's prognosis, the results revealed that the combination doxorubicin and methotrexate-loaded stimuli responsive silica based nanoparticles played a more effective role in the healing of the tumor than a free drug.[31]

Milane et al evaluated the effect of nanodrug chemotherapy on breast cancer. The study used EGFR marker to study the effects of the nanodrug. The results validated that EGFR markers and tumor sizes in the groups receiving nanodrug reduced sharply in comparison with the groups receiving the simple form drug. Since the EGFR is considered the prognostic factor, it validated that the combination doxorubicin and methotrexate-loaded stimuli responsive silica based nanoparticles is more effective in the treatment of tumors,[32] which is consistent with the results of this study. In this study, Ki -67 expression in the groups receiving oral doxorubicin plus methotrexate loaded stimuli responsive silica based nanoparticles were significantly lower than the groups receiving the commercial drug ($p < 0.001$).

Conclusion

Based on the investigative results of this study, the combination of the orally prescribed medication, doxorubicin plus methotrexate-loaded stimuli responsive silica based nanoparticles, were used for the treatment of oral squamous cell carcinoma. This combination medication demonstrated a significant reduction in the cell proliferation and severity of the malignancy, when compared with the commercial formulary form presently available for treatment of oral squamous cell carcinoma. However, it is the recommendation of this study that further research and investigative work be continued on the side effects and efficacy of the combination drug doxorubicin plus methotrexate-loaded stimuli responsive silica based nanoparticles, as compared to other pharmaceutical forms presently available for treatment of squamous cell carcinoma.

Acknowledgments

This research project with license number of 56\4537 was approved by the Research Council and School of Dentistry, Tabriz University of Medical Sciences. The researchers would like to render their deepest gratitude to the research deputy of Tabriz University of Medical Sciences for the financial support.

Conflict of Interest

Authors declare no conflict of interest.

References

1. Mehrotra R, Yadav S. Oral squamous cell carcinoma: etiology, pathogenesis and prognostic value of genomic alterations. *Indian J Cancer* 2006;43(2):60-6. doi: 10.4103/0019-509x.25886

2. Neville BW, Damm DD, Allen CM, Bouquot JE. Oral and maxillofacial pathology. 3rd ed. Philadelphia: WB Saunders co; 2009.
3. McEvoy GK, Snow EK, Kester L, Litvak K, Miller J, Welsh OH. AHFS Drug Information 2008. 1st ed. USA: American society of health system pharmacists.Bethesda. AHFS drug information; 2008.
4. Da Silva SD, Ferlito A, Takes RP, Brakenhoff RH, Valentin MD, Woolgar JA, et al. Advances and applications of oral cancer basic research. *Oral Oncol* 2011;47(9):783-91. doi: 10.1016/j.oraloncology.2011.07.004
5. Petersen PE. Oral cancer prevention and control--the approach of the World Health Organization. *Oral Oncol* 2009;45(4-5):454-60. doi: 10.1016/j.oraloncology.2008.05.023
6. Joensuu H. Systemic chemotherapy for cancer: from weapon to treatment. *Lancet Oncol* 2008;9(3):304. doi: 10.1016/s1470-2045(08)70075-5
7. Rafii-tabar E. Creation and development of nanotechnology in Iran. *Quarterly Journal of Research and Planning in Higher Education* 2002;25:188-205.
8. Kalaria DR, Sharma G, Beniwal V, Ravi Kumar MN. Design of biodegradable nanoparticles for oral delivery of doxorubicin: in vivo pharmacokinetics and toxicity studies in rats. *Pharm Res* 2009;26(3):492-501. doi: 10.1007/s11095-008-9763-4
9. Couvreur P, Vauthier C. Nanotechnology: intelligent design to treat complex disease. *Pharm Res* 2006;23(7):1417-50. doi: 10.1007/s11095-006-0284-8
10. Malekpour M, Jalali Nadushan M, Mansuri S, Hajihosseini R, Mirzaii M, Jamali D. Comparision of the cytotoxic effect of doxorubicin drug in free from and enclosed in liposomes with a negative charge and no charge in MDA-MB-231 cell line (brest cancer). *Daneshvar Journal of Shahed University* 2009;17(85):67.
11. Mudshinge SR, Deore AB, Patil S, Bhalgat CM. Nanoparticles: Emerging carriers for drug delivery. *Saudi Pharm J* 2011;19(3):129-41. doi: 10.1016/j.jsps.2011.04.001
12. Deng Z, Zhen Z, Hu X, Wu S, Xu Z, Chu PK. Hollow chitosan-silica nanospheres as pH-sensitive targeted delivery carriers in breast cancer therapy. *Biomaterials* 2011;32(21):4976-86. doi: 10.1016/j.biomaterials.2011.03.050
13. Sohrabi M, Soleimani J, Roshangar L, Vatansever S, Arbabi F, Khaki AA, et al. The effect of dietary and topical celecoxib on 4-nitroquinoline-1-oxide-induced lingual epithelium alternations in rat. *J Pak Med Assoc* 2009;59(11):769-74.
14. Shiotani H, Denda A, Yamamoto K, Kitayama W, Endoh T, Sasaki Y, et al. Increased expression of cyclooxygenase-2 protein in 4-nitroquinoline-1-oxide-induced rat tongue carcinomas and chemopreventive efficacy of a specific inhibitor, nimesulide. *Cancer Res* 2001;61(4):1451-6.
15. Arbabi Kalati F, Mesgari Abbasi M, Akbari N. Evaluation the effect of topical and systemic celecoxib on serum antioxidant in induction of tongue neoplasm in rat. *Zahedan Journal of Research in Medical Sciences* 2010;12(4):11-6.
16. Salehi R, Hamishehkar H, Eskandani M, Mahkam M, Davaran S. Development of dual responsive nanocomposite for simultaneous delivery of anticancer drugs. *J Drug Target* 2014;22(4):327-42. doi: 10.3109/1061186x.2013.876645
17. Benival DM, Devarajan PV. Lipomer of doxorubicin hydrochloride for enhanced oral bioavailability. *Int J Pharm* 2012;423(2):554-61. doi: 10.1016/j.ijpharm.2011.11.035
18. Tan Bay BH, Yip G, Selvarajan S, Tan P, Wu J, et al. Immunohistochemical detection of Ki67 in breast cancer correlates with transcriptional regulation of genes related to apoptosis and cell death. *Mod Pathol* 2005;18(3):374-81. doi: 10.1038/modpathol.3800254
19. Trihia H, Murray S, Price K, Gelber RD, Golouh R, Goldhirsch A, et al. Ki-67 expression in breast carcinoma: its association with grading systems, clinical parameters, and other prognostic factors--a surrogate marker? *Cancer* 2003;97(5):1321-31. doi: 10.1002/cncr.11188
20. Arima Y, Nishigori C, Takeuchi T, Oka S, Morimoto K, Utani A, et al. 4-Nitroquinoline 1-oxide forms 8-hydroxydeoxyguanosine in human fibroblasts through reactive oxygen species. *Toxicol Sci* 2006;91(2):382-92. doi: 10.1093/toxsci/kfj161
21. Kitakawaa D, Cabrala LAG, Marquesb MEA, Salvadorib DMF, Ribeiro DA. Medium-term tongue carcinogenesis assays: A comparative study between 4-nitroquinoline 1-oxide (4NQO)-induced rat and dimethylbenzanthracene (DMBA)-induced hamster carcinogenesis. *J Exp Anim Sci* 2006;43(3):219-27. doi: 10.1016/j.jeas.2006.09.001
22. Vered M, Yarom N, Dayan D. 4NQO oral carcinogenesis: animal models, molecular markers and future expectations. *Oral Oncol* 2005;41(4):337-9. doi: 10.1016/j.oraloncology.2004.07.005
23. Roche A, Girish BV, De Baere T, Baudin E, Boige V, Elias D, et al. Trans-catheter arterial chemoembolization as first-line treatment for hepatic metastases from endocrine tumors. *Eur Radiol* 2003;13(1):136-40. doi: 10.1007/s00330-002-1558-0
24. Endo K, Ueno T, Kondo S, Wakisaka N, Murono S, Ito M, et al. Tumor-targeted chemotherapy with the nanopolymer-based drug NC-6004 for oral squamous cell carcinoma. *Cancer Sci* 2013;104(3):369-74. doi: 10.1111/cas.12079
25. Peer D. Harnessing RNAi nanomedicine for precision therapy. *Molecular and Cellular Therapies* 2014;2:5. doi: 10.1186/2052-8426-2-5
26. Valetti S, Mura S, Stella B, Couvreur P. Rational design for multifunctional non-liposomal lipid-based nanocarriers for cancer management: theory to

practice. *J Nanobiotechnology* 2013;11(Suppl 1):S6. doi: 10.1186/1477-3155-11-s1-s6

27. Wang Q, Zhong YJ, Yuan JP, Shao LH, Zhang J, Tang L, et al. Targeting therapy of hepatocellular carcinoma with doxorubicin prodrug PDOX increases anti-metastatic effect and reduces toxicity: a preclinical study. *J Transl Med* 2013;11(1):192. doi: 10.1186/1479-5876-11-192
28. Siegal T, Horowitz A, Gabizon A. Doxorubicin encapsulated in sterically stabilized liposomes for the treatment of a brain tumor model: biodistribution and therapeutic efficacy. *J Neurosurg* 1995;83(6):1029-37. doi: 10.3171/jns.1995.83.6.1029
29. Laginha KM, Verwoert S, Charrois GJ, Allen TM. Determination of doxorubicin levels in whole tumor and tumor nuclei in murine breast cancer tumors. *Clin Cancer Res* 2005;11(19 Pt 1):6944-9. doi: 10.1158/1078-0432.CCR-05-0343
30. Steiniger SC, Kreuter J, Khalansky AS, Skidan IN, Bobruskin AI, Smirnova ZS, et al. Chemotherapy of glioblastoma in rats using doxorubicin-loaded nanoparticles. *Int J Cancer* 2004;109(5):759-67. doi: 10.1002/ijc.20048
31. Wohlfart S, Khalansky AS, Bernreuther C, Michaelis M, Cinatl J Jr, Glatzel M, et al. Treatment of glioblastoma with poly(isohexyl cyanoacrylate) nanoparticles. *Int J Pharm* 2011;415(1-2):244-51. doi: 10.1016/j.ijpharm.2011.05.046
32. Milane L, Duan Z, Amiji M. Therapeutic efficacy and safety of paclitaxel/lonidamine loaded EGFR-targeted nanoparticles for the treatment of multi-drug resistant cancer. *PLoS One* 2011;6(9):e24075. doi: 10.1371/journal.pone.0024075

Evaluation of Flavonoid Derivative and Doxorubicin Effects in Lung Cancer Cells (A549) Using Differential Pulse Voltammetry Method

Mohammad Amjadi[1], Jalal Mohammadi Khoshraj[1]*, Mir Reza Majidi[1], Behzad Baradaran[2], Miguel de la Guardia[3]

[1] *Department of Analytical Chemistry, Chemistry Faculty, Tabriz University, Tabriz, Iran.*
[2] *Immunology Research Center, Tabriz University of Medical Sciences, Tabriz, Iran.*
[3] *Department of Analytical Chemistry, University of Valencia, Valencia, Spain.*

Article info

Keywords:
- Lung neoplasms
- Doxorubicin
- Electrochemistry
- Voltammetry

Abstract

Purpose: Electrochemical measurements have prompted the progress as a consequence of their affectability, cost-affectivity and comparatively short examination time. The aim of this study was the fast evaluation of the effect of chemotherapy compounds on the viability of lung cancer cells (A549) via electrochemical methods.

Methods: Cyclic voltammetry (CV) was used as a primary method to distinguish between electrochemical behavior of normal and lung cancer cells. Differential pulse voltammetry (DPV) was employed as a complementary analyses method for the impact of doxorubicin (DOX) and Flavonoid modified drug (FMD) (US patent Application number: 62548886) on Lung cancer cells.

Results: Only one oxidative peak, at approximately -0.15 V was detected through DPV method in cancer cell line. While a significant distinguish was not seen in CV. The current intensity (I) was decreased in cancer cells with increasing the DOX and FMD levels ($t=99.027$, $\alpha=0.05$, $P=0.0000$), ($t=135.513$, $\alpha=0.05$, $P=0.0000$), respectively.

Conclusion: The movement of cancerous cells towards death through chemotherapy drugs such as DOX and FMD can make distinct and significant changes in the electrochemical behaviors of those cells.

Introduction

The intercellular communications, intracellular action and peripheral reactions of cell organelles are as yet not completely comprehended and ensemble averaged measurement of millions of cells together, being not able to give point by point data at single cell level. To evaluate the cell action, single cell analysis can be made by joining capillary electrophoresis with laser induced fluorescence or electrochemical detection, mass spectrometry or flow cytometry.[1] Electrochemical procedures have prompted the progress in the field of analysis, as a result of their affectability, low cost, and comparatively short examination time, when compared to other methods. Extra utilization of electro-analytical procedures incorporates the assurance of response mechanisms. Redox properties of variety of cells can give some knowledge about its metabolic activity or in vivo redox medication actions.[2] Differential Pulse voltammetry (DPV) is a form of linear sweep and staircase voltammetry, helpful to assay low levels of biological and mineral analytes in terms of redox activity. In DPV sequences of typical voltage pulses are superimposed on the potential linear sweep or stair steps. Lung cancer cells can be evaluated by DPV method under electrical field and can show the viability of the cells. In the differential pulse voltammogram, the tallness of the current peak obtained as a function of potential can be related to the concentration of analytes. The peak potential shifts being employed to recognize the detected species. DPV also give data about the chemical form of target analytes, as complexation and oxidation status. Hence, this technology has likewise been generally used for the electrochemical examination of proteins and cells.[3,4]

Lung cancer is one of the main sources of cancer related mortality around the world,[5] being the second most ordinarily recognized malignancy in men and women, that involved approximately 224,390 new cases and 158,080 deaths in 2016 as indicated by the American Cancer Society.[6] Because of that it is an important point to make an early diagnostics of lung cancer and to evaluate the affectivity of pharmaceuticals developed for its treatment.[7] Dox is a new class of chemotherapy that can increase the curative of lung cancer cells.[8] Polyphenols have assigned a special place in the nature in vivo/in vitro studies because of having multiple biological activities, such as: strong anti-oxidants, anti-inflammatory, anti-tumor. Quercetin with the chemical formula ($C_{15}H_{10}O_7$) as one of the important members of the polyphenols group, has the following characteristics:[9] Free radical scavenger,[10] inhibitor of TNF-α,[11] cyclooxygenase 2 and lipoxygenase

***Corresponding author:** Jalal Mohammadi Khoshraj, Email: j.mohammadi@tabrizu.ac.ir inhibitors,[12] and also chelator of intermediate metals such as iron ions that can initiate free radical formation[13] reducing the expression of a mutated P53 gene in human breast cancer cell line,[12,14,15] protecting DNA damage from chemicals,[16] the inhibitor of the synthesis of heat shock proteins,[17] inhibitor of cyclin D1 and survivin expression,[18] inhibitor of P21-ras expression in human colon cancer cell line.[19] The presence of other polyphenols along with quercetin in the FMD (cross linked chitosan-quercetin-other polyphenols) would have an extraordinary synergistic effect in enhancing the antioxidant power. The goal of this study has been the evaluation of A549 line cancer cell electrochemical behavior with carbon electrodes by voltammetry in treatment with FMD and DOX.

Materials and Methods

A stock solution of 1.0 $\times 10^{-2}$ M DOX (Sigma Aldrich, USA) was prepared in ethanol and diluted with water. Phosphate buffer solution (PBS) was used as the medium electrolyte in all experiments. Electrochemical analysis were made using an AUTOLAB 30 analyzer (Eco Chemie Netherlands) with a standard cell of three electrodes; a glassy carbon as working electrode, an Ag/AgCl/3M KCl reference electrode and a platinum auxiliary electrode. The alternating current (AC) voltage amplitude employed was 10 mv and the balance time was 5 s. All tests were made at optimum temperature.[20, 21] Samples were put into the detection cell and handled by DPV in the vicinity of 0.0 and 1.0 V (versus Ag/AgCl) until a stable voltammogram was acquired. Fresh PBS containing living cells was inserted into the measuring chamber immediately. All the electrochemical experiments were done at 37 ± 1°C. The DPV was also be used to quantify the effect of DOX concentration on A549 cell line as follows:

Effect of DOX = 100%× (Ap control – Ap DOX)/ Ap Control being Ap DOX and Ap control the peak areas of DPV obtained for A549 cells treated with and without DOX, respectively.

Cell examination

Lung cancer cell line A549 and L929, as a normal cell line (Pasteur Institute of Iran) were cultured in RPMI-1640 medium (Sigma Aldrich, USA) with penicillin (100 U/ml), streptomycin (100 μg/ml), FBS 10 % (v/v), and incubated at 37 °C in humidified 5 % CO_2. After culturing cells for 5 days, they were collected by trypsinization with 0.05 % (v/v) trypsin (Sigma Aldrich), centrifuged at 1200 rpm for 10 min, and then suspended in PBS. The concentration of the cells was examined by standard pour plate (PPC) technique. For drug tests, cells were admitted to proliferate and stick for 24 h in culture medium before exposure to DOX. A similar amount of alcohol was supplemented to the control cells to exclude the impact of ethanol on the lung cancer cells. Morphological changes of the cells, before and afterwards of the presence to DOX, were seen with a Nikon Eclipse optical microscope TE-300 (Japan). Cell viability was checked by the 3- (4, 5-dimethyl thiazol-2-yl)-2, 5-diphenyl-2H tetrazolium bromide (MTT) colorimetric assay. Cells (15×10^3 cells/well in 96 wells) were handled with various concentrations of DOX (0-600 μg/mL) for 24 hours, then 0.5 mg/mL in dimethyl sulfoxide (DMSO) was added to each well. After incubation at 37 °C for two hours, an equal volume of 90 % isopropanol and 0.5 % sodium dodecyl sulfate (SDS) (400 μL) was added to dissolve the MTT formazan crystals, and the absorbance was measured at 570 nm using an ELISA microplate reader (State Fax 2100, USA). The percentage of cell viability was calculated as: (A549 of treated cells/ A549 of untreated cells) ×100. A549 cell viability was accomplished at the same time by treating the cells with different concentrations of DOX.[22]

Statistical analysis

The data were subjected to standard one-way analysis of variance (ANOVA). The means were compared using Duncan Multiple Range test at the 5% confidence level also t-test was used to test the statistical difference between two group means at the 5% confidence level. Data was analyzed in SPSS19 and MSTATC software.

Results and Discussion

Electrochemistry examinations

Comparison between cyclic voltammetry (CV) outcomes of lung cancer and normal cells in PBS are illustrated in Figure 1 at a scan rate of 50 mV s^{-1}, while reductive peak was detected under the same position. In Figure 2 an apparent peak around -0.15 V was detected when the cells were added to the PBS. No peak was found in the blank solution, normal cell line and also PBS solution. The mean difference between the various groups along with normal cell line was significant in comparison with A549 (F=3.227 E15, α=0.05, P=0.0004). However, this difference was not statistically significant among all groups except A549.

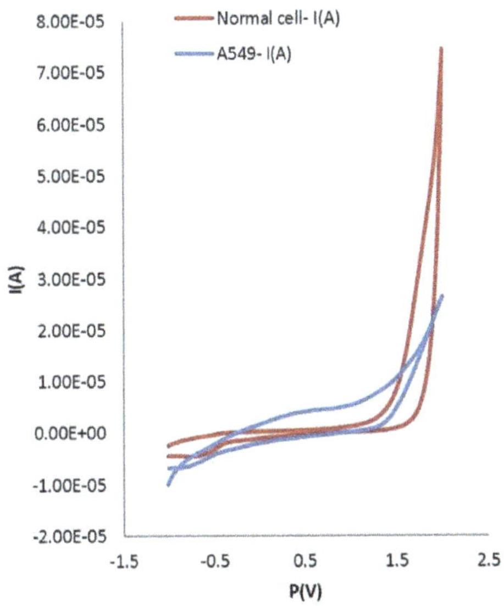

Figure 1. Comparison between CV results of lung cancer cells and normal cells in PBS at glassy carbon electrode; for the oxidative peak (upper line) and the reductive peak (lower line). Cell density, 3×10^6 cells mL^{-1}; scan rate, 50 mV s^{-1}. (t=0.677: α=0.05, P=0.5)

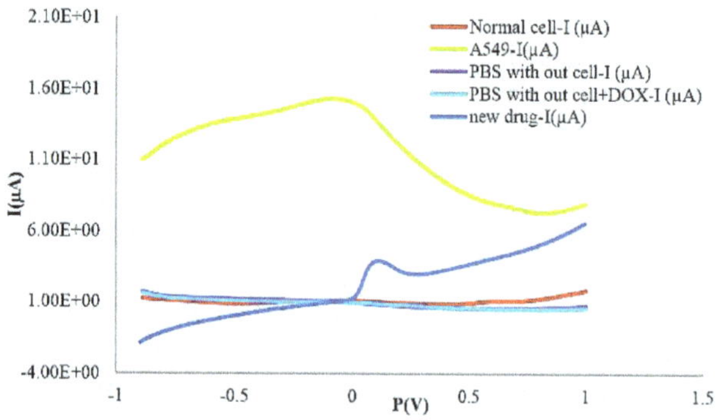

Figure 2. Comparison between DPV responses of lung cancer cells and normal cells in PBS and presence of FMD. Cell density: 3×10^6 cells mL^{-1}; scan rate, 50 mV s^{-1}.

Figure 3 and 4 show the DPV method of different concentrations of DOX on the A549 cell line. For DOX concentration from 0.02to 0.08 mg, the I index was decreased (t=99.027, α=0.05, P=0.0000). It needs to be mentioned that the I index was as same as A549 cell line around 0.08 mg. No crucial difference was seen when the concentration of DOX was higher than 100 μM. From 0.08 to 2 mg, the rate of decreasing was continued. Figure 5 and 6 show the impact of various concentrations of FMD on lung cancer cells which A549 cell line without any drug had the highest I (10.9 μA) among different concentration of FMD (t=135.513, α=0.05, P=0.0000). As FMD concentration was increased the I index decreased regularly up to 8.92μA.

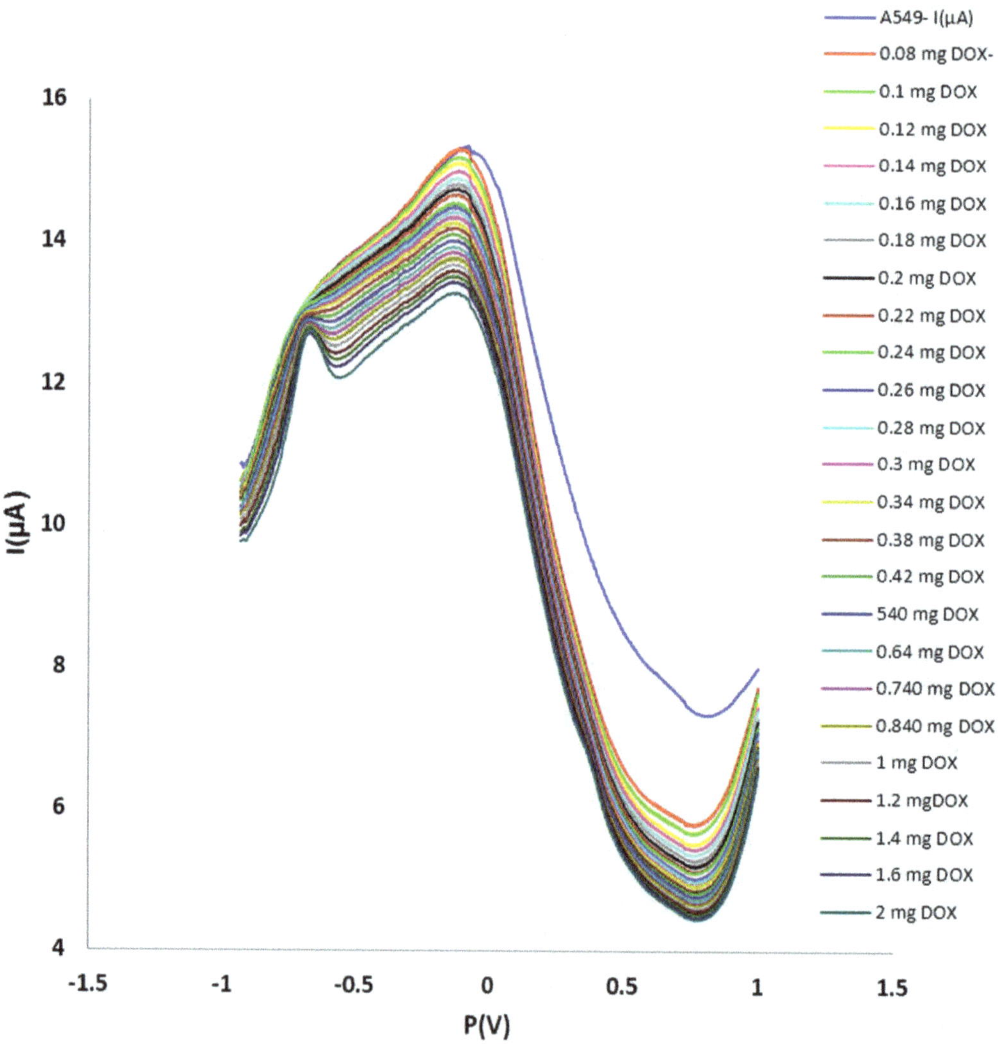

Figure 3. Effect of different concentrations of DOX on lung cancer cells A549. Cell density: 3×10^6 cells mL^{-1}; scan rate, 50 mV s^{-1}.

Electrochemical techniques have been confirmed as a sensitive way for detection of biological molecules.[23] With simple, rapid, sensitive and easily operated features, DPV has been applied to evaluate cell viability in the presence of pharmaceuticals.[4] The electrochemical behavior of A549 cancer cell line in relation with DOX and FMD at glassy carbon electrode was assembled and examined for the first-time through this study. Feng *et al.* studied electrochemical behavior of U937 cells and its performance in evaluating the effect of caffeic acid. They exploited the electrochemical procedure to investigate the effectiveness of caffeic acid on the treatment of cancer cells. This finding was parallel to the hindrance effect of caffeic acid on the viability of U937 explored by the trypan blue test,[24] which are also in agreement with the results of this study.

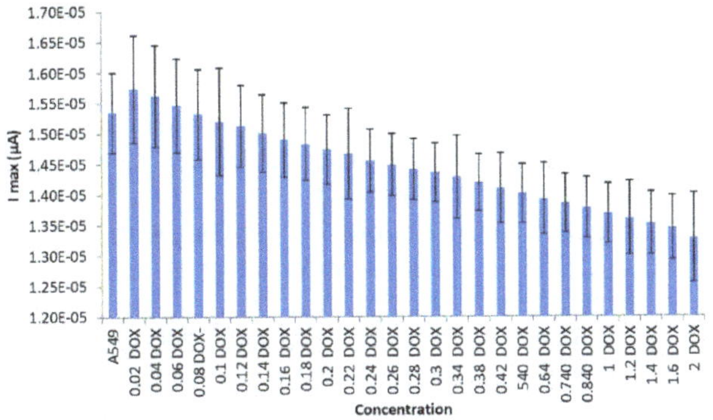

Figure 4. Effect of different concentrations of DOX on lung cancer cells A549.

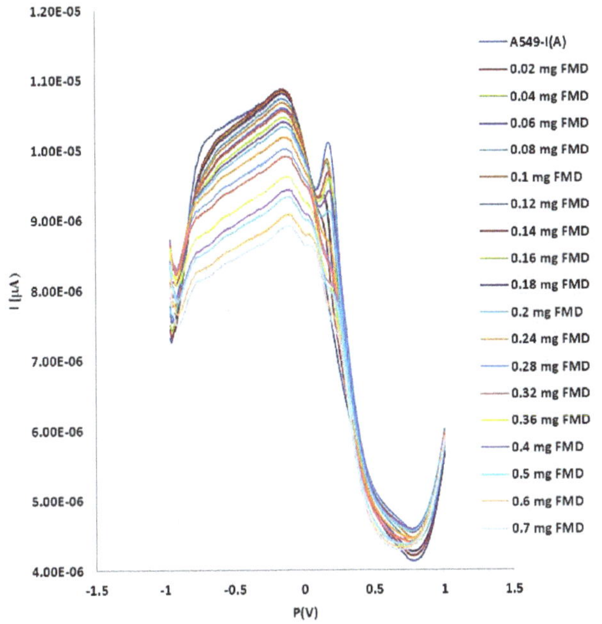

Figure 5. Effect of different concentrations of FMD on lung cancer cells. Cell density: $3{\times}10^6$ cells mL^{-1}; scan rate, 50 mV s^{-1}.

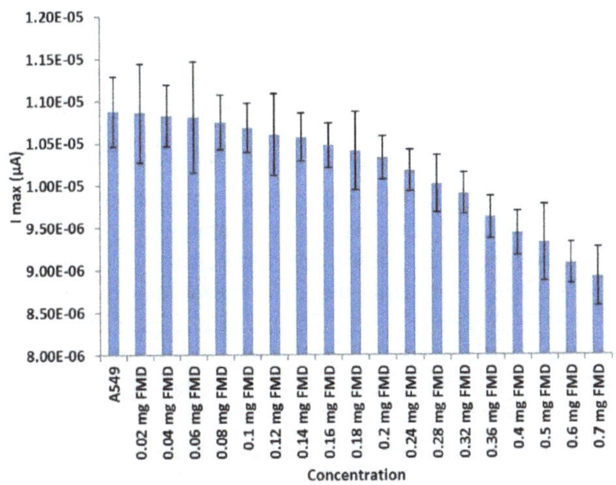

Figure 6. Effect of different concentrations of FMD on lung cancer cells A549. I max based on mg FMD

In a study of Chunmei Yu *et al.*[25] by modified electrode on K562 cancer cell line treated with arsenic trioxide and cyclophosphamide through CV and DPV exhibited that increasing the drug concentration induced the decrease of electrochemical responses significantly. In another works by João G. Pacheco et al. and Kun Wang et al.,[26,27] the preparation of a new biosensor with modified electrodes for breast cancer cells and the use of CV-DPV electrochemical methods to determine the amount and number of cancer cells by plotting the calibration curve allowed the detection of the number of cancer cells in the unknown sample.

In 2005 the electrochemical action of breast tumor cells (MCF-7) was assessed by CV and potentiometric stripping analysis (PSA) by Li and co-workers.[3] The MCF-7 cells were found to generate a PSA signal. The influence of diosgenin on the MCF-7 cells was also successfully evaluated by PSA. In the present study, CV was used for introductory experiments for distinguishing normal and lung cancer cells. Because of its high efficiency, DPV was used for complementary survey of the effect of pharmaceuticals on cell lines viability. The peaks obtained from electrochemical analyses of normal and cancer cells were different. Methods as MTT were already employed for exploiting the effects of medication on cancer cells. The effects of drugs on normal and cancer cells were inspected by the electrochemistry measurements, including CV and DPV. As shown in Figure 3, at concentrations of approximately 0.08 mg of DOX, it may be able to activate the potential pathway of apoptosis.[28] There is a peak around -0.5 V, and that is related to the DOX drug.[29]

Rising redox in the estimated limit of -0.15V in A549 cancer cell line seems to be due to the formation of pyruvate and lactate in the context of the Warburg phenomenon. The impact of doxorubicin dose providing a strong reduction of carcinoma cells, and as a result, we could be faced with the probable decline of pyruvate and lactate.[30-32] However, the use of DPV requires about one minute, while MTT test needs about 7 days to be finished. The FMD drug showed better results in cell death compared to DOX, while both drugs standard concentration were the same. For probably apoptosis of 3 million cells, a dose of 2 mg of DOX was required, but for FMD only 0.7 mg was used.[33]

Conclusion

In this study, the effects of two different drugs on cancer cells were investigated through CV and DPV. Results show that FMD (US patent Application number: 62548886) to treat the cancer, has a much better effect than DOX. Additionally, since in this survey unmodified carbon glassy electrode was exploited, this technique can be considered highly reproducible and could be used in clinical trials.

Conflict of Interest

The authors declare that they have no conflicts of interest.

References

1. Tseng F-G, Santra TS. Essentials of Single-Cell Analysis: Concepts, Applications and Future Prospects. Germany: Springer; 2016.
2. Kalanur SS, Seetharamappa J, Mamatha GP, Hadagali MD, Kandagal PB. Electrochemical behavior of an anti-cancer drug at glassy carbon electrode and its determination in pharmaceutical formulations. *Int J Electrochem Sci* 2008;3(7):756-67.
3. Li J, Liu X, Guo M, Liu Y, Liu S, Yao S. Electrochemical study of breast cancer cells mcf-7 and its application in evaluating the effect of diosgenin. *Anal Sci* 2005;21(5):561-4.
4. Li G, Miao P. Electrochemical analysis of proteins and cells. Berlin Heidelberg: Springer Science & Business Media; 2012.
5. Devarakonda S, Masood A, Govindan R. Next-generation sequencing of lung cancers: Lessons learned and future directions. *Hematol Oncol Clin North Am* 2017;31(1):1-12. doi: 10.1016/j.hoc.2016.08.008
6. Zukotynski KA, Gerbaudo VH. Molecular imaging and precision medicine in lung cancer. *PET Clin* 2017;12(1):53-62. doi: 10.1016/j.cpet.2016.08.008
7. Rossi A, Maione P, Colantuoni G, Gaizo FD, Guerriero C, Nicolella D, et al. Screening for lung cancer: New horizons? *Crit Rev Oncol Hematol* 2005;56(3):311-20. doi: 10.1016/j.critrevonc.2005.04.007
8. Gabizon A, Shmeeda H, Barenholz Y. Pharmacokinetics of pegylated liposomal doxorubicin. *Clin Pharmacokinet* 2003;42(5):419-36. doi: 10.2165/00003088-200342050-00002
9. Sak K. Site-specific anticancer effects of dietary flavonoid quercetin. *Nutr Cancer* 2014;66(2):177-93. doi: 10.1080/01635581.2014.864418
10. Di Meo F, Lemaur V, Cornil J, Lazzaroni R, Duroux JL, Olivier Y, et al. Free radical scavenging by natural polyphenols: Atom versus electron transfer. *J Phys Chem A* 2013;117(10):2082-92. doi: 10.1021/jp3116319
11. Gupta SC, Tyagi AK, Deshmukh-Taskar P, Hinojosa M, Prasad S, Aggarwal BB. Downregulation of tumor necrosis factor and other proinflammatory biomarkers by polyphenols. *Arch Biochem Biophys* 2014;559:91-9. doi: 10.1016/j.abb.2014.06.006
12. Upadhyay S, Dixit M. Role of polyphenols and other phytochemicals on molecular signaling. *Oxid Med Cell Longev* 2015;2015:504253. doi: 10.1155/2015/504253
13. Perron NR, Brumaghim JL. A review of the antioxidant mechanisms of polyphenol compounds related to iron binding. *Cell Biochem Biophys* 2009;53(2):75-100. doi: 10.1007/s12013-009-9043-x
14. Soleas GJ, Goldberg DM, Grass L, Levesque M, Diamandis EP. Do wine polyphenols modulate p53 gene expression in human cancer cell lines? *Clin Biochem* 2001;34(5):415-20.
15. Abdal Dayem A, Choi HY, Yang GM, Kim K, Saha SK, Cho SG. The anti-cancer effect of polyphenols against breast cancer and cancer stem cells: Molecular mechanisms. *Nutrients* 2016;8(9): pii: E581. doi: 10.3390/nu8090581
16. Liu CM, Ma JQ, Xie WR, Liu SS, Feng ZJ, Zheng GH, et al. Quercetin protects mouse liver against nickel-induced DNA methylation and inflammation associated with the nrf2/ho-1 and p38/stat1/nf-kappab pathway. *Food Chem Toxicol* 2015;82:19-26. doi: 10.1016/j.fct.2015.05.001
17. Lee SH, Lee EJ, Min KH, Hur GY, Lee SH, Lee SY, et al. Quercetin enhances chemosensitivity to gemcitabine in lung cancer cells by inhibiting heat shock protein 70 expression. *Clin Lung Cancer* 2015;16(6):e235-43. doi: 10.1016/j.cllc.2015.05.006
18. Fu SM, Xu MX, Lin SM, Liang Z, Cai JH. Association of cyclin d1 and survivin expression with sensitivity to radiotherapy in patients with nasopharyngeal carcinoma. *Genet Mol Res* 2014;13(2):3502-9. doi: 10.4238/2014.February.14.6
19. Raja SB, Rajendiran V, Kasinathan NK, P A, Venkatabalasubramanian S, Murali MR, et al. Differential cytotoxic activity of quercetin on colonic cancer cells depends on ROS generation through COX-2 expression. *Food Chem Toxicol* 2017;106(Pt A):92-106. doi: 10.1016/j.fct.2017.05.006
20. Supalkova V, Petrek J, Havel L, Krizkova S, Petrlova J, Adam V, et al. Electrochemical sensors for detection of acetylsalicylic acid. *Sensors* 2006;6(11):1483-97. doi:10.3390/s6111483
21. Hasanzadeh M, Sadeghi S, Bageri L, Mokhtarzadeh A, Karimzadeh A, Shadjou N, et al. Poly-dopamine-beta-cyclodextrin: A novel nanobiopolymer towards sensing of some amino acids at physiological ph. *Mater Sci Eng C Mater Biol Appl* 2016;69:343-57. doi: 10.1016/j.msec.2016.06.081
22. Chang CT, Korivi M, Huang HC, Thiyagarajan V, Lin KY, Huang PJ, et al. Inhibition of ros production, autophagy or apoptosis signaling reversed the anticancer properties of antrodia salmonea in triple-negative breast cancer (MDA-MB-231) cells. *Food Chem Toxicol* 2017;103:1-17. doi: 10.1016/j.fct.2017.02.019
23. Bukkitgar SD, Shetti NP. Electrochemical behavior of anticancer drug 5-fluorouracil at carbon paste electrode and its analytical application. *J Anal Sci Technol* 2016;7(1):1-9. doi: 10.1186/s40543-015-0080-3
24. Feng J, Luo GA, Jian HY, Wang RG, An CC. Voltammetric behavior of tumor cells U937 and its

usefulness in evaluating the effect of caffeic acid. *Electroanal* 2000;12(7):513-6.doi: 10.1002/(SICI)1521-4109(200005)12:7<513::AID-ELAN513>3.0.CO;2-D

25. Yu C, Zhu Z, Wang L, Wang Q, Bao N, Gu H. A new disposable electrode for electrochemical study of leukemia k562 cells and anticancer drug sensitivity test. *Biosens Bioelectron* 2014;53:142-7. doi: 10.1016/j.bios.2013.09.044
26. Wang K, He MQ, Zhai FH, He RH, Yu YL. A novel electrochemical biosensor based on polyadenine modified aptamer for label-free and ultrasensitive detection of human breast cancer cells. *Talanta* 2017;166:87-92. doi: 10.1016/j.talanta.2017.01.052
27. Pacheco JG, Silva MS, Freitas M, Nouws HP, Delerue-Matos C. Molecularly imprinted electrochemical sensor for the point-of-care detection of a breast cancer biomarker (CA 15-3). *Sensor Actuat B Chem* 2018;256:905-12. doi: 10.1016/j.snb.2017.10.027
28. Farhane Z, Bonnier F, Howe O, Casey A, Byrne HJ. Doxorubicin kinetics and effects on lung cancer cell lines using in vitro raman micro-spectroscopy: Binding signatures, drug resistance and DNA repair. *J Biophotonics* 2018;11(1). doi: 10.1002/jbio.201700060
29. Hashemzadeh N, Hasanzadeh M, Shadjou N, Eivazi-Ziaei J, Khoubnasabjafari M, Jouyban A. Graphene quantum dot modified glassy carbon electrode for the determination of doxorubicin hydrochloride in human plasma. *J Pharm Anal* 2016;6(4):235-41. doi: 10.1016/j.jpha.2016.03.003
30. Keizer HG, Pinedo HM, Schuurhuis GJ, Joenje H. Doxorubicin (adriamycin): A critical review of free radical-dependent mechanisms of cytotoxicity. *Pharmacol Ther* 1990;47(2):219-31.
31. Berg JM, Tymoczko JL, Stryer L. Biochemistry (Loose-Leaf). San Francisco: Freeman; 2008.
32. Tannock IF, Rotin D. Acid PH in tumors and its potential for therapeutic exploitation. *Cancer Res* 1989;49(16):4373-84.
33. Mizutani H, Tada-Oikawa S, Hiraku Y, Kojima M, Kawanishi S. Mechanism of apoptosis induced by doxorubicin through the generation of hydrogen peroxide. *Life Sci* 2005;76(13):1439-53. doi: 10.1016/j.lfs.2004.05.040

Effects of NDRG2 Overexpression on Metastatic Behaviors of HCT116 Colorectal Cancer Cell Line

Ali Golestan[1], Abbas Ghaderi[2], Zahra Mojtahedi[2]*

[1] *Autophagy Research Center, Shiraz University of Medical Sciences, Shiraz, Iran.*
[2] *Institute for Cancer Research, Shiraz University of Medical Sciences, Shiraz, Iran.*

Article info

Keywords:
· Colorectal cancer
· NDRG2
· Invasion
· Migration
· Matrix metalloproteinase

Abstract

Purpose: N-myc downstream-regulated gene 2 (NDRG2) is frequently down-regulated in cancer, and plays an important role in the control of tumor growth and metastasis. Its manipulation has been suggested as a therapy in cancer. Here, we examined the outcome of NDRG2 overexpression on proliferation, invasion, migration and MMP activity of HCT116 colorectal cancer cell line.

Methods: The HCT116 cell line (human colorectal cancer) was transfected with pCMV6-AC-GFP-NDRG2. 2,5diphenyltetrazolium bromide (MTT) assay was used to detect cell proliferation. The invasion and migration of the transfected cells were examined through transwell chambers while the MMP-9 activity was detected by the ability of the cells to digest gelatin.

Results: Overexpression of NDRG2 by stable NDRG2 transfection decreased cell proliferation, migration and invasion ability, along with decreasing MMP-9 activity.

Conclusion: Our data indicate that NDRG2 overexpression can suppress several aspect of tumorigenesis. Further investigations are necessitated to verify if NDRG2 molecule can be a therapeutic target in colorectal cancer.

Introduction

Colorectal cancer is a top-cancer killer worldwide, and its incidence is rising in several countries including Iran.[1] Novel therapeutic targets remain the choice to overcome the advanced disease and treatment failure. N-myc downstream-regulated gene 2 (NDRG2) belongs to a family of differentiation-related molecules.[2] NDRG2 has shown tumor suppressor activities in certain cancer models, and its manipulation has attracted much attention as a therapeutic target in cancer.[3]

NDRG2 is mainly expressed in skeletal muscles, the heart, brain, liver and kidney under physiological conditions.[4] It is reported that NDRG2 is under expressed in certain types of cancer (e.g., liver, thyroid, and breast cancers), suggesting a possible role for NDRG2 in tumor suppression,[5,6] In vitro assays in several cancers such as colon have shown that tumor migration and invasion were diminished after NDRG2 overexpression.[7] An important mechanism which links the overexpression of NDRG2 to compromising invasion is the downregulation of matrix metalloproteinases (MMPs), a group of zinc-dependent endo-proteinases with remarkable roles in tissue remodeling and homeostasis.[3,8] MMPs are main culprit molecules in advancing invasion and metastasis through digestion of extracellular matrix (ECM) and basement membrane components[3]. In addition to invasion ability, NRGD2 overexpression has been demonstrated to inhibit cell proliferation and upregulate tumpr suppressor p53.[9] These findings point out NDRG2 as a potential tumor suppressor gene in the studied models.

Emerging evidence demonstrates the involvement of NDRG2 in colon cancer. In recent studies, NDRG2 was found to decrease in colorectal carcinoma.[10] Furthermore, NDRG2 expression inhibited colon cancer cell proliferation by down regulation of AP-1 activity.[11]

Whether NDRG2 expression plays different roles in different types of colon cancer needs more clarification. Mutation in the Kirsten Ras (KRAS) oncogene occurs in up to 30% of colorectal cancer patients which has been associated with poorer survival.[12] We have previously investigated how NDRG2 overexpression affects cell proliferation and invasion in SW48 cells,[13] a highly invasive colon cell line with no KRAS mutation.[14] We found that overexpression of NDRG2 reduced SW48 cell proliferation as well as migration and invasion, possibly through suppressing MMP-9 activity. Here, we investigated the outcome of NDRG2 overexpression on proliferation, invasion, migration, and MMP-9 activity in HCT116 cells, a model of colon cancer with a KRAS mutation.

***Corresponding author:** Zahra Mojtahedi, Email: mojtahediz@sums.ac.ir

Materials and Methods

The human colorectal cancer cell line HCT116 (ATCC^{R} CCL-231^{TM}) was purchased from Pasteur institute of Iran. Cells were grown under standard conditions.[13] Shuttle vector pCMV6-AC-GFP plasmid (Origene), with and without NDRG2 gene, was amplified with manual amplification protocol as described previously.[13] E.coli competent cells were prepared and transformed with the plasmid, then plasmid was purified using PureLink™ HiPure Plasmid Filter Purification Kit (Invitrogen). Lipofectamine (Invitrogen) was used to transfect HCT116 cells with the plasmid pCMV6-AC- GFP-NDRG2 (NDRG2 group) or pCMV6-AC-GFP vector alone (mock group).

Stable transfected HCT116 cells were produced. Cell growth following stable transfection was evaluated by MTT assay. The ability of cells for invasion and migration was measured through the number of cells penetrating transwell membrane of Boyden chambers. In vitro wound healing was analyzed using scratch assay. The activity of MMP-9 was detected using gelatin zymography. These assays were applied to each of the three groups: WT group (non infected cells), mock group (pCMV6-AC-GFP) and NDRG2 group (pCMV6-AC-GFP-NDRG2). The details of all the above experiments were previously described.[13]

Statistical analysis was done using Graphpad Prism (version5) software. One-way ANOVA calculated the differences between studied groups followed by Tukey Post Hoc multiple comparisons. For wound healing assay, student *t*-test was performed. All data are represented by the mean ± standard deviation of three independent experiments. A P value less than 0.05 was considered significant.

Results and Discussion

Here, we explored the effect of overexpression of NDRG2, a potential tumor suppressor molecule, on proliferation, migration and invasion ability of HCT116 colon cancer cell line. HCT116cells were stably transfected with either pCMV6-AC-GFP (mock) or pCMV6-AC-GFP-NDRG2 plasmid.

In order to investigate the effect of NDRG2 overexpression on cell proliferation, MTT assay was used. Our results clearly indicated that NDRG2 overexpression decreased cell proliferation rate from third day and became more obviously thereafter compared to control groups (Figure1). The reduced proliferation of cancer cell lines after NDRG2 overexpression has been shown by other investigators.[9,13] At molecular levels, it has been found that NDRG2 affects cell viability through interaction with tumor suppressor p53.[9] In addition to p53, NDRG2 has been shown to affect cell viability through autophagy pathway.[15]

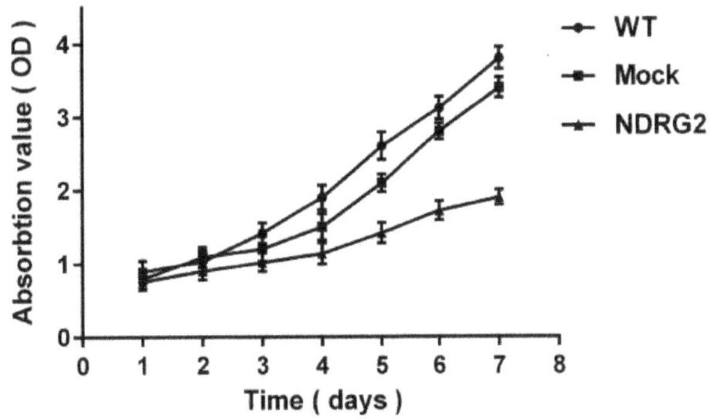

Figure 1. Overexpression of NDRG2 inhibits HCT116 cell proliferation. Cell proliferation rate was determined by MTT assay. The assays were repeated thrice, and illustrated as the mean ± SD. *=P<0.001.

The effect of NDRG2 overexpression on migration and invasion (matrigel coated transwells) revealed that forced expression of NDRG2 in HCT116 cells significantly suppressed their migration and invasion through the transwell membranes (P<0.001). Figure 2 indicates a representative of the number of traversed cells through matrigel coated transwells (data for migration assay not shown). Wound healing assay was used to determine the effect of NDRG2 overexpression on cell motility. After stable transfection, cells were stained at three interval times. This assay showed that after 24h, the NDRG2 group cells covered less than 73% of the wound, whereas mock group cells were able to close about 100% of the wound, indicating NDRG2 overexpression inhibits cell motility (Figure 3). Collectively, our results regarding migration and invasion ability of NDRG2 transfcted cells demonstrated a suppression in these activities, which is consistent with many prior publications,[13,16] but not all.[17]

Gelatin zymography of the conditioned media of cells was used for analyzing secreted MMP-9 activity. Gelatin zymographic analysis revealed that secretion of gelatinolytic MMP-9 was significantly decreased in NDRG2 transfected cells (P<0.001; data not shown), indicating that suppressive activity of the cells on migration and invasion might partly be mediated through a reduction in MMP-9 activity. There are other mechanisms through which NDRG2 overexpression can suppress tumor invasion, notably the attenuation of NF-Kβ signaling,[16] abrogation of laminin 232 pathway (a key pathway in tumor cell invasion, migration, and survival),[18] and interaction with autophagy pathway.[15]

Our results in the current study are similar to our earlier findings on another colon cancer line SW48. HCT116 cell line has a mutation in Kras gene (codon 13).[14] SW48 has no mutation in KRAS and considered a wild type in this respect. The *KRAS* is mutated in approximately 30%-50% of colorectal cancers. There are some targeted therapies in colon cancer that are administered to patients based on *KRAS* mutational status of tumor samples.[19] In two separate studies, we confirmed that NDRG2 overexpression has anti-cancer effects in both KRAS mutated and nonmutated models. Whether manipulating NDRG2 can be therapeutic in a wide range of colon cancer patients independent of KRAS mutation needs more investigations.

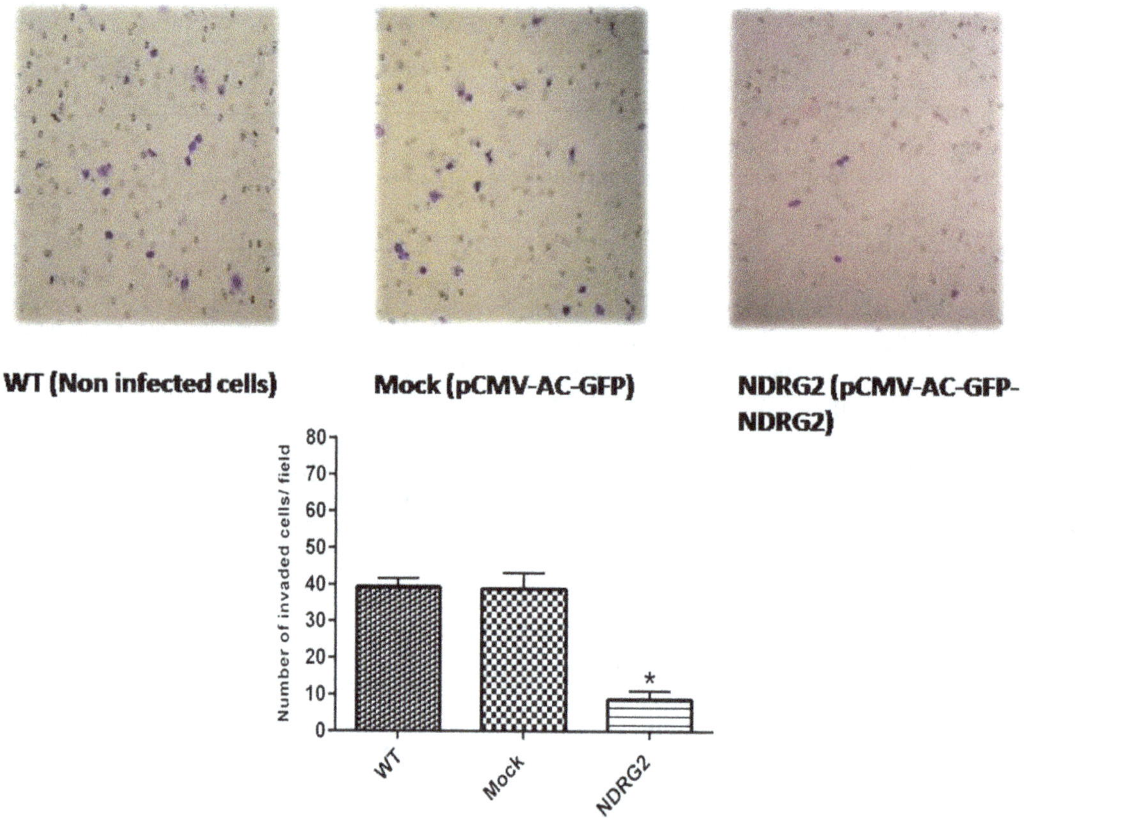

Figure 2. Invasion analysis of HCT116 cells treated using matrigel-coated transwells indicates a lower invasiveness of NDRG2 group cells than the other two groups. The assays were repeated thrice. The magnification of light microscope is 100×. *p<0.001.

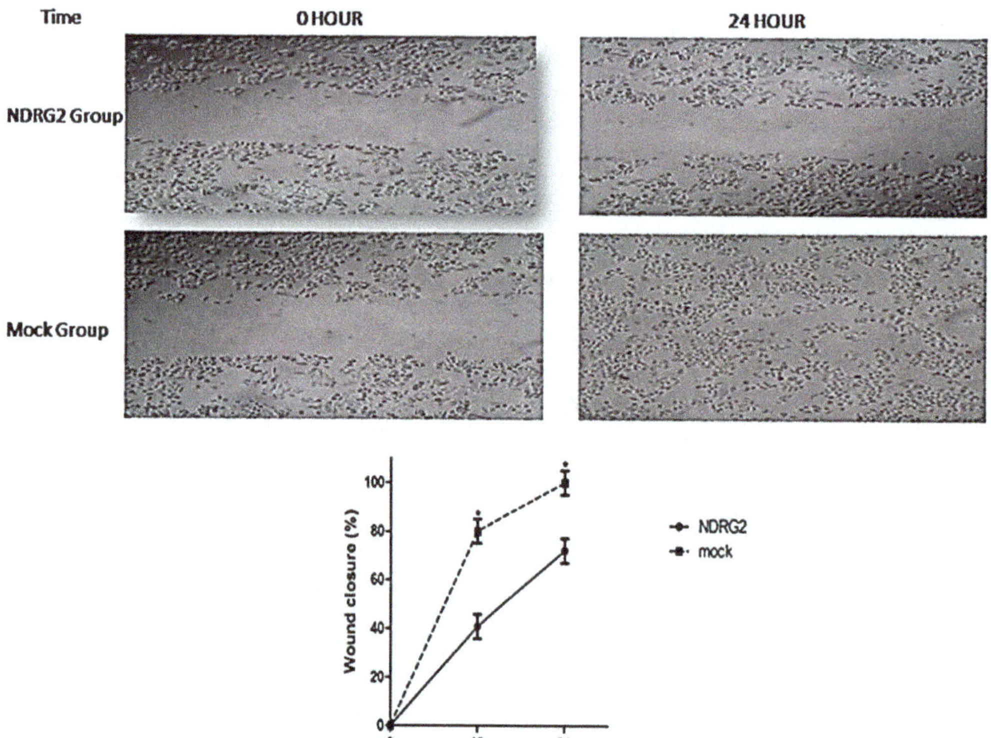

Figure 3. Wound healing assay for HCT116 cells. Photographs were taken at 40× magnification. The wound closure was quantified at 0h, and 24h post-wound by measuring the remaining unmigrated area using image J. *p<0.01.

Conclusion

Our *in-vitro* model demonstrates that the NDRG2 overexpression attenuates several aspects of tumorigenesis including the proliferation and invasive potential of human colorectal cancer cell line HCT116, a widely used model for KRAS mutated colorectal cancer. Our data in combination with our prior publications on a KRAS mutated negative cell line point to NDRG2 as a potential therapeutic target for colorectal cancer.

Acknowledgments

This work was financially supported by Shiraz Institute for Cancer Research (grant number: ICR 500). The authors declare no conflict of interest.

Conflict of Interest

The authors declare no conflict of interests.

References

1. Masoompour SM, Lankarani KB, Honarvar B, Tabatabaee SH, Moghadami M, Khosravizadegan Z. Changing epidemiology of common cancers in southern iran, 2007-2010: A cross sectional study. *PLoS One* 2016;11(5):e0155669. doi: 10.1371/journal.pone.0155669
2. Qu X, Zhai Y, Wei H, Zhang C, Xing G, Yu Y, et al. Characterization and expression of three novel differentiation-related genes belong to the human ndrg gene family. *Mol Cell Biochem* 2002;229(1-2):35-44.
3. Ma JJ, Kong LM, Liao CG, Jiang X, Wang Y, Bao TY. Suppression of mmp-9 activity by ndrg2 expression inhibits clear cell renal cell carcinoma invasion. *Med Oncol* 2012;29(5):3306-13. doi: 10.1007/s12032-012-0265-1
4. Hu XL, Liu XP, Deng YC, Lin SX, Wu L, Zhang J, et al. Expression analysis of the ndrg2 gene in mouse embryonic and adult tissues. *Cell Tissue Res* 2006;325(1):67-76. doi: 10.1007/s00441-005-0137-5
5. Kim MJ, Kim HS, Lee SH, Yang Y, Lee MS, Lim JS. Ndrg2 controls cox-2/pge(2)-mediated breast cancer cell migration and invasion. *Mol Cells* 2014;37(10):759-65. doi: 10.14348/molcells.2014.0232
6. Gao L, Wu GJ, Liu XW, Zhang R, Yu L, Zhang G, et al. Suppression of invasion and metastasis of prostate cancer cells by overexpression of ndrg2 gene. *Cancer Lett* 2011;310(1):94-100. doi: 10.1016/j.canlet.2011.06.015
7. Kim YJ, Kang HB, Yim HS, Kim JH, Kim JW. Ndrg2 positively regulates e-cadherin expression and prolongs overall survival in colon cancer patients. *Oncol Rep* 2013;30(4):1890-8. doi: 10.3892/or.2013.2642
8. Paiva KB, Granjeiro JM. Bone tissue remodeling and development: Focus on matrix metalloproteinase functions. *Arch Biochem Biophys* 2014;561:74-87. doi: 10.1016/j.abb.2014.07.034
9. Liu N, Wang L, Li X, Yang Q, Liu X, Zhang J, et al. N-myc downstream-regulated gene 2 is involved in p53-mediated apoptosis. *Nucleic Acids Res* 2008;36(16):5335-49. doi: 10.1093/nar/gkn504
10. Lorentzen A, Vogel LK, Lewinsky RH, Saebo M, Skjelbred CF, Godiksen S, et al. Expression of ndrg2 is down-regulated in high-risk adenomas and colorectal carcinoma. *BMC Cancer* 2007;7:192. doi: 10.1186/1471-2407-7-192
11. Kim YJ, Yoon SY, Kim JT, Choi SC, Lim JS, Kim JH, et al. Ndrg2 suppresses cell proliferation through down-regulation of ap-1 activity in human colon carcinoma cells. *Int J Cancer* 2009;124(1):7-15. doi: 10.1002/ijc.23945
12. Phipps AI, Buchanan DD, Makar KW, Win AK, Baron JA, Lindor NM, et al. Kras-mutation status in relation to colorectal cancer survival: The joint impact of correlated tumour markers. *Br J Cancer* 2013;108(8):1757-64. doi: 10.1038/bjc.2013.118
13. Golestan AM, Mojtahedi ZP, Ghalamfarsa GP, Hamidinia MM, Takhshid MAP. The effects of ndrg2 overexpression on cell proliferation and invasiveness of sw48 colorectal cancer cell line. *Iran J Med Sci* 2015;40(5):430-9.
14. Bonora M, Wieckowski MR, Chinopoulos C, Kepp O, Kroemer G, Galluzzi L, et al. Molecular mechanisms of cell death: Central implication of atp synthase in mitochondrial permeability transition. *Oncogene* 2015;34(12):1475-86. doi: 10.1038/onc.2014.96
15. Guo YJ, Liu JX, Guan YW. Hypoxia induced upregulation of mir-301a/b contributes to increased cell autophagy and viability of prostate cancer cells by targeting ndrg2. *Eur Rev Med Pharmacol Sci* 2016;20(1):101-8.
16. Kim A, Kim MJ, Yang Y, Kim JW, Yeom YI, Lim JS. Suppression of nf-kappab activity by ndrg2 expression attenuates the invasive potential of highly malignant tumor cells. *Carcinogenesis* 2009;30(6):927-36. doi: 10.1093/carcin/bgp072
17. O'Sullivan S, Wang J, Pigott MT, Docherty N, Boyle N, Lis SK, et al. Inhibition of matrix metalloproteinase-9 by a barbiturate-nitrate hybrid ameliorates dextran sulphate sodium-induced colitis: Effect on inflammation-related genes. *Br J Pharmacol* 2017;174(7):512-24. doi: 10.1111/bph.13712
18. Lee DC, Kang YK, Kim WH, Jang YJ, Kim DJ, Park IY, et al. Functional and clinical evidence for ndrg2 as a candidate suppressor of liver cancer metastasis. *Cancer Res* 2008;68(11):4210-20. doi: 10.1158/0008-5472.CAN-07-5040
19. Tan C, Du X. Kras mutation testing in metastatic colorectal cancer. *World J Gastroenterol* 2012;18(37):5171-80. doi: 10.3748/wjg.v18.i37.5171

Isotretinoin; A review on the Utilization Pattern in Pregnancy

Sajad Khiali[1], Afshin Gharekhani[2], Taher Entezari-Maleki[2]*

[1] *Department of Clinical Pharmacy, Faculty of Pharmacy, Tabriz University of Medical Sciences, Tabriz, Iran.*
[2] *Drug Applied Research Center, Tabriz University of Medical Sciences, Tabriz, Iran.*

Article info

Keywords:
- Isotretinoin
- Acne
- Utilization pattern
- Teratogenic effects
- Pregnancy

Abstract

Purpose: Isotretinoin is the most effective anti-acne drug with a long-term remission. However; it contains severe teratogenic effects with serious adverse drug reactions, which limits the use of medication.
Methods: To review the use of isotretinoin during pregnancy, we carried out a comprehensive search of literature in Google Scholar, Scopus and PubMed/Medline from their inception until April 2015.
Results: Database searching identified 277 records, of which, 38 articles were retrieved according to abstract and title assessment. After full-text review, 17 articles were excluded and finally, a total of 21 studies met the inclusion criteria.
Data showed an increased pattern in the use of isotretinoin. In some studies, health care providers were not fully adhered to the risk reduction programs in pregnancy. Exposing to isotretinoin among pregnant women has still occurred due to detrimental adherence to risk reduction programs which resulted in live-born infants with different kinds of abnormalities.
Conclusion: Despite the known serious adverse effect of isotretinoin, the use of drug was not based on the guidelines in some cases, which needs more attentions to prevent the severe drug related problems.

Introduction

Acne vulgaris, or simply acne is the most common disorder of skin that affects the majority of young adults.[1,2] It creates undesirable appearance with subsequent difficulties including depression and adverse effects on body image, self-stem, and quality of life.[3-6]
Several medications have been approved for the treatment of acne, but oral isotretinoin (13-cis retinoic acid) is the most clinically effective anti-acne therapy, producing long-term remission of acne symptoms by improving all the factors responsible for the generation of the disease. Based on published studies, oral isotretinoin is the gold standard treatment for serve nodulocyctic and recalcitrant acne.[7] Most studies have suggested a cumulative dose of 120 to 150 mg/kg to reduce the risk of disease relapse.[8-12] However, some newer studies found a lower rate of relapse with high-dose oral isotretinoin while others reported a comparable response rate with lower side effects using low-dose isotretinoin.[13-18] despite the well efficacy of isotretinoin in the acne therapy, several serious adverse effects including pancreatitis, depression, and suicidal thoughts have been reported. Most importantly, the teratogenicity is the major limiting factor for systemic isotretinoin use.[19-23]
Two nuclear ligand-induced receptors (retinoic acid receptors and retinoid X receptors) seems to have important role in retinoid teratogenicity through other downstream important genes in development. It has been suggested Hox gene expression causes the harmful effects of retinoic acid on the development of structures from the neural crest derivatives.[24,25]
The literature review indicated that isotretinoin use and prescription have been increasing all over the world.[26-33] For instance, a 2.5-fold increase in the use of isotretinoin was showed in the US between 1992 and 2000.[31] The Ministry of Health and Education of Iran reported a 4-fold increase in the use of isotretinoin between 2000 and 2007.[32] The well treatment efficacy of isotretinoin in the management of acne besides a higher failure rate and improper use of other therapeutic modalities may have contributed to the increased use of oral isotretinoin.[33] Due to the considerable increase in the use of isotretinoin along with its serious adverse effects on pregnancy, this study was performed to evaluate the utilization pattern of isotretinoin in pregnant women.

Methods

Data Sources and Search Strategy

A systematic search of literature was carried out in 3 major databases including PubMed/Medline, Scopus and Google Scholar from January 1980 up to April 2015. The keywords used as search terms in databases included "isotretinoin" and "pregnancy" and "prescription / use / utilization "and "isotretinoin" and "prescription / use /

***Corresponding author:** Taher Entezari-Maleki, Email: entezarim@tbzmed.ac.ir utilization". References of retrieved articles were also screened for inclusion of any additional related studies. Furthermore, a comprehensive searching of Cochornce, Science Citation Index, Embas and ISI Web of Knowledge was carried out. It is revealed that there were no additional studies.

Inclusion and Exclusion Criteria

All studies on isotretinoin concerns, awareness and its utilization in the treatment of acne were investigated. Articles published in Non-English languages, describing acne pathology or its adjuvant care as well as without full text availability were excluded.

Results and Discussion

The utilization pattern

Searching in databases identified 277 records, of which, 38 were relevant according to their title and abstract. After full-text review, 17 articles were excluded because they were irrelevant (n=5) or had no available free full-text (n=12). Finally, a total of 21 studies met the inclusion criteria.

There are a limited number of studies reporting utilization pattern of isotretinoin in the world. For example, one study in the US showed a 2.5-fold increase between 1992 and 2000.[31] Furthermore, a dramatic increase of 4-fold in the use of isotretinoin from 2000 to 2006 has been reported in developing countries such as Iran.[32]

In addition to increased use and prescription of isotretinoin, the improper use of the drug was reported in some studies. According to a study of Wysowski DK in the USA, isotretinoin rate of prescription for severe acne declined from 63% to 46%, whereas this rate for treatment of mild and moderate acne increased from 31% to 49% between 1993 and 2000.[31] Similarly, another prospective study on 274 Iranian patients indicated the improper prescriptions of isotretinoin for mild and moderate acne in 20% of patients. In this study, isotretinoin was prescribed under the usual recommended daily dose of 0.5-1 mg/kg in 51.3% of cases. Furthermore, 12.2% of cases received beyond cumulative dose of 150mg/kg and 33.5% of them were treated with less than cumulative dose of 120mg/kg.[26] In addition, based on data of Korean nationwide study, it was demonstrated that most of the physicians prescribed isotretinoin as the first-line therapy for the treatment of moderate acne.[34] A retrospective study in Dutch indicated that only 70% of patients were prescribed conventional acne therapy prior to receiving isotretinoin.[35]

Use of isotretinoin and pregnancy consideration

Due to the teratogenic effects of isotretinoin, a series of risk reduction programs including Pregnancy Prevention Program (PPP), System to Manage Accutane Related Teratogenicity (SMART) and iPLEDGE (a mandatory distribution program in the United States for isotretinoin) have been established in order to inhibit pregnant women from taking the medication and to prevent women taking the drug to get pregnant.[36,37]

In spite of implementing the PPP and Dear Healthcare Professional Letter (DHPL), a descriptive study on first-time receivers of isotretinoin also demonstrated inappropriate use of isotretinoin.[38] As well, SMART inadequate success in reducing isotretinoin-exposed pregnancies led to the development of iPLEDGE in the USA which is stricter than the other risk reduction programs.[38-42]

Reports from Middle East

Considering the lack of risk reduction programs in Iran, a drug utilization evaluation (DUE) study on 274 outpatients treated with isotretinoin, demonstrated that only 6.8% of couples used two concomitant methods of contraception.[26] Furthermore, according to a survey of 116 pharmacists' knowledge on isotretinoin teratogenic effects in Saudi Arabia, it was illustrated that community pharmacists were not sufficiently aware of its risks in female patients. Unexpectedly, 20% of pharmacists dispensed isotretinoin without any prescription. In addition, only 6.2% of them recommended two methods of contraception for females with childbearing potential.[42]

Reports from the US and North America

A study was carried out to appraise the patterns of isotretinoin use and assessed concomitant use of isotretinoin and contraceptives among females aged 13 to 45 years before and after iPLEDGE implementation between 2004 and 2008 in the USA. According to findings from Intercontinental Marketing Services (IMS) Health longitudinal prescription claims database, the number of isotretinoin prescriptions declined after iPLEDGE implementation. On the other hand, a small but significant increase in concomitant use of isotretinoin and contraceptives was observed immediately after iPlEDGE implementation. However, through the time, contraceptive utilization pattern did not significantly change before and after the implementation of iPLEDGE.[43]

A retrospective comparative study between iPLEDGE and SMART programs was done in a managed care setting. All females of childbearing potential at Kaiser Permanent Southern and Northern California with at least one prescription of isotretinoin from 1 March 2004 to 29 February 2008 were enrolled. A total of 9912 isotretinoin treatment courses and 29 fetal exposures to isotretinoin were reported. It was demonstrated that the risk of fetal exposure after iPLEDGE implementation decreased significantly in comparison with the SMART program.[44] Furthermore, a prospective Canadian population-based study on 8609 females receiving isotretinoin therapy was carried out to assess the rate of pregnancies exposed to isotretinoin from 1984 to 2002. It was demonstrated that 90 patients became pregnant among those participations. Approximately 85% of patients (n=76) terminated the pregnancy, and three spontaneous abortions and two neonatal deaths occurred. Finally, nine women had a live birth.[45]

Reports from the Europe

A systematic review of 17 studies evaluated the compliance rate with the PPP in the Europe. The findings showed that 0.2–1per 1000 women of reproduction age receiving isotretinoin became pregnant whereas 65% – 87% of these pregnancies were terminated. Furthermore, only 6–26% of prescriptions were in accordance with the PPP.[46]

According to a prospective study from 1993 to 2008 in Germany, a total of 108 pregnant women exposed to isotretinoin at the medium daily dose of 20 mg. In spite of running PPP, none of them used two complementary contraceptives. Among them, 39 pregnant women had no information about contraception usage during isotretinoin consumption. Among 69 alert subjects, contraceptives failed in 21 patients and 48 patients used no contraception methods or stopped their use too early. Approximately 81% of established pregnancies were terminated. On the other hand, one major birth defect was seen among 18 live births (with 1 pair of twins).[47]

Another study was carried out to evaluate all cases of exposure to isotretinoin during pregnancy who which was voluntarily reported to pharmacovigilance centers, the Teratogenic Agent Information Centre, and pharmaceutical companies in France and all cases who received isotretinoin during pregnancy from 1 January 2003 to 31 December 2006, were assessed. A total of 147 cases of isotretinoin exposure were reported. They divided into 3 groups; first (n=61) who get pregnant less than 1 month after isotretinoin discontinuation; second (n=23) who became pregnant during isotretinoin use and third (n=16) who were started isotretinoin while they were pregnant. Prescription of isotertinoin was done by dermatologists in 86% of cases. In addition, 19% of women did not use any contraception method.[48]

A total of 203962 pregnancies corresponding to 208161 fetuses were evaluated in a population-based study in the Netherlands between 1 January 1999 and 1 September 2007 to assess their exposure to isotretinoin. It was demonstrated that 51 women had exposure to isotretinoin. Six patients became pregnant during the last month of discontinuing isotretinoin and 45 patients exposed to isotretinoin during pregnancy. Among those potentially exposed to isotretinoin, three intrauterine deaths and two live-birth delivery with major congenital anomalies occurred.[49] In addition, a descriptive study was carried out between 2007 and 2011 to evaluate the compliance of pharmacists and dermatologists with PPP in the Netherlands. The data indicated that only 64% of dermatologists always prescribed contraception. furthermore, 22% of them prescribed it occasionally. In addition, approximately 45% of pharmacists checked the use of contraception method and 15% of them asked for a negative pregnancy test. Furthermore, Pharmacists' checks on 30-day dispensing was 82% and didn't change, whereas a check whether the prescription is out-of-date decreased from 61% to 53% from 2007 to 2011. In addition to poor compliance of pharmacists, it was demonstrated that in spite of the claim made by dermatologists regarding their compliance rate of 90% with the PPP, their compliance rate with the PPP was 25%.[50] Furthermore, a retrospective study was carried out in Dutch between 1 January 2005 and 31 December 2008 to assess the compliance with the PPP among women of reproductive age. Comprehensive information evaluating Dutch Foundation of Pharmaceutical Statistics indicated that the use of isotretinoin increased among women in reproductive age during the study period. Furthermore, the concomitant use of oral hormonal or intrauterine contraceptives and isotretinoin was low (59.3%, 95% CI: 57.6, 61.0). Also, prescription of isotretinoin by a specialist was performed in only 78.2% of the participants. In addition, only 70% of them were treated with conventional acne therapy prior to isotretinoin initiation.[35] Furthermore, a total of 500000 women were included in a drug utilization study in the Netherlands. Data of a drug prescription database from 1999 until 2006 to compare contraceptive use in isotretinoin and non-isotretinoin users was carried out. It was demonstrated that approximately 53% of the 651 patients on isotretinoin therapy were prescribed contraceptives before, during, and after discontinuation of isotretinoin in accordance with the PPP in comparison with approximately 43% in non-isotretinoin using group.[51]

A study was carried out in 2009 to collect data on performance of the coordinated PPP of isotretinoin in the Europe Union (EU) member states and Norway and Iceland. A questionnaire was sent to all of them. A total of 143 cases of isotretinoin exposures during pregnancy period were reported in 16 of 22 collaborating countries since implementation of the PPP. The PPP implementation was in force from 21th countries (Table 1).[52]

This review was conducted to evaluate isotretinoin use all over the world with a special consideration on pregnancy. This study demonstrated an increase in isotretinoin use with an improper prescription pattern.

Isotretinoin exposure during pregnancy and its consequent fetal abnormality in developed countries such as Canada, Germany, Netherlands and France is a concern.[45-49] Furthermore, a questioner based study indicated same results in the EU members, Norway and Iceland.[52]

A French study reported 127 prescriptions of isotretinoin to pregnant women by dermatologists.[6] Furthermore, it was shown that in spite of 93% of dermatologists' claim about their compliance with the PPP, there was only a compliance rate of 25% with the pooled program in Netherland in 2011.[50] In addition, according to a retrospective cohort study in Dutch, 30% of specialists didn't prescribe conventional acne therapy prior to isotretinoin initiation.[35] The data from a systematic review in Europe demonstrated a lower compliance rate of 6–26% with the PPP.[46]

Table 1. The summary of studies about use of isotretinoin during pregnancy

References	Study design	Country	Total number of patients	Results
Entezari-Maleki T, et al.[26] 2012	Prospective, drug utilization evaluation	Iran	274	6.8% of patients used two methods of contraceptive 51.3% received isotretinoin under the usual recommended daily doses
Teichert M, et al.[35] 2010	Retrospective study	Dutch	4881	Concomitant use of oral hormonal or intrauterine contraceptives and isotretinoin was 59.3%.
Pinheiro SP, et al.[43] 2013	Prospective comparative study	USA	113 578	Temporary increase in concomitant use of isotretinoin and contraceptives was observed immediately after iPlEDGE implementation
Shin J, et al.[44] 2011	Retrospective comparative study	USA	9912	The risk of fetal exposure after iPLEDGE implementation reduced significantly in comparison with the SMART program
Berard A, et al.[45] 2007	Prospective population-based study	Canada	8609	A total of 9 live births occurred.
Crijns HJ, et al.[46] 2011	Systematic review of 17 studies	Europe	141	0·2–1·0 per 1000 women of reproduction age receiving isotretinoin became pregnant whereas 65% – 87% of these pregnancies were terminated
Schaefer C, et al.[47] 2010	Observational prospective study	Germany	108	A total 18 live births occurred
Autret-Leca E. et al.[48] 2010	Prospective population-based study	France	147	A total of 147 cases of isotretinoin exposure were reported
Zomerdijk IM, et al.[49] 2014	Retrospective population-based study	Netherlands	203962	Among those potentially exposed to isotretinoin, three intrauterine deaths and two live-born infants with major congenital anomalies occurred.
Crijns I, et al.[50] 2013	Prospective descriptive study	Netherlands	556	In addition to poor compliance of pharmacists, that 25% of dermatologists were compliant with the PPP
Crijns HJ, et al.[51] 2012	Prospective drug utilization study	Netherlands	651	53% of the 651 patients on isotretinoin therapy were prescribed to use contraceptive before, during, and after discontinuation of isotretinoin in accordance to the PPP.
Crijns I, et al.[52] 2012	Prospective questionnaire- based study	Europe, Norway and Iceland	143	Exposing to isotretinoin in spite of the PPP implementation.

A study in Saudi Arabia confirmed that community pharmacists were not enough conscious about isotretinoin risks in female of childbearing potential. Furthermore, most of them didn't recommend two methods of contraception.[42] Furthermore, according to a prospective, drug utilization evaluation study in Iran, only 6.8% of couples used two methods of contraception.[26] Despite a temporary successfulness, the data showed that implementation of the iPLEDGE program in the USA in order to reduce the fetal exposure was failed.

Taken together, the results of the present study showed neither of patients nor pharmacists and dermatologists were fully adherent to the risk reduction programs. In addition, exposure to isotretinoin among women during pregnancy still occurs and leads to live-born neonates with a variety of abnormalities in all over the world.

The present mini review has some limitation. Most importantly, a total 12 revenant studies weren't included because of unavailable free full text. Furthermore, most of included studies have been carried out in developed countries. Due to lack of risk reduction programs in low-income countries, evaluating of isotretinoin pregnancy considerations are required in these countries.

Conclusion

The results of the presen1t study showed an increase in the use of isotretinoin. One of the important concerns is that the drug was not used with appropriate caution in pregnancy and in spite of development of the risk reduction programs, low adherence to these programs occurred and led to live births with congenital abnormalities.

Conflict of Interest

Authors declare no conflicts of interest.

Reference

1. Klassen AF, Newton JN, Mallon E. Measuring quality of life in people referred for specialist care of acne: Comparing generic and disease-specific measures. *J Am Acad Dermatol* 2000;43(2 Pt 1):229-33. doi: 10.1067/mjd.2000.105507
2. Ingram JR, Grindlay DJ, Williams HC. Management of acne vulgaris: An evidence-based update. *Clin Exp Dermatol* 2010;35(4):351-4. doi: 10.1111/j.1365-2230.2009.03683.x
3. Thomas DR. Psychosocial effects of acne. *J Cutan Med Surg* 2004;8(Suppl 4):3-5. doi: 10.1007/s10227-004-0752-x
4. Dalgard F, Gieler U, Holm JØ, Bjertness E, Hauser S. Self-esteem and body satisfaction among late adolescents with acne: Results from a population

survey. *J Am Acad Dermatol* 2008;59(5):746-51. doi: 10.1016/j.jaad.2008.07.013
5. Fried RG, Wechsler A. Psychological problems in the acne patient. *Dermatol Ther* 2006;19(4):237-40. doi: 10.1111/j.1529-8019.2006.00079.x
6. Yazici K, Baz K, Yazici AE, Kokturk A, Tot S, Demirseren D, et al. Disease-specific quality of life is associated with anxiety and depression in patients with acne. *J Eur Acad Dermatol Venereol* 2004;18(4):435-9. doi: 10.1111/j.1468-3083.2004.00946.x
7. Kraft J, Freiman A. Management of acne. *CMAJ* 2011;183(7):E430-5. doi: 10.1503/cmaj.090374
8. Zouboulis CC, Piquero-Martin J. Update and future of systemic acne treatment. *Dermatology* 2003;206(1):37-53. doi: 10.1159/000067821
9. Ghalamkarpour F, Nasiri S. Isotretinoin in treatment of acne: its efficacy, side effects, and recurrence rate of disease. *Arch Iran Med* 2006;9(3):228-30.
10. Haryati I, Jacinto SS. Profile of acne patients in the Philippines requiring a second course of oral isotretinoin. *Int J Dermatol* 2005;44(12):999-1001. doi: 10.1111/j.1365-4632.2005.02284.x
11. Layton AM, Dreno B, Gollnick HP, Zouboulis CC. A review of the European Directive for prescribing systemic isotretinoin for acne vulgaris. *J Eur Acad Dermatol Venereol* 2006;20(7):773-6. doi: 10.1111/j.1468-3083.2006.01671.x
12. Strauss JS, Krowchuk DP, Leyden JJ, Lucky AW, Shalita AR, Siegfried EC, et al. Guidelines of care for acne vulgaris management. *J Am Acad Dermatol* 2007;56(4):651-63. doi: 10.1016/j.jaad.2006.08.048
13. Coloe J, Du H, Morrell DS. Could higher doses of isotretinoin reduce the frequency of treatment failure in patients with acne? *J Am Acad Dermatol* 2011;65(2):422-3. doi: 10.1016/j.jaad.2010.06.025
14. Azoulay L, Oraichi D, Berard A. Isotretinoin therapy and the incidence of acne relapse: A nested case-control study. *Br J Dermatol* 2007;157(6):1240-8. doi: 10.1111/j.1365-2133.2007.08250.x
15. Neubert U, Plewig G, Ruhfus A. Treatment of gram-negative folliculitis with isotretinoin. *Arch Dermatol Res* 1986;278(4):307-13.
16. Quereux G, Volteau C, N'Guyen JM, Dreno B. Prospective study of risk factors of relapse after treatment of acne with oral isotretinoin. *Dermatology* 2006;212(2):168-76. doi: 10.1159/000090658
17. Sardana K, Garg VK. Low-dose isotretinoin in acne vulgaris: A critical review. *Br J Dermatol* 2011;165(3):698-700. doi: 10.1111/j.1365-2133.2011.10440.x
18. Sardana K, Garg VK. Efficacy of low-dose isotretinoin in acne vulgaris. *Indian J Dermatol Venereol Leprol* 2010;76(1):7-13. doi: 10.4103/0378-6323.58672
19. Amichai B, Shemer A, Grunwald MH. Low-dose isotretinoin in the treatment of acne vulgaris. *J Am Acad Dermatol* 2006;54(4):644-6. doi: 10.1016/j.jaad.2005.11.1061
20. Sladden MJ, Harman KE. What is the chance of a normal pregnancy in a woman whose fetus has been exposed to isotretinoin? *Arch Dermatol* 2007;143(9):1187-8. doi: 10.1001/archderm.143.9.1187
21. Zane LT, Leyden WA, Marqueling AL, Manos MM. A population-based analysis of laboratory abnormalities during isotretinoin therapy for acne vulgaris. *Arch Dermatol* 2006;142(8):1016-22. doi: 10.1001/archderm.142.8.1016
22. Wysowski DK, Pitts M, Beitz J. An analysis of reports of depression and suicide in patients treated with isotretinoin. *J Am Acad Dermatol* 2001;45(4):515-9. doi: 10.1067/mjd.2001.117730
23. Bigby M. Does isotretinoin increase the risk of depression? *Arch Dermatol* 2008;144(9):1197-9. doi: 10.1001/archderm.144.9.1197
24. Elmazar MM, Ruhl R, Reichert U, Shroot B, Nau H. RARα-mediated teratogenicity in mice is potentiated by an RXR agonist and reduced by an RAR antagonist: Dissection of retinoid receptor-induced pathways. *Toxicol Appl Pharmacol* 1997;146(1):21-8. doi: 10.1006/taap.1997.8221
25. Waxman JS, Yelon D. Increased Hox activity mimics the teratogenic effects of excess retinoic acid signaling. *Dev Dyn* 2009;238(5):1207-13. doi: 10.1002/dvdy.21951
26. Entezari-Maleki T, Hadjibabaie M, Dousti S, Salamzadeh J, Hayatshahi A, Javadi MR, et al. Evaluation and monitoring of isotretinoin use in Iran. *Arch Iran Med* 2012;15(7):409-12.
27. Entezari-Maleki T, Hadjibabaie M, Salamzadeh J, Javadi MR, Shalviri G, Gholami K. The evaluation of isotretinoin induced adverse drug reactions. *Afr J Pharm Pharmcol* 2011;5(16):1877-81.
28. Thielitz A, Gollnick H. Isotretinoin. How should it be used? *Hautarzt* 2013;64(4):263-8. doi: 10.1007/s00105-012-2467-z
29. Nast A, Bayerl C, Borelli C, Degitz K, Dirschka T, Erdmann R, et al. S2k-guideline for therapy of acne. *J Dtsch Dermatol Ges* 2010;8 Suppl 2:s1-59. doi: 10.1111/j.1610-0387.2010.07466.x
30. Kertzman MG, Smeets JG, Boukes FS, Goudswaard AN. Summary of the practice guideline 'Acne' (second revision) from the Dutch College of General Practitioners. *Ned Tijdschr Geneeskd* 2008;152(22):1271-5.
31. Wysowski DK, Swann J, Vega A. Use of isotretinoin (Accutane) in the United States: Rapid increase from 1992 through 2000. *J Am Acad Dermatol* 2002;46(4):505-9. doi: 10.1067/mjd.2002.120529
32. Health Ministry of Iran. The Annual Report of Drugs Prescriptions 2001 – 2007.
33. Cooper AJ. Systematic review of Propionibacterium acnes resistance to systemic antibiotics. *Med J Aust* 1998;169(5):259-61.
34. Kwon HH, Yoon HS, Suh DH, Yoon JY, Park SK, Lee ES, et al. A nationwide study of acne treatment patterns in Korea: Analysis of patient preconceived

notions and dermatologist suggestion for treatment. *Acta Derm Venereol* 2012;92(3):236-40. doi: 10.2340/00015555-1331
35. Teichert M, Visser LE, Dufour M, Rodenburg E, Straus SM, De Smet PA, et al. Isotretinoin use and compliance with the Dutch Pregnancy Prevention Programme: A retrospective cohort study in females of reproductive age using pharmacy dispensing data. *Drug Saf* 2010;33(4):315-26. doi: 10.2165/11319190-000000000-00000
36. Abroms L, Maibach E, Lyon-Daniel K, Feldman SR. What is the best approach to reducing birth defects associated with isotretinoin? *PLoS Med* 2006;3(11):e483. doi: 10.1371/journal.pmed.0030483
37. Prevost N, English JC. Isotretinoin: update on controversial issues. *J Pediatr Adolesc Gynecol* 2013;26(5):290-3. doi: 10.1016/j.jpag.2013.05.007
38. Mitchell AA, Van Bennekom CM, Louik C. A pregnancy-prevention program in women of childbearing age receiving isotretinoin. *N Engl J Med* 1995;333(2):101-6. doi: 10.1056/NEJM199507133330206
39. Honein MA, Paulozzi LJ, Erickson JD. Continued occurrence of Accutane-exposed pregnancies. *Teratology* 2001;64(3):142-7. doi: 10.1002/tera.1057
40. Brinker A, Kornegay C, Nourjah P. Trends in adherence to a revised risk management program designed to decrease or eliminate isotretinoin-exposed pregnancies: Evaluation of the accutane SMART program. *Arch Dermatol* 2005;141(5):563-9. doi: 10.1001/archderm.141.5.563
41. Azoulay L, Oraichi D, Berard A. Patterns and utilization of isotretinoin for acne from 1984 to 2003: Is there need for concern? *Eur J Clin Pharmacol* 2006;62(8):667-74. doi: 10.1007/s00228-006-0151-x
42. Alrwisan AA, Alshammari TM, Tahir KW, Aleissa FM, Aljadhey HS. Community pharmacists' knowledge of isotretinoin safety. *Saudi Med J* 2014;35(1):81-4.
43. Pinheiro SP, Kang EM, Kim CY, Governale LA, Zhou EH, Hammad TA. Concomitant use of isotretinoin and contraceptives before and after iPledge in the United States. *Pharmacoepidemiol Drug Saf* 2013;22(12):1251-7. doi: 10.1002/pds.3481
44. Shin J, Cheetham TC, Wong L, Niu F, Kass E, Yoshinaga MA, et al. The impact of the iPLEDGE program on isotretinoin fetal exposure in an integrated health care system. *J Am Acad Dermatol* 2011;65(6):1117-25. doi: 10.1016/j.jaad.2010.09.017
45. Berard A, Azoulay L, Koren G, Blais L, Perreault S, Oraichi D. Isotretinoin, pregnancies, abortions and birth defects: A population-based perspective. *Br J Clin Pharmacol* 2007;63(2):196-205. doi: 10.1111/j.1365-2125.2006.02837.x
46. Crijns HJ, Straus SM, Gispen-de Wied C, de Jong-van den Berg LT. Compliance with pregnancy prevention programmes of isotretinoin in Europe: A systematic review. *Br J Dermatol* 2011;164(2):238-44. doi: 10.1111/j.1365-2133.2010.09976.x
47. Schaefer C, Meister R, Weber-Schoendorfer C. Isotretinoin exposure and pregnancy outcome: An observational study of the Berlin Institute for Clinical Teratology and Drug Risk Assessment in Pregnancy. *Arch Gynecol Obstet* 2010;281(2):221-7. doi: 10.1007/s00404-009-1112-2
48. Autret-Leca E, Kreft-Jais C, Elefant E, Cissoko H, Darrouzain F, Grimaldi-Bensouda L, et al. Isotretinoin exposure during pregnancy: Assessment of spontaneous reports in France. *Drug Saf* 2010;33(8):659-65. doi: 10.2165/11536250-000000000-00000
49. Zomerdijk IM, Ruiter R, Houweling LM, Herings RM, Sturkenboom MC, Straus SM, et al. Isotretinoin exposure during pregnancy: A population-based study in The Netherlands. *BMJ Open* 2014;4(11):e005602. doi: 10.1136/bmjopen-2014-005602
50. Crijns I, Mantel-Teeuwisse A, Bloemberg R, Pinas E, Straus S, de Jong-van den Berg L. Healthcare professional surveys to investigate the implementation of the isotretinoin Pregnancy Prevention Programme: A descriptive study. *Expert Opin Drug Saf* 2013;12(1):29-38. doi: 10.1517/14740338.2013.745850
51. Crijns HJ, van Rein N, Gispen-de Wied CC, Straus SM, de Jong-van den Berg LT. Prescriptive contraceptive use among isotretinoin users in the Netherlands in comparison with non-users: A drug utilisation study. *Pharmacoepidemiol Drug Saf* 2012;21(10):1060-6. doi: 10.1002/pds.3200
52. Crijns I, Straus S, Luteijn M, Gispen-de Wied C, Raine J, de Jong-van den Berg L. Implementation of the harmonized EU isotretinoin Pregnancy Prevention Programme: A questionnaire survey among European regulatory agencies. *Drug Saf* 2012;35(1):27-32. doi: 10.2165/11595570-000000000-00000

20

Potential of Peptide Nucleic Acids in Future Therapeutic Applications

Soheila Montazersaheb[1,2,3]*, Mohammad Saeid Hejazi[2,3], Hojjatollah Nozad Charoudeh[4]

[1] *Stem Cell Research Center, Tabriz University of Medical Sciences, Tabriz, Iran.*
[2] *Molecular Medicine Research Center, Tabriz University of Medical Sciences, Tabriz, Iran.*
[3] *Department of Pharmaceutical Biotechnology, Faculty of Pharmacy, Tabriz University of Medical Sciences, Tabriz, Iran.*
[4] *Anatomical Sciences Department, Faculty of Medicine, Tabriz University of Medical Sciences, Tabriz, Iran.*

Article info

Keywords:
- Antigene
- Antisense
- Cancer
- Gene Therapy
- Peptide Nucleic Acid
- Splicing

Abstract

Peptide nucleic acids (PNA) are synthetic analog of DNA with a repeating N-(2-aminoethyl)-glycine peptide backbone connected to purine and pyrimidine nucleobases via a linker. Considering the unique properties of PNA, including resistance to enzymatic digestion, higher biostability combined with great hybridization affinity toward DNA and RNA, it has attracted great attention toward PNA- based technology as a promising approach for gene alteration. However, an important challenge in utilizing PNA is poor intracellular uptake. Therefore, some strategies have been developed to enhance the delivery of PNA in order to reach cognate site. Although PNAs primarily demonstrated to act as an antisense and antigene agents for inhibition of transcription and translation of target genes, more therapeutic applications such as splicing modulation and gene editing are also used to produce specific genome modifications. Hence, several approaches based on PNAs technology have been designed for these purposes.

This review briefly presents the properties and characteristics of PNA as well as different gene modulation mechanisms. Thereafter, current status of successful therapeutic applications of PNA as gene therapeutic intervention in different research areas with special interest in medical application in particular, anti-cancer therapy are discussed. Then it focuses on possible use of PNA as anti-mir agent and PNA-based strategies against clinically important bacteria.

Introduction

Peptide nucleic acid (PNA) is a non-charged DNA-like molecule that is remarkably similar to DNA and RNA both in intramolecular spacing and geometry (Figure 1). Unlike DNA or other DNA analogues, the entire sugar-phosphodiester is replaced by a neutral charge and achiral pseudopeptide backbone to which the bases are attached via a methyl carbonyl linker.[1] One consequence of this neutrality is the lower intrinsic electrostatic repulsion against complementary oligonucleotides, resulting in greater hybridization strengths. PNA has the capability to hybridize with high affinity and sequence specificity to complementary DNA or RNA sequence, obeying the Watson-Crick hydrogen-bonding scheme in which adenine pairs with thymine via two hydrogen bonds and cytosine forms three hydrogen bonds with guanine. PNA molecules with mixed sequences form duplexes with complementary DNA and RNA based on Watson–Crick rule. In addition, PNA can form conventional triplex structure through Hoogsteen binding in the major groove of helix of the double stranded DNA. Homo-pyrimidine PNA can form triplex invasion structure with DNA when targeting to homopurine sequence in duplex DNA (Figure 2). In this structure, one PNA strand hybridizes to its complementary DNA through Watson-Crick hydrogen bonds via antiparallel orientation, while the second PNA strand binds to the same sequence through Hoogsteen hydrogen bonds in parallel form.[2] Because of sufficient inherently flexible polyamide structure, PNA oligomers display higher affinity and specificity when targeting DNA and RNA strands (or PNA itself) compared to natural DNA or RNA.[3]

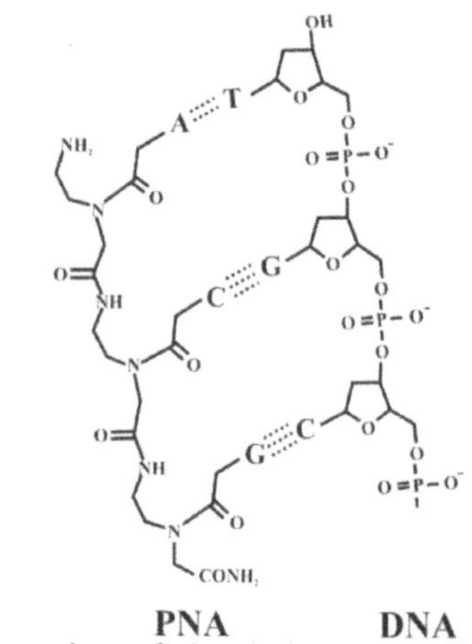

Figure1. Comparison of chemical structure of PNA and DNA backbones.[2]

***Corresponding author:** Soheila Montazersaheb, Email: montazersahebs@tbzmed.ac.ir

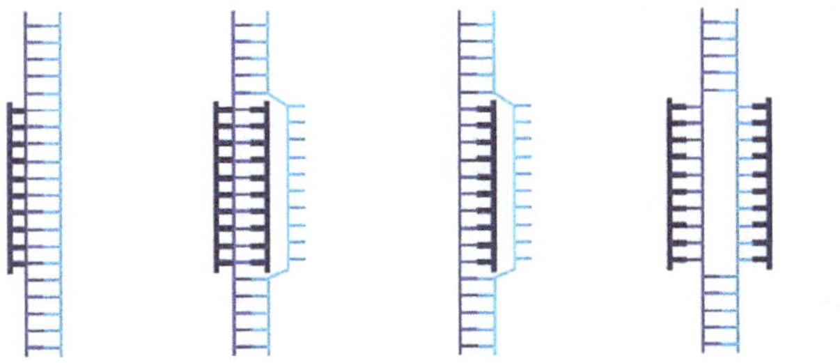

Figure 2. Schematic drawing of PNA binging modes, targeting to dsDNA. DNA is drawn as a ladder and PNA molecules are in thick structures. Triplex complex is formed by cytosine rich PNA targeting to homopurine target. Triplex invasion structure leads to the formation of a loop. In this structure, one strand of PNA binds based on Watson-Crick rule, and another strand binds through Hoogsteen bond. Duplex invasion has no sequence constraints. Double duplex invasion is formed by PNAs containing modified bases.[3]

Since the introduction of PNA by Nielsen, Buchardt, Egholm and Berg (1991),[4] it has caught attention in many fields, including molecular biology, biotechnology, biosensor systems,[5] drug discovery, genetic diagnosis and development of gene therapeutic agents.[6] In addition, PNA can be used as a diagnostic tool for detection of oncogenes through distinction between the wild type and the mutant target.[7] Owing to the peptide-like chemical structure, the synthesis of PNA is similar to peptide protocols. In this way, PNA molecules are easily synthesized by well-established solid-phase manual or automated methods using either tBoc (tert-butyloxycarbonyl group) or Fmoc (9-fluorenylmethoxycarbonyl group) solid phase and purification with high-performance liquid chromatography (HPLC).[8]

Attractive properties of PNA

PNA possesses several peculiar and unique physicochemical properties as compared to the natural counterparts. The unnatural backbone of PNAs renders charge neutrality, eliminating electrostatic repulsion which has a negative effect on binding affinity, and causes excellent hybridization affinity to target sequence. An additional outcome is that PNAs bind independently of medium salt concentration, whereas low ionic strength reduces the stability of DNA–DNA duplexes. Also, PNAs show stability at acidic pH (pH 4.5~6.5), while DNA is prone to depurinate at lower pH. Detailed results have revealed that PNAs have higher thermal melting temperature (Tm) compared to corresponding DNA–DNA or DNA–RNA duplexes as Tm of a PNA/DNA duplex for per base pair is 1° C higher than DNA–DNA duplex.

As stated above, one crucial consequence of unnatural backbone is resistance to nuclease and protease-mediated degradation in serum and cell extracts, extending the life time of this oligomer both *in vitro* and *in vivo*.[2] Noticeably, PNAs display very good mismatch sequence discrimination,[9,10] and strong binding affinity towards DNA and RNA, making this oligonucleotide mimic an interesting third generation oligonucleotide analogue with potential therapeutic applications.[11] PNA is capable of blocking the activity of DNA and RNA polymerases, telomerase, reverse transcriptase, endonucleases and transcription factors. Commensurate with these statements, the DNA/RNA recognition capacity has made PNA indeed a promising candidate for therapeutic application through modulation of gene expression via antigene and antisense mechanism (Table 1).[12,13]

Limitations of PNA Technology

Despite the remarkable properties of PNA along with simplicity of synthesis and high chemical and biological stability which make PNA as a potential candidate to develop effective gene therapeutic agents, there are basic challenges still remaining for clinical application. Poor water solubility of this oligomer due to neutral character makes it to have a tendency to form globular structures. To improve the low water solubility of PNA oligomer, some modifications should be applied including addition of positively charged residues (at the terminals) and conjugation to negative charge molecules such as DNA.

Another significant challenge of this hydrophilic oligomer is the poor cellular uptake. To combat limitations in crossing of PNAs and achieving sufficient intracellular delivery, several modifications can be performed to enhance cellular delivery. Without passing cell membrane, PNAs cannot interact with target sequence and therefore have no biological activity.[14]

PNA delivery approaches

To make a successful PNA-based technology, there is a need to find effective methods to enhance the access of PNAs into intracellular space.[15] A variety of methods such as spontaneous uptake in some type of nerve cells, electroporation, membrane permeabilization with streptolysin O, cationic lipids, and attachment of PNAs to cationic cell-penetrating peptides (CPPs) have been used for delivery of PNAs into the target cells.[16] The latter approach is an extremely efficient transport carrier for moving across cell membranes. It has been shown that CPP has no significant additional cellular toxicity especially for therapeutic application. Most known examples of CPPs are positively charged amino acids including arginine and lysine which interact with glycoproteins having negative charge on the cell surface. Of note, due to guanidine moiety in arginine residue which can interact with negative groups, this amino acid is more effective than lysine. Although the mechanism of CPP-mediated delivery is still not very clear, CPPs can release their cargo into cells using two distinct mechanisms including endocytosis and direct translocation. Since PNA needs to reach the target site for modulating gene expression, the internalized cargo must be released from endosomal compartments into the cytoplasm. It is noteworthy that co-treatment with endosome disruptive agents such as chloroquine can enhance the release of entrapment cargo, and thus dramatically increase the effects of PNA-conjugates.[17]

In vivo delivery of PNA still has many limitations. As the target site of PNA molecule is located within the cells, so PNA must enter into the cytoplasm or nucleus with assuring circulation time and reasonable excretion until reach to the target site. As noted, PNAs are hydrophilic compound and do not cross cell membranes, therefore are excreted very rapidly with half-life of approximately less than one hour. As a result, to achieve sufficient bioavailability of PNA molecules, it must be chemically modified to assure *In vivo* delivery efficacy. Detailed reports revealed that conjugation to CPP peptides can improve *in vivo* efficacy. For instance, it has been shown that PNA conjugated to oligoarginine has moderate activity in muscles in the mdx mice. Notably, nanoparticle PNA-based strategies can be used for efficient delivery of PNA to target sites.[18,19]

Advantage and disadvantage of PNA in gene-based therapy

Gene therapy uses foreign genes or short oligonucleotide sequences as therapeutic agents. Several approaches can be used for correcting of defect genes such as addition of functional alleles and correction via homologous recombination, introduction of suicide genes and prodrugs and inhibition of gene expression through synthetic oligonucleotides. There is particular interest in using oligonucleotides due to specificity to cognate site and non viral-based strategies. In conventional gene therapy, viral vectors are often used for gene delivery that may cause some risks including, stimulation of immune reaction and more importantly insertion of oncogene.[20]

PNAs are more efficient in terms of gene modulation, compared to traditional oligonucleotides such as phosphorothioate. For instance, one study showed that higher concentration of PNA is required for inhibition of gene expression than propyne-phosphorothioate oligonucleotides. Even supposing that higher concentrations of PNA is necessary to obtain reasonable antisense effects, the unique properties of PNA such as resistance to enzymatic digestion, higher stability, and specificity of PNA molecule to target sequence make it a powerful choice for gene therapy.[1]

Gene modulation mechanisms of PNA molecules

Antigene applications of PNA

PNAs have the ability to hybridize to complementary sequences at the DNA and interfering with the transcription of the target gene and as a consequence, reducing the mRNA level (Figure 3). In fact, PNA is capable of arresting transcriptional processes by virtue of its ability to form different complexes with dsDNA such as a stable triplex structure, strand invasion or strand displacement complexes leading to structural hindrance of RNA polymerase, as depicted in Figure 2.[21] Triplex-forming PNA can hamper the initiation of transcription by preventing duplex DNA unwinding or inhibition of transcription factor binding to the promoter region of target genes. Moreover, triplex-invasion structures within the transcribed region on the template strand can block the elongation of RNA polymerase along with the appearance of truncated RNA transcripts, inducing transcriptional inhibition.[22] Targeting chromosomal DNA is less effective due to difficult access to target sequence under physiological conditions. For instance, the presence of cations has potential to stabilize the DNA double strands, resulting in the reduction of helix invasion by the PNA. On the other hand, specific gene modulation via antigene mechanism is advantageous over antisense approaches, in that one (or two) copy of target sequence is evoked compared to many targets of mRNAs present in the cell.[23]

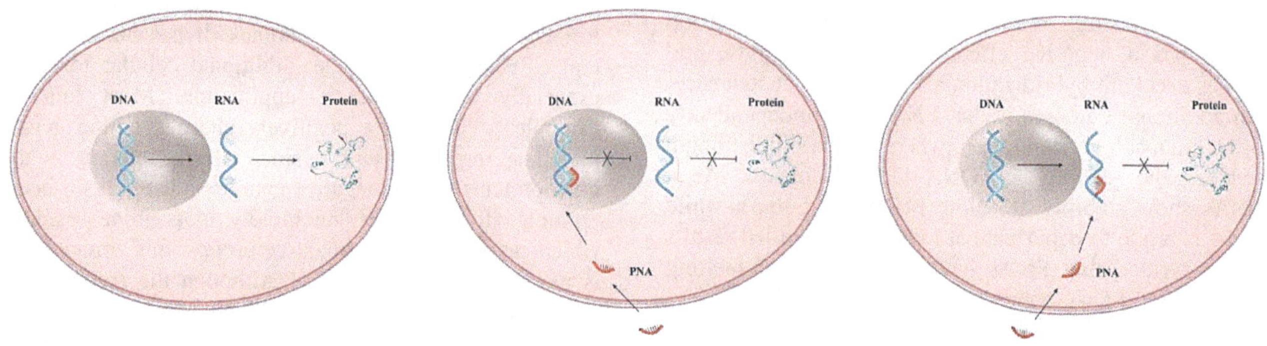

Figure 3. Schematic illustration of PNA-based strategy as antigene and antisense agents. Antigene PNA binds to complementary sequence in DNA and inhibits transcriptional process while antisense PNA hybridize to target sequence in mRNA and prevent translation procedure.

Antisense applications of PNA

In the case of RNA interference, PNA molecules mediate inhibitory effects on translational process via steric blocking mechanisms. Since PNA oligomers neither activate ribonuclease H (RNase H) nor enter RNA-induced silencing complexes (RISC) (Figure 4A), thus, antisense role of PNA may rely on mechanistic interference via different mechanisms rather than degradation of mRNA. PNAs hamper translation process through RNA transport to cytoplasm, elongation process, and translation initiation such as ribosome assembly.[24] Of note, inhibitory effects depend on hybridization strength and good accessible sequence on the mRNA molecule. Interestingly, it has been observed that duplex-forming PNAs with mixed sequence have the highest potency when targeted to AUG regions (translational start codon) or 5′terminus of mRNA (5′UTR), where ribosomal assembly occurs. Alternatively, homopyrimidine triplex-forming PNAs inhibit elongation process, leading to truncated products, whereas as noted above, duplex PNA can efficiently prevent the ribosomal assembly rather than arresting elongation (Figure 4B). Detailed data demonstrated that complete blockage of translation can be efficiently achieved by applying two or more duplex-forming PNAs. Overall, a crucial rule is considering the 5′UTR and AUG as suitable regions to obtain good antisense activity for duplex forming PNA.[25,26]

Certainly, ribosomes of eukaryotic cells recognize the translation initiation codon through scanning the mRNA sequence from the 5′-cap site to AUG codon. During the scanning process and before recognition of start codon, the assembly of ribosome has not completely occurred and is most likely not connected with the mRNA. As a result, the translation machinery is a good target to block due to accessibility of PNAs to cognate regions.

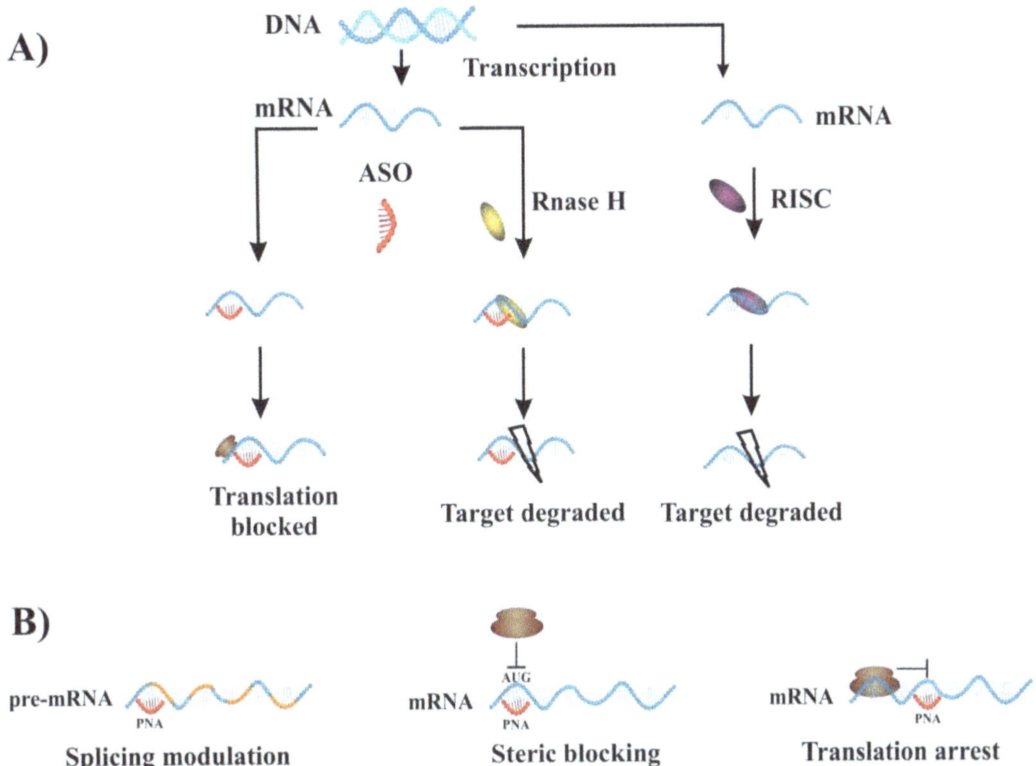

Figure 4. Some mechanisms involved in modulation of gene suppression: A) Antisense activity and RNA interference mechanisms. B) Inhibitory effect of antisense PNA via different approaches. PNAs have the ability to target AUG regions (translational start codon) or 5′UTR, where the starting point of ribosomal assembly occurs and block process, whereas triplex forming PNAs can inhibit elongation process via targeting to coding region. ASO: antisense oligonucleotide.

Modulation of splicing with PNA-based strategy

Interfering the splicing pattern is another important application of antisense PNAs, targeting and blocking specific intron-exon splice junctions within the pre-mRNA molecule. Upon targeting a PNA molecule to intron–exon junction sites, splicing machinery (spliceosome) either skips one exon (or more) or may retains intron sequence. As depicted in Figure 5, intron retention leads to the production of nonfunctional mRNA containing an intron, which is susceptible to destabilization. On the other hand, exon skipping produces an alternative protein similar to alternative splicing procedure. Since several diseases result from shifting in the splicing patterns of pre-mRNA, so interference with splicing procedure may create novel possibilities for drug development.[27] The process of pre-mRNA splicing is carried out by a very large ribonucleoprotein (RNP) complex through the removal of the intronic sequences accompanied by joining the exons at intron-exon junctions. This process is mediated by directing the spliceosome to correct splice sites at the intron-exon junctions including the 5′ and 3′ junction sites and the branch point. Employment of PNA-based technology can block correct splicing sites, which is critical for splicing mechanism.[28]

Alternative splicing can produce multiple mRNA isoforms from one gene and thus, leads to the generation of proteins with different functions. Many studies demonstrated that alternative splicing can be used to alter gene production based on physiological condition. For instance; human genes containing introns can undergo alternative splicing to adjust the desired output.[29] In addition, numerous therapeutic approaches are available to correct aberrant splicing in many disorders. Altering the splicing pattern of pre-mRNA can be done by antisense oligonucleotides in various disorder-related genes such as tau, c-myc, IL-5R, bcl-x, dystrophin, and ß-globin for obtaining therapeutically favorable results.[30,31] Overall, PNA targeting pre-mRNA sequences can efficiently modulate splicing process to obtain desirable outcome.[32,33]

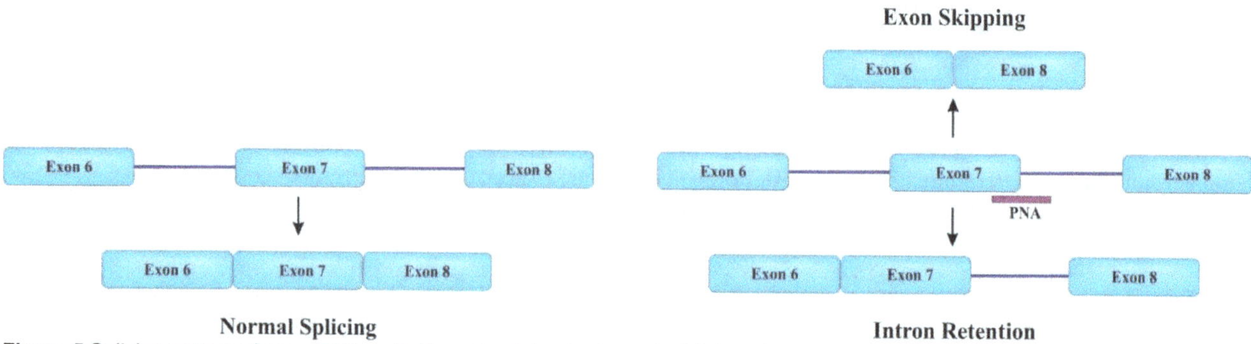

Figure 5. Splicing pattern of pre mRNA. Left: Normal splicing is shown by joining of exons to generate a spliced mRNA transcript. Right: Modification of splicing by antisense PNAs leading to exon skipping or intron retention. Blue rectangles, exons; lines, introns.

PNA-based Gene Editing Approach

Triplex-forming PNAs are effective tools to induce homologous recombination in the presence of donor DNA. For achieving this process, two PNA molecules are attached together by a linker, forming a bis-PNA. One strand of bis-PNA binds in the anti-parallel orientation based on Watson-Crick rule, and the other strand is attached via Hoogsteen bond in the parallel direction to dsDNA, making triplex formation. This structure leads to distortion of DNA helical, which has the ability to provoke DNA repair system, and results in the recombination of "donor" DNA into the desired target near binding site of PNA (Figure 6). This technology for *in vivo* site-specific gene modification is a novel approach to treat human disease. Other gene editing technologies are based on exogenous nucleases activity such as CRISPR/Cas, they may possibly create breaks in dsDNA, whilst PNA-mediated gene editing relies on repair pathways with high fidelity, thus reducing the error of end-joining which can cause additional mutations.[14]

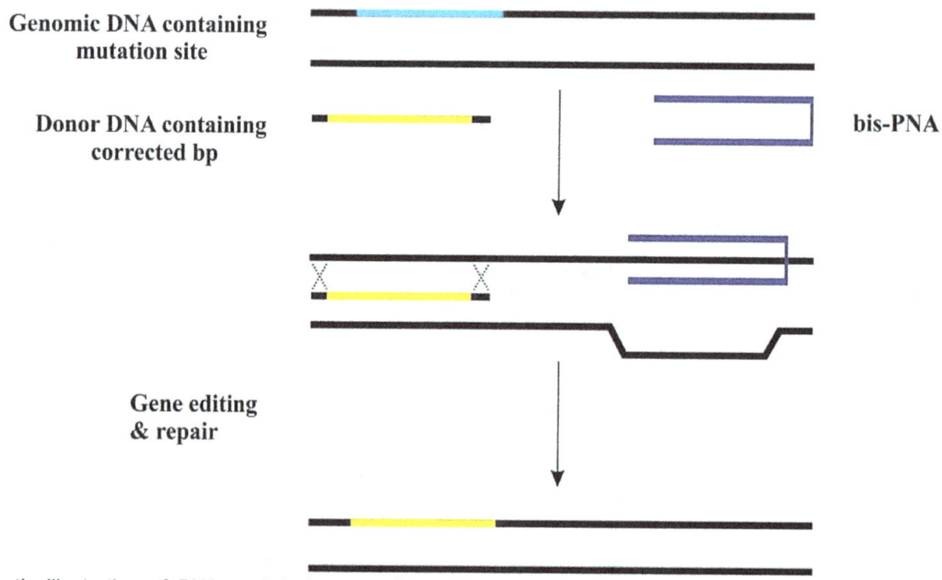

Figure 6. Schematic illustration of PNA-mediated gene editing. Triplex forming PNA can distort helical structure of DNA, inducing endogenous DNA repair in presence of DNA donor containing corrected nucleobases. The ability of PNAs in gene editing and repair comes directly from binding to cognate sites, provoking endogenous editing system.[81]

PNA as a potential therapeutic agent for cancer therapy

Cancer is a major health problem in the world and is recognized mainly as genetic disease resulting from mutations of oncogene and tumor suppressor genes. The goal of cancer therapy is to find and develop novel strategies for modulating the expression of cancer-related genes using selective anticancer agents with no cytotoxic effects as observed in conventional chemotherapy.[34] It has been shown that antigene and antisense strategies can be used to modulate transcription and translation of tumor genes. Moreover, numerous *in vitro* and *in vivo* experiments have already demonstrated the ability of PNA in controlling the dynamics of tumor gene expression. In accordance with a plethora of experiments, telomerase is found overexpressed in approximately 90% of human cancers, thereby being responsible for the immortalized cell phenotype. Of note, the modulation of this enzyme can be touted as an attractive target for cancer therapy. Besides, PNA *per se* has potential to hybridize to the RNA template region of telomerase and inhibit the catalytic activity of the enzyme.[35] Overall, these results point out PNAs may be valuable tools for target-directed anticancer agents.

Bcl-2 is a 26-kD protein, which has a key role in the dynamic of apoptosis. Overexpression of Bcl-2 correlates with prolonged survival of cells, tumor development, poor prognosis and resistance to anticancer therapies. With this background, the control of bcl-2 expression is an interesting approach in cancer therapy. They examined various PNAs targeted to different regions of mRNA sequences. *In vitro* investigations further showed that the synthesis of bcl-2 protein was blocked through PNA targeted to 5′UTR and the AUG codon of human B-cell lymphoma in a dose-dependent pattern. Moreover, the combined use of both PNAs produced complete inhibition, whereas partial translation inhibition was seen with single PNA usage. Also, a triplex forming bis-PNA was capable of binding to the template DNA strand of the bcl-2 gene and specifically suppressed the transcription of the gene with the presence of truncated product. Overall, PNA-based approach was able to selectively manipulate both translation and transcription of bcl-2 gene *in vitro*.[36]

Chronic myeloid leukemia (CML) is a malignancy, resulted from translocation of chromosomes 9q and 22q, the Philadelphia chromosome (Ph), and generate the bcr/abl oncogene. This gene produces a protein ($p210^{BCR/ABL}$) with high tyrosine kinase activity, leading to cell proliferation and malignant behavior. Thus, the unique sequence of *bcr/abl* is an attractive target for antisense therapy in CML disease. The incubation of CML cells with13 mer antisense PNA targeted to b2a2 junction in mRNA contributed to 35% decline in the level of $p210^{BCR/ABL}$ protein compared to control group. Also, anti-b2a2 PNAs have a strong antiproliferative effect in a dose dependent manner from 26% to 50% at 5 and 10 µM, respectively, displaying cell growth arrest.[37]

Acute promyelocytic leukemia (APL) is characterized by expression of the promyelocytic leukemiahetinoic acid receptor alpha gene (PML/RARa;PR). Fusion protein PML/RARα exists in all cases of APL and is generated by translocation of t (15; 17) chromosome. In this cancer model, the possibility of translation inhibition of the fused oncogene was tested by three different antisense PNAs targeting to first AUG start codon and second AUG and 5′UTR region of the fused oncogene sequence. Data showed PNAs directed against 5′UTR had the highest inhibitory activity compared to other ones. In fact, the limited effect of blocking was observed when PNAs used separately and a complete inhibition was achieved by the combination of these PNAs.[38,39]

Myc proteins play a key role in cancer. Overexpression of this protein is often correlated with DNA hypermethylation, higher cell growth rate, genomic instability and immortalization which lead to aggressive behavior of tumors.[40] Commensurate with these statements, MYCN gene can be considered as an important target for cancer therapy with novel therapeutic inhibitors such as PNA to manage proliferation and apoptosis pathways and reduce the malignant behavior of the tumor.[39,41] The possibility of PNA-based strategy for inhibition of MYCN transcription was previously examined by Tonelli and colleagues. They used an antigene PNA linked with nuclear localization signal peptide (NLS) targeted against a unique sequence of MYCN DNA (antisense DNA strand of exon 2) in six different cell lines of human neuroblastoma. The *in vitro* data showed a significant inhibition of MYCN expression by the antigene PNA in MYCN-amplified and MYCN-unamplified/low-expressed cell lines, leading to a reduction in cell proliferation rate, although no decrease was seen in MYCN-unamplified/unexpressed cell lines Compared with an antisense PNA, the inhibitory effect of the antigene PNA on MYCN gene expression showed stronger and longer inhibitory effect.[42]

Burkitt's Lymphoma (BL) cell is characterized by upregulation of the c-myc oncogene due to translocation of chromosome 8 to chromosome 14, proximal to Eµ enhancer within the Ig heavy chain locus that can induce transformed features. Therfore downregulation of translocated c-myc with a specific PNA, can reduce transformed properties in BL. Given that translocated c-myc is under Eµ enhancer control, PNAEµ targeting to enhancer sequence seem to be a potential therapeutic agent. In a preliminary experiment, evaluation of pharmacokinetic parameters for PNA to an in vivo model system in severe combined immunodeficiency mice (SCID) demonstrated that after administration of PNA, it can persist intact in an *in vivo* system for prolonged time about 600 minutes. In this regard, PNA targeted to the Eµ enhancer region located on chromosome 14 caused selective downregulation of only translocated c-myc not the normal allele.[43] Furthermore, using mice inoculated with the BL system demonstrated the potential capacity of PNAs to specifically and selectively block BL cells expansion and downregulation of c-myc expression.[44]

In addition, in a study, Cutrona and co-workers showed the effect of an anti-gene anti-myc PNA conjugated to a NLS in (BL) cell line. The authors used a 17-mer anti-myc PNA targeted to a unique sequence at the beginning of the second exon of the gene. The results indicated that PNA with 10 mM concentration achieved maximum inhibition of MYC expression (75%) and approximately (25%) reduction in cell viability, demonstrating that PNA specifically down-regulates the transcription of c-myc via binding to the double-stranded DNA *in vitro*. In consequence, PNAs are capable of inhibiting transcription of the targeted gene *in vitro* as well as *in vivo*, offering new specific therapeutic approaches to cure neoplasia.[45]

PNA as a splicing modulator in clinically relevant approaches

The erbB2 gene is amplified in approximately 20–35% of human breast cancers and other cancer types. Several studies indicated that overexpression of this gene is accompanied by the higher aggressiveness of the tumor and more importantly development of resistance to anti-estrogen treatment and chemotherapeutic strategies.[46] It has been shown that the application of antisense technology may be a useful approach towards treatment of breast cancers by targeting the translation start codon or the 3'-UTR region of the Her-2 mRNA to suppress the expression of Her-2 oncoprotein.[47] In line with this hypothesis, Nielsen et al. examined several antisense PNA oligomers targeted to intron-exon junction sites to interfere with correct splicing of erbB-2 pre-mRNA in two cancer cell lines. Since exon 19 codes ATP catalytic domain of Her-2, PNA oligomers are targeted to the 5' exon-intron junction site to induce skipping of exon 19 which harbors many of the Her-2 cancer-related mutations. Considering the flexibility of the splicing machinery,[48] obstruction of the 5' site could shift the spliceosome to another available splice site such as the 5' splice site of exon 20. Although the mechanism of skipping by PNA is not clear, it can be due to steric hindrance of pre-mRNA along with misleading of spliceosome through obstructing the correct splice site. The result demonstrated splicing redirection of Her-2 pre-mRNA by full-matched antisense PNA via skipping of erbB-2 exon 19. PNA-mediated activity can potentially be developed as anticancer strategies.[49]

The mdm2 oncogene encodes a nuclear phosphoprotein that inactivates the function of the p53 tumor suppressor protein. This oncogene is overexpressed in a wide variety of cancers.[50] In cancer therapy, mdm2 down-regulation is a promising strategy which might lead to the induction of p53. In agreement with this claim, Nielsen et al. obtained inhibition of mdm2 mRNA translation by PNA targeting to initiation site (AUG), whereby p53 levels increased.[51] Therefore, the mdm2 oncogene is an interesting antisense target for developing novel therapeutic agents and anticancer drugs. As mentioned above, PNA molecules were found to have a potent capability to target intron-exon junction sites. Again, Nielsen *et al.* designed several PNA molecules to down-regulate full-length mRNA of mdm2 or alter splice variants in human JAR cells through modulating splicing patterns. PNA oligomers tested toward the 5' or 3' splice sites in intron2 of mdm2 pre-mRNA inhibit splicing by generating a larger mRNA having retained intron 2. Among the PNAs, the most efficient is a complement to 4 bases in intron2 and 11 bases in exon3. Interestingly, another PNA which targets the 3' splice site of intron3 and is complementary to 4 bases in intron3 and 11 bases in exon4, exhibited both exon skipping as well as intron retention.[52]

Duchenne muscular dystrophy (DMD) is a lethal disease caused by point mutations in the dystrophin gene due to stop codon in exon 23 out of 79 exons. This early termination leads to complete loss of the functional muscle protein dystrophin throughout the body, which induces muscle complications. Although two FDA-approved drugs are in clinical use to treat DMD pateints, exon-skipping antisense oligonucleotide is still a promising approach in restoring reading frame and functional dystrophin protein. Preclinical studies revealed that PNAs are very promising method to induce splice correction by exon skipping in pre-mRNA of the DMD in mdx mice through intramuscular and systemic PNA delivery. PNA target to the intron22/exon23 junction site can induce skipping of exon 23 and produce a shortened protein still in reading frame shift with adequate activity to restore muscle function in a mouse (mdx) model. Also, it has been shown that single intramuscular administration of PNA could efficiently trigger exon-skipping, inducing dystrophin expression along with significant numbers of dystrophin-positive fibers in muscles in the mdx muscular dystrophy mouse model.[53] In parallel, identically designed experiment, intravenously repeated injections of high dose of PNA in mdx mice, elicited exon skipping accompanied by systemic therapeutic level of dystrophin expression and functional improvement with phenotypic rescue of mdx mice without major detectable toxicity. Based on the findings, PNA-base strategy is indeed a potent and promising applicable approach for DMD exon-skipping therapeutics, achieving restoration of functional dystrophin protein.[54]

Therapeutic approach of PNA as a gene editing agent

Available treatment for monogenic blood disorders such as sickle cell anemia and thalassemia is allogenic transplantation. However, limited accessibility of histocompatible donors along with associated side effects offers alternative strategies such as gene-targeted oligonucleotides with therapeutic potential.[55] In support of this statement, Rogers and his colleague tested the possibility of PNA as a gene editing agent in hematopoietic progenitor cells in a mice model to stimulate site-specific mutations while retaining differentiation capability of Hematopoietic stem cell (HSC). For systemic administration, PNA was linked to transport peptide Antp to target gene in murine. Intraperitoneally injected PNAs were targeted to reporter gene (supFG1) which was chromosomally integrated in transgenic mice. Results showed mutations in the supFG1 gene and higher mutation frequencies were observed within the PNA-binding site, demonstrating that HSCs can be chromosomally changed by systemically administered PNA. It shoud be adresssed that gene modification was observed in all the hematopoietic progenitors, including erythroid, myeloid and lymphoid cell lineages. These findings clearly revealed the clinical importance of *in vivo* HSCs gene therapy with a PNA-mediated approach in a stem cell population. This approach can be a new applicable therapeutic agent providing gene therapy in systemic diseases that cannot be manipulated outside the body.[56]

As mentioned above, triplex-forming PNAs can correct the mutant gene by engaging the cell's own DNA repair machinery via triggering recombination in the presence of a single stranded DNA template.[57] In an analogous study, gene-targeting strategy through intravenous injection of biodegradable nanoparticle containing triplex forming PNA (PNA-DNA-PNA) plus donor DNAs were used to edit hematopoietic stem cells in HSC engrafted mice. The results demonstrated modification of the human CCR5 gene in multiple organs in the mice, which is clinically relevant to human cells. To demonstrate the versatility of this approach, they administered nanoparticles carrying triplex forming PNAs which were targeted to β- globin, a gene associated with thalassemia disease. Analysis showed single base-pair modification in the second intron of the b-globin gene in a transgenic mice.[58] These findings are in line with *in vitro* study in which triplex forming PNAs could modify the human CCR5 gene, thus producing human immunodeficiency virus (HIV) resistant cells, as well as correcting single base-pair mutation at the intron of the *b*-globin gene, a common site of thalassemia-associated mutation.

Since PNAs can not readily cross the cell membrane and are excreted within 10–30 min after intravenous or intraperitoneal administration, hence, a delivery tool is required to access the target for *in vivo* gene editing. It has been shown that PNA and donor DNA could be efficiently encapsulated in poly (lactic-co-glycolic acid) (PLGA) nanoparticle, a FDA-approved polymer for *in vivo* drug delivery. This carrier can lead to higher efficiency in terms of gene editing both in vitro and in vivo.[59]

Bahal and McNeer reported related results by injection of nanoparticles containing next generation PNA chemistry (γPNAs) and donor DNAs targeted haematopoietic stem cells (HSCs) in a mouse model of human b-thalassemia. They observed *in vivo* gene editing of a b-thalassemia mutation in transgenic mice by simple intravenous injection of nanoparticles containing γPNA/donor DNA. In this way, the phenotype of the disease was ameliorated via elevation of blood haemoglobin levels, reduction of reticulocytosis, and reversal of splenomegaly.[60] Taken together, these findings encourage the development of *in vivo* gene editing through PNA mediated approaches as a novel therapeutic strategy for the treatment of inherited human disorders. In a similar research, two PNAs form a bis- PNA and bind to double stranded DNA forming triplex structure by Watson-crick and hoogsteen bond. In this process, γ position of regular PNA is attached to a mini-polyethylene glycol chain to enhance solubility and binding efficacy for the DNA target. Nanoparticles containing γPNAs and 60 bp donor DNAs were administered intravenously and intra amnioticly to fetal mouse tissues in order to correct IVS2-654 mutation in the β-globin gene in a mouse model of human β-thalassemia. Obtained result revealed that this strategy can cure anemia in thalassemic mice. The result revealed that PNA-mediated gene editing is an attractive method of gene editing during pregnancy, providing higher advantage compared to after birth therapy due to accessibility to progenitor cells (HSCs), which can result in propagation of the corrected gene in all progeny cells.[61]

Therapeutic Application of PNAs as Anti-miR agent

MicroRNAs (miRNAs) have important regulatory role in gene expression at post transcriptional stage. Additionally, upregulation of miRNAs expression is seen in several diseases remarkably in cancer, therefore they can be considered as important therapeutic targets.[62] Notably, anti-miR PNAs can bind miR and inhibit interaction with the RISC complex through steric hindrance, thus reducing miR expression.[63] It has been shown that PNAs have the capability to efficiently inhibit miR-155 which is expressed in the haematopoietic system in primary B cells as well as in mice model of lymphoma.[64,65] Additionally, it has been reported that PNA can be used as an inhibitor of miR-509-3p, which is cystic fibrosis transmembrane regulating miRNA.[66] Moreover, various MicroRNAs such as miR-210 are considerably upregulated in response to hypoxia condition, which is common in tumors development. MiR-210 may play a key role in survival and proliferation of tumor cells; it can be a good target for anti-cancer therapy. In a recently published study, γPNAs was used as a modified version of PNA to overcome limitations such as insolubility and tendency of globular formation. A regular PNA, a gamma PNA, and a control (mismatched) of 22 mer PNA were designed to target miR-210 in tumor Hela cell which grows as xenografts in immune-deficient nude mice using nanoparticle as a delivery system. Histopathological evidence showed that gamma PNAs targeted to miR-210, significantly suppressed tumor growth as well as increased the rate of apoptosis, compared to a regular PNA. Furthermore, expression of miR-210 is evaluated by RT-PCR in RNA extracted from the Hela tumor cells. There was a reduction in miR-210 expression levels compared to the control group. Under hypoxic condition, increase level of miR-210 is accompanied by suppression of ISCU protein which is downstream target of miR-210. Thus upon inhibition of miR-210, expression of ISCU is increased. Overall, PNA can inhibit microRNAs, offering novel approach in cancer therapy.[67]

Application of PNAs as anti-infective agent

In recent years, the rate of multi-drug resistant bacteria has increased, so it is required to treat these bacteria via developing novel drugs. Since PNA can inhibit gene expression of target gene, it can be used as antibacterial compounds to treat patients suffering from multidrug resistant bacteria. It has been reported that antisense PNA can target a variety of genes in *Pseudomonas aeruginosa*, the most clinically common and is resistant to a wide range of antibiotics.[68] Recent findings also addressed that antisense PNAs have potential to manupulate gene expression in *Plasmodium falciparum* through down regulation of an essential gene (PfSec13) which is responsible for viability in parasite. This alternative approach can be used to develop a novel and specific antimalarial drugs.[69,70] Of note, PNAs have no antibacterial activity without sequence-based homology with target site. PNA can selectively bind to the conserved sequence in variety of bacterial genus and inhibit growth in broad-spectrum of bacteria. It has been revealed that PNA targeted to translation initiation region of specific genes including *Bacillus subtilis* (gram-positive bacteria) and *Escherichia coli, Klebsiella pneumoniae and Salmonella Typhimurium* (gram negative bacteria) in a mixed culture, selectively kills bacteria, so these findings open a novel opportunities for designing new therapeutic intervention for the treatment of pathogen bacteria.[71]

Table 1. Several examples of PNA-mediated gene therapy

PNA	Target site	In vivo / in vitro	Disorder	Observed Effects	Ref.
Antigene PNA	COL1A1 gene	Normal human fibroblast cell line	Fibroproliferative Disorders	Reduction of mRNA level	72
Antigene PNA	RAD51 gene	Human MM cell line H929 & a SCID-rab mouse model	Multiple Myeloma (MM)	Inhibition of RAD51 expression	73
Antigene PNA	MYCN gene	Rhabdomyosarcoma cell line	Rhabdomyosarcomas	Reduction of MYCN expression	74
Antisense PNA	COL7A1 gene	in vitro/ Primary adult fibroblast cultures	Dominant Dystrophic Epidermolysis Bullosa	Inhibition of the transcription of a mutant COL7A1	75
Antisense PNA	miR-155	Mice	Lymphomas	Inhibition of oncomiR-155	76
Antisense PNA	miR-221	Human breast cancer MCF-7 & MDA-MB-231 cell lines	Breast Tumors	Inhibition of onco miR-221	77
Antisense PNA	miR-509-3p	A549 cell lines	Cystic Fibrosis	Inhibition of miR-509-3p	66
Antisense PNA	Targeting LTR Direct Repeats of HBV RNA	HEPG2 cell line& an acute hepatitis B mouse model	Hepatitis B	Decline in HBV DNA	78
γPNA and donor DNA	Intron containing Mutation(the IVS2-654)	in vivo (β-globin/eGFP transgenic mouse)	β-thalassaemia	Induce DNA repair in mutaded gene	79
Antigene	Dystrophin Gene in Muscle Stem Cells	ex vivo/ in mdx mice, a mouse model of DMD	Duchenne muscular dystrophy	Permanently correct single-point mutations at the genomic level in stem cells	80

Conclusion

Since the invention of PNA, several applications have been developed based on the unique properties of this oligomer; in particular, exploiting alteration of gene expression with focus on the antisense and antigene activity of PNA. Much attention has recently been given for possible clinical applications of PNAs in combination with drugs which are used in the clinic in cancer therapy based on *in vivo* experimental systems and clinical trials. However, in practice, great consideration is still needed in terms of *in vivo* administration such as immunogenicity, biodistribution, and other problems related to drug development.

Acknowledgments

This review is a part of Ph.D thesis of Soheila Montazersaheb (Thesis No. : 102) at Faculty of Pharmacy, Tabriz University of Medical Sciences, Tabriz, Iran. The authors would like to acknowledge Prof. Peter Nielsen (University of Copenhagen, Denmark) for helpful comments on the manuscript.

Conflict of Interest

There is no conflict of interest in this study.

References

1. Dean DA. Peptide nucleic acids: Versatile tools for gene therapy strategies. *Adv Drug Deliv Rev* 2000;44(2-3):81-95. doi: 10.1016/S0169-409X(00)00087-9
2. Pellestor F, Paulasova P. The peptide nucleic acids (PNAs), powerful tools for molecular genetics and cytogenetics. *Eur J Hum Genet* 2004;12(9):694-700. doi: 10.1038/sj.ejhg.5201226
3. Nielsen PE. Peptide nucleic acids (PNA) in chemical biology and drug discovery. *Chem Biodivers* 2010;7(4):786-804. doi: 10.1002/cbdv.201000005
4. Nielsen PE, Egholm M, Berg RH, Buchardt O. Sequence-selective recognition of DNA by strand displacement with a thymine-substituted polyamide. *Science* 1991;254(5037):1497-500. doi: 10.1126/science.1962210
5. Raoof JB, Ojani R, Golabi SM, Hamidi-Asl E, Hejazi MS. Preparation of an electrochemical PNA biosensor for detection of target DNA sequence and

single nucleotide mutation on p53 tumor suppressor gene corresponding oligonucleotide. *Sens Actuators B Chem* 2011;157(1):195-201. doi: 10.1016/j.snb.2011.03.049

6. Sharma C, Awasthi SK. Versatility of peptide nucleic acids (PNAs): Role in chemical biology, drug discovery, and origins of life. *Chem Biol Drug Des* 2017;89(1):16-37. doi: 10.1111/cbdd.12833
7. Metaferia B, Wei JS, Song YK, Evangelista J, Aschenbach K, Johansson P, et al. Development of peptide nucleic acid probes for detection of the HER2 oncogene. *PloS One* 2013;8(4):e58870. doi: 10.1371/journal.pone.0058870
8. Braasch DA, Nulf CJ, Corey DR. Synthesis and purification of peptide nucleic acids. *Curr Protoc Nucleic Acid Chem* 2002;9(1):4.11.1-4. 8. doi: 10.1002/0471142700.nc0411s09
9. Hejazi MS, Pournaghi-Azar MH, Alipour E, Abdolahinia ED, Arami S, Navvah H. Development of a novel electrochemical biosensor for detection and discrimination of DNA sequence and single base mutation in dsDNA samples based on PNA-dsDNA hybridization-a new platform technology. *Electroanalysis* 2011;23(2):503-11. doi: 10.1002/elan.201000413
10. Ahour F, Pournaghi-Azar MH, Alipour E, Hejazi MS. Detection and discrimination of recombinant plasmid encoding hepatitis C virus core/E1 gene based on PNA and double-stranded DNA hybridization. *Biosens Bioelectron* 2013;45:287-91. doi: 10.1016/j.bios.2013.01.063
11. Siddiquee S, Rovina K, Azriah A. A review of peptide nucleic acid. *Adv Tech Biol Med* 2015;3(2). doi: 10.4172/2379-1764.1000131
12. Nielsen PE. Modulating gene function with peptide nucleic acids (PNA). In: Crooke ST, editor. Antisense drug technology. Taylor & Francis; 2008. P. 507-18.
13. Nielsen PE. Peptide nucleic acid: A versatile tool in genetic diagnostics and molecular biology. *Curr Opin Biotechnol* 2001;12(1):16-20. doi: 10.1016/S0958-1669(00)00170-1
14. Quijano E, Bahal R, Ricciardi A, Saltzman WM, Glazer PM. Therapeutic peptide nucleic acids: Principles, limitations, and opportunities. *Yale J Biol Med* 2017;90(4):583-98.
15. Nielsen PE. Addressing the challenges of cellular delivery and bioavailability of peptide nucleic acids (PNA). *Q Rev Biophys* 2005;38(4):345-50. doi: 10.1017/S0033583506004148
16. Shiraishi T, Nielsen PE. Enhanced delivery of cell-penetrating peptide-peptide nucleic acid conjugates by endosomal disruption. *Nat Protoc* 2006;1(2):633-6. doi: 10.1038/nprot.2006.92
17. Said Hassane F, Saleh AF, Abes R, Gait MJ, Lebleu B. Cell penetrating peptides: Overview and applications to the delivery of oligonucleotides. *Cell Mol Life Sci* 2010;67(5):715-26. doi: 10.1007/s00018-009-0186-0
18. Nielsen PE, Shiraishi T. Peptide nucleic acid (PNA) cell penetrating peptide (CPP) conjugates as carriers for cellular delivery of antisense oligomers. *Artif DNA PNA XNA* 2011;2(3):90-9. doi: 10.4161/adna.18739
19. Margus H, Padari K, Pooga M. Cell-penetrating peptides as versatile vehicles for oligonucleotide delivery. *Mol Ther* 2012;20(3):525-33. doi: 10.1038/mt.2011.284
20. Gonçalves GAR, Paiva RMA. Gene therapy: Advances, challenges and perspectives. *Einstein (Sao Paulo)* 2017;15(3):369-75. doi: 10.1590/S1679-45082017RB4024
21. Shakeel S, Karim S, Ali A. Peptide nucleic acid (PNA)—a review. *J Chem Technol Biotechnol* 2006;81(6):892-9. doi: 10.1002/jctb.1505
22. Hu J, Corey DR. Inhibiting gene expression with peptide nucleic acid (PNA)--peptide conjugates that target chromosomal DNA. *Biochemistry* 2007;46(25):7581-9. doi: 10.1021/bi700230a
23. Janowski BA, Kaihatsu K, Huffman KE, Schwartz JC, Ram R, Hardy D, et al. Inhibiting transcription of chromosomal DNA with antigene peptide nucleic acids. *Nat Chem Biol* 2005;1(4):210-5. doi: 10.1038/nchembio724
24. Zaffaroni N, Villa R, Folini M. Therapeutic uses of peptide nucleic acids (PNA) in oncology. In: Janson CG, During MJ, editors. Peptide nucleic acids, morpholinos and related antisense biomolecules. Springer; 2006. P. 171-80.
25. Järver P, Coursindel T, Andaloussi SE, Godfrey C, Wood MJ, Gait MJ. Peptide-mediated cell and in vivo delivery of antisense oligonucleotides and sirna. *Mol Ther Nucleic Acids* 2012;1:e27. doi: 10.1038/mtna.2012.18
26. Nielsen E. RNA targeting using peptide nucleic acid. In: Erdmann V, Barciszewski J, Brosius J, editors. RNA towards medicine. Berlin: Springer; 2006. P. 395-403.
27. Nielsen PE. Gene targeting using peptide nucleic acid. In: Herdewijn P, editor. Oligonucleotide synthesis. New Jersey: Humana Press; 2005. P. 343-58.
28. Wahl MC, Will CL, Lührmann R. The spliceosome: Design principles of a dynamic RNP machine. *Cell* 2009;136(4):701-18. doi: 10.1016/j.cell.2009.02.009
29. Sazani P, Kole R. Therapeutic potential of antisense oligonucleotides as modulators of alternative splicing. *J Clin Invest* 2003;112(4):481-6. doi: 10.1172/JCI19547
30. Yang SP, Song ST, Song HF. Advancements of antisense oligonucleotides in treatment of breast cancer. *Acta Pharmacol Sin* 2003;24(4):289-95.
31. Aartsma-Rus A, Van Ommen GJ. Antisense-mediated exon skipping: A versatile tool with therapeutic and research applications. *RNA* 2007;13(10):1609-24. doi: 10.1261/rna.653607
32. Garcia-Blanco MA. Alternative splicing: Therapeutic target and tool. *Prog Mol Subcell Biol* 2006;44:47-64.

33. Garcia-Blanco MA, Baraniak AP, Lasda EL. Alternative splicing in disease and therapy. *Nat Biotechnol* 2004;22(5):535-46. doi: 10.1038/nbt964
34. Mologni L, Gambacorti-Passerini C. PNAs as novel cancer therapeutics. *Lett Pept Sci* 2003;10(3-4):297-308. doi: 10.1007/bf02484565
35. Nielsen PE. Gene targeting and expression modulation by peptide nucleic acids (PNA). *Curr Pharm Des* 2010;16(28):3118-23. doi: 10.2174/138161210793292546
36. Mologni L, Nielsen PE, Gambacorti-Passerini C. In vitro transcriptional and translational block of the bcl-2 gene operated by peptide nucleic acid. *Biochem Biophys Res Commun* 1999;264(2):537-43. doi: 10.1006/bbrc.1999.1548
37. Rapozzi V, Burm BE, Cogoi S, van der Marel GA, van Boom JH, Quadrifoglio F, et al. Antiproliferative effect in chronic myeloid leukaemia cells by antisense peptide nucleic acids. *Nucleic Acids Res* 2002;30(17):3712-21. doi: 10.1093/nar/gkf451
38. Mologni L, leCoutre P, Nielsen PE, Gambacorti-Passerini C. Additive antisense effects of different PNAs on the in vitro translation of the PML/RARα gene. *Nucleic Acids Res* 1998;26(8):1934-8. doi: 10.1093/nar/26.8.1934
39. Vita M, Henriksson M. The Myc oncoprotein as a therapeutic target for human cancer. *Semin Cancer Biol* 2006;16(4):318-30. doi: 10.1016/j.semcancer.2006.07.015
40. Lee TI, Young RA. Transcriptional regulation and its misregulation in disease. *Cell* 2013;152(6):1237-51. doi: 10.1016/j.cell.2013.02.014
41. Wang LL, Teshiba R, Ikegaki N, Tang XX, Naranjo A, London WB, et al. Augmented expression of MYC and/or MYCN protein defines highly aggressive MYC-driven neuroblastoma: A children's oncology group study. *Br J Cancer* 2015;113(1):57-63. doi: 10.1038/bjc.2015.188
42. Tonelli R, Purgato S, Camerin C, Fronza R, Bologna F, Alboresi S, et al. Anti-gene peptide nucleic acid specifically inhibits MYCN expression in human neuroblastoma cells leading to cell growth inhibition and apoptosis. *Mol Cancer Ther* 2005;4(5):779-86. doi: 10.1158/1535-7163.MCT-04-0213
43. Boffa LC, Cutrona G, Cilli M, Mariani MR, Matis S, Pastorino M, et al. Therapeutically promising PNA complementary to a regulatory sequence for c-myc: Pharmacokinetics in an animal model of human burkitt's lymphoma. *Oligonucleotides* 2005;15(2):85-93. doi: 10.1089/oli.2005.15.85
44. Boffa LC, Cutrona G, Cilli M, Matis S, Damonte G, Mariani MR, et al. Inhibition of burkitt's lymphoma cells growth in SCID mice by a PNA specific for a regulatory sequence of the translocated c-myc. *Cancer gene ther* 2007;14(2):220-6. doi: 10.1038/sj.cgt.7701002
45. Cutrona G, Carpaneto EM, Ulivi M, Roncella S, Landt O, Ferrarini M, et al. Effects in live cells of a c-myc anti-gene PNA linked to a nuclear localization signal. *Nat Biotechnol* 2000;18(3):300-3. doi: 10.1038/73745
46. Roskoski R Jr. The ErbB/HER receptor protein-tyrosine kinases and cancer. *Biochem Biophys Res Commun* 2004;319(1):1-11. doi: 10.1016/j.bbrc.2004.04.150
47. Roh H, Pippin J, Drebin JA. Down-regulation of HER2/neu expression induces apoptosis in human cancer cells that overexpress HER2/neu. *Cancer Res* 2000;60(3):560-5.
48. Mercatante DR, Kole R. Control of alternative splicing by antisense oligonucleotides as a potential chemotherapy: Effects on gene expression. *Biochim Biophys Acta* 2002;1587(2-3):126-32. doi: 10.1016/S0925-4439(02)00075-3
49. Pankratova S, Nielsen BN, Shiraishi T, Nielsen PE. PNA-mediated modulation and redirection of Her-2 pre-mRNA splicing: Specific skipping of erbB-2 exon 19 coding for the ATP catalytic domain. *Int J Oncol* 2010;36(1):29-38. doi: 10.3892/ijo_00000472
50. Zhao Y, Yu H, Hu W. The regulation of MDM2 oncogene and its impact on human cancers. *Acta Biochim Biophys Sin (Shanghai)* 2014;46(3):180-9. doi: 10.1093/abbs/gmt147
51. Shiraishi T, Nielsen PE. Down-regulation of MDM2 and activation of p53 in human cancer cells by antisense 9-aminoacridine-PNA (peptide nucleic acid) conjugates. *Nucleic Acids Res* 2004;32(16):4893-902. doi: 10.1093/nar/gkh820
52. Shiraishi T, Eysturskarð J, Nielsen PE. Modulation of mdm2 pre-mRNA splicing by 9-aminoacridine-PNA (peptide nucleic acid) conjugates targeting intron-exon junctions. *BMC Cancer* 2010;10:342. doi: 10.1186/1471-2407-10-342
53. Yin H, Lu Q, Wood M. Effective exon skipping and restoration of dystrophin expression by peptide nucleic acid antisense oligonucleotides in mdx mice. *Mol Ther* 2008;16(1):38-45. doi: 10.1038/sj.mt.6300329
54. Gao X, Shen X, Dong X, Ran N, Han G, Cao L, et al. Peptide nucleic acid promotes systemic dystrophin expression and functional rescue in dystrophin-deficient mdx mice. *Mol Ther Nucleic Acids* 2015;4:e255. doi: 10.1038/mtna.2015.27
55. Hoban MD, Orkin SH, Bauer DE. Genetic treatment of a molecular disorder: Gene therapy approaches to sickle cell disease. *Blood* 2016;127(7):839-48. doi: 10.1182/blood-2015-09-618587
56. Rogers FA, Lin SS, Hegan DC, Krause DS, Glazer PM. Targeted gene modification of hematopoietic progenitor cells in mice following systemic administration of a PNA-peptide conjugate. *Mol Ther* 2012;20(1):109-18. doi: 10.1038/mt.2011.163
57. Chin JY, Glazer PM. Repair of DNA lesions associated with triplex-forming oligonucleotides. *Mol Carcinog* 2009;48(4):389-99. doi: 10.1002/mc.20501
58. McNeer NA, Schleifman EB, Cuthbert A, Brehm M, Jackson A, Cheng C, et al. Systemic delivery of triplex-forming PNA and donor DNA by

nanoparticles mediates site-specific genome editing of human hematopoietic cells in vivo. *Gene Ther* 2013;20(6):658-69. doi: 10.1038/gt.2012.82

59. Chin JY, Kuan JY, Lonkar PS, Krause DS, Seidman MM, Peterson KR, et al. Correction of a splice-site mutation in the beta-globin gene stimulated by triplex-forming peptide nucleic acids. *Proc Natl Acad Sci U S A* 2008;105(36):13514-9. doi: 10.1073/pnas.0711793105
60. Bahal R, McNeer NA, Quijano E, Liu Y, Sulkowski P, Turchick A, et al. In vivo correction of anaemia in β-thalassemic mice by γPNA-mediated gene editing with nanoparticle delivery. *Nat Commun* 2016;7:13304. doi: 10.1038/ncomms13304
61. Ricciardi AS, Bahal R, Farrelly JS, Quijano E, Bianchi AH, Luks VL, et al. In utero nanoparticle delivery for site-specific genome editing. *Nat Commun* 2018;9(1):2481. doi: 10.1038/s41467-018-04894-2
62. Rupaimoole R, Slack FJ. Microrna therapeutics: Towards a new era for the management of cancer and other diseases. *Nat Rev Drug Discov* 2017;16(3):203-22. doi: 10.1038/nrd.2016.246
63. Marchelli R, Corradini R, Manicardi A, Sforza S, Tedeschi T, Fabbri E, et al. Gene Modulation by Peptide Nucleic Acids (PNAs) Targeting microRNAs (miRs). In: You Y, editor. Targets in Gene Therapy. InTech; 2011. P. 29-46.
64. Fabani MM, Abreu-Goodger C, Williams D, Lyons PA, Torres AG, Smith KG, et al. Efficient inhibition of miR-155 function in vivo by peptide nucleic acids. *Nucleic Acids Res* 2010;38(13):4466-75. doi: 10.1093/nar/gkq160
65. Cheng CJ, Bahal R, Babar IA, Pincus Z, Barrera F, Liu C, et al. MicroRNA silencing for cancer therapy targeted to the tumour microenvironment. *Nature* 2015;518(7537):107-10. doi: 10.1038/nature13905
66. Amato F, Tomaiuolo R, Borbone N, Elce A, Amato J, D'Errico S, et al. Design, synthesis and biochemical investigation, by in vitro luciferase reporter system, of peptide nucleic acids as new inhibitors of mir-509-3p involved in the regulation of cystic fibrosis disease-gene expression. *MedChemComm* 2014;5(1):68-71. doi: 10.1039/C3MD00257H
67. Gupta A, Quijano E, Liu Y, Bahal R, Scanlon SE, Song E, et al. Anti-tumor activity of miniPEG-γ-modified PNAs to inhibit microRNA-210 for cancer therapy. *Mol Ther Nucleic Acids* 2017;9:111-9. doi: 10.1016/j.omtn.2017.09.001
68. Maekawa K, Azuma M, Okuno Y, Tsukamoto T, Nishiguchi K, Setsukinai K, et al. Antisense peptide nucleic acid-peptide conjugates for functional analyses of genes in Pseudomonas aeruginosa. *Bioorg Med Chem* 2015;23(22):7234-9. doi: 10.1016/j.bmc.2015.10.020
69. Kolevzon N, Nasereddin A, Naik S, Yavin E, Dzikowski R. Use of peptide nucleic acids to manipulate gene expression in the malaria parasite Plasmodium falciparum. *PLoS One* 2014;9(1):e86802. doi: 10.1371/journal.pone.0086802
70. Amit-Avraham I, Pozner G, Eshar S, Fastman Y, Kolevzon N, Yavin E, et al. Antisense long noncoding RNAs regulate var gene activation in the malaria parasite Plasmodium falciparum. *Proc Natl Acad Sci U S A* 2015;112(9):E982-91. doi: 10.1073/pnas.1420855112
71. Mondhe M, Chessher A, Goh S, Good L, Stach JE. Species-selective killing of bacteria by antimicrobial peptide-PNAs. *PloS One* 2014;9(2):e89082. doi: 10.1371/journal.pone.0089082
72. Imamura Y, Tsuboi S, Sugiyama T, Kittaka A, Shin Y. A peptide nucleic acid to reduce type I collagen production by fibroblast cells. *Open J Med Chem* 2015;5(1):1-8. doi: 10.4236/ojmc.2015.51001
73. Alagpulinsa DA, Yaccoby S, Ayyadevara S, Shmookler Reis RJ. A peptide nucleic acid targeting nuclear RAD51 sensitizes multiple myeloma cells to melphalan treatment. *Cancer Biol Ther* 2015;16(6):976-86. doi: 10.1080/15384047.2015.1040951
74. Tonelli R, McIntyre A, Camerin C, Walters ZS, Di Leo K, Selfe J, et al. Antitumor activity of sustained N-myc reduction in rhabdomyosarcomas and transcriptional block by antigene therapy. *Clin Cancer Res* 2012;18(3):796-807. doi: 10.1158/1078-0432.CCR-11-1981
75. Amato J, Stellato MI, Pizzo E, Petraccone L, Oliviero G, Borbone N, et al. PNA as a potential modulator of COL7A1 gene expression in dominant dystrophic epidermolysis bullosa: A physico-chemical study. *Mol BioSyst* 2013;9(12):3166-74. doi: 10.1039/c3mb70283a
76. Babar IA, Cheng CJ, Booth CJ, Liang X, Weidhaas JB, Saltzman WM, et al. Nanoparticle-based therapy in an in vivo microRNA-155 (miR-155)-dependent mouse model of lymphoma. *Proc Natl Acad Sci U S A* 2012;109(26):E1695-704. doi: 10.1073/pnas.1201516109
77. Brognara E, Fabbri E, Aimi F, Manicardi A, Bianchi N, Finotti A, et al. Peptide nucleic acids targeting miR-221 modulate p27Kip1 expression in breast cancer MDA-MB-231 cells. *Int J Oncol* 2012;41(6):2119-27. doi: 10.3892/ijo.2012.1632
78. Zeng Z, Han S, Hong W, Lang Y, Li F, Liu Y, et al. A Tat-conjugated Peptide Nucleic Acid Tat-PNA-DR Inhibits Hepatitis B Virus Replication In Vitro and In Vivo by Targeting LTR Direct Repeats of HBV RNA. *Mol Ther Nucleic Acids* 2016;5:e295. doi: 10.1038/mtna.2016.11
79. Bahal R, Quijano E, McNeer NA, Liu Y, Bhunia DC, Lopez-Giraldez F, et al. Single-stranded γPNAs for in vivo site-specific genome editing via Watson-Crick recognition. *Curr Gene Ther* 2014;14(5):331-42.

Synergic Antibacterial Effect of Curcumin with Ampicillin; Free Drug Solutions in Comparison with SLN Dispersions

Faezeh Alihosseini[1], Shirzad Azarmi[2,3], Solmaz Ghaffari[1,4,*], Setareh Haghighat[5], Seyed Mahdi Rezayat Sorkhabadi[6,7]

[1] *Department of Medical Nanotechnology, Pharmaceutical Sciences Branch, Islamic Azad University (IAUPS), Tehran, Iran.*
[2] *Faculty of Pharmacy and Pharmaceutical Sciences, University of Alberta, Edmonton, Alta, Canada.*
[3] *Research Center for Pharmaceutical Nanotechnology, Faculty of Pharmacy, Tabriz University of Medical Sciences, Tabriz, Iran.*
[4] *Young Researchers and Elite Club, Pharmaceutical Sciences Branch, Islamic Azad University, (IAUPS), Tehran, Iran.*
[5] *Department of Microbiology, Faculty of Advanced Sciences and Technology, Pharmaceutical Sciences Branch, Islamic Azad University (IAUPS), Tehran, Iran.*
[6] *Department of Medical Nanotechnology, School of Advanced Sciences and Technology in Medicine, Tehran University of Medical Sciences (TUMS), Tehran, Iran.*
[7] *Department of Pharmacology and Toxicology, Pharmaceutical Sciences Branch, Islamic Azad University, (IAUPS), Tehran, Iran.*

Article info

Keywords:
- Solid Lipid Nanoparticles
- Curcumin
- Synergy
- Ampicillin

Abstract

Purpose: This study was designed to investigate benefit of using nanotechnology on increasing of synergic antibacterial effect of natural and chemical antibacterial agents.
Methods: At first the MIC and MBC of Curcumin and Ampicillin as selected antibacterial agents was determined, after that Solid Lipid Nanoparticles (SLNs) of each active ingredients as well as Curcumin-Ampicillin loaded SLNs were prepared using high pressure homogenization technique. Characterization of prepared SLNs was done, then MIC, MBC and contact killing time were investigated for Curcumin-Ampicillin loaded SLNs in comparison with free Curcumin and Ampicillin solutions as well as Ampicillin and Curcumin SLNs.
Results: Based on results nanoparticles with the size of 150 nm show much more decreased MIC and MBC when Ampicillin and Curcumin were loaded together on SLNs than solutions in which free Ampicillin and Curcumin were mixed.
Conclusion: It seems that using nanotechnology could cause decrease the dosage of antibiotics and risk of having antibiotic resistance bacteria strains.

Introduction

Todays increased resistance to antibiotics and decreasing of effective antibiotics has resulted in a challenge in the treatment of infections in the world.[1]

Curcuma longa as a plant of Zingiberaceae family has antimicrobial effect against many microorganisms with different mechanisms.[2-3] Ampicillin as a β-lactam could inhibit bacteria cell wall synthesis to kill the bacteria.[4] Beta-lactam antibiotics are the most preferred antibiotic group in the treatment of infections due to their wide spectrum and minimal side effects but bacteria go to be resistance against them.[5] Some studies have previously demonstrated that curcumin potentiates the effects of chemical antibiotics against bacteria strains.[6]

Our previous studies showed that loading of antibiotics on SLNs could cause to decrease MIC and MBC against S.aureus, Ecoli and P.aeroginosa significantly.[7,8]

The aim of this study was to investigate the synergistic effect of curcumin and ampicillin against P.aeroginosa, S.aureus, Ecoli, C.diphtheria, B.Subtilis and MRSA as well as to determine the antibacterial activity of their combination when loaded on SLNs.

Materials and Methods

Preparation of Solutions

Solution A

A stock solution of free ampicillin was prepared in sterile water that was further diluted in Muller–Hinton broth to reach a concentration of 0.125 µg/mL.

Solution B

A stock solution of free curcumin was prepared in sterile water that was further diluted in Muller–Hinton broth to reach a concentration of 0.125 µg/mL.

Solution C

Then a stock solution of free ampicillin and curcumin was prepared by mixing of 50-50% of the two above solutions.

***Corresponding author:** Solmaz Ghaffari, Email: ghaffari.s@iaups.ac.ir

Preparation of SLNs

Curcumin and ampicillin loaded SLNs were prepared separately using high pressure homogenization method based on the Varshosaz et al method in which hot oily phase was added to aqueous phase under homogenization.[9] Table 1 shows the formulations.

Table 1. SLN formulations.

Formulation name	Amount of curcumin(mg)	Amount of Ampicillin(mg)	Amount of cholesterol(mg)	Amount of tween 80(mg)	Distilled water(ml)	Ethanol/acetone (ml)	Homogenization (minutes)
A	726	----	80. 605	1.5	121	22/7.5	7
B	----	218	605	1.5	121	22/7.5	7
C	726	218	605	1.5	121	22/7.5	7
D	363	109	605	1.5	121	22/7.5	7
E	Mixture of formulation A and B in 50-50% ratio, formulation E was designed to compare that is it better that active ingredients load together on SLNs or each of them load separately and then prepared drug loaded SLNs mix in 50-50% ratio (comparison of formulation D and E).						

Determination of particle size of SLNs

All SLNs, were investigated to determine particle size distribution by Malvern instrument.

Morphology studies

Morphology of the nanoparticles was characterized by scanning electron microscopy.

Antibacterial studies

Inhibitory zone Determination

The "well diffusion test" was carried out using P.aueroginosa (ATCC 27853), S.aureus (ATTC 25923), Ecoli (ATCC 25922), C.diphtheria (ATCC 39255), B.Subtilis (PTCC 1720) and MRSA 252.[8]

MIC and MBC Detection

The conventional broth macrodilution tube method was used to determine MIC and MBC of all above solutions and formulations with respect to P.aueroginosa, S.aureus, Ecoli, C.diphtheria, B.subtilis and MRSA in vitro.[7,10]

killing contact time Determination

In this procedure, 0.1 ml of bacteria suspension equivalent to 0.5 McFarland standards were added to tubes contain 9.9 ml Muller-Hilton broth with MIC concentration of formulations A, B, C, D and E Muller-Hilton broth as control, and incubation was done at 37°C. Then samples were taken from growing bacteria cultures in desired times and spread on Muller-Hilton agar and colonies were count after incuation.

Results and Discussion

Particle size of SLNs

Results (Z-average) showed that the particle size of formulations A,B,C and D were 159, 149, 163 and 145 nm respectively. Poly Dispersity Indexes were less than 0.5 for all formulations.

Morphology studies

All desired SLN formulations were spherical.

Antibacterial studies

Determination of inhibition zone

Table 2 shows the result of inhibition zone of formulation A-D. Results show that although MRSA and C.diphtheria are resistant against curcumin SLNs (formulation A) but these SLNs could increase inhibition zone when is combine with ampicillin on SLNs (formulation C), so a synergy could be seen. There are not significant differences between formulation D and E for none of bacteria strains except S.aureus, MRSA and P.aueroginosa in which seems that it will be better if drugs load together in formulation process (formulation D) instead of preparing of each formulation (A and B) and then mix them in 50-50% ratio (formulation E).

Table 2. Results of measurement of inhibition zone of formulations A-E for six bacterial strains

Bacteria strain	Formulations				
	A	B	C	D	E
S.aureus	1.5 cm	2.5 cm	3 cm	3 cm	2.5 cm
Ecoli	0.5 cm	3 cm	2 cm	1.5 cm	1.5 cm
B.Subtilis	1 cm	1.5 cm	2.5 cm	2 cm	2 cm
P.aueroginosa	0	1 cm	1 cm	0.75 cm	0.5 cm
C.diphtheria	0	2 cm	2.25 cm	2 cm	2 cm
MRSA	0	1.5 cm	2 cm	1.5 cm	1.25 cm

MIC and MBC studies

Results were shown in Tables 3 and 4. The enhancement of antibacterial effect when curcumin used with ampicillin was obtained as reported in Table 3 for free drugs solutions especially for MIC regarding to B.subtilis, C.diphteria and MRSA. Comparisons of data series of Table 3 and 4, show that MIC and MBC of ampicillin and curcumin which were loaded together on SLNs (formulation C) were much more decreased than solution C in which free ampicillin and curcumin was mixed together. About B.subtilis MIC of formulation C is practically the same as solution C but the resistancy of bacteria to free drugs in MBC was broken by using SLNs. P.aueroginosa is resistant against free drug mixture of ampicillin and curcumin but formulation C is effective on this strain and MBC is two times larger than MIC in this situation. For C.diphteria, no significant changes were observed in MIC of Solution C and formulation C but MBC decreased 4 times when drugs loaded on SLNs in comparison with free drugs. About MRSA MIC decreased 2 times with using SLNs and the resitancy of MRSA about MBC was broken. The increasing of antibacterial effect of ampicillin SLNs in comparison with free ampicillin against Ecoli, S.aureus and P.aueroginosa was reported by Alihoseyni et al.[8] Previously the efficacy of SLNs to decrease MIC and MBC of Curcumin was demonstrated.[11]

Killing contact time

Table 5 shows killing contact time results. Formulation C after 10 hours contact with S.aureus, Ecoli, P.aueroginosa, C.diphtheria, B.subtilis show the highest killing percentage in comparison with formulations A, B, D and E. The efficacy of all formulations against all bacteria strains is time dependent and the most bacteria killing percentage was reported after 10 hours, may be due to sustained drug release profiles.

Presented results demonstrated the probability of benefits of using nanotechnology to decrease the dosage of antibiotics and decrease risk of having antibiotic resistance bacteria strains.

Table 3. MIC and MBC results for desired solutions against six bacteria strains

Bacterial Strains	MBC (µg/ml)			MIC (µg/ml)		
	Solutions			Solutions		
	A	B	C	A	B	C
S.aureus	8	Resistance	7.5 (ampi) 125 (cur)	2	125	2(ampi) 31.25(cur)
Ecoli	30	Resistance	30 (ampi) 500(cur)	8	500	7.5(ampi) 125(cur)
B.Subtilis	Resistance	Resistance	Resistance	30	Resistance	15(ampi) 250(cur)
P.aueroginosa	Resistance	Resistance	Resistance	Resistance	Resistance	Resistance
C.diphtheria	30	Resistance	30 (ampi) 500(cur)	8	250	7.5(ampi) 125(cur)
MRSA	Resistance	Resistance	Resistance	30	Resistance	15(ampi) 250(cur)

Table 4. MIC and MBC results for desired formulations against six bacteria strains

Bacterial Strains	MBC (µg/ml)				MIC (µg/ml)			
	Formulations Name				Formulations Name			
	A	C	D	E	A	C	D	E
S.aureus	250	4(ampi) 62.5(cur)	4(ampi) 62.5(cur)	4(ampi) 62.5(cur)	125	0.5(ampi) 7.8 (cur)	4(ampi) 62.5(cur)	1 (ampi) 15.62 (cur)
Ecoli	500	8(ampi) 125(cur)	16(ampi) 250(cur)	16(ampi) 250(cur)	250	4(ampi) 62.5(cur)	16(ampi) 250(cur)	8(ampi) 125(cur)
B.Subtilis	1000	32(ampi) 500(cur)	64(ampi) 1000(cur)	32(ampi) 500 (cur)	500	16(ampi) 250(cur)	32(ampi) 500(cur)	16(ampi) 250 (cur)
P.aueroginosa	resistant	32(ampi) 500(cur)	64(ampi) 1000(cur)	32(ampi) 500 (cur)	resistant	16(ampi) 250(cur)	32(ampi) 500(cur)	16 (ampi) 250 (cur)
C.diphtheria	500	8(ampi) 125(cur)	16(ampi) 250(cur)	16(ampi) 250(cur)	250	8(ampi) 125	16(ampi) 250(cur)	8(ampi) 125 (cur)
MRSA	resistant	16(ampi) 250(cur)	32(ampi) 500(cur)	32(ampi) 500(cur)	resistant	8(ampi) 125(cur)	32(ampi) 500(cur)	8(ampi) 125(cur)

Table 5. Results of killing contact time studies for SLNs

Bacteria Strain	Formulation Name	Percentage of decreasing on bacteria count (%)		
		4 hrs	8 hrs	10 hrs
S.aureus	A	80	86	96
	B	0	0	100
	C	88	100	100
	D	50	70	100
	E	75	95	100
Ecoli	A	68	60	81
	B	66	73	83
	C	50	73	85
	D	0	11	72
	E	50	70	83
P.aueroginosa	A	0	12	25
	B	9	18	54
	C	0	25	62.5
	D	0	9	45
	E	0	20	60
C.diphtheria	A	0	50	70
	B	66	66	66
	C	60	85	93
	D	25	60	70
	E	0	20	60
B.Subtilis	A	0	0	0
	B	0	70	70
	C	83	80	100
	D	25	75	100
	E	150	50	70
MRSA	A	0	33	86
	B	0	28	64
	C	44	72	83
	D	0	53	76
	E	25	65	90

Acknowledgments

The authors would like to acknowledge the research vice chancellor of Pharmaceutical Sciences Branch, Islamic Azad University for technical support of this project.

Conflict of Interest

The Authors report no declaration of interest.

References

1. Teow SY, Ali SA. Synergistic antibacterial activity of Curcumin with antibiotics against Staphylococcus aureus. *Pak J Pharm Sci* 2015;28(6):2109-14.
2. Choudhary N, Sekhon BS. Potential therapeutic effect of curcumin an update. *J Pharm Edu Res* 2012;3(2):64-71.
3. Sun J, Bi C, Chan HM, Sun S, Zhang Q, Zheng Y. Curcumin-loaded solid lipid nanoparticles have prolonged in vitro antitumour activity, cellular uptake and improved in vivo bioavailability. *Colloids Surf B Biointerfaces* 2013;111:367-75. doi: 10.1016/j.colsurfb.2013.06.032

4. Zhang L, Pornpattananangku D, Hu CM, Huang CM. Development of Nanoparticles for Antimicrobial Drug Delivery. *Curr Med Chem* 2010;17(6):585-94. doi: 10.2174/092986710790416290
5. Gunez H, Dogan M, Gumus A, Mutly R, Topkaya AE. Investigation of Synergistic Effects of Curcumin with some Antibiotics in Extended Spectrum Beta Lactamase Positive or Negative Escherichia Coli and Klebsiella Pneumoniae Isolates. *Acta Med Mediterr* 2013;29:761-5.
6. Mun SH, Kim SB, Kong R, Choi JG, Kim YC, Shin DW, et al. Curcumin Reverse Methicillin Resistance in Staphylococcus aureus. *Molecules* 2014;19(11):18283-95. doi: 10.3390/molecules191118283
7. Ghaffari S, Varshosaz J, Saadat A, Atyabi F. Stability and antimicrobial effect of amikacin-loaded solid lipid nanoparticles. *Int J Nanomedicine* 2011;6:35-43. doi: 10.2147/IJN.S13671
8. Alihoseyni F, Ghaffari S, Dabirsiaghi AR, Haghighat S. Preparation and evaluation of ampicillin solid lipid nanoparticles. *World J Pharm Sci* 2014;2(9):914-20.
9. Varshosaz J, Ghaffari S, Khoshayand MR, Atyabi F, Azarmi S, Kobarfard F. Development and optimization of solid lipid nanoparticles of amikacin by central composite design. *J Liposome Res* 2010;20(2):97-104. doi: 10.3109/08982100903103904
10. Siddiqi SH, Heifets LB, Cynamon MH, Hooper NM, Laszlo A, Libonati JP, et al. Rapid broth macrodilution method for determination of MICs for Mycobacterium avium isolates. *J Clin Microbiol* 1993;31(9):2332-8.
11. Jourghanian P, Ghaffari S, Ardjmand M, Haghighat S, Mohammadnejad M. Sustained release Curcumin loaded Solid Lipid Nanoparticles. *Adv Pharm Bull* 2016;6(1):17-21. doi: 10.15171/apb.2016.004

An Experimental Study on the Mechanical and Biological Properties of Bio-Printed Alginate/Halloysite Nanotube/Methylcellulose/Russian Olive-Based Scaffolds

Babak Roushangar Zineh[1], **Mohammad Reza Shabgard**[1], **Leila Roshangar**[2*]

[1] *Mechanical Engineering Department, University of Tabriz, Tabriz, Iran.*
[2] *Stem Cell Research Center, Tabriz University of Medical Sciences, Tabriz Iran.*

Article info

Keywords:
· Halloysite nanotube
· Alginate
· Methylcellulose
· Scaffold
· Bioprint
· WST assay

Abstract

Purpose: Cartilage shows neither repairs nor regenerative properties after trauma or gradual wear and causes severe pain due to bones rubbing. Bioprinting of tissue-engineered artificial cartilage is one of the most fast-growing sciences in this area that can help millions of people against this disease.

Methods: Bioprinting of proper bioscaffolds for cartilage repair was the main goal of this study. The bioprinting process was achieved by a novel composition consisting of alginate (AL), Halloysite nanotube (HNT), and methylcellulose (MC) prepared in bio-ink. Also, the effect of Russian olive (RO) in chondrocytes growth on bioscaffolds was also investigated in this work. Compressive, hardness and viscosity tests, Energy-Dispersive X-Ray Spectroscopy (EDX), Fourier-Transform Infrared Spectroscopy (FT-IR), Differential Scanning Calorimetry (DSC), water-soluble Tetrazolium (WST) assay, and also transmission electron microscopy (TEM) and scanning electron microscopy (SEM) were carried out.

Results: The results show that in constant concentrations of AL, MC, and RO (20 mg/ml AL, 20 mg/ml MC, and 10 mg/ml RO) when concentration of HNT increased from 10 mg/ml (T-7) to 20 mg/ml (T-8) compressive stiffness increased from 241±45 kPa to 500.66±19.50 kPa. Also, 20 mg/ml of AL in composition saved proper water content for chondrocyte growth and produced good viscosity properties for a higher printing resolution.

Conclusion: RO increased chondrocytes living cell efficiency by 11% on bioprinted scaffolds in comparison with the control group without RO. Results obtained through in-vivo studies were similar to those of in-vitro studies. According to the results, T-7 bio-ink has good potential in bioprinting of scaffolds in cartilage repairs.

Introduction

The goal of tissue engineering is to produce bioscaffolds with good tolerance against existing mechanical forces and biocompatible properties such as living tissues without any toxicity.[1-3] Bioprinting process is one of the best methods to produce bioscaffolds with living cells. High accuracy in printing dimensions, homogenous dispersion of cells through the scaffold, and excellent control during the printing process make the bioprinting favorable to tissue engineering scientists.[4] The bioprinting idea is based on the printing of biomaterials and living cells together. Today, the challenges in bioprinting are producing proper biomaterial that can increase the cell living efficiency besides its good mechanical properties similar to living tissues and suitable properties for high-resolution printing such as proper viscosity.[5] Alginate (AL) as a compound with good properties during the bioprinting process such as satisfactory mechanical properties and proper compressive modulus can be used in knee cartilage repairs.[6] AL changes to a stable hydrogel through ionic interaction between carboxyl groups of alginate and Ca^{2+}.[7,8] Biocompatibility of AL and its controllable viscosity improve its applications in scaffolding and bioprinting.[9] Halloysite is a biocompatible nanoclay.[10] The main advantage of halloysite is that it can be used easily after washing and sterilization in bioprinting and cell culture structures, making it much cheaper than other nanofillers.[11] Addition of 4-5 wt.% halloysite nanoclay can increase material mechanical strength between 50-80%, suggesting its perfect potential for an appropriate additive in bioscaffolds and bioprinting.[10] Nanofibers of cellulose are beneficial in scaffolding because of their biocompatibility and good mechanical characteristics. Methylcellulose (Mc) as a favorable material for cell culture and scaffolding could increase bioprinting efficiency.[12] Russian olive (Elaeagnus angustifolia L.) fruit and seed powder are traditionally used for the healing of knee and cartilage defects.[13,14] Russian olive (RO) fruit contains sugar, vitamins (such as

***Corresponding author:** Leila Roshangar, Email: roshangarl@tbzmed.ac.ir tocopherol, vitamin C, B1), and minerals such as (calcium, magnesium, potassium, and iron). These vitamins and minerals are very beneficial for chondrocytes growth and their proliferation.[15] Ming Xian Liu et al.[16] studied several compositions consisting of alginate/halloysite nanotube (HNTs) composite bioscaffolds produced by the freeze-drying method. HNTs is mixed with alginate for enhancing both the mechanical and biological properties of freeze-dried bioscaffolds. HNTs that are partly oriented in a zigzag form in the composite scaffolds increase the density and water-swelling ratio of the composition. The results revealed that fibroblast cells of the mice attach effectively to the alginate/HNT scaffolds surface and the pure alginate and shows potential for tissue engineering applications. Afshar et al.[17] investigated Aminated chitosan/alginate scaffold containing halloysite nanotubes composition for improving cell attachments to the freeze-dried scaffolds. The results show that the scaffolds compared of chitosan/alginate/halloysite have a high cell proliferation and cell attachments with L929 cells to the scaffolds. Huijun Li et al.[18] studied alginate/methylcellulose composition to increase the adhesion between three-dimensional bioprinted layers of bioscaffolds and revealed that the novel Alg/MC composition has a potential to be used in bioprinting of tissues. Biao Huang et al.[19] studied sodium alginate (SA)/halloysite nanotubes (HNTs) composites and reported that HNTs can improve the mechanical properties of composite hydrogels. Their results also revealed that the SA/HNTs biomaterial with 80% HNTs has a compressive stress of 2.99 MPa, while the compressive stress of pure sodium alginate hydrogel is 0.8 MPa at 80% strain. Anuj Kumar et al.[20] studied the effects of CNCs and/or HNTs on alginate based bioscaffolds and reported the improved mechanical, thermal, and cytocompatibility properties of scaffolds. Yildirim et al.[21] studied alginate and single-walled carbon nanotube (SWCNT) scaffolds produced by a freeform fabrication technique. They reported some mechanical improvements in the alginate when mixed with SWCNT and suggested the great potential of alginate/SWCNT bioscaffolds for bioscaffolding.

According to previous studies, bioprinting with AL/HNT/MC has not yet been performed. We added RO fruit and seed powder to bio-ink for studying its effect on cells living performance. AL can increase the water content and formability of biomaterial. Addition of MC not only increases mechanical properties of biomaterial but also produce micropores during cell cultivation period. HNT also increases the mechanical endurance of biomaterial. Finally, RO due to its specific composition could increase the biological performance of bioscaffolds. Different mechanical and biological tests such as compressive, hardness and viscosity tests, scanning electron microscopy (SEM), inverted microscopy, Energy-Dispersive X-Ray Spectroscopy (EDS), Fourier-Transform Infrared Spectroscopy (FT-IR), Differential Scanning Calorimetry (DSC), vital staining of cells via cell tracer, and WST assay were carried out to characterize the properties of the developed bio-ink.

Materials and Methods

Alginic acid sodium salt with a molecular weight of 150-250 kda, methylcellulose with a molecular weight of 90 kda, phosphate buffered saline (PBS-containing sodium chloride (8 g/L), sodium phosphate (0.24 g/L), potassium chloride (0.2 g/L) and potassium phosphate (1.42 g/L)), trypsin, and WST were purchased from Sigma Aldrich (Munich, Germany). Halloysite nanotube with a molecular weight of 294 kda was purchased from natural-nano (Rochester, NY, USA). Lipophilic vital dye Dil (Biottium, INC, Hayward, USA) and Human chondrocytes were purchased from Pasteur Institute Tehran (Iran). Dried RO powder was purchased from Biology Institute of Tabriz Medical University (Iran). Fetal bovine serum was purchased from Life Technologies (Grand Island, NY, USA) and phosphate buffer was purchased from Proscitech, Thuringowa (Australia). Araldite, uranyl acetate, lead citrate, and aqueous osmium tetroxide were purchased from TAAB, Berkshire (UK). HEPES buffered saline (HBS-10 g/L HEPES, 16 g/L NaCl, 0.74 g/L KCl, 0.27 g/L $Na_2HPO_4.2H_2O$ and 2.0 g/L dextrose), Paraformaldehyde (PFA), uranyl acetate and Araldite purchased from Sigma Aldrich (Munich, Germany). Glutaraldehyde was purchased from Proscitech (Munich, Germany). Dulbecco's Modified Eagle's Medium (DMEM), Ham's F12, fetal bovine serum, L-ascorbate, penicillin, streptomycin, and fungizone were purchased from Gibco (UK). Lipophilic vital dye Dil was purchased from Biottium (INC, Hayward, USA). Finally, toluidine blue, acetone, BSA plus, and 2-(4-Amidinophenyl)-6-indole carb amidine dihydrochloride (DAPI) were purchased from Sigma Aldrich (Munich, Germany).

Preparation of biomaterial

Alginate and MC solutions were prepared in the concentrations of 10 mg/ml and 20 mg/ml for AL and 10 mg/ml and 20 mg/ml for MC in phosphate buffered saline (PBS). Then, different percentages of AL and MC solutions were mixed in a ratio of 1:1 and stirred for 4 h. Afterward, 10 mg/ml and 20 mg/ml of HNT powder were prepared in deionized water and added to these solutions and incubated under stirring overnight. The prepared bio-inks (with different compositions) were added to the solutions of fruit and seed powder of RO with a concentration of 10 mg/ml. All experiments were performed at room temperature (37 °C). Table 1 shows prepared bio-inks with different compositions.

Table 1. Prepared bio-inks with different compositions

BIO-INK	Alginate (mg/ml)	Methylcellulose (mg/ml)	Halloysite (mg/ml)	RO (mg/ml)
T-1	10	10	10	10
T-2	10	10	20	10
T-3	10	20	10	10
T-4	10	20	20	10
T-5	20	10	10	10
T-6	20	10	20	10
T-7	20	20	10	10
T-8	20	20	20	10

Bioprinting of cartilage scaffolds and experimental tests
Injection based bioprinter manufactured in our lab and used for scaffold bioprinting. The bioprinter shown in Figure 1 has a high accuracy, trustable sterile cartridge, and filtering fans for clean air circulation. Chondrocytes were dissociated into single cells and gently mixed with prepared bio-inks. The final concentration was 5 $\times 10^6$ cells/ml. The mixture was sterilized using ultraviolet radiation. Layers were Perpendicular to each other. The thickness of printing layers was 0.5 mm without line spacing. Bioprinting was done using a 0.5 mm needle. Bioprinting speed of 10 mm/s and feed rate of 5mm^3/s were selected. Scaffolds were printed with 5 layers, 20 rows, and 20 columns. Bioprinted scaffolds were then transferred into glass plates and placed in an incubator. Next, a 100 mM $CaCl_2$ solution was added over scaffolds for 8 min and ionic interaction occurred between the alginate chains and Ca^{2+}.

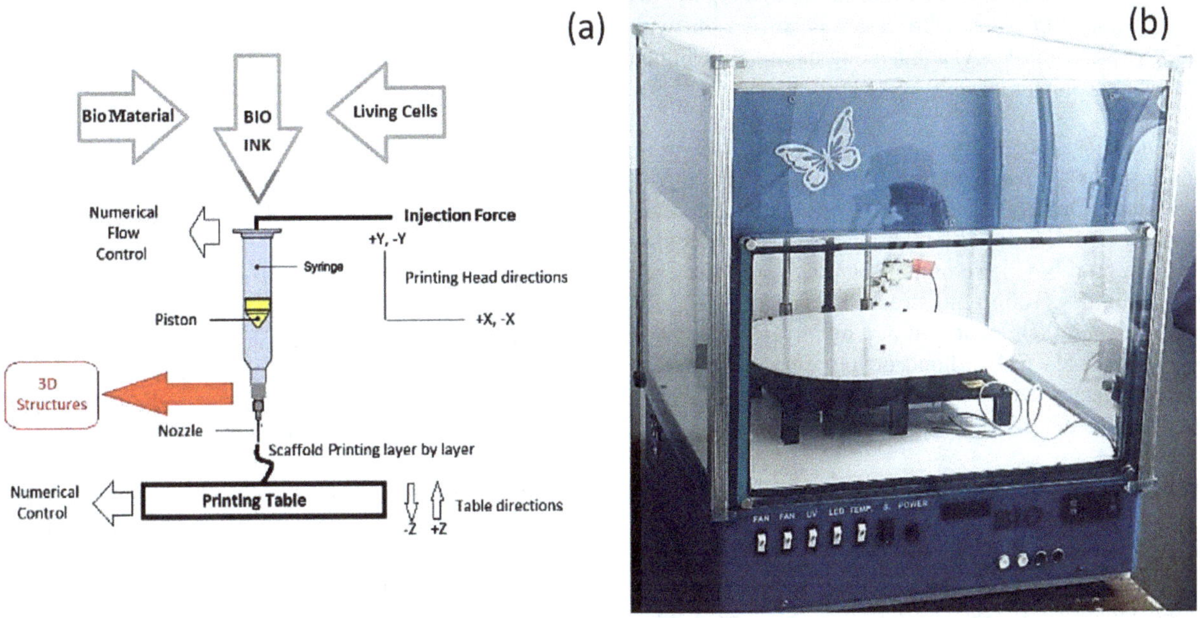

Figure 1. Bioprinter used during the tests (a) A schematic of bioprinter (b) The bioprinter used for experimental tests

Viscosity investigation
The solutions with different composition of bio-inks and cells were used for measurement of viscosity. The kinematic viscosity of different solutions was measured using ATAGO viscometer BASE plus (Japan) at room temperature with three repetitions. The viscosity of the bio-inks without living cells was identified in the same condition.

Scanning electron microscopy
Scaffolds were subjected to SEM using a Mira3 TESCAN (Czech). Before the SEM analysis, the specimens were washed twice with HEPES buffered saline (HBS) and dried samples were coated with gold for 300 seconds with sputtering coater and prepared for imaging.

Energy-Dispersive X-Ray Spectroscopy
In order to prepare biomaterials for EDS (Mira3 TESCAN), dried samples were placed in the EDX equipment to determine the elemental composition of biomaterials.

Transmission electron microscopic analysis
For ultrastructural studies, cultured chondrocytes were fixed in 2.5% glutaraldehyde in a 0.1M phosphate buffer and post-fixed in 1% aqueous osmium tetroxide. The samples were then dehydrated in the graded concentration of ethanol and embedded in Araldite. Ultra-thin sections from selected blocks were treated with uranyl acetate and lead citrate and observed in (LEO 906) TEM (Oberkochen, Germany).

Differential Scanning Calorimetry
The thermal characterization of composition was obtained with a differential scanning calorimeter (DSC), Linseis PT100 (Germany). The samples heating rate was 10 °C/min–1 from 0 °C to 120 °C. The N_2 atmosphere with a flow rate of 20 ml/min was used for tests.

Compressive characterization
Compressive tests were performed by GOTECH AI-7000M (Taiwan) on freeze-dried solid scaffolds at a 2.00 mm/min loading speed by averaging of three repetitions (n=3). Samples were cut into 40 mm diameter and 20 mm height. The unconfined compressive tests were performed according to ASTM D695 at 90% strain at 37 °C.

Hardness determination
The solid model was used to determine the hardness of material at 37 °C. In each sample shore, a hardness was calculated according to ASTM D2240 with five repetitions.

Fourier transform infrared

Bruker (Germany) spectrometer was used to take spectra of T-7 bio-ink. Next, 2 mg sample of 200 mg kbr pallets were prepared and subjected to scanning within a range of 400- 4000 cm-1.

Thermogravimetric analysis (TGA)

Thermal stability of the bio-ink gel studied in this test. Gel bio-ink was freeze at -60 °C and then dried in vacuum for 96 h. the grounded gel (8 mg in weight) was tested in platinum plate. TGA test was carried out with Linseis (L81A1750-USA) at a heating rate of 8 °C/min in nitrogen atmosphere from 20 °C to 800 °C.

Cell culture

Chondrocytes were cultured in a special media containing Dulbecco's Modified Eagle's Medium (DMEM) and Ham's F12 (1:1 mixture) supplemented with 10% fetal bovine serum, 50 μg/μl L-ascorbate, 100 μg/μl penicillin, 100 μg/ml streptomycin, and 2.5 μg/μl fungizone, and then incubated in a humidified incubator at 37 °C with 5% CO_2. Chondrocytes were expanded to 80% confluency and then dissociated. About 5×10^6 chondrocytes per ml of bio-ink were used in this study.

Cell cytotoxicity assay

Cytotoxicity assay was conducted using the WST assay. The samples were incubated for 24, 48, 72, and 96 h at 37 °C and 5% CO_2. For WST assay, the medium of the printed construct in each group was replaced with a WST for 1h. The absorbance at 480 nm wavelength was detected using an ELISA plate reader (BioTek, VT, USA) at 600 nm reference wavelength. Cells with blue stain represented viable cells and revealed their distribution in the bio-ink. Samples were transferred into PBS for light microscopy analysis (Olympus, Japan).

Cell viability study

CM-Dil staining method[22] was used to monitor the live cells. The 3D cell-tracer construct was cultured for 1, 6, and 20 days in a chondrocyte medium labeled with 2μm cell tracer TM CM-Dil. Suspended chondrocytes at a density of 1×10^6 cell/ml were labeled with 5 μl/ml of Dil construct agent. Cells were incubated with a labeled solution at 37 °C for 20 min and studied with a fluorescent microscopy apparatus (Olympus, Japan).

Histological analysis

Cultured chondrocytes were fixed in 4% paraformaldehyde and kept frozen until sectioning. Then they were sectioned using cryostat and stained with toluidine-blue and safranin 0-fast green, according to previous studies.[23] Histological analyses were carried out using light microscopy.

Transplantation of chondrocyte-seeded construct

To transport chondrocyte-seeded construct, 10 male sheep (Bergamasca–Massese) were purchased. Sheep were sedated with Xylazine hydrochloride (HCl) (0.1 mg/kg sheep) for a surgical procedure. Both knee joints were exposed via a lateral Para patellar skin incision. Two full-thickness cartilage defects (4 mm in diameter and 1 mm in depth)[24] were created in each joint. The chondrocyte-seeded construct was fashioned in the defect as much as possible. The defect in both knees was filled with hydrogel and sealed with fibrin glue (Tisseel™Baxter AG) for 6 months. Right knee was chosen as the control group and left knee was chosen as the treatment group. The sheep were maintained for 6 a month post-treatment and then the specimens were transferred to the laboratory.

Toluidine blue staining

In this step, 1% of toluidine blue was used for staining and extra dye were washed by PBS and then mounted with Canada balsam.

Immunofluorescence staining of collagen Type 2

We cut 10 μm thick sections by cryostat, fixed them using -20 °C acetone, and washed three times with PBS (10 mm sodium phosphate, 0.15 M sodium chloride, and pH 7.4). The slides were incubated with a solution of 1% BSA plus 10% goat serum for 2 h. Then, the primary antibody was added and incubated for 18 h at 4 °C. The secondary antibody was added for 1 h and then 4′,6-diamidino-2-phenylindole (DAPI) was added to each section. The slides were protected from light and incubated for 10 min at room temperature and were washed twice, 5 min each, in PBS. Morphological analyses were conducted with fluorescent microscopy.

Statistical analysis

The Mean ± standard deviation (SD) was used for data expression. Excel statistical software and GraphPad Prism 7 were used for data analysis. An independent sample t-test was used for viscosity studies. All data are the average of three repetitions in each test. Repeated measurement analysis was used to determine statistical significance in compression and WST tests results. All analyses were performed at a significance level of $p < 0.05$.

Results and Discussion

Bioprinting of 3D scaffolds containing chondrocytes

The prepared bio-inks were mixed slowly with chondrocyte in concentration of 5×10^6 /cm^2. Chondrocytes were mixed for 150 seconds and then filled in sterilized cartridge for printing. Scaffolds with different composition were printed (Figure 2). Bio-ink containing 30 mg/ml alginate, 50 mg/ml HNT, and 30 mg/ml methylcellulose solutions show the best performance in bioprinting and saved the printing shape very well. A high percentage of alginate increased the gel form of bio-ink and improved printing resolution. Existence of RO powder (10 mg/ml) had no significant effect on printing results of scaffolds.

Microstructure and composition

Using SEM images with high magnifications (Figure 3a) showed a homogenous composition, a high percentage of HNT, and RO particles at the surface of the dried samples. MC particles, Nanotubes of HNT in parallel and zigzag forms with each other and RO powder can be seen in Figure 3b. Also, dried samples of 24 h cell cultured scaffolds showed a strong attachment of cells to the surface of bioprinted scaffolds in SEM images (Figure 3c). Also, EDS results show Aluminum (Al), sodium (Na), Silicon (Si), and chlorine (Cl) in the composition sourced from a constituent of the biomaterial.

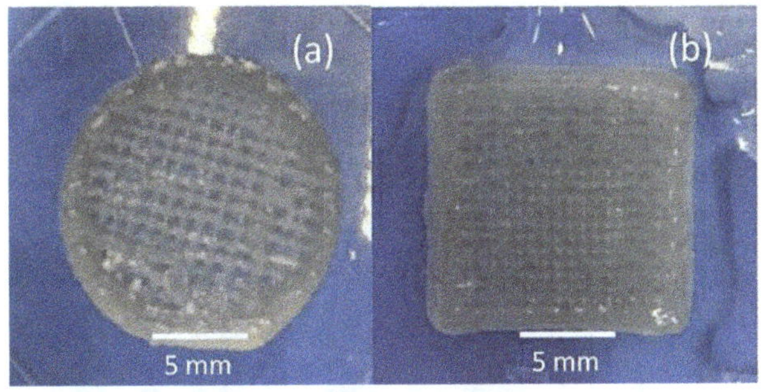

Figure 2. Printed scaffolds(a) A scaffold printed without living cells (b) A scaffold printed with living cells

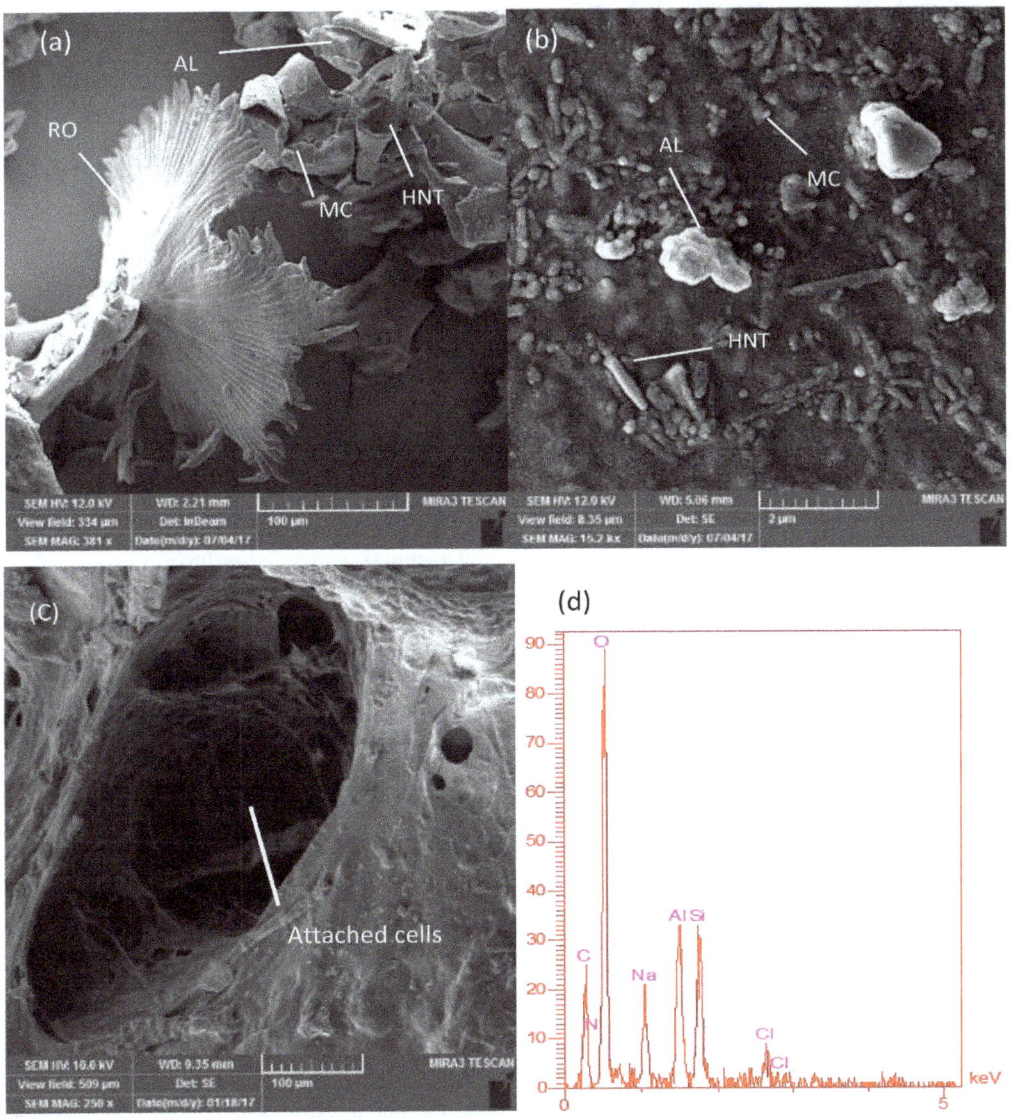

Figure 3. Scanning electron microscopy images of Methylcellulose particles, Halloysite nanotubes, and RO powder(a) RO, alginate, methylcellulose, and HNT at the surface (b) the zig-zag combination of HNT in bio-ink surface (c) cells attached at the surface of bioprinted scaffolds, and (d) Energy dispersive x-ray of T-7 biomaterial.

Compressive investigation

Different amounts of HNT and AL alter compressive properties of bioprinted scaffolds. It is seen from Figure 4 that 20 mg/ml of HNT and 20 mg/ml of AL (T-8) compressive properties are higher in comparison with 10 mg/ml of HNT and 10 mg/ml of AL (T-1). Also, the T-7 group shows a higher compressive stress (210%) in comparison to the T-1 group. Compressive stiffness continually grows by increasing the amounts of HNT and AL; however, HNT has a higher effect on compressive stiffness than AL. Results revealed that existence of methylcellulose and RO powder did not change the compressive properties of different bio-inks significantly.

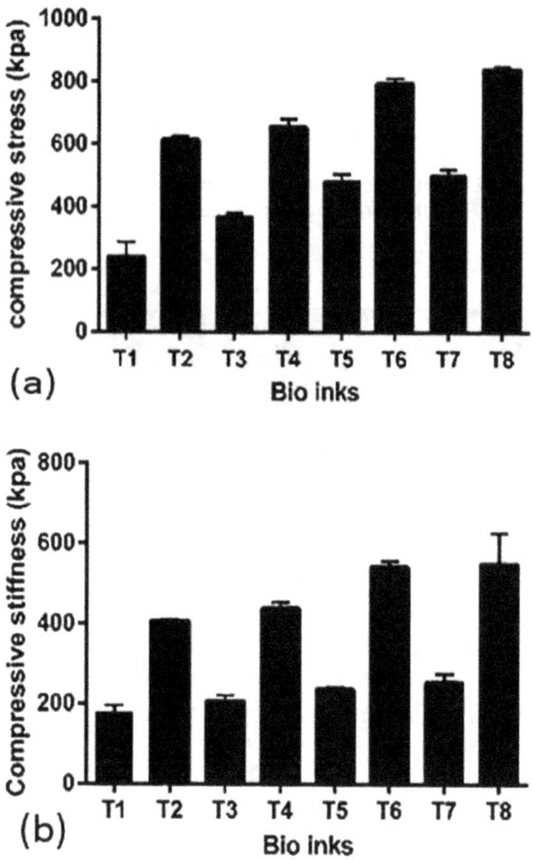

Figure 4. Compressive properties of bioprinted scaffolds
(a): Compressive stress increased from T-1 to T-8 according to alginate and halloysite Nano tube content of biomaterials.
(b): Compressive stiffness increases from T-1 to T-8 due to a different percentage of alginate and HNT in the structure.

Kinematic viscosity investigation

The kinematic viscosity of different bio-inks with different compositions is shown in Table 2. The kinematic viscosity decreases by adding cells to each group. Best results of bioprinting were achieved in viscosities between 2000-2400 mm^2/s.

Table 2. Kinematic viscosity of bio-inks with and without living cells

Bio-ink	Kinematic Viscosity (mm^2/s) Without cells	Kinematic Viscosity (mm^2/s) With cells
T-1	1200	1100
T-2	1400	1300
T-3	1600	1500
T-4	1800	1700
T-5	1900	1800
T-6	2100	2100
T-7	2300	2200
T-8	2500	2300

Hardness investigation

The hardness of different composition of solid materials was measured at different points of each sample (n=5) and the mean hardness for each one was calculated (Table 3). By increasing the amounts of alginate and HNT in the composition of bio-inks shore A, hardness increases continually.

Table 3. Different results of shore A hardness test from bio-ink samples (n=5)

Bio-ink	Shore A hardness
T-1	53.6± 0.894
T-2	57.8± 0.836
T-3	60± 0.707
T-4	60.8± 0.836
T-5	65.6± 0.547
T-6	68.4 ± 1.140
T-7	71±1.000
T-8	77± 1.581

Differential Scanning Calorimetry (DSC)

The DSC tests were taken between 0 and 120 °C. This range was chosen because of working temperature of bioscaffolds. It is seen that there is no exothermic or endothermic peak in working range but an endothermic peak seen in 104.8 °C due to a water loss of the samples. Figure 5a presents the DSC analysis of T-7 biomaterial.

Thermogravimetric analysis

Figure 5b shows the TGA curves of T-7 bio-ink in a nitrogen atmosphere from ambient temperature to 800 °C. The TGA curve of T-7 shows three mass losses and degradation steps. The first step was about 13% before 100 °C due to evaporation of physically bound water in alginate and bio-ink structure. The mass loss of about 35% around 190 °C for bio-ink was related to the decomposition of alginate macromolecular chains in bio-ink composition. eventually, The TGA curve of T-7 shows almost constant decreasing from 500 to 800 °C.

Fourier transform infrared (FT-IR)

FT-IR results (Figure 5c) show that the peaks at 3400-3900 cm^{-1} (3435.03 cm^{-1} for T-7) are related to O-H stretching bonds of Alginate and Methylcellulose. Also, in the range from 2850 to 3000 cm^{-1} (2930.00 cm^{-1} for T-7), stretching vibration C–H can be seen. A peak at 2144.63 cm^{-1} is indexed to Si-H bonds related to the existence of HNTs in the structure. Peaks at 1646.71, 1735.74, and 1561.93 cm^{-1} provide an evidence for existence of carboxylic acid salt (-COO asymmetric stretch, 1500-1650 cm^{-1}).[25] In addition, a peak at 1426.40 is related to C–C stretching; peak at 1458.22 is attributed to CH2 and CH3 bonds; and the peaks at 1038.46 indexed to C–O, 816.75 and 914.01 are indexed to C–C–H, and 673.84 cm^{-1} is indexed to C–O–H stretching vibration bonds.[26]

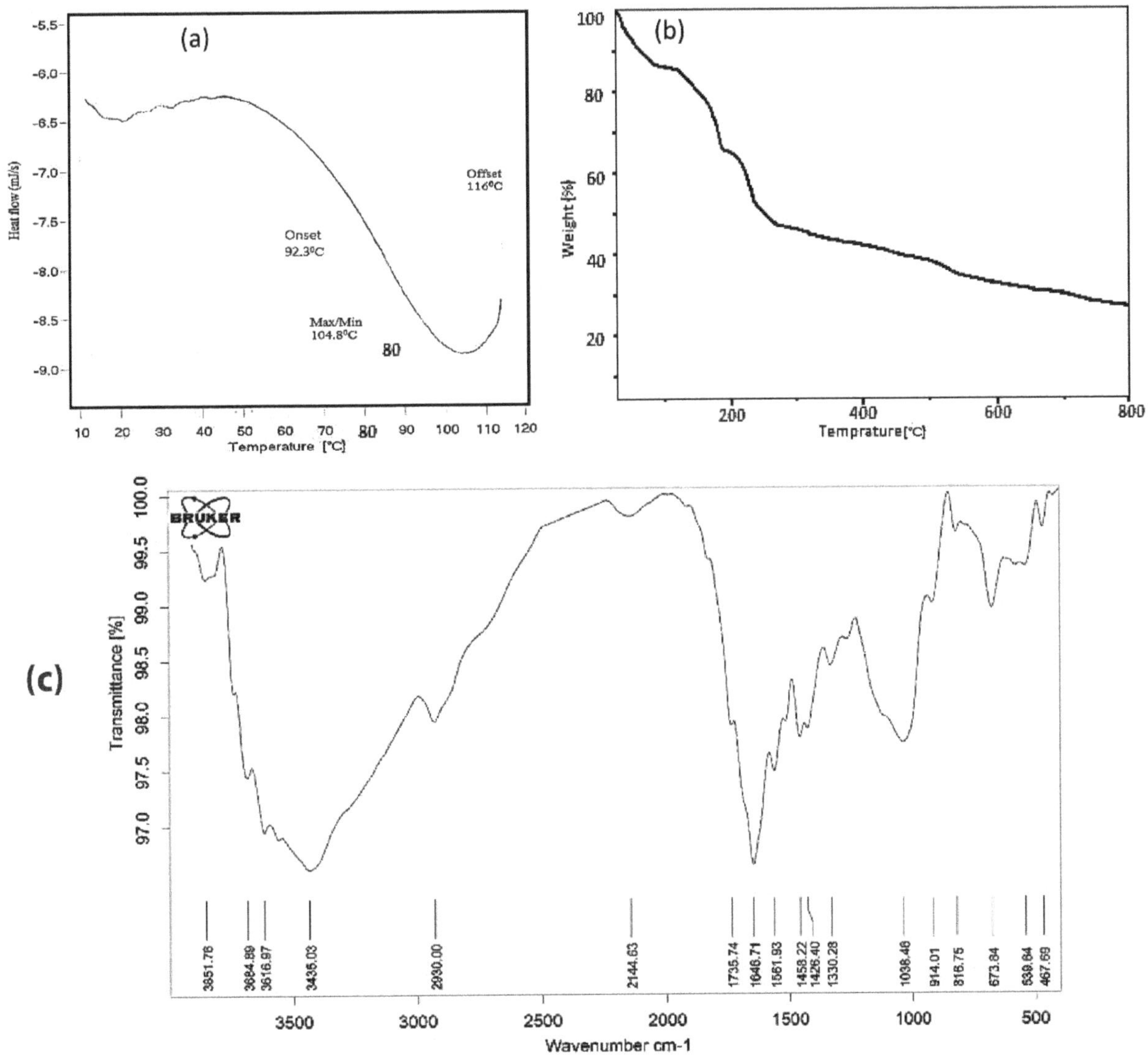

Figure 5. (a): Differential Scanning Calorimetry results of T-7 Bio-ink, (b): Thermogravimetric analysis curves of T-7 bio-ink (c): Fourier transform infrared results of T-7 Bio-ink.

Histological analysis

Histological evaluation of different chondrocyte-seeded constructs was carried out for 20 days of in-vitro culture. After 20 days, they were sectioned and stained for proteoglycan deposition using safranin-o. In each group, the culture positively stained for 20 days was compared with 0 and 6-day cultures and then the results were compared with those of 8 different constructs. The high positively stained proteoglycan deposition observed in the T-7 group is shown in Figure 6a. The morphological study showed that in 0-day cultures, chondrocytes appeared as flattened cells without capsule and show a uniform distribution. A pericellular region of GAG-rich extracellular matrix, approximately 1 to 5 μm in width surrounded most cells on day 0. However, in 20-days culture, the cells had a rounded shape surrounded by a capsule and minimal cell division was observed. A glycosaminoglycan (GAG-rich) pericellular matrix, approximately 5 to 8 μm in width surrounded most cell groups. It appeared that the surrounding pericellular matrix in the T-7 group was obviously wider than the other groups (Figure 6a). The chondrocytes appeared to be increased in size by passing time and they had the largest size on day 20. Besides, the comparison between groups showed that the cell in the T-7 group had numerous cells with a larger size than the other groups (Figure 6b).

Ultrastructural study

Transmission electron microscopy (TEM) revealed that the cells from different groups have similar ultrastructure. As shown in Figure 6a, in day 20, the cells within the constructs displayed all characteristics of chondrocyte (nucleus, lipid droplets, mitochondria, rough endoplasmic reticulum, and free ribosomes). Sparse and thin collagen type 2 fibers were found in ECM of 20-days culture. However, in 0-day culture (Figure 7), compared to 20-days culture, there were no collagen fibers in the ECM. Moreover, in 0-day, cells were morphologically flattened in the chondrocyte-seeded constructs.

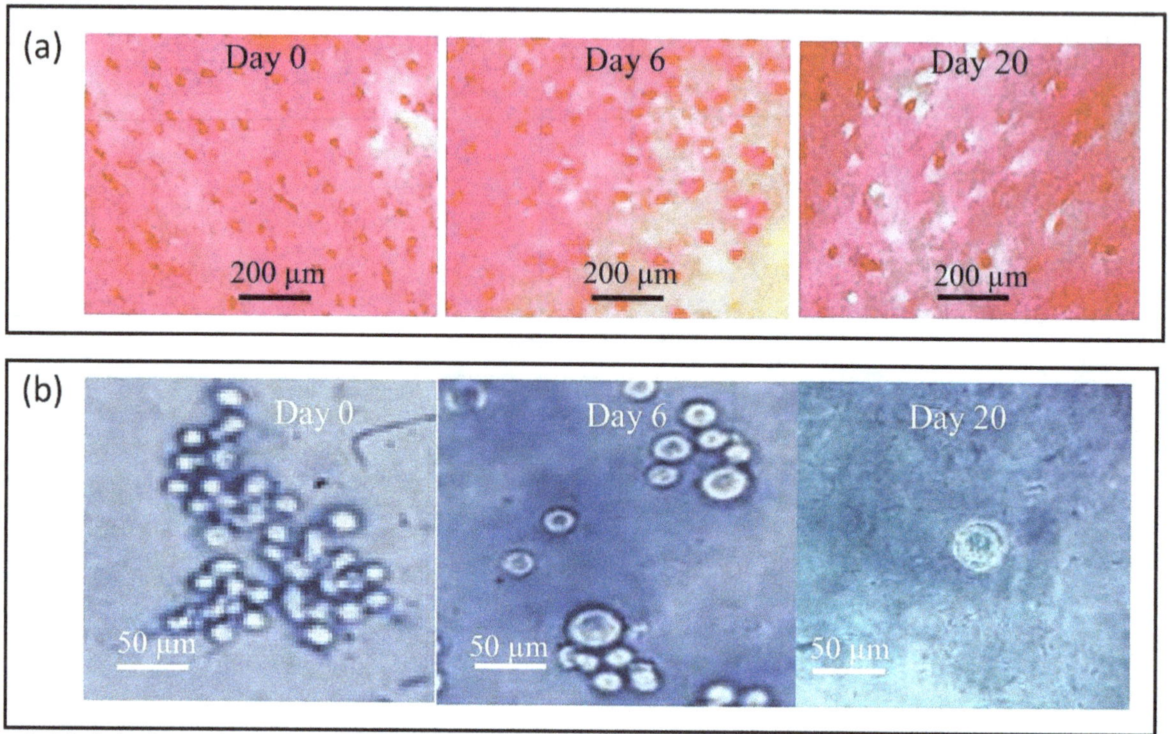

Figure 6. (a): Safranin-o staining of printed chondrocyte-seeded constructs in 0, 6, and 20 days' culture from the T-7 group. Note the increase in cell size and highly positive stain for safranin-o in day 20 culture as compared with 0 and 6 days' cultures, (b): Photomicrographs of chondrocyte-seeded constructs at different days of culture from the T-7 group; Note the increase in cell size with the progress of culture, Toluidine blue staining.

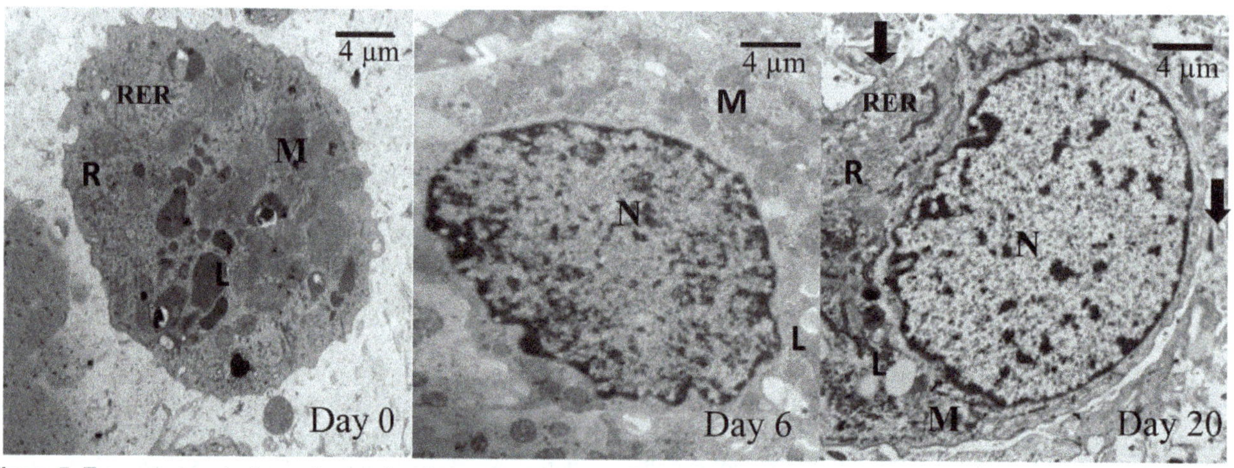

Figure 7. Transmission electron micrographs of chondrocytes at a different day of culture from the T-7 group; Note the appearance of collagen fiber (arrow) in the 20-days culture. Also, note chondrocyte characterized by Nucleus (N), Mitochondria (M), Rough endoplasmic reticulum (RER), Lipid droplet (L), Free ribosomes(R).

Cell Viability

To determine cell viability after bio-ink extrusion, survival of chondrocytes was assessed using Dil dye. The chondrocyte viability and patterning were conducted by labeling with red fluorescent cell linker Dil dye. The viability of chondrocyte for a longer term in printed construct was assessed in 1-, 6-, and 20-days cultures (Figure 8). The printed cells continued to proliferate for 20 days after printing, with no significant difference when compared to the 1 and 6 days. Assessment of live cells by morphological studies showed $\geq$ 90% cell viability for 1-, 6-, and 20-days cultures after extrusion. Homogeneous red signals from the live/dead graph after 20 days of culture indicate that cells were populating the whole bioprinted construct. Figure 6b show viable cells on the bioprinted tracts immediately after printing. After 6 days of culture, the constructs were still filled with live cells (Figure 8). These results show that the printed construct preserved cell viability during the bioprinting process and provided a favorable microenvironment for cell proliferation. The highest live cells number were observed in the T-7 group (Table 4).

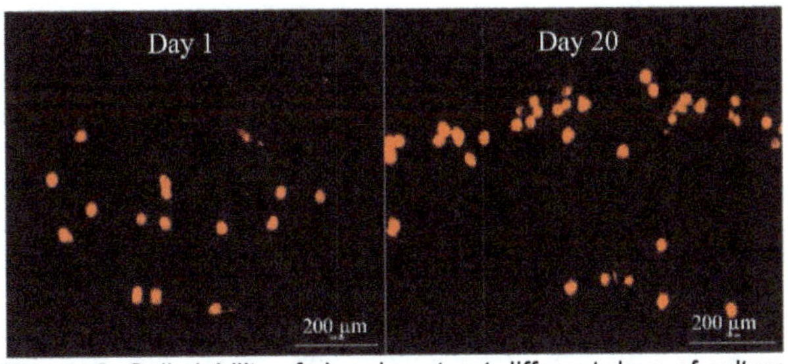

Figure 8. Cell viability of chondrocyte at different days of culture after printing by CM-Dil staining.

Table 4. Number of the viable cell after printing by day of culture in the T-7 group

Culture	Live cell number
1 day	108± 12.08
6 day	110.20±8.23
20 day	121.01±10.37

WST assay and Cytotoxicity

Cell toxicity and proliferation in the bio-ink were tested by WST assay technique. A higher amount of alginate correlated with an increased cell viability percentage while a higher amount of HNT is associated with decreased cell viability percentage. The higher amount of alginate and lower amount of HNT in bio-ink correlated with better biological performance and showed a higher living percentage in WST assay tests. Presence of RO powder had a positive effect on cell viability percentage by 11%. To evaluate the effect of different composition on chondrocyte survival rate, the biomaterials were added to DMEM. Figure 9 shows the effects of different composition on viability that were cultured in DMEM for 24, 48, 72, and 96 h. All the experiments were performed in triplicate.

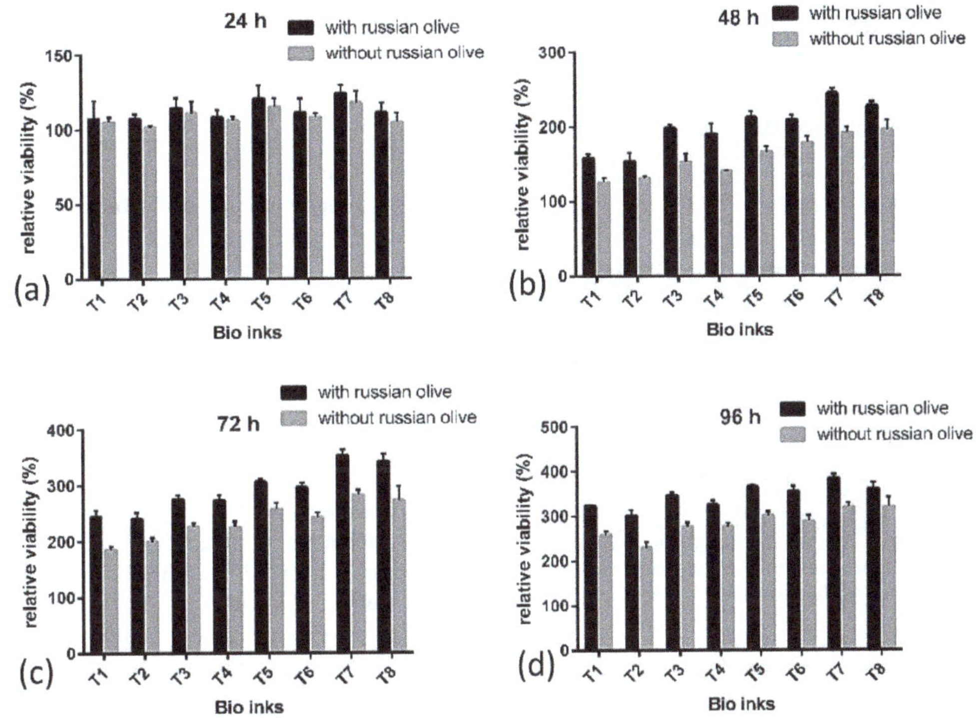

Figure 9. Relative viability percentage in a different composition cultured for a) 24 h, b) 48 h, c) 72 h, and d) 96 h.

In vivo study

The in-vivo study was carried out based on in-vitro studies and the cells from the best responding group (T-7 group) were selected for the in-vivo study. Grossly, the repaired tissue in the artificial defect (Figure 10a) is hyaline cartilage-like when compared with normal hyaline cartilage (Figure 10b). The repaired cartilage tissue that resulted from a chondrocyte-seeded construct in treated sheep knees revealed hyaline cartilage-like tissue (Figure 11b) compared with normal hyaline cartilage (Figure 11a). Immunofluorescence staining exhibited a strong collagen type 2 positive staining and an increase in collagen type 2 in the chondrocyte-seeded construct (Figures 12a and 12b). Moreover, the negative control did not show any collagen type 2 expressions (Figures 13a and 13b).

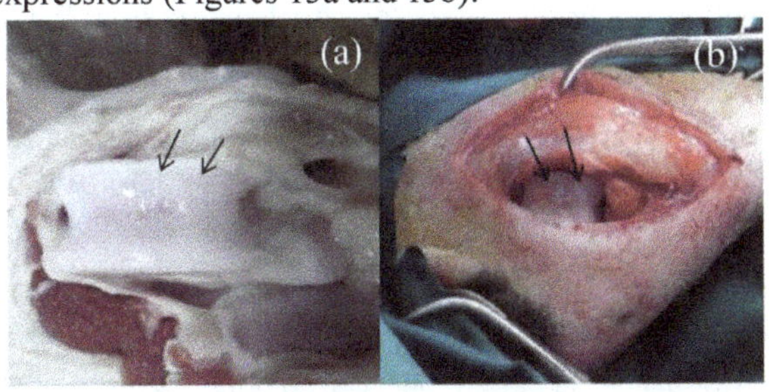

Figure 10. Post-surgical knee joint in implanted chondrocyte-seeded construct on cartilage defects after 6 months(a): The articular defects were repaired with cartilaginous tissues (b): Small amount of cartilage-like white color tissues at the defects in the control group after 6 months.

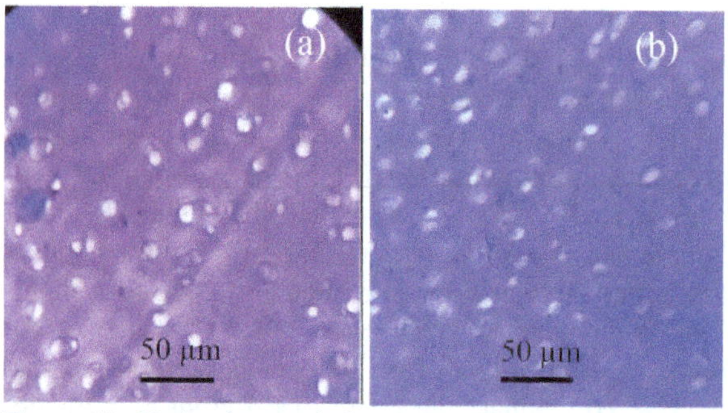

Figure 11. Photomicrograph from normal hyaline cartilage (a): Repaired tissue in implanted chondrocyte-seeded construct on cartilage defects after 6 months and (b): Toluidine blue staining.

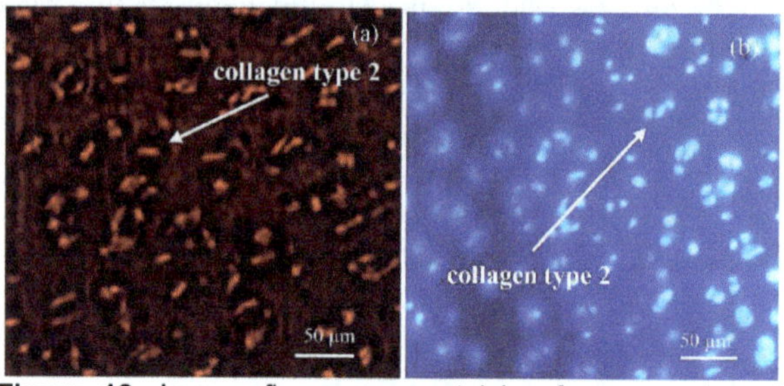

Figure 12. Immunofluorescence staining for expression of collagen type 2: (a): the chondrocyte-seeded constructs in articular defect after 6 months. (b): DAPI staining.

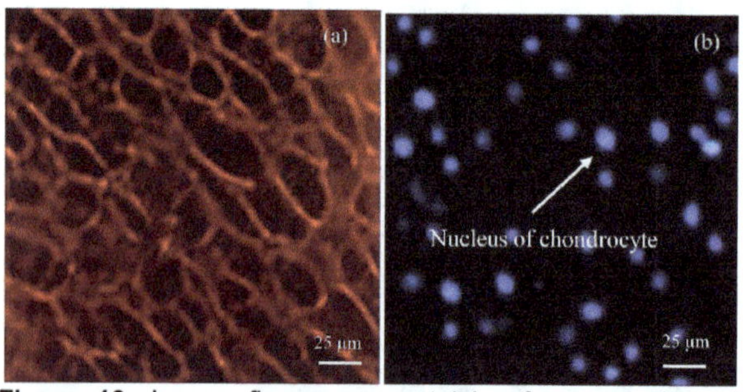

Figure 13. Immunofluorescence staining for expression of collagen Type 2 (a): In the negative control, (b): DAPI staining.

Bio-inks with different compositions were printed, among which T-7 bio-ink showed the best results with chondrocytes. Different mechanical factors such as hardness, viscosity, and compressive properties influence the efficiency of bioprinted scaffolds. The proper hardness of bioprinted scaffolds should meet the hardness of natural cartilage. This range is from 0.5 to 4.0 MPa in microhardness tests.[6,27] By increasing the amount of HNT in structure, shore A hardness of samples increases, probably due to the high mechanical characteristics of halloysite nanotubes and structure of halloysite.[28] The high density of halloysite nanotubes and homogenous distribution of tubes along the applied force increase the hardness of biomaterials.[29] The best results of hardness due to the mechanical and biological performance achieved in T-7 bio-ink. The bio-ink viscosity of biomaterials affects both printing and cell proliferation.[30,31] From the printing aspect, the best kinematic viscosity for bioprinting of alginate-based bio-inks is between 2000 and 2400 mm^2/s.[9] A higher viscosity is required for a higher extrusion force, which in turn negatively affects living cells and causes problems such as printing needle blockage and lower resolution.[32] In T-7 Bio-ink with proper viscosity, cell viability increases and leads to a higher bioprinting resolution. Alginate, HNT, and methylcellulose affect the bio-ink viscosity. Results of viscosity tests revealed that higher amounts of alginate and HNT increase the viscosity of bio-ink (Table 2). Alginate gel-like structure after crosslinking by $CaCl_2$ and crosslink of halloysite nanotubes with each other and alginate are the reasons for a higher viscosity.[10] Methylcellulose is added to bio-inks in cartilage scaffolds to adjust the viscosity of biomaterials.[12] In higher viscosities, there are high pressures over cell-laden biomaterial for extruding from the needle; so the cells are harmed and cell viability is decreased. Results show that a proper viscosity that meets both biological and mechanical properties is T-7. In addition, when the viscosity is too low, the bioprinting resolution reduces significantly. By an increase in viscosity, printing resolution increased but the cell viability decreased. Hence, the viscosities from 2000 to 2400 mm^2/s are the best choices in AL/MC/HNT/RO composition for using as a biomaterial in bioprinting process. The IR spectra of the bio-ink show the presence of all continents (AL, MC, HNT, and RO). The –OH peak at 3435.03 cm^{-1} is probably because of the presence of AL (20 mg/ml) in the composition.[33] High concentration of HNT leads to a –C=O band at 1646.71, 1735.74, and 1561.93 cm-1.[33] A peak at 2,930.00 cm^{-1} in the T-7 bio-ink is indexed to the aliphatic –CH groups existing in Alginate and MC. As mentioned earlier, MC was washed during the cell culture period and it produces a porous structure in scaffolds.[7] These micro size porosities increase the cell living efficiency and improve cell attachments to bioscaffolds. Actually, the micropores produced along cell cultivation improves the surface potential of bioscaffolds for better cell adhesion.[34] Compressive properties of bioscaffolds in T-7 Bio-ink meet the natural cartilage for achieving the best results.[35] The human natural cartilage had a strength of 240-850 kPa in compression.[36,37] Accordingly, bio-inks prepared in this study had a compressive stress between 241±45 kPa (T-1) to 839.66±10.01 kPa (T-8) and compressive stress for T-7 was 500.66±19.50 kPa. Compressive test results established that HNT had a remarkable role in increasing compressive properties and the bio-inks containing higher amounts of HNT had more desired compressive properties.[38] As mentioned earlier, this phenomenon is due to the tubular structure of HNT and homogenous distribution of these tubules in all directions, which improve the strength of biomaterial. The effect of alginate is lower than that of the HNT on compressive properties because its gel-like structure after crosslinking and cross-linked Ca chains had lower compressive properties in comparison with HNT.[6] WST assay tests results show high a percentage of living cells after 24, 48, 76, and 96 h according to compatible bio-

inks composition with chondrocytes. Test results showed that cell viability increased from the first day of cell culture up to 96 h after bioprinting. It is evident from Figure 8 that relative viability is always higher in lower amounts of HNT and increases by increasing alginate in the composition. Additionally, the metabolic activity of chondrocytes is also increased in low HNT. Besides, as can be seen from GAG production, collagen type 2 is synthesized and grown in size by the passage of time. In the T-7 bio-ink that contains 30 mg/ml alginate and 30 mg/ml HNT, a higher percentage of cell viability (Figure 7) was achieved, suggesting the optimal property of prepared bio-ink for chondrocyte culture. Alginate is a well-known biomaterial used for bioscaffolding. On the other hand, HNT increases the printing and mechanical performance of bioprinted scaffolds.[30] RO powder did not affect the mechanical properties of bioscaffolds but its fibrous structure changed the cell viability rate.[13] Traditionally, RO fruit and seed powder are used to relieve pains in joints and knee. The sugar, vitamins such as tocopherol, vitamins C and B1, and minerals like calcium, magnesium, potassium, and iron existing in RO are essential for chondrocytes' growth.[15] These properties of RO are the reason for a higher number of living cells 11% after 96 h.
when it is added to bio-ink. As can be seen from the WST results, RO affects the bioprinting cell viability by
Another challenge with cartilage repair is that the proliferating chondrocytes tend to become fibrous cartilage, which is characteristically different from hyaline cartilage.[39] Interestingly, in the present study, the cells maintained their hyaline cartilage property by producing collagen type 2 on 20 days of culture. From the mechanical and biological aspects, the T-7 bio-ink showed best results for bioprinting. The best bio-ink should meet both the mechanical and biological characteristics. Although mechanical properties of T-8 bio-ink was better than the T-7, higher amounts of HNT in its structure decreased the survival rate and bioactivity of seeded chondrocytes. T-7 bio-ink shows good mechanical properties and provides a proper medium for chondrocyte proliferation and bioactivity as shown by WST assay and morphological studies.

Conclusion

Bioprinting of alginate/HNT/methylcellulose with RO powder was performed in this study. Mechanical and biological characterizations showed that composition containing 20 mg/ml alginate, 20 mg/ml methylcellulose, and 10 mg/ml halloysite nanotube solutions mixed with 10 mg/ml RO fruit and seed powder increased chondrocyte viability by 11%. Also, the compressive stress of bioprinted structures was increased by 210% in T-7 bio-ink in comparison with T-1 bio-ink, which contains lower amounts of alginate and HNT in its structure. Based on our results, it can be concluded that T-7 bio-ink has a high potential for usage in cartilage repairs and bioprinting process.

Acknowledgments

This research did not receive any specific grant from funding agencies in the public, commercial, or not-for-profit sectors.

Conflict of Interest

The authors declare that they have no conflict of interest.

References

1. Savkovic V, Li H, Seon JK, Hacker M, Franz S, Simon JC. Mesenchymal stem cells in cartilage regeneration. *Curr Stem Cell Res Ther* 2014;9(6):469-88.
2. Samiei M, Aghazadeh M, Alizadeh E, Aslaminabadi N, Davaran S, Shirazi S, et al. Osteogenic/odontogenic bioengineering with co-administration of simvastatin and hydroxyapatite on poly caprolactone based nanofibrous scaffold. *Adv Pharm Bull* 2016;6(3):353. doi: 10.15171/apb.2016.047
3. Mohammadi F, Mohammadi Samani S, Tanideh N, Ahmadi F. Hybrid scaffolds of hyaluronic acid and collagen loaded with prednisolone: An interesting system for osteoarthritis. *Adv Pharm Bull* 2018;8(1):11-19. doi: 10.15171/apb.2018.002
4. Rhee S, Puetzer JL, Mason BN, Reinhart-King CA, Bonassar L. 3d bioprinting of spatially heterogeneous collagen constructs for cartilage tissue engineering. *Acs Biomater Sci Eng* 2016;2(10):1800-5. doi: 10.1021/acsbiomaterials.6b00288
5. Kang HW, Lee SJ, Ko IK, Kengla C, Yoo JJ, Atala A. A 3d bioprinting system to produce human-scale tissue constructs with structural integrity. *Nat Biotechnol* 2016;34(3):312-9. doi: 10.1038/nbt.3413
6. Camarero-Espinosa S, Rothen-Rutishauser B, Foster EJ, Weder C. Articular cartilage: From formation to tissue engineering. *Biomater Sci* 2016;4(5):734-67. doi: 10.1039/c6bm00068a
7. Markstedt K, Mantas A, Tournier I, Martínez Ávila H, Hägg D, Gatenholm P. 3d bioprinting human chondrocytes with nanocellulose–alginate bioink for cartilage tissue engineering applications. *Biomacromolecules* 2015;16(5):1489-96. doi: 10.1021/acs.biomac.5b00188
8. Lotfipour F, Mirzaeei S, Maghsoodi M. Evaluation of the effect of cacl2 and alginate concentrations and hardening time on the characteristics of lactobacillus acidophilus loaded alginate beads

using response surface analysis. *Adv Pharm Bull* 2012;2(1):71-8. doi: 10.5681/apb.2012.010
9. Jia J, Richards DJ, Pollard S, Tan Y, Rodriguez J, Visconti RP, et al. Engineering alginate as bioink for bioprinting. *Acta Biomater* 2014;10(10):4323-31. doi: 10.1016/j.actbio.2014.06.034
10. Fakhrullin RF, Lvov YM. Halloysite clay nanotubes for tissue engineering. *Nanomedicine (Lond)* 2016;11(17):2243-6. doi: 10.2217/nnm-2016-0250
11. Huang B, Liu M, Zhou C. Cellulose–halloysite nanotube composite hydrogels for curcumin delivery. *Cellulose* 2017;24(7):2861-75. doi: 10.1007/s10570-017-1316-8
12. Schütz K, Placht AM, Paul B, Brüggemeier S, Gelinsky M, Lode A. Three-dimensional plotting of a cell-laden alginate/methylcellulose blend: Towards biofabrication of tissue engineering constructs with clinically relevant dimensions. *J Tissue Eng Regen Med* 2017;11(5):1574-87. doi: 10.1002/term.2058
13. Farzaei MH, Bahramsoltani R, Abbasabadi Z, Rahimi R. A comprehensive review on phytochemical and pharmacological aspects of elaeagnus angustifolia. *J Pharm Pharmacol* 2015;67(11):1467-80. doi: 10.1111/jphp.12442
14. Amiri Tehranizadeh Z, Baratian A, Hosseinzadeh H. Russian olive (elaeagnus angustifolia) as a herbal healer. *BioImpacts* 2016;6(3):155-67. doi: 10.15171/bi.2016.22
15. Hamidpour R, Hamidpour S, Hamidpour M, Shahlari M, Sohraby M, Shahlari N, et al. Russian olive (elaeagnus angustifolia l.): From a variety of traditional medicinal applications to its novel roles as active antioxidant, anti-inflammatory, anti-mutagenic and analgesic agent. *J Tradit Complement Med* 2017;7(1):24-9. doi: 10.1016/j.jtcme.2015.09.004
16. Liu M, Dai L, Shi H, Xiong S, Zhou C. In vitro evaluation of alginate/halloysite nanotube composite scaffolds for tissue engineering. *Mater Sci Eng C Mater Biol Appl* 2015;49:700-12. doi: 10.1016/j.msec.2015.01.037
17. Amir Afshar H, Ghaee A. Preparation of aminated chitosan/alginate scaffold containing halloysite nanotubes with improved cell attachment. *Carbohydr Polym* 2016;151:1120-31. doi: 10.1016/j.carbpol.2016.06.063
18. Li H, Tan YJ, Leong KF, Li L. 3d bioprinting of highly thixotropic alginate/methylcellulose hydrogel with strong interface bonding. *Acs Appl Mater Interfaces* 2017;9(23):20086-97. doi: 10.1021/acsami.7b04216
19. Huang B, Liu M, Long Z, Shen Y, Zhou C. Effects of halloysite nanotubes on physical properties and cytocompatibility of alginate composite hydrogels. *Mater Sci Eng C Mater Biol App*l 2017; 70(pt 1):303-10. doi: 10.1016/j.msec.2016.09.001
20. Kumar A, Rao KM, Han SS. Development of sodium alginate-xanthan gum based nanocomposite scaffolds reinforced with cellulose nanocrystals and halloysite nanotubes. *Polym Test* 2017;63:214-25. doi: 10.1016/j.polymertesting.2017.08.030
21. Yildirim ED, Yin X, Nair K, Sun W. Fabrication, characterization, and biocompatibility of single-walled carbon nanotube-reinforced alginate composite scaffolds manufactured using freeform fabrication technique. *J Biomed Mater Res B Appl Biomater* 2008;87(2):406-14. doi: 10.1002/jbm.b.31118
22. Ahmadi M, Rahbarghazi R, Aslani MR, Shahbazfar AA, Kazemi M, Keyhanmanesh R. Bone marrow mesenchymal stem cells and their conditioned media could potentially ameliorate ovalbumin-induced asthmatic changes. *Biomed Pharmacother* 2017;85:28-40. doi: 10.1016/j.biopha.2016.11.127
23. Suvarna KS, Layton C, Bancroft JD. Bancroft's theory and practice of histological techniques. United Kingdom: Elsevier Health Sciences; 2012.
24. Guo X, Park H, Young S, Kretlow JD, Van den Beucken JJ, Baggett LS, et al. Repair of osteochondral defects with biodegradable hydrogel composites encapsulating marrow mesenchymal stem cells in a rabbit model. *Acta Biomater* 2010;6(1):39-47. doi: 10.1016/j.actbio.2009.07.041
25. Daemi H, Barikani M. Synthesis and characterization of calcium alginate nanoparticles, sodium homopolymannuronate salt and its calcium nanoparticles. *Sci Iran* 2012;19(6):2023-8. doi: 10.1016/j.scient.2012.10.005
26. Lai C, Zhang S, Sheng L, Liao S, Xi T, Zhang Z. Tempo-mediated oxidation of bacterial cellulose in a bromide-free system. *Colloid Polym Sci* 2013;291(12):2985-92. doi:10.1007/s00396-013-3033-7
27. Grellmann W, Berghaus A, Haberland EJ, Jamali Y, Holweg K, Reincke K, et al. Determination of strength and deformation behavior of human cartilage for the definition of significant parameters. *J Biomed Mater Res A* 2006;78 (1):168-74. doi: 10.1002/jbm.a.30625
28. Liu M, Jia Z, Jia D, Zhou C. Recent advance in research on halloysite nanotubes-polymer nanocomposite. *Prog Polym Sci* 2014;39(8):1498-525
29. Li X, Dunne N, Li X, Aifantis KE. Scaffolds reinforced by fibers or tubes for tissue repair. *BioMed Res Int* 2014:501275. doi: 10.1155/2014/501275
30. Chung JH, Naficy S, Yue Z, Kapsa R, Quigley A, Moulton SE, et al. Bio-ink properties and printability for extrusion printing living cells. *Biomater Sci* 2013;1(7):763-73. doi:10.1039/C3BM00012E

31. Ferris CJ, Gilmore KJ, Beirne S, McCallum D, Wallace GG. Bio-ink for on-demand printing of living cells. *Biomater Sci* 2013;1(2):224-30. doi: 10.1039/C2BM00114D
32. Panwar A, Tan LP. Current status of bioinks for micro-extrusion-based 3d bioprinting. *Molecules* 2016;21(6): pii: E685. doi:10.3390/molecules21060685
33. Jana S, Trivedi MK, Tallapragada RM, Branton A, Trivedi D, Nayak G, et al. Characterization of physicochemical and thermal properties of chitosan and sodium alginate after biofield treatment. *Pharmaceut Anal Acta* 2015;6(10). doi: 10.4172/2153-2435.1000430
34. Schütz K, Placht AM, Paul B, Brüggemeier S, Gelinsky M, Lode A. Three-dimensional plotting of a cell-laden alginate/methylcellulose blend: Towards biofabrication of tissue engineering constructs with clinically relevant dimensions. *J Tissue Eng Regen Med* 2017;11(5):1574-87. doi: 10.1002/term.2058
35. Wan Y, Chen X, Xiong G, Guo R, Luo H. Synthesis and characterization of three-dimensional porous graphene oxide/sodium alginate scaffolds with enhanced mechanical properties. *Mater Express* 2014;4(5):429-34. doi: 10.1166/mex.2014.1188
36. Akizuki S, Mow VC, Müller F, Pita JC, Howell DS, Manicourt DH. Tensile properties of human knee joint cartilage: I. Influence of ionic conditions, weight bearing, and fibrillation on the tensile modulus. *J Orthop Res* 1986;4(4):379-92. doi: 10.1002/jor.1100040401
37. Roth V, Mow V. The intrinsic tensile behavior of the matrix of bovine articular cartilage and its variation with age. *J Bone Joint Surg Am* 1980;62(7):1102-17.
38. Low IM, Hakamy A, Shaikh F. High performance natural fiber-nanoclay reinforced cement nanocomposites. Berlin: Springer; 2017.
39. Pritzker KP, Gay S, Jimenez SA, Ostergaard K, Pelletier JP, Revell PA, et al. Osteoarthritis cartilage histopathology: Grading and staging. *Osteoarthritis Cartilage* 2006;14(1):13-29. doi: 10.1016/j.joca.2005.07.014

Oleoylethanolamide Supplementation Reduces Inflammation and Oxidative Stress in Obese People

Laleh Payahoo[1], Yaser Khajebishak[2], Mohammad Asghari Jafarabadi[3], Alireza Ostadrahimi[4]*

[1] Talented Student Center, Student Research Committee, Nutrition Research Center, Faculty of Nutrition and Food Science, Tabriz University of Medical Sciences, Tabriz, Iran.

[2] Student Research Committee, Faculty of Nutrition and Food Science, Tabriz University of Medical Sciences, Tabriz, Iran.

[3] Road Traffic Injury Research Center, Department of Statistics and Epidemiology, Faculty of Health, Tabriz University of Medical Sciences, Tabriz, Iran.

[4] Nutrition Research Center, Faculty of Nutrition and Food Science, Tabriz University of Medical Sciences, Tabriz, Iran.

Article info

Keywords:
- Inflammation
- Endocannabinoids
- Obesity
- Oleoylethanolamide
- Oxidative stress

Abstract

Purpose: Obesity as a serious public health problem worldwide, results in the incidence of many chronic diseases. Obesity has been recognized as a chronic low-grade inflammation disorder. Altered endocannabinoid system tone is also involved in the pathogenesis of obesity. The present study aimed to investigate the effects of oleoylethanolamide supplementation on inflammatory biomarkers and oxidative stress in obese people.

Methods: This randomized, double-blind, placebo-controlled clinical trial was carried out on 60 healthy obese people in 2016 in Tabriz, Iran. Eligible subjects were randomly divided into intervention (received daily, two 125 mg OEA capsules) and control groups (the same amounts of starch) and treated for 8 weeks. Blood samples (5 ml) were taken in fasting state at the baseline and at the end of the study. The concentrations of MDA and TAS were measured using a spectrophotometer. A high sensitive-C reactive protein level was measured by Immunoturbidimetry assay using the commercial kit. IL-6 and TNF-α levels were assayed by the ELISA method. The differences between groups were assessed by ANCOVA and statistical significance was determined at $p<0.05$.

Results: Analysis was done on 56 participants who continued intervention until the end of the study. A significant decrease in the IL-6 and TNF-α serum concentrations was observed in the intervention group ($p<0.001$). Changes in other variables were undetectable ($p>0.05$).

Conclusion: The use of OEA as a complementary pharmacotherapy agent could be effective in improving inflammation and oxidative stress in obese people. Future studies are needed to confirm the obtained results.

Introduction

Obesity as a serious public health problem, results from an imbalance between energy intake and energy expenditure.[1] Growing evidences have shown that there is an increase in the prevalence of obesity in the world.[2] Iran is no exception in this regard. According to the second national integrated micronutrient survey in 2011 to 2015, about 40.3 and 19.2% of the Iranian population were overweight and obese, respectively.[3] Obesity was recognized as a chronic low-grade inflammation.[4] Chronic inflammation participates in the appearance of many adverse disorders such as diabetes, metabolic syndrome, some kinds of cancer and nonalcoholic fatty liver disease.[5-8] It has been shown that the levels of pro-inflammatory cytokines and acute phase proteins such as C-reactive protein (CRP), interleukin-6 (IL-6) and tumor necrosis factor–alpha (TNF-α) increase in obese people.[9-11]

Besides inflammation, an altered endocannabinoid system tone is involved in the pathogenesis of obesity.[12] Endocannabinoids exert their physiological functions in the body mainly via two receptors: cannabinoid receptors 1 and 2 (CB1 amd CB2).[13] Some endocannabinoids-like compounds including oleoylethanolamide (OEA) are structurally similar to endocannabinoids but are incapable of binding to cannabinoid receptors.[14]

Oleoylethanolamide as an endogenous ethanolamide fatty acid is synthesized in the small intestine cells and adipose tissues,[15,16] neurons[17] and astrocytes[18] and exerts its biological functions through other pathways instead of cannabinoid receptors.[19] Oatmeal, nuts, and cocoa powder are the major foods sources of OEA in meals. However, the amount of OEA found in these foods is low (fewer than 2 μg/g).[20,21] In addition to the protective effects of OEA in the many metabolic diseases including neurodegenerative disorders, anti-atherosclerosis effects,

***Corresponding author:** Alireza Ostadrahimi, Email: ostadrahimi@tbzmed.ac.ir

apoptosis, relieving pain, enhancement of lipid metabolism, cytoprotective actions on the pancreatic beta cells,[22-34] decreasing inflammation and body weight are considered as other beneficial effects of OEA.[25-35] In obese people, OEA can regulate the energy homeostasis and appetite mainly by activation of various receptors including proximal proliferator-activated receptor-α (PPAR-α), G-protein-coupled receptor 119 (GPR119) and transient receptor potential cation channel subfamily V (TRPV1). Indeed, OEA activates these receptors and delays meal initiation, reduces meal size, decreases intervals between meals and finally modulates body weight.[23,36-38]

According to experimental studies, OEA also suppresses the expression of IL-6, interleukin-8 (IL-8), intercellular adhesion molecule-1 (ICAM-1) and vascular cell adhesion molecule-1 (VCAM-1) in TNF-α induced inflammation in human umbilical vein endothelial cells through the activation of inflammatory receptors. OEA also inhibited the nuclear factor kappa-B (NF-kB) pathway in the body.[39] In YT *et al's* survey, OEA (50 µmol/L) inhibited the TNF-α induced VCAM-1 expression in HUVEC.[40]

Considering the high prevalence of obesity and due to the lack of clinical studies assessing OEA´s potential in reducing inflammatory biomarkers and oxidative stress in obese people, the present study was aimed at investigating the effects of OEA supplementation on the inflammation and oxidative stress biomarkers in obese people.

Materials and Methods

This randomized, double-blind, controlled clinical trial was done on 60 healthy obese people from November to May 2016 in Tabriz, Iran. Individuals between the ages of 18 and 59 years and with a body mass index (BMI) between 30 and 40 kg/m2 were defined as inclusion criteria. All participants were informed through the announcement and poster invitation and were recruited from clinics and healthcare centers of Tabriz University of Medical Science. Exclusion criteria were participants with current clinical problems including kidney diseases, liver and heart failure, gastrointestinal and rheumatic disorders, cigarette, smoking, pregnancy, and breastfeeding and menopause in women, participants taking antibiotics, probiotics and prebiotics supplements, weight loss drugs, omega 3 supplements, and multivitamin and mineral supplements during one month prior to the study.

The sample size was calculated according to the same variable (body mass) as a previous study.[41] By considering the confidence interval 95%, power 90%, two-tailed test, and taking into account the 0.9% changes, the minimum sample size was calculated to be 26 healthy obese people in each group. Given that losses were possible in the follow-up period, 30 individuals were included in each group.

A written consent form completed by eligible participants at baseline. Demographic questionnaires including age, sex, occupational status, and educational level were completed by participants at baseline.All participants were randomly allocated to an intervention or a placebo group. The intervention group received two 125 mg OEA capsules daily 30-minutes before lunch and dinner meals (synthesized at the Nutrition Research Center, Tabriz University of Medical Science, Iran); the materials for synthesis were obtained from the Sigma-Aldrich Company (in detail was explained in our previous study)[42] for 8 weeks. The placebo group received the same amount of placebo (starch). A third person who labeled capsules with identical shapes and colors with 2 codes remained unknown to the researchers until the end of the assays. Figure 1 shows how people were recruited and followed until the end of the study. All subjects were followed by weekly phone call to confirm that they consumed the capsules regularly. The data on those who consumed more than 90% of the capsules were analyzed.

Anthropometric and biochemical assessments

At baseline, anthropometric measurements were taken in the fasting state. Body weights and heights were measured without shoes and with light clothing using a Seca scale (precision 100 g, Seca, Hamburg, Germany) and a stadiometer (Seca, Germany), respectively. The BMI was calculated by dividing weight/height2 (kg/m2). Blood samples (5mL) were collected in vacuum collection tubes containing EDTA in the fasting state (10-12 hour, water permitted) at baseline and at the end of the study. The serums were isolated by high-speed centrifugation and were frozen immediately at −70 °C until assay. The concentration of malondialdehyde (MDA) and the total antioxidant status (TAS) were measured with a spectrophotometer using a commercial kit (Merck chemicals and Randox Laboratories, Ltd, Crumlin, UK, respectively). The Immunoturbidimetry assay and commercial kit were used to measure the high sensitive-C reactive protein level (Biosystems, Barcelona Spain COD 31927). The levels of IL-6 and TNF-α were also assayed using ELISA kits, according to the manufacturer's instructions (IBL (REF BE53061 and REF BE55001, International GmbH, Hamburg, Germany).

Statistical analysis

SPSS software was used to analysis of data (version 20; SPSS Inc., Chicago, IL). The normal distribution of variables was assessed by the Kolmogorov-Smirnov test. Numerical data was presented as mean (Standard deviation) and categorical data was presented as frequency (percentage). The baseline characteristics were compared by independent sample t tests (for quantitative variables) and the chi-squared test (for qualitative variables) in both groups. The within-group changes of IL-6, TNF-α, hs-CRP, MDA, and TA concentrations were assessed by paired sample t-test. We used analysis of covariance (ANCOVA) to detect difference between the intervention and placebo groups after adjusting for baseline measurements and confounder factors including age, sex, occupational and educational status. $p< 0.05$ was defined as statistically significant.

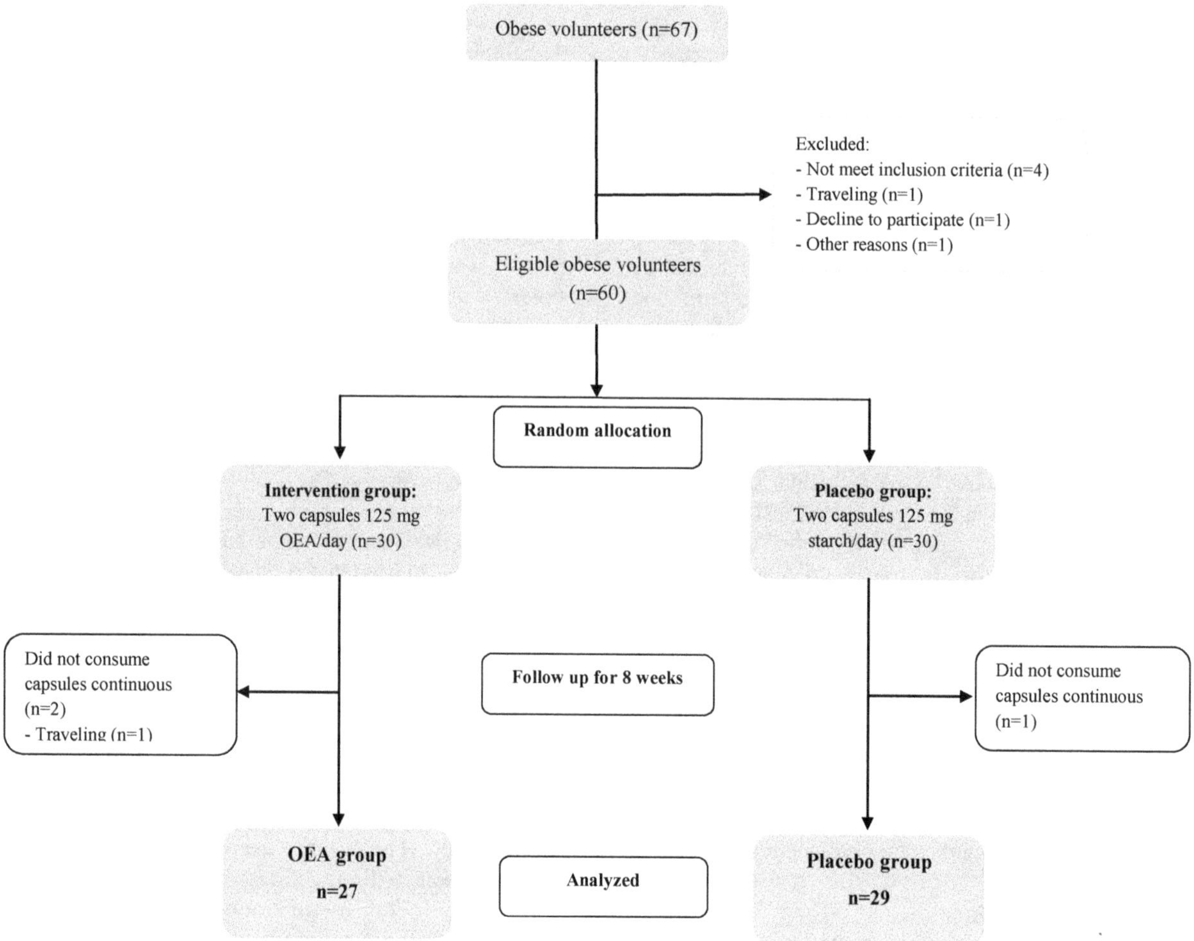

Figure 1. The flowchart of the study from baseline until the end of study

Results and Discussion

Table 1 presents the baseline characteristics of participants in both groups. The analysis was performed on data from 56 participants who completed the intervention. Mean (SD) ages of subjects in the intervention group were 37.37 (8.74) and in the placebo group was 38.13 (9.28) years. About 55% and 65% of subjects in the intervention and placebo groups were females. No significant differences detected for all baseline variables with the exception of educational level ($p>0.05$). Participants reported no side effect or symptoms either during OEA treatment or at the end of the intervention.

Figure 2 shows the changes in the inflammatory biomarkers and oxidative stress indices before and after the intervention in both groups. The levels of IL-6 decreased significantly in the intervention group (before Mean (SD) = 6.51 (0.95), after Mean (SD) = 5.99 (0.72); $p=0.011$). Changes in the placebo group were not significant ($p>0.05$). According to the ANCOVA test, there was a significant difference between groups regarding the IL-6 variable, after adjusting for baseline value and demographic characteristics ($p<0.001$). TNF-α decreased significantly in the OEA group in comparison with baseline (before Mean (SD)=6.44 (3.19), after Mean (SD)=4.20 (2.19); $p=0.007$) and this result was confirmed by ANCOVA test ($p=0.001$).

The levels of hs-CRP in the OEA group decreased significantly at the end of the study ($p=0.044$) and a non-significant increase of this variable was detected in the placebo group ($p>0.05$). However, the ANCOVA test did not attain statistical significance. Changes in other biomarkers (MDA and TAS) were not significant ($p>0.05$). Table 2 presents the mean difference between inflammatory biomarkers and oxidative stress indices between groups after adjusting for baseline value and demographic characteristics.

Different dietary interventions have been identified to reduce inflammatory cytokines in chronic disorders.[43] Indeed, dietary components act as ligands of the receptors for the activation of genes involved in the regulation of inflammatory responses.[44] Oleoylethanolamide, a lipid mediator component, is a structural analog of the endocannabinoids with several beneficial effects in metabolic status.[41,45]

The present study investigated the potential anti-inflammatory effects of OEA in obesity. At the end of the study, the concentrations of IL-6 and TNF-α decreased significantly. However, the level of other biomarkers did not show significant changes between groups. Higher levels of IL-6 in obese people increases the expression of other acute phase proteins and systemic inflammation markers such as CRP.[46] In agreement with this study, Anton *et al* investigated the anti-inflammatory effects of OEA in 87 rats exposed to alcohol. Supplementation of male Wistar rats (n=4-6 per group) with 5mg/kg OEA, resulted in a decrease of interleukin-1 β (IL-1 β), monocyte chemoattractant protein 1 (MCP-1), TNF-α levels and inhibition of pro-inflammatory enzymes including cyclooxygenase-2 (COX-2) and inducible nitric oxide syntheses (iNOS). Also, it has been reported that OEA had anti-depression effects and neuroprotective effects on alcohol intoxicated rats.[35] In the study of Sun *et al*, the neuroprotective effects of OEA through the activation of PPAR-α receptors were reported. Supplementation of OEA (10mg/kg) increased the expression of I_kB as NF_kB-inhibitory protein in cortex cerebral mouse and inhibited the expression of COX-2 as NF_kB-regulated protein.[26] Zolese *et al* investigated the effects of OEA on lipid peroxidation and high-density lipoprotein (HDL)-associated paraoxonase activity (as an enzyme involved in antioxidant and anti-inflammatory pathways) in plasma samples derived from 13 healthy people. The results showed that incubation of plasma with 1μM OEA and 20-70μM $CuSO_4$ and 10 mM (2,2 -Azobis-(2-amidinopropane) hydrochloride (AAPH) for 7 h protected plasma lipids and paraoxonase 1 enzyme activity against AAPH and copper-induced oxidation.[47]

Table 1. The demographic characteristics of obese people in the onset of study (n=56)

Variables	OEA group (n=27)	Placebo group (n=29)	P[a]
Age (year)	37.37 (8.74)	38.13 (9.28)	0.572
Gender			
- Female	15 (55.6)	19 (65.5)	0.109
- Male	12 (44.4)	10 (34.5)	
Education level			
- Illiterate	13 (48.1)	15 (51.7)	
- Diploma	3 (11.1)	11 (37.9)	0.010
- Bachelor degree and above	11 (40.7)	3(10.3)	
Occupation			
- Clerk	8 (29.6)	4 (13.8)	
- Housewife	14 (51.9)	19 (65.5)	0.438
- Worker	5 (18.5)	6 (20.7)	
Weight (kg)	93.02 (13.22)	91.23 (13.61)	0.628
Height (cm)	163.73 (9.41)	160.96 (8.91)	0.340
BMI (kg/m^2)	34.69 (2.41)	35.11 (2.82)	0.552
IL-6 (pm/mL)	6.51 (0.95)	6.43 (0.64)	0.698
TNF-α (pm/mL)	6.44 (3.19)	5.86 (1.85)	0.412
Hs-CRP (pm/mL)	7.04 (3.12)	7.28 (2.23)	0.666
TAS (mmol/L)	1.56 (0.37)	1.52 (0.37)	0.682
MDA (μmol/L)	1.79 (0.49)	1.72 (0.30)	0.533

[a] Independent sample t-Test/ Chi2 test
Data presented as Mean (SD)/ frequency (%)

In another study, the anti-inflammatory and neuroprotective properties of OEA were assessed in neuro-inflamed Wistar Hannover rats induced by lipopolysaccharide (LPS) (n=94, 5-6/group). OEA (10 mg/kg) prevented the significant up-regulation of NF_kB and significantly reduced lipopolysaccharide-induced oxidative/nitrosative stress ($p<0.001$). Also, OEA disrupted lipopolysaccharide-induced anhedonia as the main symptom of a depressive-like state ($p<0.001$).[48] In the study of Ma *et al*, the antioxidant and anti-inflammatory properties of OEA in 20 male mice were investigated. OEA (10 mg/kg/day) was administered orally for 8 weeks. The results showed that OEA prevented oxidative stress and endothelial cell damage, and inhibited early atherosclerotic plaque formation.[49] Table 3 summarized the results of studies regarding OEA supplementation on the inflammatory biomarkers and oxidative stress.

OEA exert its antioxidant and anti-inflammatory effects through different mechanisms. OEA acts as an endogenous ligand of the PPAR-α.[42,50] PPAR-α is a member of the nuclear receptor proteins family and exerts effective roles in many metabolic pathways such as adipocytes differentiation and lipid metabolism.[51] Regulating inflammatory responses was also attributed to the PPAR-α function. In macrophages, PPAR-α inhibits the scavenger receptor and nitric oxide synthesis.[39] Also, PPAR-α reduces leukocyte adhesion to the activated endothelial cells and controls the migration of transendothelial leukocytes.[52] Agonists of PPAR-α suppress the expression of IL-6 and COX-2 involved in the inflammatory pathways.[53] OEA as a ligand of PPAR-α binds to the PPAR-α receptors and reduces the production of reactive oxygen species (ROS) and pro-inflammatory cytokines.[54] OEA also inhibits the expression of VCAM-1 and ICAM-1 as molecules involved in the inflammatory responses.[55] Other mechanisms involved in the cytoprotective and anti-inflammatory effects of OEA include the increasing activity of the anti-oxidative enzyme, reducing lipid peroxidation, and apoptosis-related proteins expression.[49] To the best of the authors′ knowledge, this was the first clinical study to evaluate the unique effects of oleoylethanolamide on the inflammatory biomarkers and oxidative stress in obese people. The main limitations of this study include the insufficient purity of the synthesized OEA (~ 85%), not measuring OEA concentrations in the serum samples and the shorter duration of the supplementation.

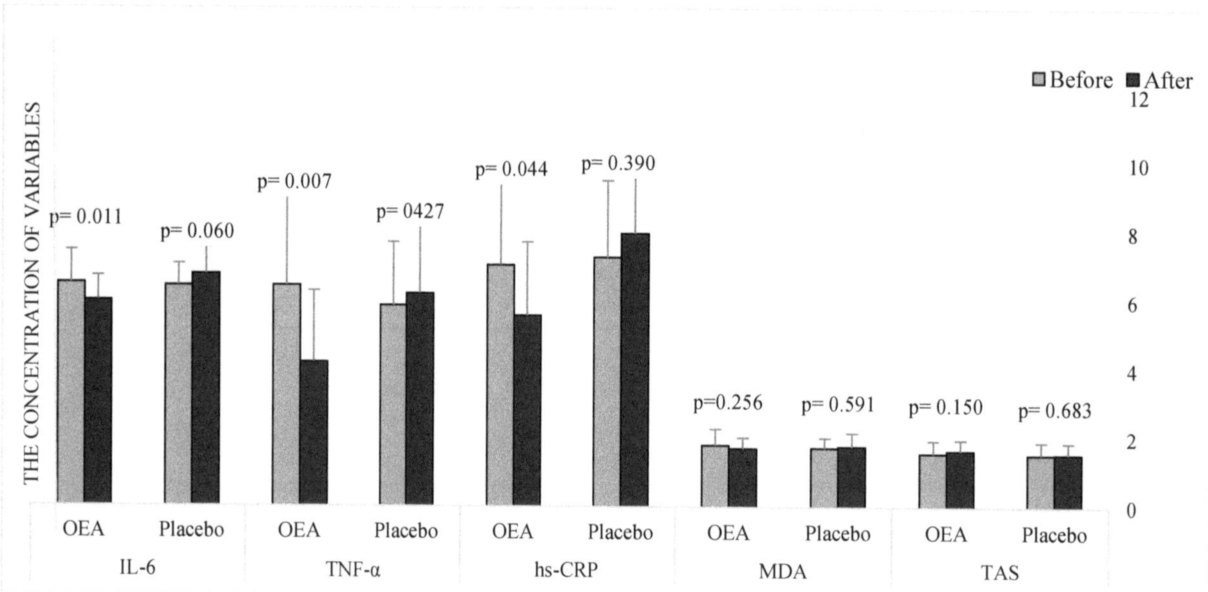

Figure 2. The Mean (SD) of inflammatory biomarkers and oxidative stress indices in the OEA and placebo groups (n=56)

Table 2. The effects of OEA supplementation on the inflammatory biomarkers and oxidative stress in obese people (n=56)

Variables	OEA group (n=27)	Placebo group (n=29)	Mean Diff (95% CI) P[a]
IL-6 (pm/mL)			
Before	6.51 (0.95)	6.43 (0.64)	0.853 (0.447-1.258)
After	5.99 (0.72)	6.77 (0.78)	<0.001
TNF-α (pm/mL)			
Before	6.44 (3.19)	5.86 (1.85)	2.127 (0.935-3.319)
After	4.20 (2.09)	6.21 (2.20)	0.001
hs-CRP (pm/mL)			
Before	7.04 (3.12)	7.28 (2.23)	1.590 (-0.242-3.422)
After	5.56 (2.16)	7.97 (2.41)	0.087
MDA (μmol/L)			
Before	1.79 (0.49)	1.72 (0.30)	0.108 (-0.085-0.300)
After	1.70 (0.33)	1.76 (0.41)	0.267
TAS (mmol/L)			
Before	1.56 (0.37)	1.52 (0.37)	0.093 (-0.210-0.025)
After	1.63 (0.32)	1.53 (0.34)	0.119

Data were presented as Mean (SD)
[a] Mean Diff (95% CI)P for ANCOVA test (Adjusting on Baseline values, age, gender, education, and occupation variables)

Table 3. The results of studies about the effects of oleoylethanolamide on the inflammatory biomarkers and oxidative stress

Samples	Dose, Duration	Results	Reference
Wild-type mice (C57BL/6)	OEA (10mg/kg) for 3 days	- The expression of IkB as NFkB-inhibitory protein in cortex cerebral of mouse increased - The expression of COX-2 as NFkB-regulated protein inhibited	Sun et al. (2007)
Healthy people (n=13)	OEA (1μM) CuSO4 (20-70μM) (2,2 -Azobis-(2-amidinopropane) hydrochloride (AAPH) (10 mM) for 7 hours	- Plasma lipids and paraoxonase 1 enzyme activity protected against AAPH and copper-induced oxidation by OEA	Zolese et al. (2008)
Vascular endothelial cell, healthy HUVEC and TNF-alpha induced HUVECs	OEA (10, 50 and 100 μmol.L) cultured at 37 degrees C for 7 h	- OEA (10 and 50 μmol.L) induced the CB2 protein and mRNA expression, but not 100 μmol.L. - TNF-alpha induced VCAM-1 expression and THP-1 adhere to HUVEC inhibited	YT et al, (2014)
Male mice (n=20)	OEA (10 mg/kg) administered orally 8 weeks	- Oxidative stress and endothelial cell damage prevented - Early atherosclerotic plaque formation inhibited	Ma et al. (2015)
Wistar Hannover rats (n=94, 5-6 /group) terated by LPS	OEA (10 mg/kg) 8 weeks	- Up-regulation of NFkB/ lipopolysaccharide-induced oxidative/nitrosative stress inhibited significantly ($p<0.001$) - Lipopolysaccharide-induced anhedonia as a core symptom of a depressive-like state disrupted ($p<0.001$)	Sayd et al, (2015)
Wistar rats exposed to alcohol (n=87, n=4-6 per groups)	OEA (5mg/kg)	- The levels of IL-1β, MCP-1, TNF-α decreased - Pro-inflammatory enzymes including COX-2 and iNOS inhibited - OEA had anti-depression effects and neuroprotective effects on alcoholic rats	Anton et al. (2017)

Conclusion

In summary, daily supplementation of two 125 mg oleoylethanolamide in 56 healthy obese people for 8 weeks significantly decreased the levels of IL-6 and TNF-α; however, changes in MDA, TAS, and hs-CRP were insignificant. Considering the many beneficial effects of OEA, its use as a complementary agent could be effective in improving inflammation in obese people. However, future studies are needed to confirm the current results.

Acknowledgments

The authors thank the Department of Nutrition, Faculty of Health and Nutrition. This is a part of a database from Ph.D. thesis entitled "The effect of oleoylethanolamide supplementation on PPAR-α gene expression, some inflammatory biomarkers and the abundance of Akkermansia muciniphila bacteria in the stool of obese people: A double-blind randomized placebo-controlled clinical trial".

Conflict of Interest

The authors declare there is no conflict of interest in the content of this study.

References

1. Fallah-Fini S, Rahmandad H, Huang TT, Bures RM, Glass TA. Modeling us adult obesity trends: A system dynamics model for estimating energy imbalance gap. *Am J Public Health* 2014;104(7):1230-9. doi: 10.2105/AJPH.2014.301882
2. Aekplakorn W, Inthawong R, Kessomboon P, Sangthong R, Chariyalertsak S, Putwatana P, et al. Prevalence and trends of obesity and association with socioeconomic status in thai adults: National health examination surveys, 1991-2009. *J Obes* 2014;2014:410259. doi: 10.1155/2014/410259
3. Pouraram H, Djazayery A, Mohammad K, Parsaeian M, Abdollahi Z, Dorosty Motlagh A, et al. Second national integrated micronutrient survey in Iran: Study design and preliminary findings. *Arch Iran Med* 2018;21(4):137-44.
4. Calder PC, Ahluwalia N, Brouns F, Buetler T, Clement K, Cunningham K, et al. Dietary factors and low-grade inflammation in relation to overweight and obesity. *Br J Nutr* 2011;106(S3):S5-78. doi: 10.1017/S0007114511005460
5. Lumeng CN, Saltiel AR. Inflammatory links between obesity and metabolic disease. *J Clin Invest* 2011;121(6):2111-7. doi: 10.1172/JCI57132

6. Vucenik I, Stains JP. Obesity and cancer risk: Evidence, mechanisms, and recommendations. *Ann N Y Acad Sci* 2012;1271:37-43. doi: 10.1111/j.1749-6632.2012.06750.x
7. Jung UJ, Choi MS. Obesity and its metabolic complications: The role of adipokines and the relationship between obesity, inflammation, insulin resistance, dyslipidemia and nonalcoholic fatty liver disease. *Int J Mol Sci* 2014;15(4):6184-223. doi: 10.3390/ijms15046184
8. Onuora S. Rheumatoid arthritis: Obesity skews markers of inflammation. *Nat Rev Rheumatol* 2017;13(6):323. doi: 10.1038/nrrheum.2017.62
9. Lukic L, Lalic NM, Rajkovic N, Jotic A, Lalic K, Milicic T, et al. Hypertension in obese type 2 diabetes patients is associated with increases in insulin resistance and il-6 cytokine levels: Potential targets for an efficient preventive intervention. *Int J Environ Res Public Health* 2014;11(4):3586-98. doi: 10.3390/ijerph110403586
10. Derosa G, Fogari E, D'Angelo A, Bianchi L, Bonaventura A, Romano D, et al. Adipocytokine levels in obese and non-obese subjects: An observational study. *Inflammation* 2013;36(4):914-20. doi: 10.1007/s10753-013-9620-4
11. Maachi M, Pieroni L, Bruckert E, Jardel C, Fellahi S, Hainque B, et al. Systemic low-grade inflammation is related to both circulating and adipose tissue TNFalpha, leptin and IL-6 levels in obese women. *Int J Obes Relat Metab Disord* 2004;28(8):993-7. doi: 10.1038/sj.ijo.0802718
12. Geurts L, Lazarevic V, Derrien M, Everard A, Van Roye M, Knauf C, et al. Altered gut microbiota and endocannabinoid system tone in obese and diabetic leptin-resistant mice: Impact on apelin regulation in adipose tissue. *Front Microbiol* 2011;2:149. doi: 10.3389/fmicb.2011.00149
13. Roche R, Hoareau L, Bes-Houtmann S, Gonthier MP, Laborde C, Baron JF, et al. Presence of the cannabinoid receptors, CB1 and CB2, in human omental and subcutaneous adipocytes. *Histochem Cell Biol* 2006;126(2):177-87. doi: 10.1007/s00418-005-0127-4
14. Bellocchio L, Cervino C, Pasquali R, Pagotto U. The endocannabinoid system and energy metabolism. *J Neuroendocrinol* 2008;20(6):850-7. doi: 10.1111/j.1365-2826.2008.01728.x
15. Schmid PC, Wold LE, Krebsbach RJ, Berdyshev EV, Schmid HH. Anandamide and other N-acylethanolamines in human tumors. *Lipids* 2002;37(9):907-12. doi: 10.1007/s11745-002-0978-z
16. Hansen HS, Moesgaard B, Hansen HH, Petersen G. N-acylethanolamines and precursor phospholipids - relation to cell injury. *Chem Phys Lipids* 2000;108(1-2):135-50. doi: 10.1016/S0009-3084(00)00192-4
17. Di Marzo V, Fontana A, Cadas H, Schinelli S, Cimino G, Schwartz JC, et al. Formation and inactivation of endogenous cannabinoid anandamide in central neurons. *Nature* 1994;372(6507):686-91. doi: 10.1038/372686a0
18. Walter L, Franklin A, Witting A, Möller T, Stella N. Astrocytes in culture produce anandamide and other acylethanolamides. *J Biol Chem* 2002;277(23):20869-76. doi: 10.1074/jbc.M110813200
19. Rodriguez de Fonseca F, Navarro M, Gomez R, Escuredo L, Nava F, Fu J, et al. An anorexic lipid mediator regulated by feeding. *Nature* 2001;414(6860):209-12. doi: 10.1038/35102582
20. Astarita G, Rourke BC, Andersen JB, Fu J, Kim JH, Bennett AF, et al. Postprandial increase of oleoylethanolamide mobilization in small intestine of the burmese python (Python molurus). *Am J Physiol Regul Integr Comp Physiol* 2006;290(5):R1407-12. doi: 10.1152/ajpregu.00664.2005
21. Premkumar LS. Fascinating facts about phytonutrients in spices and healthy food: Scientifically proven facts. Xlibris Corporation; 2014.
22. Gonzalez-Aparicio R, Blanco E, Serrano A, Pavon FJ, Parsons LH, Maldonado R, et al. The systemic administration of oleoylethanolamide exerts neuroprotection of the nigrostriatal system in experimental parkinsonism. *Int J Neuropsychopharmacol* 2014;17(3):455-68. doi: 10.1017/S1461145713001259
23. Fu J, Gaetani S, Oveisi F, Lo Verme J, Serrano A, Rodriguez De Fonseca F, et al. Oleylethanolamide regulates feeding and body weight through activation of the nuclear receptor PPAR-alpha. *Nature* 2003;425(6953):90-3. doi: 10.1038/nature01921
24. Sanchis-Segura C, Spanagel R. Behavioural assessment of drug reinforcement and addictive features in rodents: An overview. *Addict Biol* 2006;11(1):2-38. doi: 10.1111/j.1369-1600.2006.00012.x
25. Lo Verme J, Fu J, Astarita G, La Rana G, Russo R, Calignano A, et al. The nuclear receptor peroxisome proliferator-activated receptor-α mediates the anti-inflammatory actions of palmitoylethanolamide. *Mol Pharmacol* 2005;67(1):15-9. doi: 10.1124/mol.104.006353
26. Sun Y, Alexander SP, Garle MJ, Gibson CL, Hewitt K, Murphy SP, et al. Cannabinoid activation of PPARα; a novel neuroprotective mechanism. *Br J Pharmacol* 2007;152(5):734-43. doi: 10.1038/sj.bjp.0707478
27. Mazzola C, Medalie J, Scherma M, Panlilio LV, Solinas M, Tanda G, et al. Fatty acid amide hydrolase (FAAH) inhibition enhances memory acquisition through activation of PPAR-α nuclear receptors. *Learn Mem* 2009;16(5):332-7. doi: 10.1101/lm.1145209
28. Hill MN, Miller GE, Carrier EJ, Gorzalka BB, Hillard CJ. Circulating endocannabinoids and N-acyl ethanolamines are differentially regulated in major depression and following exposure to social stress.

Psychoneuroendocrinology 2009;34(8):1257-62. doi: 10.1016/j.psyneuen.2009.03.013
29. Murillo-Rodríguez E, Vázquez E, Millán-Aldaco D, Palomero-Rivero M, Drucker-Colin R. Effects of the fatty acid amide hydrolase inhibitor URB597 on the sleep-wake cycle, c-fos expression and dopamine levels of the rat. *Eur J Pharmacol* 2007;562(1-2):82-91. doi: 10.1016/j.ejphar.2007.01.076
30. Lambert DM, Vandevoorde S, Jonsson KO, Fowler CJ. The palmitoylethanolamide family: A new class of anti-inflammatory agents? *Curr Med Chem* 2002;9(6):663-74. doi: 10.2174/0929867023370707
31. Lueneberg K, Domínguez G, Arias-Carrión O, Palomero-Rivero M, Millán-Aldaco D, Morán J, et al. Cellular viability effects of fatty acid amide hydrolase inhibition on cerebellar neurons. *Int Arch Med* 2011;4(1):28. doi: 10.1186/1755-7682-4-28
32. Di Marzo V, Sepe N, De Petrocellis L, Berger A, Crozier G, Fride E, et al. Trick or treat from food endocannabinoids? *Nature* 1998;396(6712):636-7. doi: 10.1038/25267
33. Stone VM, Dhayal S, Smith DM, Lenaghan C, Brocklehurst KJ, Morgan NG. The cytoprotective effects of oleoylethanolamide in insulin-secreting cells do not require activation of GPR119. *Br J Pharmacol* 2012;165(8):2758-70. doi: 10.1111/j.1476-5381.2011.01755.x
34. Martinez de Ubago M, Garcia-Oya I, Perez-Perez A, Canfran-Duque A, Quintana-Portillo R, Rodriguez de Fonseca F, et al. Oleoylethanolamide, a natural ligand for PPAR-alpha, inhibits insulin receptor signalling in HTC rat hepatoma cells. *Biochim Biophys Acta* 2009;1791(8):740-5. doi: 10.1016/j.bbalip.2009.03.014
35. Antón M, Alén F, Gómez de Heras R, Serrano A, Pavón FJ, Leza JC, et al. Oleoylethanolamide prevents neuroimmune HMGB1/TLR4/NF-kB danger signaling in rat frontal cortex and depressive-like behavior induced by ethanol binge administration. *Addict Biol* 2017;22(3):724-41. doi: 10.1111/adb.12365
36. Contreras AV, Torres N, Tovar AR. PPAR-α as a key nutritional and environmental sensor for metabolic adaptation. *Adv Nutr* 2013;4(4):439-52. doi: 10.3945/an.113.003798
37. Hansen KB, Rosenkilde MM, Knop FK, Wellner N, Diep TA, Rehfeld JF, et al. 2-Oleoyl glycerol is a GPR119 agonist and signals GLP-1 release in humans. *J Clin Endocrinol Metab* 2011;96(9):E1409-17. doi: 10.1210/jc.2011-0647
38. Zhang LL, Yan Liu D, Ma LQ, Luo ZD, Cao TB, Zhong J, et al. Activation of transient receptor potential vanilloid type-1 channel prevents adipogenesis and obesity. *Circ Res* 2007;100(7):1063-70. doi: 10.1161/01.RES.0000262653.84850.8b
39. Xu X, Guo H, Jing Z, Yang L, Chen C, Peng L, et al. N-Oleoylethanolamine Reduces Inflammatory Cytokines and Adhesion Molecules in TNF-alpha-induced Human Umbilical Vein Endothelial Cells by Activating CB2 and PPAR-alpha. *J Cardiovasc Pharmacol* 2016;68(4):280-91. doi: 10.1097/FJC.0000000000000413
40. Gai YT, Shu Q, Chen CX, Lai YL, Li WJ, Peng L, et al. Anti-atherosclerosis role of N-oleoylethanolamine in CB2. *Yao Xue Xue Bao* 2014;49(3):316-21.
41. Mangine GT, Gonzalez AM, Wells AJ, McCormack WP, Fragala MS, Stout JR, et al. The effect of a dietary supplement (n-oleyl-phosphatidyl-ethanolamine and epigallocatechin gallate) on dietary compliance and body fat loss in adults who are overweight: A double-blind, randomized control trial. *Lipids Health Dis* 2012;11:127. doi: 10.1186/1476-511X-11-127
42. Payahoo L, Khajebishak Y, Barzegari A, Alipour SH, Asghari Jafarabadi M, Farrin N, et al. Oleoylethanolamide increases the expression of PPAR-α and reduces appetite and body weight in obese people: A clinical trial. *Appetite* 2018;128:44-9. doi: 10.1016/j.appet.2018.05.129
43. Payahoo L, Ostadrahimi A, Mobasseri M, Jafarabadi MA, Mahdavi AB, Mahluji S. Anethum graveolens L. Supplementation has anti-inflammatory effect in type 2 diabetic patients. *IJTK* 2014;13(3):461-5.
44. Patterson E, Wall R, Fitzgerald GF, Ross RP, Stanton C. Health implications of high dietary omega-6 polyunsaturated fatty acids. *J Nutr Metab* 2012;2012:539426. doi: 10.1155/2012/539426
45. Barbaro D, Menasci A, Baldini B, Pasquini C, Lapi P. The Dietary Supplement EGCG: NOPE (N-Oleyl-Phosphatidyletathanolamine and Epigallocatechin-3-Gallato Formula) Helps Patients to Follow a Flexible Dietary Regimen and Induces Loss of Weight in Patients who had Previously Experienced No Response to Other Weight Loss Intervention. *J Obes Weig Los Ther* 2011;1(1):105. doi: 10.4172/2165-7904.1000105
46. Visser M, Bouter LM, McQuillan GM, Wener MH, Harris TB. Low-grade systemic inflammation in overweight children. *Pediatrics* 2001;107(1):E13. doi: 10.1542/peds.107.1.e13
47. Zolese G, Bacchetti T, Masciangelo S, Ragni L, Ambrosi S, Ambrosini A, et al. Effect of acylethanolamides on lipid peroxidation and paraoxonase activity. *Biofactors* 2008;33(3):201-9.
48. Sayd A, Antón M, Alén F, Caso JR, Pavón J, Leza JC, et al. Systemic administration of oleoylethanolamide protects from neuroinflammation and anhedonia induced by lps in rats. *Int J Neuropsychopharmacol* 2015;18(6). doi: 10.1093/ijnp/pyu111
49. Ma L, Guo X, Chen W. Inhibitory effects of oleoylethanolamide (OEA) on H(2)O(2)-induced human umbilical vein endothelial cell (HUVEC) injury and apolipoprotein E knockout (ApoE-/-) atherosclerotic mice. *Int J Clin Exp Pathol* 2015;8(6):6301-11.

50. Fu J, Oveisi F, Gaetani S, Lin E, Piomelli D. Oleoylethanolamide, an endogenous PPAR-α agonist, lowers body weight and hyperlipidemia in obese rats. *Neuropharmacology* 2005;48(8):1147-53. doi: 10.1016/j.neuropharm.2005.02.013
51. Barger PM, Kelly DP. PPAR signaling in the control of cardiac energy metabolism. *Trends Cardiovasc Med* 2000;10(6):238-45. doi: 10.1016/S1050-1738(00)00077-3
52. Duval C, Chinetti G, Trottein F, Fruchart JC, Staels B. The role of PPARs in atherosclerosis. *Trends Mol Med* 2002;8(9):422-30. doi: 10.1016/S1471-4914(02)02385-7
53. Delerive P, Gervois P, Fruchart JC, Staels B. Induction of IκBα expression as a mechanism contributing to the anti-inflammatory activities of peroxisome proliferator-activated receptor-α activators. *J Bioll Chem* 2000;275(47):36703-7. doi: 10.1074/jbc.M004045200
54. Fan A, Wu X, Wu H, Li L, Huang R, Zhu Y, et al. Atheroprotective effect of oleoylethanolamide (OEA) targeting oxidized LDL. *PloS One* 2014;9(1):e85337. doi: 10.1371/journal.pone.0085337
55. Chen C, Jin X, Meng X, Zheng C, Shen Y, Wang Y. Inhibition of TNFα-induced adhesion molecule expression by (Z)-(S)-9-octadecenamide, N-(2-hydroxyethyl,1-methyl). *Eur J Pharmacol* 2011;660(2-3):305-9. doi: 10.1016/j.ejphar.2011.04.009

Eryngium Billardieri Induces Apoptosis via *Bax* Gene Expression in Pancreatic Cancer Cells

Neda Roshanravan[1], Parina Asgharian[2,3], Hassan Dariushnejad[4], Naimeh Mesri Alamdari[5], Behzad Mansoori[6], Ali Mohammadi[6], Shahriar Alipour[7], Meisam Barati[8], Abed Ghavami[9], Vajihe Ghorbanzadeh[10], Fatemeh Aamazadeh[9], Alireza Ostadrahimi[9]*

[1] *Cardiovascular Research Center, Tabriz University of Medical Sciences, Tabriz, Iran.*
[2] *Drug Applied Research Center, Tabriz University of Medical Sciences, Tabriz, Iran.*
[3] *Department of Pharmacognosy, Tabriz University of Medical Sciences, Tabriz, Iran.*
[4] *Department of Medical Biotechnology, Faculty of Medicine, Lorestan University of Medical Sciences, Khorramabad, Iran.*
[5] *Students Research Committee, School of Health, Iran University of Medical Science, Tehran, Iran.*
[6] *Immunology Research Center, Tabriz University of Medical Sciences, Tabriz, Iran.*
[7] *Department of Molecular Medicine, Connective Tissue Disease Research Center, Tabriz University of Medical Sciences, Tabriz,Iran.*
[8] *Students Research Committee, Cellular and Molecular Nutrition Department, Shahid Beheshti University of Medical Sciences, Tehran, Iran.*
[9] *Nutrition Research Center, School of Nutrition, Tabriz University of Medical Science, Tabriz, Iran.*
[10] *Razi Herbal Medicine Research Center, Lorestan University of Medical Sciences, Khorramabad, Iran.*

Article info

Keywords:
· Adenocarcinoma
· *Bax*
· Cyclin D1
· *Eryngium*
· Pancreas

Abstract

Purpose: Pancreatic adenocarcinoma has a high prevalence all over the world. Most of the therapeutic approaches failed as a result of tumor invasion and rapid metastasis. Several natural plants have been shown to have promising therapeutic effects. Thus, the aim of this study was to investigate the cytotoxic activity of *Eryngium billardieri* against PANC-1 cancer cell lines.

Methods: Dimethylthiazole diphenyltetrazolium bromide assay (MTT assay) and flow cytometry were used to assess the cytotoxicity of *E. billardieri* extracts against PANC-1 cancer cell lines. Quantitative Polymerase Chain Reaction (qPCR) was conducted to investigate the expression levels of Bcl2- associated X protein (*BAX*) and *cyclin D1*.

Results: The results of the MTT assay showed that *E. billardieri* extracts had cytotoxic effects on PANC- 1 cancer cell lines. Moreover, the findings from the gene expression confirmed the over expression of *Bax*, and under expression of *cyclin D1* following treatment with dichloromethane (DCM) and n-hexane (n- hex) extracts in cancer cells ($P < 0.05$). Interestingly, the flow cytometry results showed that DCM and n- hex extracts of *E. billardieri* induced apoptosis in PANC- 1 cancer cell lines.

Conclusion: The results of this study demonstrated that DCM and n- hex extracts of *E. billardieri* significantly induce apoptosis by increasing *Bax* and decreasing *cyclin D1* mRNA expression. Therefore, *E. billardieri* may be regarded as a novel approach for treatment of pancreatic cancer as a result of its promising apoptotic and cytotoxic properties.

Introduction

Pancreatic adenocarcinoma is one of the most lethal malignant neoplasms across the world, and is associated with the lowest 5-year survival rate.[1] According to the GLOBOCAN 2012 estimates, pancreatic cancer accounts for more than 331000 deaths per year, making it the third leading cause of cancer death in both sexes together.[2] The major barrier to positive clinical outcomes for this type of cancer is delayed diagnosis and resistance to existing malignancy therapeutics.[3]

Apoptosis, as a major mechanism which regulates pathways to control cell proliferation and death, is suggested for consideration as one of the targeted therapy strategies for tumor cells.[4] In recent years, a number of investigations have been carried out that show novel strategies for more successful prevention and therapy of pancreatic cancer. Previous studies demonstrated that *cyclin D1* and *Bax* genes are the most important regulators in controlling the proliferation and apoptosis of cells.[5]

Cyclin D1 protein plays a crucial role in regulating the progress of the cell during the G1 phase of the cell cycle. The *cyclin D1* gene is intensified in pancreatic carcinomas.[6] Proapoptotic *Bax* protein can induce apoptosis via the intrinsic signaling pathway (also known

***Corresponding author:** Alireza Ostadrahimi, Email: ostadrahimi@tbzmed.ac.ir

as mitochondrial apoptosis).[7,8] Previous findings suggest that enhanced apoptosis-promoting *Bax* gene expression may have therapeutic application in pancreatic cancer cells.[9,10]

Pioneering clinical studies have reported that medicinal herbs and their derivative phytocompounds can be considered as useful complementary treatments for cancer.[11,12] *E. billardieri* (Figure 1) belongs to the Umbelliferae family which is used extensively as a medicinal plant worldwide for the treatment of various inflammatory disorders.[13] In Iranian folk medicine, various parts of this plant are used for a wide range of ailments; such as various inflammatory disorders, rheumatism, sinusitis, wound healing, urinary infections, scorpion bites, goiter etc.[13,14] Extracts obtained from the root and aerial parts of *E. billardieri* previously showed anti-inflammatory and anti-hyperglycemic effects.[15,16]

The dim prognosis of pancreatic adenocarcinoma is due to a lack of molecular pathways regarding disease development. PANC-1 cell lines (Pancreatic cancer cell lines) are currently used as *in vitro* models to assay pancreatic ductal adenocarcinoma carcinogenesis. The morphological and genetic characteristics of these cell lines are well- known already.[17] In continuation of our scientific works on the evaluation of the anti-proliferative activity of the Iranian Medicinal plants,[18-25] this study investigated the cytotoxic activity of n-hex, DCM and methanol (Met) extracts of the aerial parts of *E. billardieri* against PANC-1 cancer cell lines via *Bax* and *cyclin D1* mRNA expression.

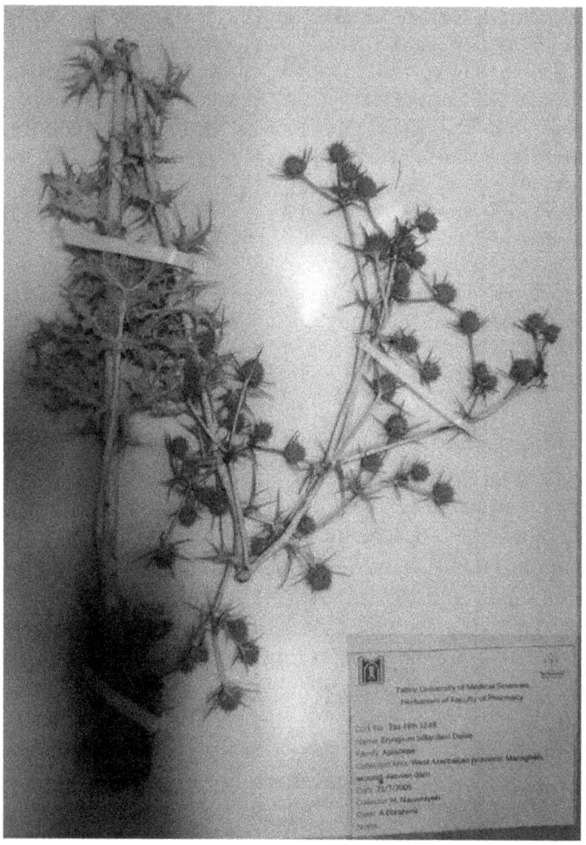

Figure 1. *Eryngium billardieri.*

Materials and Methods

Materials

Methanol, L-glutamine, Penicillin-Streptomycin, MTT, Phosphate-buffered saline (PBS), Trypsin-Ethylenediaminetetraacetic acid (EDTA) solution, and RPMI 1640 were purchased from Sigma (Sigma, St. Louis, MO, USA). Fetal bovine serum (FBS) (HyClone, Logan, UT, USA), Dimethyl sulfoxide (DMSO), Diethyl pyrocarbonate (DEPC) water (Merck, Germany), AnnexinV-FITC/PI apoptosis kit (Invitrogen, USA), SYBR Green PCR master mix (Takara Bio Inc., Tokyo, Japan) were used in this study.

Plant materials were collected from Maragheh-Mountains (Eastern Azerbaijan Province, Iran). Voucher specimens were authenticated by Herbarium of Faculty of Pharmacy, Tabriz University of Medical Sciences. The fresh aerial parts of *E. billardieri* (100 g) were extracted with 1.1 L of n-hex, DCM and MeOH solvents by Soxhlet apparatus, respectively. Then, to reach the highest purity percentage, the extract was filtered by Whatman filter paper no.40 and was placed in the temperature of 36°C. To yield a dry and concentrated extract, rotary vacuum evaporator was used. Extracts were kept in sterile screw-capped containers and were stored at 6°C until use.

PANC-1 and human embryonic kidney normal cell line (KDR/293) were obtained from the Pasteur Institute, National cell bank, Tehran, Iran. The cells were grown in RPMI 1640 medium (Sigma, St. Louis, MO, USA) which were supplemented with 10% FBS, penicillin G (100 U/ml), and streptomycin (100 µg/ml). Cells were cultured in 25 cm2 culture T- flasks at 37°C in humidified air with 5% CO2.

MTT assay, gene expression and flow cytometry

In-vitro, cytotoxicity was assessed by 3-[4, 5-dimethylthiazol-2-yl]-3, 5-diphenyl tetrazolium bromide for treated and untreated PANC- 1 and KDR/293 cell lines. MTT assay is a high accuracy colorimetric method that is widely used to determine cell viability and cell cytotoxicity, particularly in the expansion of new drugs. The cells were seeded in 96-well plates at a density of 15,000 cells per well in their respective RPMI 1640 media. When the cells were approximately more than 80% confluent were left untreated or treated with DCM, MeOH and n-hex extracts of_*E. billardieri.* The half maximal inhibitory concentration (IC_{50}) was determined by MTT test in the range of 0 to 1600 µg/mL at 24 and 48 hours (Figure 2).

Analyses of *Bax* and cyclin D1 genes expression were all performed after 48 hours of *E. billardieri* treatment by reverse transcription-polymerase chain reaction. Total RNA was extracted from cultured cell lines using TRIzol reagent (Invitrogen, USA) according to the manufacturer's instructions. *β- actin* was considered as an internal control. The relative absorbance ratio at A260/280 and A260/230 on a spectrophotometer (NanoDrop One/Onec, Thermo Scientific) was used to confirm RNA quality and quantity. Total RNA was then converted to cDNA by reverse transcription using Prime Script RT Reagent kit (Takara, RR037Q, Japan) according to manufacturer's recommendations for cDNA synthesis. For qRT-PCR, three replicates of each sample were amplified in a 20 µL reaction mixture containing SYBR Green reaction mix (Takara, Japan) and 0.5 mM of primer and analyzed using real-time PCR (Mic – qPCR, Australia). The amount of the *Bax* and cyclin D1 mRNA were normalized against that of the *β- actin* mRNA and the relative mRNA abundance was analyzed using $-2^{\Delta\Delta CT}$ method.[26] The primer sequences were designed through the use of PrimerBank and summarized in supplementary appendix (Table 1). PANC- 1 and KDR/293 cells were seeded into six-well culture plates (1.0×106 cells/well) with RPMI 1640 media and incubated at growth condition for 48 h. After that, the cells were washed with pre-warmed culture media and were carefully replaced with a prepared fixative solution (pre-warmed RPMI containing 4% formaldehyde). Cells were treated with 50, 100 and 200 µg/mL of DCM, Met, and n-hex extracts of *E. billardieri*. After treatment time point (48 h), the untreated and treated cells were separated by Trypsin-EDTA, and supernatants were thrown away after centrifugation at 900 rpm for 10 min at 28°C. According to the AnnexinV-FITC/PI apoptosis kit (Invitrogen, USA) instructions, the cell pellets were washed once in PBS, then once in 1X Binding Buffer and were centrifuged and disposed supernatant in each phase. After this stage, the cells were resuspended in 100 µl of 1X binding buffer and were transferred into a new 5 ml tube. Then, 5 µl of FITC-conjugated Annexin V was added to 100 µL of the cell suspension and incubated for 15 min under a dark condition at room temperature. After incubation time, the cells were washed with 1X binding buffer and resuspended in 200 µL of 1X binding buffer again. At the final stage, 5 µl of propidium iodide (PI) staining solution was added to the cells and was analyzed by flow cytometry. Quadrant settings were fixed with untreated controls and copied to dot plots of the treated cells. Data analysis was done using FlowJo (Treestar, Inc., San Carlos, CA). The experiment was repeated triplicate.

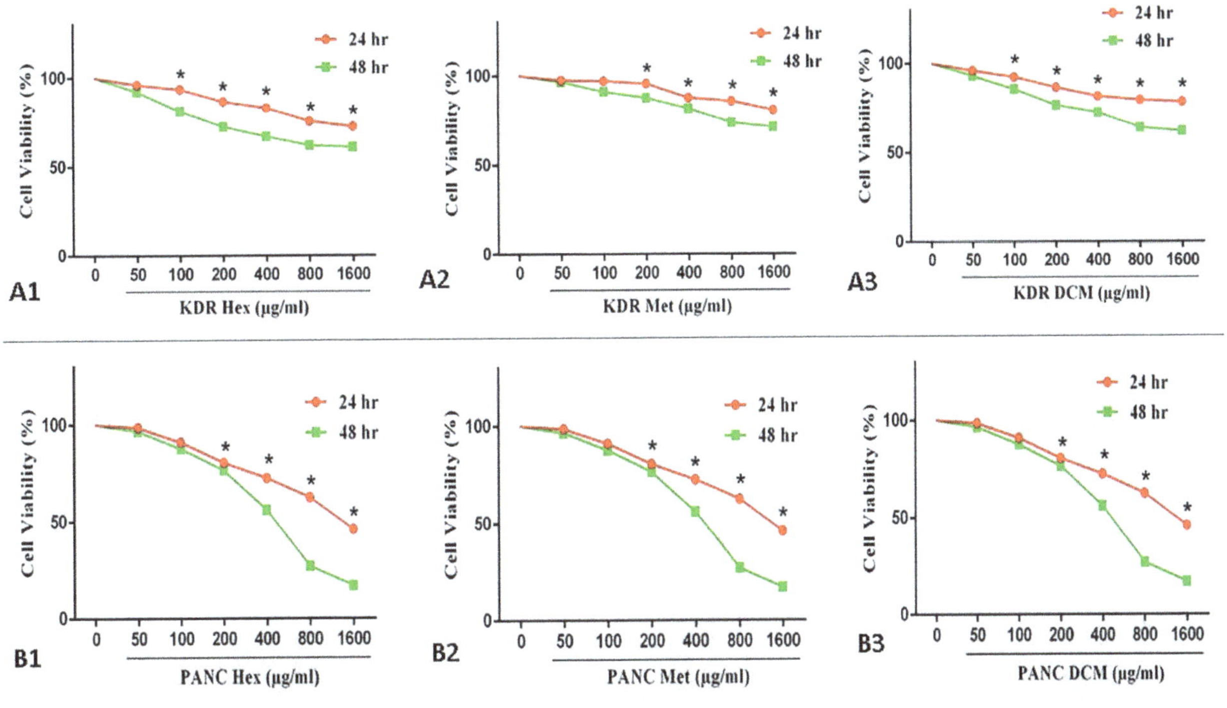

Figure 2. Diagram representing the cytotoxic effect of the *Eryngium billardieri* extract on PANC-1 and KDR/293 cells at 24 & 48 h. A1: KDR Hex, A2: KDR Met, A3: KDR DCM; B1: PANC Hex, PANC Met, PANC DCM.*p < 0.05. Hex: n-hexane extracts; DCM: dichloromethane extracts; Met: methanol extracts.

Table 1. Sequence of Genes primers for qRT-PCR

Gene	Primers	
Bax	Forward	TTCTGACGGCAACTTCAACT
	Reverse	CAGCCCATGATGGTTCTGAT
Cyclin- D1	Forward	CCACTCCTACGATACGCTACTA
	Reverse	CCAGCATCTCATAAACAGGTCA
β-actin	Forward	GGTGAAGGTGACAGCAGT
	Reverse	TGGGGTGGCTTTTAGGAT

Statistical analysis

Graph Pad Instat 6 software (GraphPad Instant biostatistics, San Diego, CA, USA) was used to test significant differences between various treatment groups. All data are expressed as means ± SD. Analysis of the experimental data was done by using the one-way ANOVA analysis of variance; following Tukey's post hoc using SPSS (SPSS Inc. Chicago, IL, USA version 16.0). *P*-values less than 0.05 were considered to be significant.

Results

E.billardieri extracts had cytotoxic effects on PANC- 1 cancer cell lines

To determine the cytotoxic effects of *E. billardieri* extracts on PANC-1 and KDR/293 cells MTT assay was performed. Data analysis of cells treated with plant extract at 0- 1600 µg/mL concentrations in 24 & 48 h is illustrated in Figure 2. Moreover, the half-maximal inhibitory concentrations (IC_{50}) after treatment by various concentrations of DCM, Met and n-hex extracts of *E. billardieri* were determined and presented in Table 2. As seen in Figure 2, due to the treatment by Met, DCM and n-hex extracts of *E. billardieri* the survival rates of PANC- 1 cells were significantly decreased compared with untreated cell lines ($p<0.05$) in time and dose dependent manner. However, as shown in Figure 2, the extracts had growth inhibitory effect on the KDR/293 normal cell only in high concentrations which IC_{50} could not be defined from the responses.

Table 2. The IC_{50} dose of *E. billardieri* extracts on PANC-1 and KDR/293 cells at 24 & 48 h.

Time	24h		48h	
Cell line	PANC-1	KDR	PANC-1	KDR
n-hex	836.2	-	217.3	-
DCM	1128	-	306.8	-
Met	1329	-	448.5	-

n-hex: n-hexane extracts; DCM: dichloromethane extracts; Met: methanol extracts

DCM and n-hex extracts of E. billardieri influenced on the Bax and Cyclin- D1 mRNA expression in PANC- 1 cancer cell lines

We used a QRT-PCR to evaluate the *Bax* and *cyclin D1* expression in PANC- 1 and KDR/293 normal cell lines. According to the results of qRT-PCR (the obtained data are presented in Figure 3), the expression levels of *Bax* were significantly increased in PANC-1 cells after treatment with DCM and n-hex extracts with 100 and 200 µg/ mL concentration compared to untreated control cells and KDR/293 ($p<0.05$). Interestingly, the expression level of *cyclin D1* mRNA decreased after treatment with DCM and n-hex extracts in the treated cancer cells compared to untreated control cells ($p<0.05$). Furthermore, there were not any significant differences in the expression levels of investigated genes subsequent to exposure KDR/293 normal cells ($p>0.05$). Unexpectedly, we did not see any difference in the expression levels of *Bax* and *cyclin D1* genes subsequent to exposure cell lines with Met extract of *E. billardieri* ($p>0.05$). Upon to the results of QRT-PCR, it is obvious that none of the extracts at the concentration of 50µg/ mL had effects on genes expression in PANC-1 and KDR/293 cell lines ($p>0.05$).

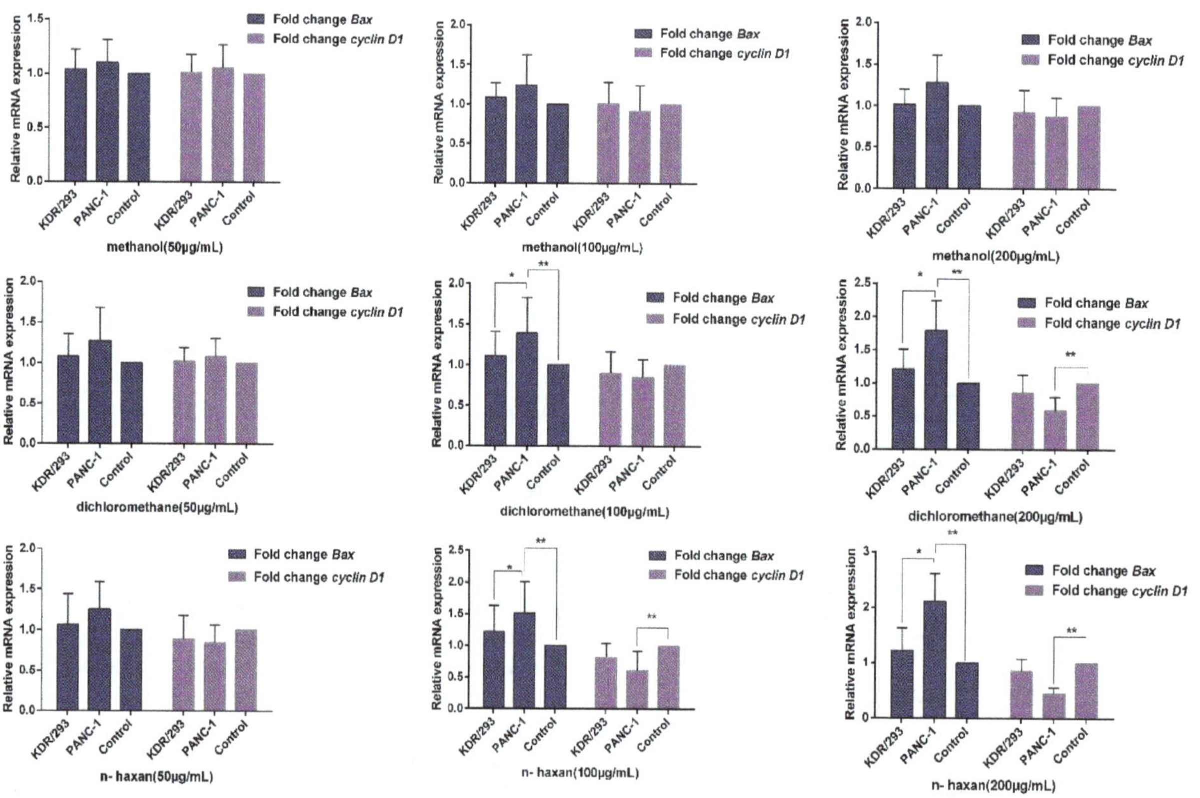

Figure 3. Changes in genes expression in PANC-1 and KDR/293 cell lines treated with the IC_{50} concentration of the *Eryngium billardieri* extracts compared to control group (untreated cell lines). *p< 0.05, **p < 0.05 versus control one (Untreated cells).

DCM and n-hex extracts of E. billardieri induced apoptosis in PANC- 1 cancer cell lines

Figures 4 showed the representative FACS plots._The flow cytometry results represented that the untreated control KDR/293 and PANC-1 cells that primarily incubated by Annexin V and PI were approximately viable and no apoptosis and no necrosis occurred (97.8% & 85.2% respectively: Annexin V-/ PI-). Meanwhile, treatment with DCM and n-hex extracts in the highest determined dose (200 *µg/ mL)* for 48 h increased the percentage of PANC-1 cells in late (Annexin V+/PI+) apoptosis compared to the untreated control and normal KDR/293 cells. Our results revealed that Met extract of *E. billardieri* couldn't be able to trigger apoptosis pathway in PANC-1 and KDR/293 cell lines (Annexin V-/PI-). However, DCM and n-hex extracts of *E. billardieri* might initiate apoptosis in KDR/293 cells at slow rate with highest determined dose (200 *µg/ mL)*. In addition, after treatment with DCM and n-hex extracts of *E. billardieri* in three doses four groups including viable cells (Annexin V and PI negative), necrosis (Annexin V negative and PI positive), cells undergoing early apoptosis (Annexin V positive and PI negative), and cells in the late stage of apoptosis (Annexin V and PI positive) appeared. As a result, we can conclude that DCM and n-hex extracts of *E. billardieri* can induce a high level of apoptosis in treated cells ($p<0.05$).

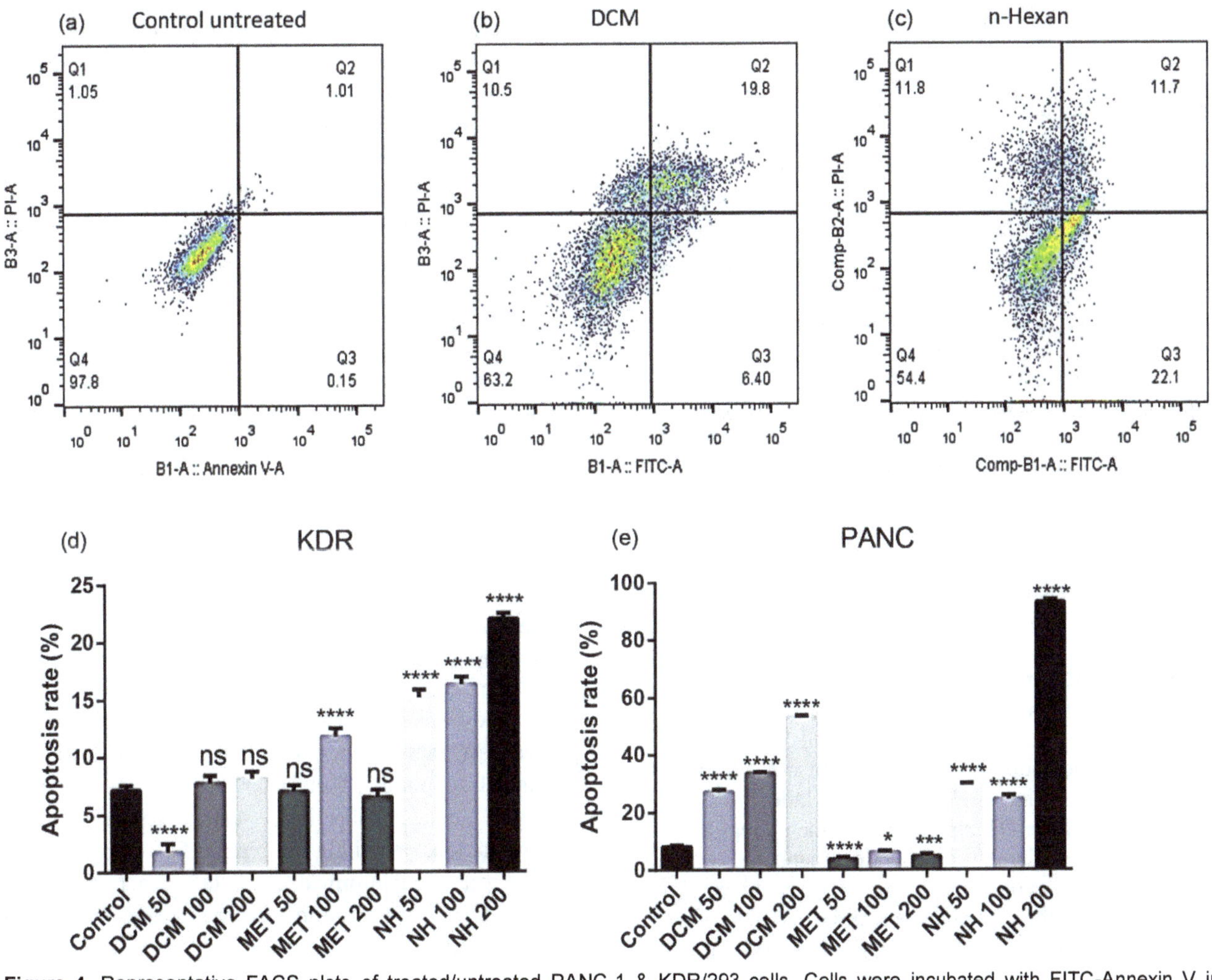

Figure 4. Representative FACS plots of treated/untreated PANC-1 & KDR/293 cells. Cells were incubated with FITC-Annexin V in combination with PI to detect apoptosis and necrosis and classified as necrotic cells (the upper left quadrant (Q1); Annexin −/PI +), late apoptotic cells (the upper right quadrant (Q2); Annexin +/PI +), early apoptotic cells (the lower right quadrant (Q3); Annexin +/PI −) or intact cells (the lower left quadrant (Q4); Annexin −/PI −). (a): control untreated KDR cells, (b): DCM 50 µg/mL on PANC-1 cells, (c): n-hexan 50 µg/mL on PANC-1 cells. (d): Apoptosis rate in KDR cells. (e): Apoptosis rate in PANC-1 cells. *<0.05, ***<0.01, ****<0.001. NH: n-hexane; Met: methanol; DCM: dichloromethane.

Discussion

Pancreatic adenocarcinoma is the third leading cause of cancer-related death. Its highly lethal rate can be attributed to its poor prognosis and despite the advances in surgical intervention and chemotherapy; little effect has been made on the mortality rate of this disease. There is a serious need for complementary therapies with better efficacy. Previous *in vitro* studies about medicinal plants revealed that different species of *Eryngium* have demonstrated biological activities including cytotoxic, apoptotic, antimicrobial and anti-inflammatory.[27] The focus of the present work was to investigate the molecular pathways including cell cycle arrest and apoptosis of *E. billardieri* and its antitumor cytotoxic effect.

In this study, it was found that DCM and n-hex extracts of *E. billardieri* could induce a high level of apoptosis in PANC-1 treated cells and kept the ratio of necrosis negligible. Moreover, these extracts increased the expression level of *Bax* mRNA in PANC-1 cell lines whereas the *cyclin D1* expression was decreased in the treated cancer cells. As it was expected, the elevated expression of *Bax* mRNA was in line with apoptosis in PANC-1 treated cells.

Cell cycle progression is regulated at both the G to S and G to M transition states as a result of the activation and inactivation of specific protein kinases family and their regulatory subunits including cyclins and catalytic subunits which are termed cyclin-dependent kinases (Cdks). Till now, 11 members of the cyclins have been identified including cyclins A, B1±2, C, D1±3, E, F, G and H. The *cyclin D1* plays a vital role in orchestrating cell progression through the G1 phase of the cell cycle and determines whether a cell will progress towards mitogenesis. Several observational studies have suggested that *cyclin D1* plays a key role in promoting the growth of certain human malignancies.[6,28] By considering various findings, nowadays it has been established that deregulation of *cyclin D1* expression has contributed to the loss of cell cycle control and enhance tumorigenesis.[29] A correlation has previously been pointed out between increased *cyclin D1* and cancer formation.[30,31] Based on the results of this study, the DCM and n-hex extracts of *E. billardieri* reduced *cyclin D1*expression in treated cancer cells with no effect on the normal cells.

We also confirmed that both *E. billardieri* extracts can stimulate *Bax* mRNA expression in PANC-1 cancer cells. *Bax* as a pro-apoptotic protein can trigger apoptosis by increasing the opening of the mitochondrial voltage-dependent anion channels, which induce the loss in its membrane potential.[32] Our results suggest that the apoptotic mechanisms of n-hex extracts of *E. billardieri* in PANC-1 cells include the down regulation of *cyclin D1* expression and the up regulation of *Bax* expression in a dose-dependent manner.

Our results replicate the findings of Esmaeili et al.[14] who indicated the cytotoxic potential effects of *E. billardieri* on MCF-7, A549, HepG-2 and HT-29 cell lines. The main components of *Eryngium* species such as essential oils, sterols, saponin, and sanicula saponin are responsible for its cytotoxic activities. These compounds have shown potent and highly selective inhibition against PANC-1, HL-60, A549, PC-3, and MRC-5 tumor cell lines with almost no cytotoxicity against normal human cells.[33,34]

The hexane extract of various species of *Eryngium* exhibited anti-inflammatory and antioxidant activities in animal models.[35] It has been mentioned that these effects may be due to a decrease in nitric oxide, inflammatory cytokines and TNF-α synthesis.[36] In line with several investigations which attempted to find bioactive natural anticancer compounds, that induce apoptosis in cancer cells without cytotoxic effects against normal human cells, we indicated that the cytotoxic dose of DCM and n-hex extracts of *E. billardieri* did not cause a significant change in the survival rate of KDR/293 normal cells. The results of this study indicated that nonpolar extracts of *E. billardieri* were generally more effective than the methanolic ones. Similarly, Roumy et al[37] showed the high cytotoxic/antiplasmodial effects of the DCM and n-hex extracts of some Amazonian plants. Therefore, the effective inhibition of PANC-1 cancer cells *in vitro* suggests that DCM and n-hex extracts of *E. billardieri* may be potentially promising anticancer agents for the effective treatment of pancreatic cancer cells. In this study, there are some limitations: 1) the examination of anticancer effects on PANC-1 cancer cells results to its effect to be unknown on other pancreatic cancer cell lines. 2) Lack of isolation and investigation of *E. billardieri* constituents.

Conclusion

In conclusion, the results of the current study are the first to indicate that DCM and n-hex extracts of *E. billardieri* significantly induce apoptosis by increasing *Bax* and decreasing *cyclin D1* mRNA expression. However, more molecular studies for investigating the probable apoptotic pathways of the cytotoxic activity of *E. billardieri* should be conducted to achieve a definite conclusion.

Acknowledgments

The authors would like to thank the Nutrition Research Center of Tabriz University of Medical Sciences.

This study was funded by Tabriz University of Medical Sciences (grant number: IR.TBZMED.5.553473). The financial supporter of the study had no role in study design, data collection, data analysis, data interpretation, or writing the report. The corresponding author was well informed of all the data in the study and had final responsibility for the decision to submit for publication.

Conflict of Interest

The authors declare that they have no conflict of interest.

Abbreviations

Dimethylthiazole diphenyltetrazolium bromide assay: MTT assay; Quantitative Polymerase Chain Reaction: qPCR; Bcl2- associated X protein: BAX; Phosphate-buffered saline: PBS; Ethylenediaminetetraacetic acid: EDTA; Fetal bovine serum: FBS; Dimethyl sulfoxide:

DMSO; Diethyl pyrocarbonate: DEPC; half maximal inhibitory concentration: IC50; Cyclin-dependent kinases: Cdks

References

1. Li D, Xie K, Wolff R, Abbruzzese JL. Pancreatic cancer. *Lancet* 2004;363(9414):1049-57. doi: 10.1016/S0140-6736(04)15841-8
2. Ferlay J, Soerjomataram I, Dikshit R, Eser S, Mathers C, Rebelo M, et al. Cancer incidence and mortality worldwide: Sources, methods and major patterns in GLOBOCAN 2012. *Int J Cancer* 2015;136(5):E359-86. doi: 10.1002/ijc.29210
3. Al-Wadei MH, Al-Wadei HA, Schuller HM. Pancreatic cancer cells and normal pancreatic duct epithelial cells express an autocrine catecholamine loop that is activated by nicotinic acetylcholine receptors α3, α5, and α7. *Mol Cancer Res* 2012;10(2):239-49. doi: 10.1158/1541-7786.MCR-11-0332
4. Réjiba S, Bigand C, Parmentier C, Hajri A. Gemcitabine-based chemogene therapy for pancreatic cancer using ad-dck:: Umk gdept and ts/rr sirna strategies. *Neoplasia* 2009;11(7):637-50.
5. Abdullah JM, Ahmad F, Ahmad KA, Ghazali MM, Jaafar H, Ideris A, et al. Molecular genetic analysis of bax and cyclin d1 genes in patients with malignant glioma. *Neurol Res* 2007;29(3):239-42. doi: 10.1179/016164107X158965
6. Kornmann M, Ishiwata T, Itakura J, Tangvoranuntakul P, Beger HG, Korc M. Increased cyclin d1 in human pancreatic cancer is associated with decreased postoperative survival. *Oncology* 1998;55(4):363-9. doi: 10.1159/000011879
7. Staibano S, Mignogna MD,Lo Muzio Lo, Di Alberti L, Di Natale E, Lucariello A, et al. Overexpression of cyclin-d1, bcl-2, and bax proteins, proliferating cell nuclear antigen (pcna), and DNA-ploidy in squamous cell carcinoma of the oral cavity. *Hum Pathol* 1998; 29(11):1189-94.
8. Mansoori B, Mohammadi A, Hashemzadeh S, Shirjang S, Baradaran A, Asadi M, et al. Urtica dioica extract suppresses mir-21 and metastasis-related genes in breast cancer. *Biomed Pharmacother* 2017;93:95-102. doi: 10.1016/j.biopha.2017.06.021
9. Xu ZW, Friess H, Büchler MW, Solioz M. Overexpression of bax sensitizes human pancreatic cancer cells to apoptosis induced by chemotherapeutic agents. *Cancer Chemother Pharmacol* 2002;49(6):504-10. doi: 10.1007/s00280-002-0435-5
10. Mohammadi A, Mansoori B, Aghapour M, Baradaran B. Urtica dioica dichloromethane extract induce apoptosis from intrinsic pathway on human prostate cancer cells (pc3). *Cell Mol Biol (Noisy-le-grand)* 2016;62(3):78-83.
11. Yin SY, Wei WC, Jian FY, Yang NS. Therapeutic applications of herbal medicines for cancer patients. *Evid Based Complement Alternat Med* 2013; 2013: 302426. doi: 10.1155/2013/302426
12. Mohammadi A, Mansoori B, Goldar S, Shanehbandi D, Khaze V, Mohammadnejad L, et al. Effects of urtica dioica dichloromethane extract on cell apoptosis and related gene expression in human breast cancer cell line (MDA-Mb-468). *Cell Mol Biol (Noisy-le-grand)* 2016; 62(2):62-7.
13. Sefidkon F, Dabiri M, Alamshahi A. Chemical composition of the essential oil of eryngium billardieri f. Delaroche from iran. *J Essent Oil Res* 2004;16(1):42-3. doi: 10.1080/10412905.2004.9698648
14. Esmaeili S, Irani M, Zehan HM, Keramatian B, Harandi ZT, Hamzeloo-Moghadam M. Cytotoxic activity of some ethnic medicinal plants from southwest of Iran. *Res J Pharmacogn* 2016;3(1):43-7.
15. Yesilada E, Tanaka S, Tabata M, Sezik E. The antiinflammatory activity of the fractions from eryngium billardieri in mice. *Phytother Res* 1989;3(1):38-40. doi: 10.1002/ptr.2650030111
16. Küpeli E, Kartal M, Aslan S, Yesilada E. Comparative evaluation of the anti-inflammatory and antinociceptive activity of turkish eryngium species. *J Ethnopharmacol* 2006;107(1):32-7. doi: 10.1016/j.jep.2006.02.005
17. Gradiz R, Silva HC, Carvalho L, Botelho MF, Mota-Pinto A. Mia paca-2 and panc-1–pancreas ductal adenocarcinoma cell lines with neuroendocrine differentiation and somatostatin receptors. *Sci Rep* 2016;6:21648. doi: 10.1038/srep21648
18. Tofighi Z, Asgharian P, Goodarzi S, Hadjiakhoondi A, Ostad SN, Yassa N. Potent cytotoxic flavonoids from iranian securigera securidaca. *Med Chem Res* 2014; 23(4): 1718-24. doi: 10.1007/s00044-013-0773-3
19. Asnaashari S, Delazar A, Asgharian P, Lotfipour F, Bamdad Moghaddam S, Heshmati Afshar F. In-vitro bioactivity and phytochemical screening of extracts from rhizomes of eremostachys azerbaijanica rech. F. Growing in iran. *Iran J Pharm Res* 2017; 16(1):306-14.
20. Asgharian P, Delazar A, Lotfipour F, Asnaashari S. Bioactive properties of eremostachys macrophylla montbr. & auch.Rhizomes growing in iran. *Pharm Sci* 2017;23(3):238-43.doi: 10.15171/PS.2017.35
21. Yaripour S, Delnavazi MR, Asgharian P, Valiyari S, Tavakoli S, Nazemiyeh H. A survey on phytochemical composition and biological activity of zygophyllum fabago from iran. *Adv Pharm Bull* 2017;7(1):109-14. doi: 10.15171/apb.2017.014
22. Asgharian P, Afshar FH, Asnaashari S, Lotfipour F, Baradaran B, Zolali E, et al. Evaluation of various biological activities of the aerial parts of scrophularia frigida growing in iran. *Iran J Pharm Res* 2017;16(1):277-89.

23. Goodarzi S, Nateghpour M, Asgharian P, Hadjiakhoondi A, Yassa N, Tavakoli S, et al. Antimalarial and cytotoxic activities of roots and fruits fractions of astrodaucus persicus extract. *Iran J Basic Med Sci* 2017;20(12):1318-23. doi: 10.22038/IJBMS.2017.9554
24. Afshar FH, Asgharian P, Khodaie L, Delazar A, Lotfipour F, Baradaran B. Anti-proliferative and antimicrobial activity of methanolic extract and SPE fractions of artemisia spicigera. *Jundishapur J Nat Pharm Prod* 2016; in press: e36903. doi: 10.5812/jjnpp.36903
25. Delazar A, Asgharian P, Asnaashari S. Biological and phytochemical screening of eremostachys azerbaijanica rech.F. Aerial parts. *Jundishapur J Nat Pharm Prod* 2017;12(3) (Supp); e64312 .doi:10.5812/jjnpp.64312
26. Livak KJ, Schmittgen TD. Analysis of relative gene expression data using real-time quantitative pcr and the 2(- Delta Delta c(T)) method. *Methods* 2001;25(4):402-8. doi: 10.1006/meth.2001.1262
27. Erdem SA, Nabavi SF, Orhan IE, Daglia M, Izadi M, Nabavi SM. Blessings in disguise: A review of phytochemical composition and antimicrobial activity of plants belonging to the genus eryngium. *Daru* 2015;23-53. doi: 10.1186/s40199-015-0136-3
28. Graña X, Reddy EP. Cell cycle control in mammalian cells: Role of cyclins, cyclin dependent kinases (cdks), growth suppressor genes and cyclin-dependent kinase inhibitors (ckis). *Oncogene* 1995; 11 (2):211-19.
29. Motokura T, Arnold A. Cyclins and oncogenesis. *Biochim Biophys Acta* 1993;1155(1):63-78.
30. Yu Q, Geng Y, Sicinski P. Specific protection against breast cancers by cyclin d1 ablation. *Nature* 2001;411(6841):1017-21. doi: 10.1038/35082500
31. Gansauge S, Gansauge F, Ramadani M, Stobbe H, Rau B, Harada N, et al. Overexpression of cyclin d1 in human pancreatic carcinoma is associated with poor prognosis. *Cancer Res* 1997; 57 (9):1634-7.
32. Wolter KG, Hsu YT, Smith CL, Nechushtan A, Xi XG, Youle RJ. Movement of Bax from the Cytosol to Mitochondria during Apoptosis. *J Cell Biol* 1997;139(5)1281-91.
33. Wang P, Su Z, Yuan W, Deng G, Li S. Phytochemical constituents and pharmacological activities of eryngium l.(apiaceae). *pharma crops* 2012;3:99-120.
34. Kartal M, Mitaine-Offer AC, Paululat T, Abu-Asaker M, Wagner H, Mirjolet JF, et al. Triterpene saponins from eryngium campestre. *J Nat Prod* 2006;69(7):1105-8. doi: 10.1021/np060101w
35. Garcia MD, Saenz MT, Gomez MA, Fernandez MA. Topical antiinflammatory activity of phytosterols isolated from eryngium foetidum on chronic and acute inflammation models. *Phytother Res* 1999; 13(1):78-80. doi: 10.1002/(SICI)1099-1573(199902)13:1<78::AID-PTR384>3.0.CO;2-F
36. Strzelecka M, Bzowska M, Koziel J, Szuba B, Dubiel O, Riviera Nunez D, et al. Anti-inflammatory effects of extracts from some traditional mediterranean diet plants. *J Physiol Pharmacol Supplement* 2005;56(suppl 1):139-56.
37. Roumy V, Garcia-Pizango G, Gutierrez-Choquevilca AL, Ruiz L, Jullian V, Winterton P, et al. Amazonian plants from peru used by quechua and mestizo to treat malaria with evaluation of their activity. *J Ethnopharmacol* 2007;112(3):482-9. doi: 10.1016/j.jep.2007.04.009

Construction and Development of a Cardiac Tissue-Specific and Hypoxia-Inducible Expression Vector

Shahrooz Ghaderi[1,2,3#], Neda Alidadiani[1#], Jafar Soleimani Rad[4], Hamid Reza Heidari[5], Nafi Dilaver[6], Behzad Mansoori[1], Reza Rhabarghazi[7,8], Rezayat Parvizi[9], Vahid Khaze Shahgoli[1], Behzad Baradaran[1*]

[1] *Immunology Research Center, Tabriz University of Medical Sciences, Tabriz, Iran.*
[2] *Department of Molecular Medicine, Faculty of Advanced Medical Sciences, Tabriz University of Medical Sciences, Tabriz, Iran.*
[3] *Student research committee, Tabriz University of Medical Sciences, Tabriz, Iran.*
[4] *Department of Anatomy, Faculty of Medicine, Tabriz University of Medical Sciences, Tabriz, Iran.*
[5] *Department of Pharmaceutical Biotechnology, Faculty of Pharmacy, Tabriz University of Medical Sciences, Tabriz, Iran.*
[6] *Swansea University Medical School, Swansea University, Swansea, UK.*
[7] *Stem cell Research Center, Tabriz University of Medical Sciences, Tabriz, Iran.*
[8] *Department of Applied Cell Sciences, Faculty of Advanced Medical Sciences, Tabriz University of Medical Sciences, Tabriz, Iran.*
[9] *Department of Cardiothoracic Surgery, Faculty of Medicine, Tabriz University of Medical Sciences, Tabriz, Iran.*

Article info

Keywords:
· Hypoxia
· Hypoxia response element
· *Cis* regulatory elements

Abstract
Purpose: Cardiovascular gene therapy is a sophisticated approach, thanks to the safety of vectors, stable transgene expression, delivery method, and different layers of the heart. To date, numerous expression vectors have been introduced in biotechnology and biopharmacy industries in relation to genetic manipulation. Despite the rapid growth of these modalities, they must be intelligently designed, addressing the cardiac-specific transgene expression and less side effects. Herein, we conducted a pilot project aiming to design a cardiac-specific hypoxia-inducible expression cassette.
Methods: We explored a new approach to design an expression cassette containing cardiac specific enhancer, hypoxia response elements (HRE), cardiac specific promoter, internal ribosome entry site (IRES), and beta globin poly A sequence to elicit specific and inducible expression of the gene of interest. Enhanced green fluorescent protein (eGFP) was sub-cloned by *BglII* and *NotI* into the cassette. The specificity and inducible expression of the cassette was determined in both mouse myoblast C2C12 and mammary glandular tumor 4T1 as 'twin' cells. eGFP expression was evaluated by immunofluorescence microscope and flow cytometry at 520 nm emission peak.
Results: Our data revealed that the designed expression cassette provided tissue specific and hypoxia inducible (O_2<1%) transgene expression.
Conclusion: It is suggested that cardiac-specific enhancer combined with cardiac-specific promoter are efficient for myoblast specific gene expression. As well, this is for the first time that HRE are derived from three well known hypoxia-regulated promoters. Therefore, there is no longer need to overlap PCR process for one repeated sequence just in one promoter.

Introduction

Since identification and description of hypoxia-inducible factor 1 (HIF-1) by Wang *et al.*,[1] more than 200,000 articles have been published in scientific literatures. HIF-1 is an inducible transcription factor, which binds to hypoxia response elements (HREs) or enhancer elements during hypoxia. HREs are located in the upstream of promoter region. HIF-1 regulates several genes, such as vascular endothelial growth factor (VEGF) and erythropoietin (EPO).[2] hypoxia inducible factor-1 alpha (HIF-1) is comprised of a heterodimer basic helix-loop-helix (bHLH) transcriptional complex and is divided into distinct subsets, including HIF-1α and aryl hydrocarbon receptor nuclear translocator (ARNT), encoding a protein that is referred to beta (β) subunit. HIF-1 belongs to a conserved subfamily of PER-ARNT-SIM (PAS), which functions as oxygen sensors. The PAS domain is a subfamily of bHLH, which is a transcription factor. The HIF family consists of HIF-1α, -1β, -2α, -2β, -3α, -3β.[3,4] In normoxia, HIF-1α is degraded by ubiquitin-mediated proteolysis activity, while being transcribed into mature RNA under hypoxic conditions, leading to an increase in oxygen delivery to the tissues. Therefore, HIF-1α has an essential role both in physiologic and pathologic conditions, including, but not limited to, myocardial ischemia, coronary artery disease, organ rejection and some cancers.[5,6]

***Corresponding author:** Behzad Baradaran, Email: baradaranb@tbzmed.ac.ir, # These authors contributed equally to this work.

Among all the above-mentioned circumstances, HIF-1α plays a great role in cardiovascular diseases. Lack of oxygen contributes to augmented hypoxia in coronary and cardiac tissue, subsequently leading to a cardiac stroke. Despite the emergence of novel surgical and medical approaches, cardiac infarction is set to become the leading cause of death up to the year 2020.[7] Several reports have indicated that cardiac function, if not completely, then partially, can be ameliorated following gene or cell therapy in experimental models of infarction.[8,9] However, ectopic gene expression has its disadvantages, such as hemangioma or uncontrolled vascular formation. It is, therefore, essential to regulate gene expression via the modulation of upstream elements of promoters like HREs. It should also be noted that hypoxia may subsequently exist in other tissues as a result of physiologic statement. Hence, tissue specific gene expression is essential to develop suitable vectors for gene therapy. This approach is also considered to be useful for sophisticated studies in the field of biomedical research such as cellular imaging and tracking,[10] genome editing,[11] stem cell engineering,[12] and the study of signaling pathways.[13-15]

In this study, we investigated the cardiac specific promoter and cardiac specific enhancer combined with HREs consensus sequence.

Materials and Methods

Expression cassette designing and cloning

In order to construct the expression cassette, all the elements were synthesized by Generay Biotechnology Company (Shanghai, China) and sub-cloned into pGH cloning vector by *NdeI* and *NheI* restriction enzymes (Fermentas, Germany) (Figure 1). eGFP was sub-cloned into the cassette by *BglII* and *NotI* (Figure 2). Briefly, 1 µg plasmid DNA was digested by *BglII and NotI* (Fermentas, Germany) and the relevant buffer was added up to the final volume of 20 µl in 37 °C for 1 h. Enzymatic reaction was inactivated by chloroform and the cloning procedure was confirmed by *HindIII* digestion.

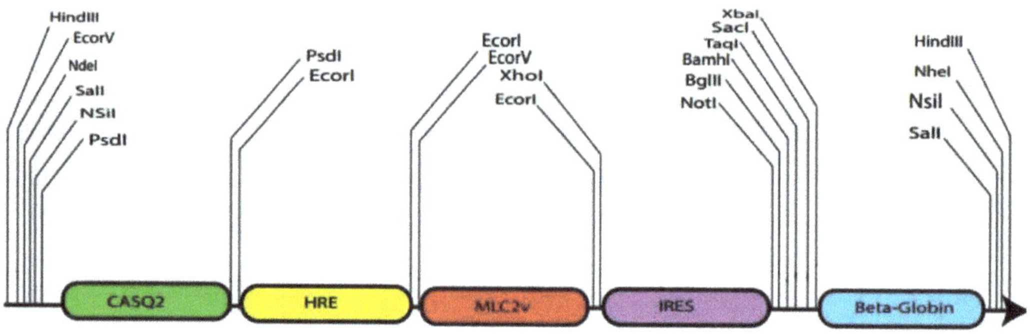

Figure 1. Schematic view of expression cassette. Expression cassette contains CASQ2 enhancer, HRE, MLC2v promoter, IRES, and β-globin poly A sequence.

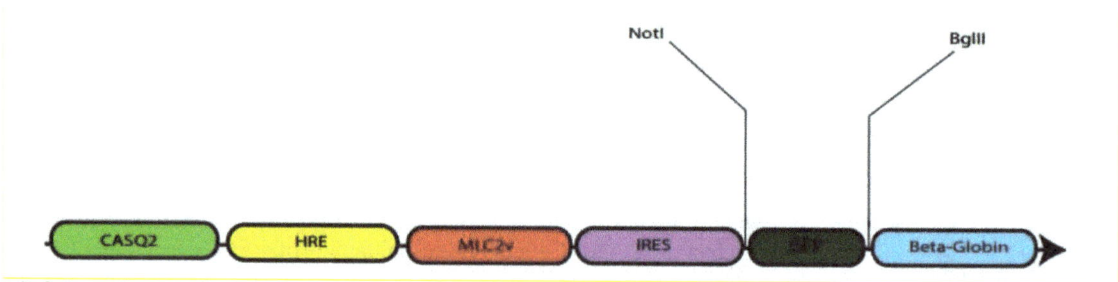

Figure 2. Schematic view of eGFP cloning into the cassette. eGFP was cloned into the cassette by *NotI* and *BglII* restriction enzymes.

Bacterial strains and plasmid preparation

Two strains of *Escherichia Coli* (E. *coli*) were used including DH5α and DH10β (Top10, Invitrogen, Thermo Fisher Scientific, USA). The plasmid was transformed into cells using the calcium chloride ($CaCl_2$) method.[16] *E. coli* bearing the desired plasmid was cultured in lysogeny broth (LB) media for 16 hrs at 37 °C in a shaker incubator. Cells with a density of 3-4×10⁹ cells/ml with OD_{600}=3 were harvested and DNA was extracted by plasmid DNA extraction kit (Qiagen, Midiprep Plasmid DNA Extraction Kit).

Cell Culture

The mouse myoblast cell line C2C12 (CRL-1772) and the mouse mammary gland cell line 4T1 (CRL-2539) was purchased from American Type Culture Collection (ATCC, Rockville, MD, USA). C2C12 cells were cultured in high glucose Dulbecco's Modified Eagle's Medium (DMEM) with 10% fetal bovine serum (FBS, Invitrogen, USA) and 0.584 g/L L-glutamine (Sigma-Aldrich, USA) in 37°C incubator and humidified 5% CO_2 and 95% air.[17] 4T1 cells, a 6-thioguanine resistant cell line,[18] were cultured in RPMI-1640 (Sigma-

Aldrich, USA) and 10% FBS (Invitrogen Gibco) in 37°C incubator and humidified atmosphere with 5% CO_2 and 95% air. Cell lines were passaged after 80% confluence.

The induction of hypoxic condition

To create hypoxia, C2C12 and 4T1 cell lines were incubated for 90 min in a hypoxic condition, containing 94% N_2, 4% CO_2 and 1% O_2, and hanks buffer. As a normoxia control "twin" cells were kept in a normoxic incubator.

Plasmid Transient Transfection

For achieving transient transfection, Gene Pulser XcellTM electroporation system (Bio-Rad, USA) was used. Following 60% confluence, media was removed and cells were harvested using 0.25% Trypsin-EDTA solution. Approximately 4-5 $\times 10^6$ cells were harvested by adding 3 ml complete media and then centrifuged for 5 min at 1000g and 4°C.[19] Thereafter, cells were re-suspended in 400μl opti-MEM (buffer O).[20] Then, 10μg of *supercoiled* DNA was overlaid to the cell suspension and mixed in wells. The cuvette was placed on ice for 5 min. Then, cells were transfected with the optimized exponential protocol (one shock for 18 seconds, at a voltage 120).

Fluorescence microscopy

Slides were visualized with a Zeiss Axioplan using 485 band pass filters set to view eGFP. All images were analyzed with AxioCam digital camera and Zeiss proprietary software (Axiovision Ver. 3.0.6.0). Images were manipulated in Adobe Photoshop 5.5.

Flow cytometry

eGFP expression was detected 48 hrs after transfection. Myocyte cells were harvested by trypsin/EDTA. Cells were centrifuged at 1000g for 10 min at 4°C. The cells were then washed three times with 500 μl of PBS. Fluorescence-activated cell sorting (FACS) caliber-micro flow cytometer (Becton Dickinson, NJ, USA) was used to analyze eGFP expression. GFP was excited by an argon laser and fluorescence's at 485/520 nm band pass filter in the FL1 channel. All raw data were analyzed using FlowJo software version 7.6.1.

Western Blotting

Cells in the both hypoxia and normoxia groups were collected from the wells and their protein contents were detected using an extraction Kit (Santa Cruz, USA) following the manufacturer's protocol. Total protein concentration was measured using a Nanodrop (Thermo-Scientific, USA). Samples were prepared for western blotting by adding loading buffer to each sample. Proteins were electrophoresed on 12% SDS-polyacrylamide gel and transferred to PVDF membranes. The membranes were blocked by incubating with 0.3 g bovine serum albumin in 10 ml of washing buffer at 4°C overnight. Membranes were then washed three times with PBS for 10 min. Then, the membranes were incubated with anti-HIF-1α antibody (dilution: 1:500; Santa-Cruz) for 4 hrs at 4°C. The membranes were then washed three times for 10 min each and incubated with the secondary antibody for 2 hrs. Roche ECL kit and semi-dry X-ray were used for imaging of immunoreactive protein bands.

Results

eGFP Cloning confirmation with HindIII digestion

To confirm eGFP cloning, the expression cassette was digested by *HindIII* and positive colony was determined by three sharp plasmid DNA band, including 3000, 2000 and 1500 bps on gel electrophoresis. Meanwhile, empty expression cassette was digested into two bands on 2500 and 1500 bps (Figure 3A and B).

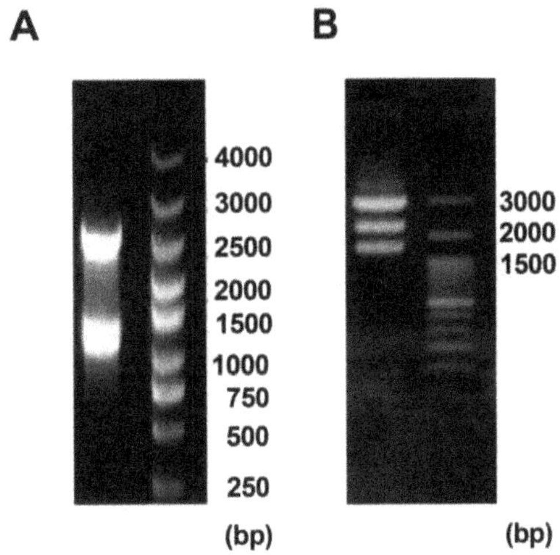

Figure 3. A; Confirmation of eGFP cloning into the cassette. Expression cassette was linearized by *HindIII* two sharp plasmid DNA band on 2500 and 1500 bps (Ladder 4000bps). B; Confirmation of eGFP cloning into the cassette by *HindIII* digestion three sharp plasmid DNA band on 3000, 2000 and 1500bps (Ladder 3000bps).

Exploration of the CASQ2 enhancer and cardiac tissue specific promoter

Calsequestrin 2 (CASQ2) as a cardiac specific enhancer plus myosin light chain-2 (MLC_{2v}) cardiac specific promoter provided tissue specificity. Thanks to highly cardiac specific sequence expression, eGFP was detected in myoblast C2C12 cell line, but not in 4T1 'twin' cell.

Exploring of HRE

In this study, 35 putative sites, including 9 ARNT, HIF-1, and 26 sp1 from EPO, VEGF-A, and phosphoglycerate kinase 1 (PGK-1) promoters were driven (Figure 4A and B, Table 1). HRE sequence was analyzed for insulator boundary elements to prevent enhancer and promoter interaction (Table 2). The elements provided hypoxia inducible expression. eGFP was detected under hypoxia and was not expressed under normoxia condition.

Hypoxia induction in C2C12 and 4T1 cell lines

HIF-1α at transcriptional and translational levels was stabilized under hypoxic condition. Then, we detected HIF-1α protein in hypoxic condition. Notably, we could not detect any HIF-1α protein in normoxia (Figure 5C).

Table 1. 35 Putative sites that is existing on Hypoxia Responses Elements (HRE) including 9 ARNT and 26 sp1.

The JASPAR database							
35 putative sites were predicted with these settings (80%) in sequence named 1							
Model ID	**Model name**	**Score**	**Relative score**	**Start**	**End**	**Strand**	**predicted site sequence**
MA0079.2	SP1	6.736	0.800936630165687	27	36	1	CCCCGGCGAC
MA0079.3	SP1	1.668	0.802126030842755	38	48	1	CTTCCTGCTCC
MA0079.3	SP1	14.558	0.964296987823859	44	54	1	GCTCCGCCCCT
MA0079.2	SP1	9.501	0.870571327605649	45	54	1	CTCCGCCCCT
MA0079.1	SP1	6.122	0.800408014237765	46	55	-1	TAGGGGCGGA
MA0259.1	ARNT::HIF1A	8.788	0.928072894030867	81	88	1	CGGCGTGC
MA0259.1	ARNT::HIF1A	9.817	0.958770479367351	90	97	1	GGACGTGA
MA0259.1	ARNT::HIF1A	10.396	0.976043464702457	110	117	-1	AGACGTGC
MA0259.1	ARNT::HIF1A	9.025	0.935143183364926	145	152	1	ATACGTGG
MA0259.1	ARNT::HIF1A	10.321	0.973806031368894	174	181	1	CTACGTGC
MA0079.1	SP1	7.476	0.847637728498468	188	197	-1	CAGGCTGTGT
MA0079.2	SP1	6.736	0.800936630165687	212	221	1	CCCCGGCGAC
MA0079.3	SP1	1.668	0.802126030842755	223	233	1	CTTCCTGCTCC
MA0079.3	SP1	14.558	0.964296987823859	229	239	1	GCTCCGCCCCT
MA0079.2	SP1	9.501	0.870571327605649	230	239	1	CTCCGCCCCT
MA0079.1	SP1	6.122	0.800408014237765	231	240	-1	TAGGGGCGGA
MA0259.1	ARNT::HIF1A	6.391	0.856564524690194	266	273	1	GAGCGTGT
MA0259.1	ARNT::HIF1A	4.936	0.813158318019073	281	288	-1	CTACGGGC
MA0259.1	ARNT::HIF1A	8.854	0.930041835364402	306	313	-1	AAACGTGC
MA0259.1	ARNT::HIF1A	8.575	0.921718583363548	316	323	1	CCGCGTGC
MA0079.1	SP1	6.765	0.822836896268513	344	353	1	CAGGGGCGGT
MA0079.2	SP1	7.611	0.822972926823903	345	354	-1	CACCGCCCCT
MA0079.3	SP1	10.560	0.913997570755554	345	355	-1	GCACCGCCCCT
MA0079.1	SP1	7.289	0.841114865450646	346	355	1	GGGGCGGTGC
MA0079.3	SP1	3.163	0.820934842377801	350	360	-1	CTCCCGCACCG
MA0079.2	SP1	13.214	0.964080778453597	357	366	-1	CCCCGCCTCC
MA0079.3	SP1	13.420	0.949979644996513	357	367	-1	ACCCCGCCTCC
MA0079.1	SP1	11.046	0.972165113956893	358	367	1	GAGGCGGGGT
MA0079.3	SP1	3.129	0.820507083453258	362	372	-1	CCCACACCCCG
MA0079.2	SP1	8.685	0.850020906950673	364	373	-1	CCCCACACCC
MA0079.3	SP1	7.096	0.870416485031539	364	374	-1	GCCCCACACCC
MA0079.2	SP1	7.202	0.812672532157377	368	377	-1	CCCGCCCCAC
MA0079.2	SP1	8.757	0.851834179361406	369	378	-1	TCCCGCCCCA
MA0079.3	SP1	10.509	0.913355932368739	369	379	-1	ATCCCGCCCCA
MA0079.1	SP1	9.870	0.931144328158824	370	379	1	GGGGCGGGAT

Table 2. Insulator sequences have been located on HRE sequence.

Motif PWM	Motif Sequence	Input Sequence Name	Motif Start Location	Motif Length	Motif Orientation	Score
REN_20	CCTACGGGCACAGGGGACAC	1	87	20	+	-12.4488
MIT_LM2	GCGTCGCCGGGGGGCCCAC	1	153	19	+	-13.4637
MIT_LM2	GCGTCGCCGGGGGGCCCAC	1	338	19	+	-13.4637
MIT_LM7	GAGACAGCACGTAGGGCAAG	1	189	20	+	-7.41144
MIT_LM23	GAGACAGCACGTAGGGCAAG	1	189	20	+	-5.62159

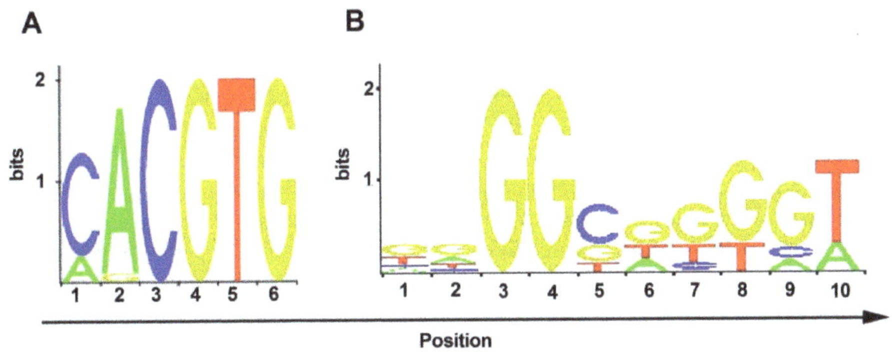

Figure 4. A; ARNT consensus sequence has been repeated 9 times in HRE. B; sp1 consensus sequence has been repeated 26 times in HRE

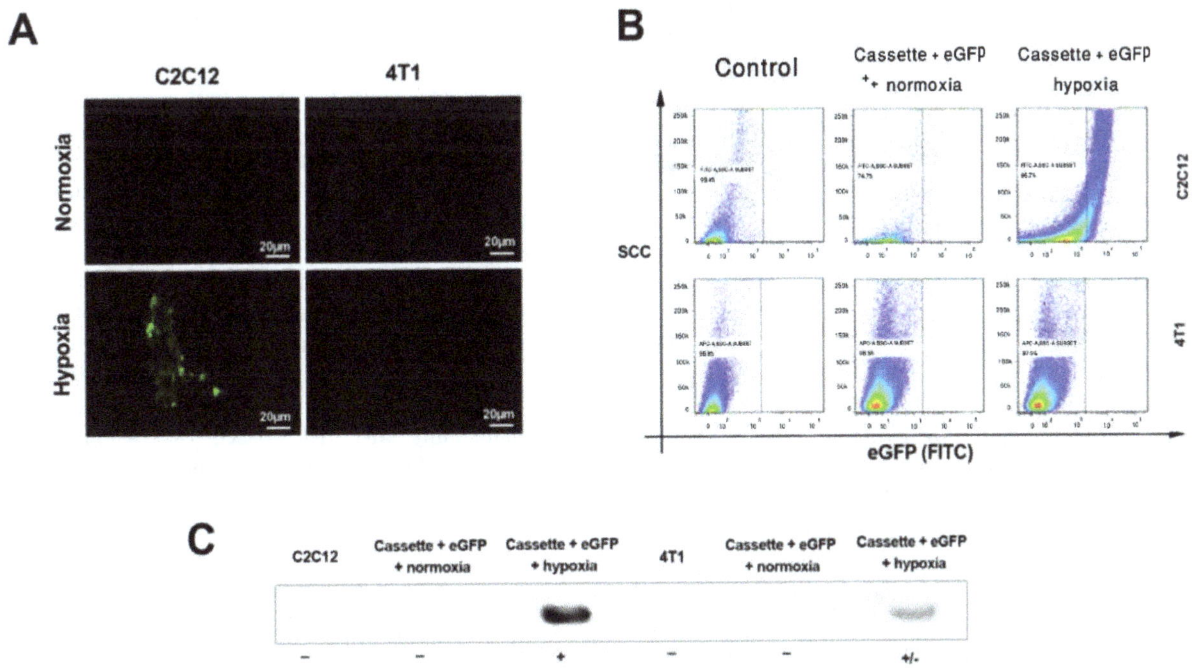

Figure 5. A; The results of immunofluorescence microscopy 48 hrs post transfection presented the specific expression of eGFP in the hypoxic condition at C2C12 myoblast cell line. eGFP was not detected in 4T1 cells in both hypoxic and normoxic condition. B; Flow cytometry results indicate the expression of eGFP under hypoxic condition in C2C12 cell line. C; Confirmation of hypoxia induction in both C2C12 and 4T1 cell lines by western blotting.

Expression cassette optimization

After subsequent transfection (48 h and 72 h), HREs exhibited the most intense fluorescence 48 hrs after transient transfection only in the hypoxic condition. Both cell lines were incubated under normoxic and hypoxic conditions to determine the function of HREs, including

HIF-1α and sp1 transcription factor binding site. The expression vector generated a sharp eGFP expression, which was detected by immunofluorescence microscope 48 hrs after transfection in the C2C12 cell line under hypoxic conditions. On the other hand, No significant eGFP was detected in 4T1 cells. eGFP was expressed in C2C12 cell line but not 4T1 under hypoxic (O_2<1%) condition. Moreover, we cannot detect any significant eGFP signals in C2C12 under normoxia. Flow cytometry results showed that myoblast cells expressed eGFP in hypoxia. However, eGFP was not express in 4T1 cells in both hypoxia and normoxia. Overall, experiments demonstrated that our designed cassette was expressed and, hence, functioned appropriately (Figure 5A and B).

eGFP measured 72h after transient transfection

After confirmation of hypoxia inducible and tissue specific expressions in expression cassette, the green fluorescence signals were analyzed 72 h and 96 h after transient transfection. eGFP signals were detected after 72h of transient transfection by the immune fluorescence microscopy at 520 band pass filter. However, we could not detect eGFP signals after 96 h after transfection (Figure 6).

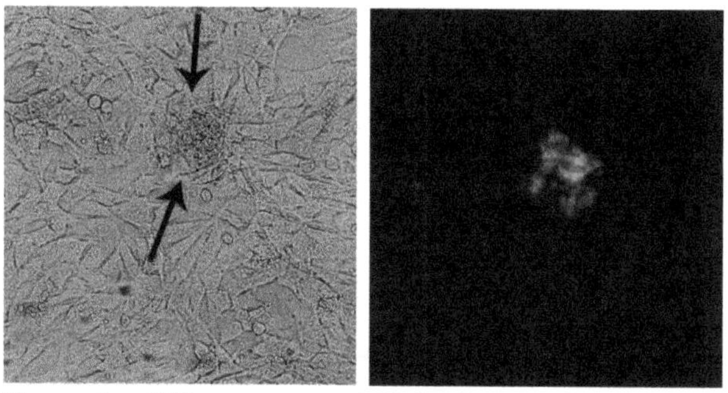

Figure 6. eGFP measurement 72 h after transfection. Arrow indicated the eGFP expression in C2C12.

Discussion

The results obtained through the experiments support some of our hypotheses. The current study explored the application of bioinformatics to improve the efficiency of cardiac gene therapy. Based on *in silico* analysis, we chose a cardiac specific *cis*-regulatory conserved motif that belonged to *calsequestrin 2 (CASQ2)* gene. The corresponding gene is specifically expressed in the heart. Tissue-specific *cis*-regulatory elements and correlated transcription factors, including myogenic regulatory factors (MRFs) like myogenic differentiation 1 (MYOD1), myogenic factor 5 (MYF5), myogenin and myogenin regulator factor 4 (MRF4), myogenic factor 6 (MYF6) interact with other transcription factors, particularly T box protein 2 (TBX2) and NK2 homeobox 5 (Nkx2.5).,[21-24] which play a pivotal role in the correct differentiation and progressive formation of cardiac muscle (Table 3). This summary helps us to understand the role of specific *cis*-regulatory elements in designing tissue-specific expression cassettes. Both CASQ2 and MLC_{2v} have a specific transcription factor binding site (TFBSs), which is efficient for cardiac-specific transgene expression.

Rincon *et al.*, [25] previously showed that *CASQ2* had a strong specificity for cardiac muscle. They made a construct consisting of *CASQ2* and myosin heavy chain α (MHCα) as a cardiac specific promoter. In this study, we used MLC_{2v} because of its cardiac-specific regulatory elements (Table 4). For inducible expression under hypoxic conditions, we used HREs derived from phosphoglycerate kinase (PGK1), VEGF-165, and EPO promoter. However, it was shown that HRE was a conserved sequence itself, but the most noted HRE sequence was derived from the EPO promoter.[26] To make copies of inducible elements obtained from one promoter, overlap PCR must be performed. For easier construct production of the desired elements, we used promoter and 5′UTRs of three different genes.[27,28]

HIF-1α belongs to a family of transcription factor with dimeric helices, containing basic amino acid residues that simplify DNA binding. bHLH proteins usually bind to a consensus sequence, well-known as HREs. Additionally, Sp1 is a zinc finger transcription factor that binds to GC-rich motifs of some promoters.[29,30] Sp1 binding sites are located near the HRE regions on the promoter. More studies have shown that sp1 protein becomes overexpressed under hypoxic conditions.[31] on the other side, hypoxic conditions have dual translation models known as cap-dependent and cap-independent (IRES) mechanisms. Notably, hypoxia has a strong restrictive effect on cap-dependent mRNA translation.[32] However, cellular IRES has a significant role in adaptation to hypoxic stress but is not increased at translational level, possibly due to inhibition of protein synthesis in order to conserve energy. IRESs are natural translational enhancers and, hence, mediate internal initiation of translation when present between desired genes.

In clinical assays, bicistronic IRES-based expression vectors have fewer side effects than monocistronic based expression vectors. When we designed a vector for hypoxia-inducible expression, strong viral IRESs were used for efficient cap-independent gene expression. Fundamentally, the IRES-based expression vector is efficient for *in vitro* and *in vivo* gene expression under hypoxic conditions.[33] Encephalomyocarditis virus (EMCV) is on-route into clinical studies and will hopefully be beneficial for patients. Our research, however, focused on *in vitro* studies. It is essential to study this cassette *in vivo* to evaluate all hypoxia-specific elements, such as enhancers (sp1, ARNT, and IRES) in a heterogenic population of myoblast and adult myocytes. However, we demonstrated that these elements were efficient for gene expression on hypoxic myoblasts in an *in vitro* model.

Conclusion

In conclusion, combination of the cardiac/muscle specific cis-regulatory elements, *CASQ2*, and myosin light chain-2 (MLC_{2v}) have a significant specificity for myocytes. Both *CASQ2* and MLC_{2v} have a specific TFBS, which is efficient for cardiac-specific transgene expression. Sp1 binding sites are located near the HRE regions on the promoter. Therefore, Sp1 and HIF-1α have binding sites to a far distance of HREs derived from three promoters. Therefore, there is no longer need to overlap PCR process for one repeated sequence just in one promoter. This expression cassette well-designed for cardiac specific hypoxia inducible gene expression.

Table 3. Cardiac specific transcription binding sites located on the CASQ2 enhancer.

Model ID	Model name	Score	Relative score	Start	End	Strand	Predicted site sequence
MA0037.2	GATA3	3.279	0.820594050245556	7	14	1	AGAAAAAC
MA0052.2	MEF2A	5.498	0.801872773397612	51	65	1	TACCTTACATAGCTC
MA0052.2	MEF2A	8.618	0.843873743315264	90	104	-1	TCCTAAAAATGGAGT
MA0083.2	SRF	8.230	0.817813133982383	90	107	-1	GCATCCTAAAAATGGAGT
MA0499.1	Myod1	5.403	0.859668968902211	105	117	1	TGCAGTTGTTTCA
MA0052.2	MEF2A	17.095	0.957989840107549	118	132	1	GGCTAAAAATAAATC
MA0063.1	Nkx2-5	5.189	0.833795488710155	136	142	-1	TTCATTG
MA0035.3	Gata1	2.402	0.800738582375976	151	161	-1	GTCGTATCTAA
MA0037.2	GATA3	6.588	0.872659931082488	153	160	1	AGATACGA
MA0482.1	Gata4	2.124	0.802327146192479	176	186	-1	CTGTATCAGCG
MA0499.1	Myod1	0.838	0.800984257597511	191	203	-1	TTCACCAGTCGGA
MA0482.1	Gata4	2.114	0.802183373083414	202	212	-1	TCTTCCCTCTT
MA0482.1	Gata4	6.727	0.868505908295031	223	233	-1	TCTTGTCTTTT
MA0036.2	GATA2	7.206	0.849841616420247	224	237	-1	ACATTCTTGTCTTT
MA0035.3	Gata1	6.525	0.857230665045272	224	234	-1	TTCTTGTCTTT
MA0037.2	GATA3	6.588	0.872659931082488	226	233	1	AGACAAGA
MA0482.1	Gata4	6.776	0.869210396529448	244	254	-1	CCTTATTTCAT
MA0036.2	GATA2	5.069	0.820706175169384	245	258	-1	GCCTCCTTATTTCA
MA0035.3	Gata1	5.099	0.837692049986718	245	255	-1	TCCTTATTTCA
MA0037.2	GATA3	5.281	0.852094773556387	247	254	1	AAATAAGG
MA0482.1	Gata4	5.484	0.850634910838269	271	281	-1	CTTTCTCTTCT
MA0035.3	Gata1	2.802	0.806219259811756	272	282	-1	TCTTTCTCTTC
MA0037.2	GATA3	3.921	0.830695680797781	274	281	1	AGAGAAAG

Table 4. Specific transcription factor and their binding sites are Myosin Light Chain 2 (MLC2).

Entrez_ID	Symbol	Alias	GO_P	GO_C
4250	SCGB2A2	MGB1 UGB2	na	na
94234	FOXQ1	HFH1	transcription; regulation of transcription, DNA dependent; hair follicle morphogenesis	nucleus
6927	TCF1	HNF1 HNF1A LFB1 MODY3	Bone resorption; positive regulation of transcription from RNA polymerase II promoter	nucleus; transcription factor complex
6722	SRF	MCM1	Heart looping; transcription; signal transduction; multicellular organismal development; Heart development; positive regulation of transcription from RNA polymerase II promoter; muscle maintenance	nucleus
3170	FOXA2	HNF3B MGC19807 TCF3B	transcription; regulation of transcription, DNA dependent; lung development; epithelial cell differentiation; positive regulation of transcription from RNA polymerase II promoter; branching morphogenesis of a tube	nucleus
3169	FOXA1	HNF3A MGC33105 TCF3A	transcription; regulation of transcription, DNA dependent; lung development; epithelial cell differentiation; hormone metabolic process; glucose homeostasis; positive regulation of transcription from RNA polymerase II promoter; branching morphogenesis of a tube	nucleus
4763	NF1	DKFZp686J1293 NFNS VRNF WSS	cell cycle; Ras protein signal transduction; negative regulation of cell proliferation; regulation of glial cell differentiation; negative regulation of progression through cell cycle; regulation of small GTPase mediated signal transduction	intracellular; cytoplasm

Acknowledgments
This work was a part of Ph.D. thesis and supported by the Research Council, Tabriz University of Medical Sciences. The authors thank the personnel of Immunology Research Center, Department of Pharmaceutical biotechnology for their kind guidance.

Conflict of Interest
The authors declare "no" conflict of interest.

Abbreviations
HREs: hypoxia response elements, **HIF-1α:** hypoxia inducible factor-1 alpha, **VEGF-A:** vascular endothelial growth factor-A, **PGK-1:** phosphoglycerate kinase 1, **MLC$_{2v}$:** myosin light chain, **EPO:** erythropoietin, **ARNT:** aryl hydrocarbon receptor nuclear translocator, **eGFP:** enhanced green fluorescent protein, **CASQ2:** calsequestrin 2, **bHLH:** basic helix-loop-helix , **PAS:** PER-ARNT-SIM, **EMCV:** encephalomyocarditis virus, **UTR:** untranslated region, **IRES:** internal ribosome entry site, **MRFs:** myogenic regulatory factors, **MYOD1:** myogenic differentiation 1, **MYF5:** myogenic factor 5, **MYF6:** myogenic factor 6, **MHC-α:** myosin heavy chain- alpha, **TBX2:** T box protein 2, **NKX2-5:** NK2 homeobox 5.

References
1. Wang GL, Jiang BH, Rue EA, Semenza GL. Hypoxia-inducible factor 1 is a basic-helix-loop-helix-PAS heterodimer regulated by cellular O2 tension. *Proc Natl Acad Sci* 1995;92(12):5510-4.
2. Manalo DJ, Rowan A, Lavoie T, Natarajan L, Kelly BD, Ye SQ, et al. Transcriptional regulation of vascular endothelial cell responses to hypoxia by HIF-1. *Blood* 2005;105(2):659-69. doi: 10.1182/blood-2004-07-2958

3. Semenza GL, Agani F, Booth G, Forsythe J, Iyer N, Jiang BH, et al. Structural and functional analysis of hypoxia-inducible factor 1. *Kidney Int* 1997;51(2):553-5.
4. Hon WC, Wilson MI, Harlos K, Claridge TD, Schofield CJ, Pugh CW, et al. Structural basis for the recognition of hydroxyproline in HIF-1 alpha by pVHL. *Nature* 2002;417(6892):975-8. doi: 10.1038/nature00767
5. Semenza GL. Hypoxia-inducible factor 1 and cardiovascular disease. *Annu Rev Physiol* 2014;76:39-56. doi: 10.1146/annurev-physiol-021113-170322
6. Semenza GL. Oxygen sensing, hypoxia-inducible factors, and disease pathophysiology. *Annu Rev Pathol* 2014;9:47-71. doi: 10.1146/annurev-pathol-012513-104720
7. GBD 2013 Mortality and Causes of Death Collaborators. Global, regional, and national age-sex specific all-cause and cause-specific mortality for 240 causes of death, 1990-2013: A systematic analysis for the Global Burden Of Disease Study 2013. *Lancet* 2015;385(9963):117-71. doi: 10.1016/S0140-6736(14)61682-2
8. Su H, Joho S, Huang Y, Barcena A, Arakawa-Hoyt J, Grossman W, et al. Adeno-associated viral vector delivers cardiac-specific and hypoxia-inducible VEGF expression in ischemic mouse hearts. *Proc Natl Acad Sci U S A* 2004;101(46):16280-5. doi: 10.1073/pnas.0407449101
9. Matkar PN, Leong-Poi H, Singh KK. Cardiac gene therapy: Are we there yet? *Gene Ther* 2016;23(8-9):635-48. doi: 10.1038/gt.2016.43
10. Warlich E, Kuehle J, Cantz T, Brugman MH, Maetzig T, Galla M, et al. Lentiviral vector design and imaging approaches to visualize the early stages of cellular reprogramming. *Mol Ther* 2011;19(4):782-9. doi: 10.1038/mt.2010.314
11. Ran FA, Hsu PD, Wright J, Agarwala V, Scott DA, Zhang F. Genome engineering using the CRISPR-Cas9 system. *Nat Protoc* 2013;8(11):2281-308. doi: 10.1038/nprot.2013.143
12. Hockemeyer D, Wang H, Kiani S, Lai CS, Gao Q, Cassady JP, et al. Genetic engineering of human pluripotent cells using TALE nucleases. *Nat Biotechnol* 2011;29(8):731-4. doi: 10.1038/nbt.1927
13. Lim WA. Designing customized cell signalling circuits. *Nat Rev Mol Cell Biol* 2010;11(6):393-403. doi: 10.1038/nrm2904
14. Reyes-Juarez JL, Juarez-Rubi R, Rodriguez G, Zarain-Herzberg A. Transcriptional analysis of the human cardiac calsequestrin gene in cardiac and skeletal myocytes. *J Biol Chem* 2007;282(49):35554-63. doi: 10.1074/jbc.M707788200
15. Razi Soofiyani S, Baradaran B, Lotfipour F, Kazemi T, Mohammadnejad L. Gene therapy, early promises, subsequent problems, and recent breakthroughs. *Adv Pharm Bull* 2013;3(2):249-55. doi: 10.5681/apb.2013.041
16. Li X, Sui X, Zhang Y, Sun Y, Zhao Y, Zhai Y, et al. An improved calcium chloride method preparation and transformation of competent cells. *Afr J Biotechnol* 2010;9(50):8549-54.
17. Yaffe D, Saxel O. Serial passaging and differentiation of myogenic cells isolated from dystrophic mouse muscle. *Nature* 1977;270(5639):725-7. doi: 10.1038/270725a0
18. Aslakson CJ, Miller FR. Selective events in the metastatic process defined by analysis of the sequential dissemination of subpopulations of a mouse mammary tumor. *Cancer Res* 1992;52(6):1399-405.
19. Chen CW, Wu SY, Hu GM. Single Differentiated Neurons from Pluripotent Embryonic Stem Cells: Motor Protein Modeling and Neurodegenerative Disease. In: Tseng FG, Santra TS, editor. Essentials of Single-Cell Analysis. 1st ed. Springer-Verlag Berlin Heidelberg; 2016. PP. 383-414.
20. Flanagan M, Gimble JM, Yu G, Wu X, Xia X, Hu J, et al. Competitive electroporation formulation for cell therapy. *Cancer Gene Ther* 2011;18(8):579-86. doi: 10.1038/cgt.2011.27
21. Mansoori B, Sandoghchian Shotorbani S, Baradaran B. RNA interference and its role in cancer therapy. *Adv Pharm Bull* 2014;4(4):313-21. doi: 10.5681/apb.2014.046
22. Rindt H, Knotts S, Robbins J. Segregation of cardiac and skeletal muscle-specific regulatory elements of the beta-myosin heavy chain gene. *Proc Natl Acad Sci U S A* 1995;92(5):1540-4. doi: 10.1073/pnas.92.5.1540
23. Sheikh F, Lyon RC, Chen J. Functions of myosin light chain-2 (MYL2) in cardiac muscle and disease. *Gene* 2015;569(1):14-20. doi: 10.1016/j.gene.2015.06.027
24. Habets PE, Moorman AF, Clout DE, van Roon MA, Lingbeek M, van Lohuizen M, et al. Cooperative action of Tbx2 and Nkx2.5 inhibits ANF expression in the atrioventricular canal: Implications for cardiac chamber formation. *Genes Dev* 2002;16(10):1234-46. doi: 10.1101/gad.222902
25. Rincon MY, Sarcar S, Danso-Abeam D, Keyaerts M, Matrai J, Samara-Kuko E, et al. Genome-wide computational analysis reveals cardiomyocyte-specific transcriptional Cis-regulatory motifs that enable efficient cardiac gene therapy. *Mol Ther* 2015;23(1):43-52. doi: 10.1038/mt.2014.178
26. Lindebro MC, Poellinger L, Whitelaw ML. Protein-protein interaction via PAS domains: role of the PAS domain in positive and negative regulation of the bHLH/PAS dioxin receptor-Arnt transcription factor complex. *EMBO J* 1995;14(14):3528-39.
27. Ghaderi S, Alidadiani N, Dilaver N, Heidari HR, Parvizi R, Rahbarghazi R, et al. Role of glycogen synthase kinase following myocardial infarction and ischemia-reperfusion. *Apoptosis* 2017;22(7):887-97. doi: 10.1007/s10495-017-1376-0

28. Wang FS, Wang CJ, Chen YJ, Chang PR, Huang YT, Sun YC, et al. Ras induction of superoxide activates ERK-dependent angiogenic transcription factor HIF-1alpha and VEGF-A expression in shock wave-stimulated osteoblasts. *J Biol Chem* 2004;279(11):10331-7. doi: 10.1074/jbc.M308013200
29. Lan S, Ostberg S, Punga T, Akusjarvi G. A suppressive effect of Sp1 recruitment to the first leader 5' splice site region on L4-22K-mediated activation of the adenovirus major late promoter. *Virus Res* 2015;210:133-40. doi: 10.1016/j.virusres.2015.07.026
30. ang G, Pei Y, Teng H, Cao Q, Wang R. Specificity protein-1 as a critical regulator of human cystathionine gamma-lyase in smooth muscle cells. *J Biol Chem* 2011;286(30):26450-60. doi: 10.1074/jbc.M111.266643
31. Tan NY, Khachigian LM. Sp1 phosphorylation and its regulation of gene transcription. *Mol Cell Biol* 2009;29(10):2483-8. doi: 10.1128/MCB.01828-08
32. Richter JD, Sonenberg N. Regulation of cap-dependent translation by eIF4E inhibitory proteins. *Nature* 2005;433(7025):477-80. doi: 10.1038/nature03205
33. Fernandez-Chamorro J, Lozano G, Garcia-Martin JA, Ramajo J, Dotu I, Clote P, et al. Designing synthetic RNAs to determine the relevance of structural motifs in picornavirus IRES elements. *Sci Rep* 2016;6:24243. doi: 10.1038/srep24243

Enhanced *in Vitro* Anti-Tumor Activity of 5-Azacytidine by Entrapment into Solid Lipid Nanoparticles

Farhad Jahanfar[1,2], Akbar Hasani[2], Dariush Shanebandi[3], Mohammad Rahmati[2], Hamed Hamishehkar[4]*

[1] *Biotechnology Research Center and Student Research Committee, Tabriz University of Medical Sciences, Tabriz, Iran.*
[2] *Department of Biochemistry and Clinical Laboratories, Faculty of Medicine, Tabriz University of Medical Sciences, Tabriz, Iran.*
[3] *Immunology Research Center, Tabriz University of Medical Sciences, Tabriz, Iran.*
[4] *Drug Applied Research Center, Tabriz University of Medical Sciences, Tabriz, Iran.*

Article info

Keywords:
- 5-azacytidine
- Solid lipid nanoparticles
- SLN
- Cancer
- Cytotoxicity

Abstract

Purpose: In this study the effectiveness of encapsulating of 5-azacytidine into the lipid nanoparticles was investigated and *in vitro* effect of encapsulated 5-azacytidine studied on MCF-7 cell lines

Methods: 5-azacytidine -loaded solid lipid nanoparticles were produced by double emulsification (w/o/w) method by using stearic acid as lipid matrix, soy lecithin and poloxamer 407 as surfactant and co-surfactant respectively. Particle size, zeta potential, surface morphology, entrapment efficiency and kinetic of drug release were studied. *In vitro* effect of 5-azacytidine on MCF-7 cell line studied by MTT assay, DAPI staining, Rhodamine B relative uptake, and also Real time RT-PCR was performed for studying difference effect of free and encapsulated drug on expression of RARß2 gene.

Results: The formulation F5 with 55.84±0.46 % of entrapment efficiency shows zero order kinetic of drug release and selected for in vitro studies; the cytotoxicity of free drug and encapsulated drug in 48 h of incubation have significant difference. DAPI staining shows morphology of apoptotic nucleus in both free and encapsulated drug, Rhodamine B labeled SLNs show time dependency and accumulation of SLNs in cytoplasm. Real time qRT-PCR doesn't show any significant difference ($p>0.05$) in expression of RARß2 gene in both cells treated with free or encapsulated drug.

Conclusion: The results of the present study indicated that the entrapment of 5-azacytidine into SLNs enhanced its cytotoxicity performance and may pave a way for the future design of a desired dosage form for 5-azacytidine.

Introduction

5-azacytidine was first synthesized in 1963[1] as an effective anti-cancer agent for the treatment of leukemia.[2-4] In 2004, the FDA approved the application of 5-azacytidine in treating myelodysplastic syndrome as the first drug effective in epigenetic therapy by inhibiting DNA methyltransferase.[5] Furthermore, 5-azacytidine inhibits protein production by being incorporated into RNA and interrupting its performance.[6,7] Although a few investigations have illustrated the effectiveness of experiments,[8,9] most clinical trials of the effects of 5-azacytidine on solid tumors are disappointing.[10] Due to its short half-life, 5-azacytidine is unable to permeate solid tumors and remain long enough to affect cancer cells.[11] The primary reason for this is the deactivation of 5-azacytidine by chemical hydrolysis or enzymatic deamination which results in short plasma stability.[12,13] A second reason is the need of particular variably expressed nucleoside transporters for cellular uptake.[14] There are two main strategies to overcome these obstacles. The first is to change the drug structure by chemical reactions like esterification.[15] Although this strategy shows good results, the drug approving procedure for new drugs is time- and cost-consuming. The second strategy is to encapsulate 5-azacytidine in nanoparticles to protect it from enzymatic deamination. This concept also makes drug uptake independent of transporters by nanoparticle endocytosis into the targeted cells.[16] Nanoparticulate carriers are introduced for passive drug targeting to tumor tissues through the enhanced permeability and retention (EPR) effect.[17-19] EPR implies that nanoparticles tend to accumulate in tumor tissue much more than they do in normal tissue. However, these explored nanoparticulate delivery systems demonstrate their own disadvantages. Commonly reported drawbacks of colloidal carriers such as liposomes, nanosponges, microemulsions and nanoemulsions, polymeric nanoparticles, and nanocapsules are burst drug release, physical and chemical instability during storage,[20-23] difficulty in industrial fabrication, the presence of organic solvents applied in the production of these systems, some limitations in polymer toxicity[24,25] and many more too

***Corresponding author:** Hamed Hamishehkar, Email: Hamishehkarh@tbzmed.ac.ir numerous to mention. All of these disadvantages suggest that these colloidal drug delivery systems are not perfect.[24] Solid lipid nanoparticles (SLNs) were developed in the beginning of the 1990s as drug carriers[26] proposing the superiorities of emulsions, liposomes, and polymeric nanoparticles. The solid lipid matrix is able to protect encapsulated drugs from chemical instability and offer sustaining drug release patterns compared with nanoemulsions.[27,28] SLNs give stable nanosuspension for an extended period of time in comparison with liposomes.[29,30] Furthermore, the SLNs are made of physiologically well-tolerated and generally recognized as safe (GRAS) excipients which reduce the cytotoxicity, leading to their wide variety of applications including dermal, oral, pulmonary, and intravenous use compared with polymeric nanoparticles.[26,31] The greatest benefit of SLNs is the possibility of their industrial scale production.[32-34]

The present study aimed to formulate 5-azacytidine-loaded SLNs for the first time to a) overcome 5-azacytidine instability, and b) increase its anti-tumor performance. The stability of 5-azacytidine was studied via high performance liquid chromatography (HPLC). The cytotoxicity and uptake of the nanoparticulate system were investigated through MTT assay, DAPI staining, Rhodamine B labeling, and Real Time Quantitative Reverse Transcription PCR investigation on the expression of the retinoic acid receptor β2 (RARß2) gene of MCF-7 (human breast adenocarcinoma cell line).

Materials and Methods

Materials

MCF-7 cell line were purchased from National Cell Bank of Iran (NCBI, Tehran, Iran) 5-azacytidine, fetal bovine serum (FBS),RPMI-1640, DAPI powder, soy lecithin, Poloxamer® 407 and MTT powder were obtained from Sigma-Aldrich co. Rhodamine B, stearic acid purchased from Merck (Darmstadt, Germany). RNX-plus solution purchased from CinnaGene (CinnaGene, Tehran, Iran), cDNA synthetase kit and SYBR® Premix Ex Taq™II purchased from Takara (Takara, Japan). All other chemicals were of analytical grade. All solutions were prepared with deionized water.

Methods

Preparation of SLN

5-azacytidine (5mg) was dissolved in aqueous solution. Stearic acid and soy lecithin were melted together at 70°C. Stearic acid, a saturated monoacid triglyceride was selected as a negatively charged solid lipid and soy lecithin as a negatively charged low HLB surfactant to increase the chance of positively charged drug encapsulation. The aqueous phase (5 mL) was warmed up to 70°C and added to lipid phase under homogenization (DIAX 900, Heidolph, Germany) at 20000 rpm to form initial w/o emulsion. Then the external water phase and co-surfactant (1% Poloxamer) was added to the initial w/o emulsion under high shear homogenization to form w/o/w emulsion. SLN was finally prepared by cooling down the solution and conversion of emulsion to dispersion by lipid solidification. Since the lipid and surfactant amounts play the major role in size and drug loading capacity of SLNs,[34,35] various formulations were prepared according to change in Stearic acid and soy lecithin (Table 1) and evaluated in the points of size and drug entrapment efficiency. Blank SLN formulation was similarly prepared except that 5-azacytidine was omitted. To prepare fluorescent-labeled SLN, Rhodamine B was used in place of 5-azacytidine.

Table 1. Formulation details and characterization results of solid lipid nanoparticles. Data was presented as mean ± standard deviation (n=at least 3).

Code	Stearic acid (mg)	Soy lecithin (mg)	EE[a] (%)	LC[b] (%)	Size (nm)	PDI[c]	Zeta potential (mv)
F1	20	5	18.74±0.21	3.75±0.04	96±9.34	0.31±0.03	-18.2±0.39
F2	20	10	23.14±0.81	3.86±0.13	115±8.14	0.28±0.01	-18.7±0.72
F3	20	15	22.51±0.32	3.22±0.04	186±7.21	0.24±0.06	-17.8±0.23
F4	30	5	47.34±0.11	6.76±0.01	367±6.45	0.18±0.02	-16.3±0.21
F5	30	10	55.84±0.46	6.98±0.05	204±10.45	0.19±0.04	-18.4±0.34
F6	30	15	45.57±0.62	5.06±0.07	202±11.34	0.25±0.02	-16.2±0.43

[a] Encapsulation Efficiency
[b] Loading Capacity
[c] Polydispersity Index

Characterization of 5-azacytidine-loaded SLNs

Particles size, size distribution (polydipersity index (PDI)), and zeta potential value of formulations were measured by photon correlation spectroscopy (Nano ZS, Malvern Instruments, UK). For this determination SLN samples were diluted with phosphate buffer saline until appropriate concentration and analyzed in triplicate. Particles Morphology was investigated with scanning electron microscopy (SEM, VEGA TESCAN, Czech Republic). For this analysis, SLN formulations were diluted in de-ionized water and few drops of this diluted SLN suspension were mounted on a glass lamella, air-dried and gold coated under vacuum. The SEM experiment was carried out on the optimized formulation (F5).

The encapsulation efficiency percent (EE%) and loading capacity percent (LC%) were expressed as the percentage of entrapped 5-azacytidne to the added 5-azacytidne or to the used lipid, respectively. EE was measured by first separation of the un-entrapped 5-azacytidne by centrifugation method using of Amicon® Ultra-15 with molecular weight cutoff of 100 kDa (Millipore, Darmstadt, Germany) tube. The formulation was added to the upper chamber of the Amicon® tube and then the tube was centrifuged (Sigma 3K30, Darmstadt, Germany) at 5000 rpm for 5 min. The filtrated solution was analyzed by HPLC method under the following conditions: column 150×4.6 mm; ODS-3 5µm, room temperature, acetonitrile/water 40/60 as mobile phase, flow rate 1 ml/min, UV detection at 243 nm, and 20 µl injection volume.[36] The 5-azacytidine EE and LC values were calculated according to the following equations:

$$EE\ (\%) = \frac{W_{(\text{Initial 5-azacytidine})} - W_{(\text{Free 5-azacytidine})}}{W_{(\text{Initial 5-azacytidine})}} \times 100$$

$$LC\ (\%) = \frac{W(\text{Entrapped 5-azacytidine})}{W(\text{Total lipid})} \times 100$$

In-vitro release studies

Drug-loaded SLNs equal to 5 mg of 5-azacytidine was diluted in 5 ml of phosphate buffer (10 mM) pH 7.4, entered into dialysis bag (molecular cut-off of 12,000 Da; Sigma, Steinem, Germany) and immersed into 100 mL phosphate buffer pH 7.4 and 37±0.5°C under stirring. One milliliter of medium during the intervals 1, 2, 4, 6, 8, 12, 24 h was withdrawn and replaced with buffer. To analyze the release kinetics of 5-azacytidine from SLNs, the data of release were subjected to the following equations:

Zero order equation: $Q_t=K_0.t$ where Q_t is the percentage of drug released at time t and k_0 is the release rate constant; First order equation: $\ln(100- Qt)=\ln 100-k_1.t$ where k_1 is the release rate constant; Higuchi's equation: $Q_t=K_H.t^{1/2}$ where k_H is the Higuchi release rate constant; Hixson-Crowell: $(100- Qt)^{1/3}=100^{1/3}-k_{Hc}.t$ where k_{Hc} is the Hixson-Crowell rate constant. These samples were analyzed by HPLC method as described above.

Cell culture

the human MCF-7 (human breast adenocarcinoma cell line) were maintained in RPMI-1640 complete growth medium supplemented with 10% FBS, 1% glutamine (2 mM), 1% antibiotic-antimycotic mixture (10000 U/ml penicillin,10000mg/ml streptomycin) and bicarbonate sodium 2%. In a humidified incubator (Thermo Fisher Scientific) at 37°C under 5% CO_2 atmosphere. Cells were sub cultured every 2-4 days using Trypsin.

MTT Assay

To compare effect of encapsulated 5-azacytidine in SLNs with free form of drug and blank SLNs on viability of MCF-7 cell line, we performed MTT assay. Briefly, the MCF-7 cell was seeded in 96-well flat bottom plates. When the cells reached to 40-50% confluence, culture medium were replaced by fresh culture medium containing a range of sample concentration, after 24, 48 h of incubation in a humidified incubator (5% CO_2) at 37°C, the culture medium were removed carefully from each well, and wells were washed with 200 µl of phosphate buffer saline PBS. The 200 µl fresh culture medium containing 0.5 mg/ml MTT reagent was added to each well. After 4 h incubation at 37°C, cell culture media was replaced with 200 µl of DMSO and 25 µl of Sorenson buffer (0.1 M glycine, 0.1 M NaCl, pH 10.5). After 30 min of incubation at 37°C in shaking incubator, absorbance was measured at 570 nm using a spectrophotometric plate reader (stat fax®-2100, awareness technology). Cell viability was calculated as the percentage of absorbance in wells with the treated cells versus the control cells.

DAPI Staining Assay

For analyzing apoptosis in the MCF-7 cell line which is treated with free form of 5-azacytidin and encapsulated 5-azacytidin in SLNs, DAPI staining assay was performed. Briefly, MCF-7 and cell line were seeded in six-well culture plates (100000 cells/well) containing 12 mm sterile cover-slips which is treated with collagen I , after 24 h of incubation in humidified incubator (5% CO_2) at 37°C, culture medium were replaced with fresh culture medium containing a range of sample concentrations, and with DMSO as positive control for 48 h. then cells were fixed by 4% paraformaldehyde, and permeablized with 0.1% (w/v) Triton X-100 for 5 min,washed in PBS and stained with DAPI work solution and washed again with PBS. Fluorescence Images were obtained with Olympus BX50 microscope, selected wavelengths were 365–375 nm (DAPI, blue).

Rhodamine B uptake studies

Rhodamine B was used as a fluorescence probe to analyzing the cellular uptake of Rhodamine B loaded SLNs. After encapsulation of Rhodamine B in SLNs unencapsulated Rhodamine B was removed by centrifugal filter devices (Amicon® ultra, ultra cell-50k, Darmstadt, Germany). MCF-7 cell was seeded in six-well culture plates (100000 cells/well), which each well contain 12 mm sterile cover-slip that treated previously with collagen I. seeded cells were incubated in 37°C ,5% CO_2 at humidified incubator for overnight. Then cells were treated with 1 ml of Rhodamine B loaded SLNs and incubated for 2 h and after that period the culture medium was removed and each well washed with PBS, then cells were fixed by 4% paraformaldehyde, and permeablized with 0.1% (w/v) Triton X-100 for 5 min, washed in PBS and stained with DAPI work solution and washed again with PBS. Fluorescence Images were obtained with Olympus BX50 microscope. Selected wavelengths were 365–375 nm (DAPI, blue), 530–550 nm (Rhodamine B, red).

Real-time RT–PCR

For Real-time RT–PCR analysis, MCF-7 cells (1×10^6) were plated in 100 mm tissue culture dishes after plating for 24 h, cells were treated with 1µM of free 5-azacytidine and encapsulated 5-azacytidine in SLN for duration of 72 h, Total RNA was extracted from cultured cells with RNX Plus kit as described in the manufactory's manual. RNA concentration and purity were evaluated by agarose gel electrophoresis and determined by measurement of the absorbance at 260 nm and 280 nm with NanoDrop™ 1000 Spectrophotometer (Thermo Scientific). RNA samples were used as substrate for reverse transcription using a cDNA synthesis kit according to the manufactory's manual. The cDNA was diluted 1:10, and 2 µl were used for each reaction. Real-time PCR was performed with SYBR ® Premix Ex Taq™II kit in the Real-time Detection System (Rotor-Gene 6000, Germany). Results were normalized for expression of the housekeeping gene which is GAPDH. For Real-time PCR analysis, primers for qPCR were designed using primer 3.0 web based software with an optimal annealing temperature of 61°C.the sequences of primers for RARβ2 is (sense, 5-GACTGTATGGATGTTCTGTCAG-3; antisense, 5-ATTTGTCCTGGCAGACGAAGCA-3), for GAPGH is (sense, 5-ACTTTGGTATCGTGGAAGGACTC-3; antisense, 5-CAGGGATGATGTTCTGGAGAGC-3). Gene expression was normalized relative to GAPDH using Delta–Delta CT. Experiments were performed in triplicates.

Statistical Analysis

The experiments were repeated at least in triplicate and data was expressed as the mean ± standard deviation. Statistical analysis was performed using a one-way analysis of variance (one-way ANOVA) with multiple comparisons between deposition data using a Tukey honest significant difference test (SPSS, version 17, Chicago, IL, USA). A P value of <0.05 was considered significant.

Results and Discussion

SLN preparation

Particle size is one the most important characteristics of SLNs for successful passive targeting and cellular endocytosis.[37] Average particle sizes of 5-azacytidin-loaded SLNs in different formulations are shown in Table 1.

As can be seen, they ranged from 96 ± 9.3 to 367 ± 6.4 nm. It was claimed that the appropriate size range for the effective cytotoxic performance of nanoparticles is <200 nm.[16] Therefore, most formulations in this study were in the suitable size range. The PDI of SLNs was found to be in the range of 0.18 to 0.31 (Table 1). The narrow size distribution of the carriers guarantees uniform drug delivery to the target tissue. A PDI below 0.2 is considered as a uniform size distribution.[38] The PDI of formulations F4 and F5 were 0.18 and 0.19, respectively. The SEM image which supports the size data is shown in Figure 1.

Zeta potential is another key parameter for the colloidal stability of nanoparticles. It has been reported that zeta potential values ±30 mV are considered suitable and effective for the colloidal stability of nanosuspensions. The zeta potential of all formulations was almost in the same range (-16.2 to -18.7 mV) as shown in Table 1. Although the zeta potential of formulation were in the lower range, an appropriate size stability was found after 6 months (data not shown), probably because of the hindering effect of the polymeric co-surfactant (poloxamer) used in the external aqueous phase to stabilize nanoparticles.[39] 5-azacytidine is a hydrophilic material; therefore, it can be predicted that its effective encapsulation into lipid-based nanocarriers would be problematic. Hopefully, by using the double emulsion technique and an adequate amount of inner phase surfactant, the appropriate percent of drug entrapment can be achieved (Table 1). Furthermore, negative charge lipid (stearic acid) may be helpful in the appropriate encapsulation of a positively-charged drug. In this study, the percentages of EE and LC were 18.7 to 55.8 and 3.2 to 7.0, respectively. Because of the highest LC and zeta potential values, the almost lowest PDI value, and the appropriate size, the F5 formulation was selected as the optimized one used for in vitro cytotoxic investigations (MTT assay, Real time RT-PCR, Rhodamine B uptake and DAPI staining).

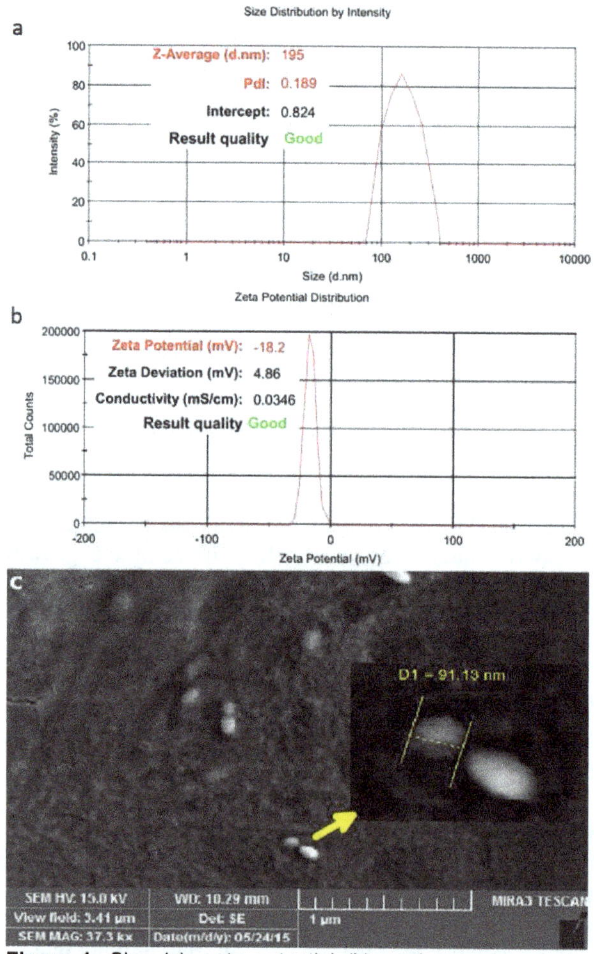

Figure 1. Size (a), zeta potential (b), and scanning electron microscopy images (c) of optimized 5-azacytidin-loaded solid lipid nanoparticles.

In vitro drug release study

The formulations prepared with high surfactant amounts (F3 and F5) presented faster drug release (Figure 2) than the others.

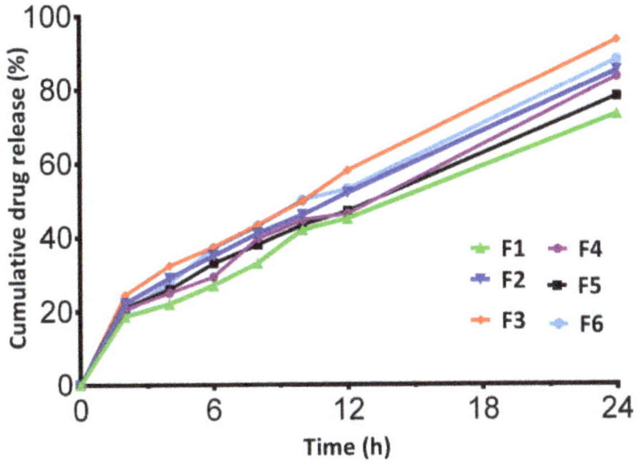

Figure 2. *In vitro* drug release profile for different formulations of 5-azacytidine-loaded solid lipid nanoparticles.

The presence of lipophilic surfactant in the lipid matrix structure might have enhanced water penetration into the matrix via emerged pores and caused drug leakage and release in higher values than the others. The SLNs fabricated with a higher lipid amount released drug in a slower pattern as well. All formulations released more than 80% of drug during 24 h, indicating potentially enough release of drug in targeted cancer tissue after formulation administration. Therefore, there was an initial 20% burst release, and the remaining 60% released during 24 h, which may be a suitable drug release pattern for efficient drug accumulation in cancer cells.[40] To define the kinetics of 5-azacytidne release from controlled release drug carriers, different mathematical models have been suggested. The zero order model defines drug delivery systems where the release of drug is not dependent on its concentration.[41] The formulators prefer to develop drug delivery systems which release drug in a zero order manner to achieve a steady release of drug.[42] The first order kinetic explains release from carriers where the release rate is concentration-dependent.[41] Drug release in the Higuchi model is directly related to a square root of time based on the Fickian diffusion.[43] The Hixson-Crowell cube root equation explains the changes of drug release by change in surface area and diameter of the particles with time and is mostly used in the case of drug carriers which dissolute or erode over time.[44] The *in vitro* drug release indicated that all formulations resulted in zero order drug release kinetics (Table 2).

Table 2. Kinetic parameters of 5-azacytidne release from the solid lipid nanoparticles

	Zero-order		First-order		Highuchi		Hixson-Crowell	
	K_0 ($\%h^{-1}$)	R^2	K_1 (h^{-1})	R^2	K_H ($\%h^{-1/2}$)	R^2	K_0 ($\%h^{-1}$)	R^2
F1	0.025	0.991	0.052	0.985	0.162	0.970	0.013	0.993
F2	0.028	0.999	0.075	0.963	0.180	0.974	0.018	0.984
F3	0.031	0.998	0.111	0.934	0.198	0.969	0.023	0.969
F4	0.029	0.992	0.072	0.954	0.182	0.955	0.017	0.975
F5	0.028	0.998	0.058	0.975	0.164	0.973	0.015	0.989
F6	0.030	0.990	0.086	0.964	0.195	0.987	0.020	0.987

MTT assay study

MTT assay has been widely used to measure cell viability. Figure 3 shows the percentage of MCF-7 cell survival after exposure to blank SLN and 5-azacytidine, either free or loaded in SLNs.

Encapsulated drug shows a higher cytotoxicity for MCF-7 in 48 hours of treatment than in 24 hours. This result may have been caused by different parameters such as drug release, drug degradation rate, and the doubling time of the MCF-7 cell line which is approximately 24-48 hours.[45] 5-azacytidine inhibits DNA methyltransferases[46] (the enzymes responsible for *de novo* methylation of the new synthesized DNA during the *S*-phase and the maintenance of methylation).[7] Therefore, prolonged exposure of cancer cells to this drug is essential for optimal efficacy. It has been reported that the elimination half-life of 5-azacytidine is about 4 hours (i.v. or s.c. administration).[47] Therefore, drug encapsulation in SLNs might increase its stability. This may explain the superiority of drug-loaded SLNs cytotoxicity performance to free drug in 48 h incubation.

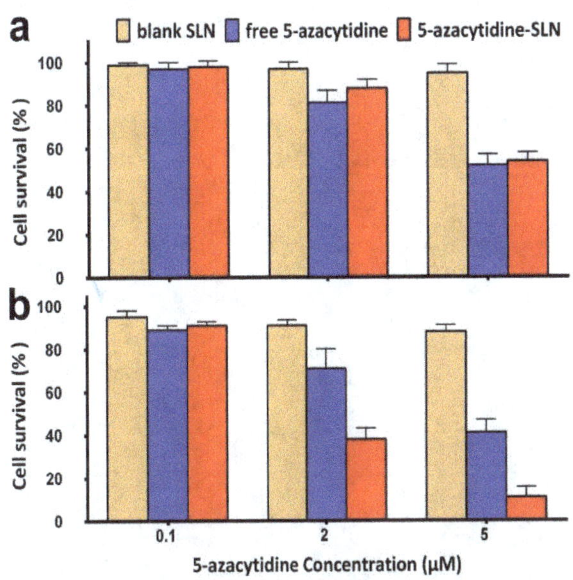

Figure 3. Dose dependent study of MCF-7 (breast cancer cell line) survival in exposure to free 5-azacytidine, encapsulated 5-azacytidin and blank solid lipid nanoparticles (SLN) in 24h (a) and 48h (b). Data is presented as mean ± standard deviation (n=6).

DAPI staining

To observe the different effects of free 5-azacytidine and loaded 5-azacytidine on the morphology of cell nuclei, DAPI staining was performed. DAPI was used for visualizing apoptotic cells for which nuclear DNA fragmentation and condensed chromosome were considered.[48] Figure 4 shows the images of untreated control cells and treated MCF-7 cells which were stained with DAPI after exposure to free 5-azacytidine and loaded 5-azacytidine in SLNs for about 48 hours. The morphological changes of the nuclear chromatin in both cells treated with free 5-azacytidine and encapsulated 5-azacytidine indicate programmed cell death (apoptosis).

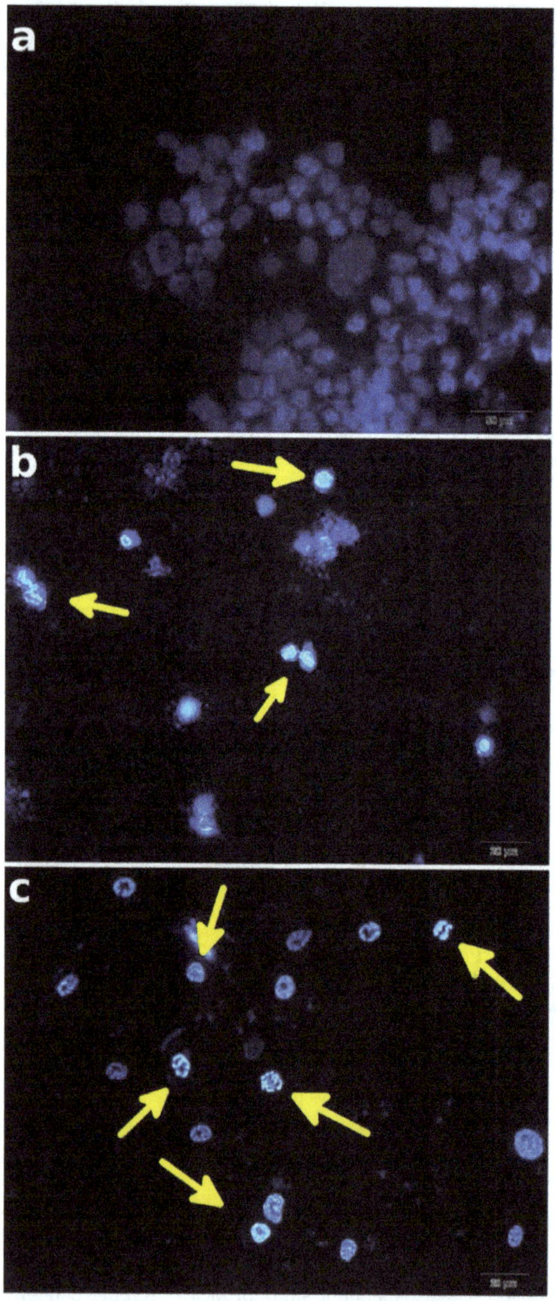

Figure 4. Fluorescent images of DAPI staining of untreated MCF-7 (a), and those treated with 5-azacytidine solution (5 μM) (b) and 5-azacytidine-loaded solid lipid nanoparticles in equivalent concentration (c).

Relative uptake of SLNs in MCF-7

To confirm the uptake of SLNs into MCF-7 cells, Rhodamine B-loaded SLNs were used to incubate cultured cell lines within 2 h and were analyzed by florescent microscope. Free form Rhodamine B and blank SLN were used as negative controls to eliminate any interference which is negligible fluorescence. As shown in Figure 5, Rhodamine B is red and the cell nucleus stained with DAPI is blue. After 2 h of incubation, a bright light appeared within the cells indicating that SLNs particles were internalized into the cells. The pictures of cells show a comparable difference among MCF-7 cells after 5 minutes and after 2 hours. The study of Rhodamine b-loaded blank SLNs clearly show the time-dependent increase in fluorescence intensity inside the MCF-7 which was caused by the uptake of Rhodamine B-loaded SLNs. SLNs accumulated in the cytoplasm after uptake by MCF-7 cells.

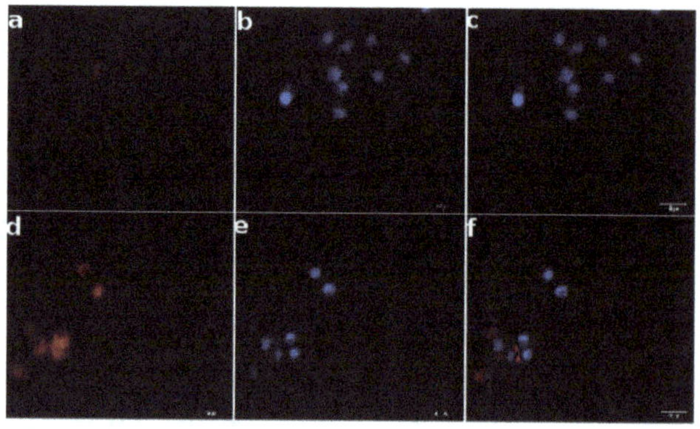

Figure 5. Fluorescence images of the cells incubated with the Rhodamine B labeled solid lipid nanoparticles (SLNs) for 5 min (a) and 2h (d) and after those visualized with DAPI (b and e). The merged Figures were used to show the cell localization of SLNs (c and f).

Real time RT–PCR

Epigenetic modification plays a crucial role on gene expression. Cancer cells use epigenetic modifications for silencing tumor suppressors. Breast cancer is greatly modified by epigenetic mechanisms, mostly the hypermethylation of CpG islands.[49] Aberrant methylation of the retinoic acid receptor β2 (RARβ2) promotor was reported in the MCF-7 cell line,[50] which is responsible for the low expression of the RARβ2 gene. In the current study, RARβ2 gene expression was measured after treatment with encapsulated 5-azacytidine and free 5-azacytidine with Real Time qRT-PCR. Figure 6 shows the expression of RARβ2 mRNA for treated cells with 1 μM free 5-azacytidine and encapsulated. The current study showed no significant difference ($p>0.05$) between free form and encapsulated 5-azacytidine. This result shows that the drug was still effective after the encapsulation procedure.

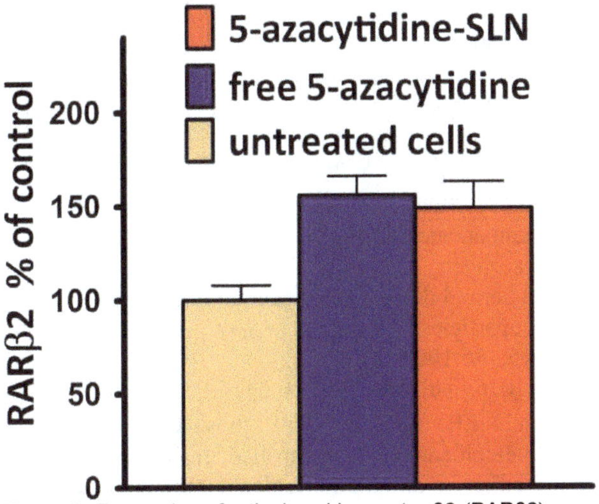

Figure 6. Expression of retinoic acid receptor β2 (RARβ2) gene after 3 days treatment of MCF-7 cells with 1 μM free 5-azacytidine and equivalent concentration of 5-azacytidineloaded solid lipid nanoparticles (SLN). Glyceraldehyde 3-phosphate dehydrogenase (GAPDH) was used as an internal control. Data were expressed as means ± standard deviation.

Conclusion

The developed SLN showed promising 5-azacytidine encapsulation probably due to the ion-pair interaction of the negatively charged lipid with the positively charged drug. *In vitro* cell cytotoxicity experiments proved the better performance of 5-azacytidine-loaded SLN than free 5-azacytidine, which may attributed to better endocytosis of nanoparticulate carriers and higher drug stability. Real Time qRT-PCR confirmed that 5-azacytidine remained stable during SLN preparation and encapsulation by almost the same performance in gene expression. The poor loading capacity, however, is a major disadvantage of SLN formulation. The results of this study pave the way for introducing an efficient formulation of 5-azacytidine for cancer therapy.

Acknowledgments

The authors would like to thank the drug applied research center, Tabriz University of Medical Sciences for financial support (93/310). This article is part of an MSc thesis (93/2-7/9) of clinical biochemistry submitted in Faculty of Medicine, Tabriz University of Medical Sciences.

Ethical Issues

Not applicable.

Conflict of Interest

The authors report no conflicts of interest.

References

1. Piskala A, Šorm F. Nucleic acids components and their analogues. LI. Synthesis of 1-glycosyl derivatives of 5-azauracil and 5-azacytosine. *Collect Czech Chem Commun* 1964;29(9):2060-76. doi: 10.1135/cccc19642060
2. Li LH, Olin EJ, Buskirk HH, Reineke LM. Cytotoxicity and mode of action of 5-azacytidine on l1210 leukemia. *Cancer Res* 1970;30(11):2760-9.
3. Karon M, Sieger L, Leimbrock S, Finklestein JZ, Nesbit ME, Swaney JJ. 5-azacytidine: A new active agent for the treatment of acute leukemia. *Blood* 1973;42(3):359-65.
4. Von Hoff DD, Slavik M, Muggia FM. 5-azacytidine. A new anticancer drug with effectiveness in acute myelogenous leukemia. *Ann Intern Med* 1976;85(2):237-45.
5. Kaminskas E, Farrell A, Abraham S, Baird A, Hsieh LS, Lee SL, et al. Approval summary: Azacitidine for treatment of myelodysplastic syndrome subtypes. *Clin Cancer Res* 2005;11(10):3604-8. doi: 10.1158/1078-0432.CCR-04-2135
6. Veselý J, Čihák A. 5-Azacytidine: mechanism of action and biological effects in mammalian cells. *Pharmacol Therapeut A* 1978;2(4):813-40. doi:10.1016/0362-5478(78)90016-5
7. Christman JK. 5-azacytidine and 5-aza-2'-deoxycytidine as inhibitors of DNA methylation: Mechanistic studies and their implications for cancer therapy. *Oncogene* 2002;21(35):5483-95. doi: 10.1038/sj.onc.1205699
8. Schaefer M, Hagemann S, Hanna K, Lyko F. Azacytidine inhibits rna methylation at dnmt2 target sites in human cancer cell lines. *Cancer Res* 2009;69(20):8127-32. doi: 10.1158/0008-5472.CAN-09-0458
9. David GL, Yegnasubramanian S, Kumar A, Marchi VL, De Marzo AM, Lin X, et al. Mdr1 promoter hypermethylation in mcf-7 human breast cancer cells: Changes in chromatin structure induced by treatment with 5-aza-cytidine. *Cancer Biol Ther* 2004;3(6):540-8.
10. Aparicio A, Weber JS. Review of the clinical experience with 5-azacytidine and 5-aza-2'-deoxycytidine in solid tumors. *Curr Opin Investig Drugs* 2002;3(4):627-33.
11. Howell PM, Liu Z, Khong HT. Demethylating agents in the treatment of cancer. *Pharmaceut* 2010;3(7):2022-44. doi:10.3390/ph3072022
12. Chan KK, Giannini DD, Staroscik JA, Sadee W. 5-azacytidine hydrolysis kinetics measured by high-pressure liquid chromatography and 13c-nmr spectroscopy. *J Pharm Sci* 1979;68(7):807-12.
13. Mahfouz RZ, Jankowska A, Ebrahem Q, Gu X, Visconte V, Tabarroki A, et al. Increased cda expression/activity in males contributes to decreased cytidine analog half-life and likely contributes to worse outcomes with 5-azacytidine or decitabine therapy. *Clin Cancer Res* 2013;19(4):938-48. doi: 10.1158/1078-0432.CCR-12-1722
14. Rius M, Stresemann C, Keller D, Brom M, Schirrmacher E, Keppler D, et al. Human concentrative nucleoside transporter 1-mediated uptake of 5-azacytidine enhances DNA

demethylation. *Mol Cancer Ther* 2009;8(1):225-31. doi: 10.1158/1535-7163.MCT-08-0743

15. Brueckner B, Rius M, Markelova MR, Fichtner I, Hals PA, Sandvold ML, et al. Delivery of 5-azacytidine to human cancer cells by elaidic acid esterification increases therapeutic drug efficacy. *Mol Cancer Ther* 2010;9(5):1256-64. doi: 10.1158/1535-7163.MCT-09-1202
16. Martins S, Costa-Lima S, Carneiro T, Cordeiro-da-Silva A, Souto EB, Ferreira DC. Solid lipid nanoparticles as intracellular drug transporters: An investigation of the uptake mechanism and pathway. *Int J Pharm* 2012;430(1-2):216-27. doi: 10.1016/j.ijpharm.2012.03.032
17. Danhier F, Feron O, Preat V. To exploit the tumor microenvironment: Passive and active tumor targeting of nanocarriers for anti-cancer drug delivery. *J Control Release* 2010;148(2):135-46. doi: 10.1016/j.jconrel.2010.08.027
18. Salehi R, Rasouli S, Hamishehkar H. Smart thermo/ph responsive magnetic nanogels for the simultaneous delivery of doxorubicin and methotrexate. *Int J Pharm* 2015;487(1-2):274-84. doi: 10.1016/j.ijpharm.2015.04.051
19. Salehi R, Hamishehkar H, Eskandani M, Mahkam M, Davaran S. Development of dual responsive nanocomposite for simultaneous delivery of anticancer drugs. *J Drug Target* 2014;22(4):327-42. doi: 10.3109/1061186X.2013.876645
20. Hamishehkar H, Rahimpour Y, Kouhsoltani M. Niosomes as a propitious carrier for topical drug delivery. *Expert Opin Drug Deliv* 2013;10(2):261-72. doi: 10.1517/17425247.2013.746310
21. Rahimpour Y, Hamishehkar H. Liposomes in cosmeceutics. *Expert Opin Drug Deliv* 2012;9(4):443-55. doi: 10.1517/17425247.2012.666968
22. Ghaderi S, Ghanbarzadeh S, Mohammadhassani Z, Hamishehkar H. Formulation of gammaoryzanol-loaded nanoparticles for potential application in fortifying food products. *Adv Pharm Bull* 2014;4(Suppl 2):549-54. doi: 10.5681/apb.2014.081
23. Mahdavi H, Mirzadeh H, Hamishehkar H, Jamshidi A, Fakhari A, Emami J, et al. The effect of process parameters on the size and morphology of poly(D, L-Lactide-Co-Glycolide) micro/nanoparticles prepared by an oil in oil emulsion/solvent evaporation technique. *J Appl Polym Sci* 2010;116(1):528-34. doi: 10.1002/app.31595
24. Selvamuthukumar S, Velmurugan R. Nanostructured lipid carriers: A potential drug carrier for cancer chemotherapy. *Lipids Health Dis* 2012;11:159. doi: 10.1186/1476-511X-11-159
25. Smith A. Evaluation of poly (lactic acid) as a biodegradable drug delivery system for parenteral administration. *Int J Pharm* 1986;30(2-3):215-20. doi:10.1016/0378-5173(86)90081-5
26. Muller RH, Mader K, Gohla S. Solid lipid nanoparticles (sln) for controlled drug delivery - a review of the state of the art. *Eur J Pharm Biopharm* 2000;50(1):161-77.
27. Ezzati Nazhad Dolatabadi J, Valizadeh H, Hamishehkar H. Solid lipid nanoparticles as efficient drug and gene delivery systems: Recent breakthroughs. *Adv Pharm Bull* 2015;5(2):151-9. doi: 10.15171/apb.2015.022
28. Ghanbarzadeh S, Hariri R, Kouhsoltani M, Shokri J, Javadzadeh Y, Hamishehkar H. Enhanced stability and dermal delivery of hydroquinone using solid lipid nanoparticles. *Colloids Surf B Biointerfaces* 2015;136:1004-10. doi: 10.1016/j.colsurfb.2015.10.041
29. Souto EB, Wissing SA, Barbosa CM, Muller RH. Development of a controlled release formulation based on sln and nlc for topical clotrimazole delivery. *Int J Pharm* 2004;278(1):71-7. doi: 10.1016/j.ijpharm.2004.02.032
30. Ezzati Nazhad Dolatabadi J, Hamishehkar H, Eskandani M, Valizadeh H. Formulation, characterization and cytotoxicity studies of alendronate sodium-loaded solid lipid nanoparticles. *Colloids Surf B Biointerfaces* 2014;117:21-8. doi: 10.1016/j.colsurfb.2014.01.055
31. Hamishehkar H, Shokri J, Fallahi S, Jahangiri A, Ghanbarzadeh S, Kouhsoltani M. Histopathological evaluation of caffeine-loaded solid lipid nanoparticles in efficient treatment of cellulite. *Drug Dev Ind Pharm* 2015;41(10):1640-6. doi: 10.3109/03639045.2014.980426
32. Müller R, Lippacher A, Gohla S. Solid lipid nanoparticles (SLN) as a carrier system for the controlled release of drugs. USA: Marcel Dekker; 2000.
33. Bhaskar K, Anbu J, Ravichandiran V, Venkateswarlu V, Rao YM. Lipid nanoparticles for transdermal delivery of flurbiprofen: Formulation, in vitro, ex vivo and in vivo studies. *Lipids Health Dis* 2009;8:6. doi: 10.1186/1476-511X-8-6
34. Severino P, Andreani T, Macedo AS, Fangueiro JF, Santana MH, Silva AM, et al. Current state-of-art and new trends on lipid nanoparticles (sln and nlc) for oral drug delivery. *J Drug Deliv* 2012;2012:750891. doi: 10.1155/2012/750891
35. Schmidts T, Dobler D, Nissing C, Runkel F. Influence of hydrophilic surfactants on the properties of multiple w/o/w emulsions. *J Colloid Interface Sci* 2009;338(1):184-92. doi: 10.1016/j.jcis.2009.06.033
36. Galloni C, Azzarà VG, Loardi G. TCH-016 Extended Chemical-Physical Stability of 25 mg/ml Azacitidine Suspension. *Eur J Hosp Pharm Sci Pract* 2013;20(Suppl 1):A74-A. doi:10.1136/ejhpharm-2013-000276.207
37. Murugan K, Choonara YE, Kumar P, Bijukumar D, du Toit LC, Pillay V. Parameters and characteristics governing cellular internalization and trans-barrier trafficking of nanostructures. *Int J Nanomedicine* 2015;10:2191-206. doi: 10.2147/IJN.S75615

38. Das S, Ng WK, Tan RB. Are nanostructured lipid carriers (nlcs) better than solid lipid nanoparticles (slns): Development, characterizations and comparative evaluations of clotrimazole-loaded slns and nlcs? *Eur J Pharm Sci* 2012;47(1):139-51. doi: 10.1016/j.ejps.2012.05.010
39. Heurtault B, Saulnier P, Pech B, Proust JE, Benoit JP. Physico-chemical stability of colloidal lipid particles. *Biomaterials* 2003;24(23):4283-300.
40. Allen TM, Cullis PR. Drug delivery systems: Entering the mainstream. *Science* 2004;303(5665):1818-22. doi: 10.1126/science.1095833
41. Desai SJ, Simonelli AP, Higuchi WI. Investigation of factors influencing release of solid drug dispersed in inert matrices. *J Pharm Sci* 1965;54(10):1459-64.
42. Hughes GA. Nanostructure-mediated drug delivery. *Nanomedicine* 2005;1(1):22-30. doi: 10.1016/j.nano.2004.11.009
43. Higuchi T. Mechanism of sustained-action medication. Theoretical analysis of rate of release of solid drugs dispersed in solid matrices. *J Pharm Sci* 1963;52:1145-9.
44. Hixson AW, Crowell JH. Dependence of reaction velocity upon surface and agitation. *Ind Eng Chem* 1931;23(10):1160-8. doi: 10.1021/ie50262a025
45. Sutherland RL, Hall RE, Taylor IW. Cell proliferation kinetics of mcf-7 human mammary carcinoma cells in culture and effects of tamoxifen on exponentially growing and plateau-phase cells. *Cancer Res* 1983;43(9):3998-4006.
46. Brueckner B, Garcia Boy R, Siedlecki P, Musch T, Kliem HC, Zielenkiewicz P, et al. Epigenetic reactivation of tumor suppressor genes by a novel small-molecule inhibitor of human DNA methyltransferases. *Cancer Res* 2005;65(14):6305-11. doi: 10.1158/0008-5472.CAN-04-2957
47. Kaminskas E, Farrell AT, Wang YC, Sridhara R, Pazdur R. Fda drug approval summary: Azacitidine (5-azacytidine, vidaza) for injectable suspension. *Oncologist* 2005;10(3):176-82. doi: 10.1634/theoncologist.10-3-176
48. Tone S, Sugimoto K, Tanda K, Suda T, Uehira K, Kanouchi H, et al. Three distinct stages of apoptotic nuclear condensation revealed by time-lapse imaging, biochemical and electron microscopy analysis of cell-free apoptosis. *Exp Cell Res* 2007;313(16):3635-44. doi: 10.1016/j.yexcr.2007.06.018
49. Jovanovic J, Ronneberg JA, Tost J, Kristensen V. The epigenetics of breast cancer. *Mol Oncol* 2010;4(3):242-54. doi: 10.1016/j.molonc.2010.04.002
50. Arapshian A, Kuppumbatti YS, Mira-y-Lopez R. Methylation of conserved cpg sites neighboring the beta retinoic acid response element may mediate retinoic acid receptor beta gene silencing in mcf-7 breast cancer cells. *Oncogene* 2000;19(35):4066-70. doi: 10.1038/sj.onc.1203734

Metformin Protects against Radiation-Induced Pneumonitis, Fibrosis and Attenuates Upregulation of Dual Oxidase Genes Expression

Rasoul Azmoonfar[1], Peyman Amini[2], Hana Saffar[3], Saeed Rezapoor[2], Elahe Motevaseli[4], Mohsen Cheki[5], Rasoul Yahyapour[6], Bagher Farhood[7], Farzad Nouruzi[8], Ehsan Khodamoradi[1], Dheyauldeen Shabeeb[9,10], Ahmed Eleojo Musa[11], Masoud Najafi[1]*

[1] *Radiology and Nuclear Medicine Department, School of Paramedical Sciences, Kermanshah University of Medical Science, Kermanshah, Iran.*
[2] *Department of Radiology, Faculty of Paramedical, Tehran University of Medical Sciences, Tehran, Iran.*
[3] *Clinical and Anatomical Pathologist at Tehran University of Medical Science, Imam Khomeini Hospital Complex, Tehran, Iran.*
[4] *Department of Molecular Medicine, School of Advanced Technologies in Medicine, Tehran University of Medical Sciences, Tehran, Iran.*
[5] *Department of Radiologic Technology, Faculty of Paramedicine, Ahvaz Jundishapur University of Medical Sciences, Ahvaz, Iran.*
[6] *School of Medicine, Jiroft University of Medical Sciences, Jiroft, Iran.*
[7] *Departments of Medical Physics and Radiology, Faculty of Paramedical Sciences, Kashan University of Medical Sciences, Kashan, Iran.*
[8] *Department of Medical Radiation Engineering, Science and Research Branch, Islamic Azad University, Tehran, Iran.*
[9] *Department of Medical Physics and Biomedical Engineering, Faculty of Medicine, Tehran University of Medical Sciences (International Campus), Tehran, Iran.*
[10] *Department of Physiology, College of Medicine, University of Misan, Misan, Iraq.*
[11] *Research Center for Molecular and Cellular Imaging, Tehran University of Medical Sciences (International Campus), Tehran, Iran.*

Article info

Keywords:
- Radiation
- Metformin
- Inflammation
- Fibrosis
- DUOX1
- DUOX2

Abstract

Purpose: Lung tissue is one of the most sensitive organs to ionizing radiation (IR). Early and late side effects of exposure to IR can limit the radiation doses delivered to tumors that are within or adjacent to this organ. Pneumonitis and fibrosis are the main side effects of radiotherapy for this organ. IL-4 and IL-13 have a key role in the development of pneumonitis and fibrosis. Metformin is a potent anti-fibrosis and redox modulatory agent that has shown radioprotective effects. In this study, we aimed to evaluate possible upregulation of these cytokines and subsequent cascades such as IL4-R1, IL-13R1, Dual oxidase 1 (DUOX1) and DUOX2. In addition, we examined the potential protective effect of metformin in these cytokines and genes, as well as histopathological changes in rat's lung tissues.
Methods: 20 rats were divided into 4 groups: control; metformin treated; radiation + metformin; and radiation. Irradiation was performed with a ^{60}Co source delivering 15 Gray (Gy) to the chest area. After 10 weeks, rats were sacrificed and their lung tissues were removed for histopathological, real-time PCR and ELISA assays.
Results: Irradiation of lung was associated with an increase in IL-4 cytokine level, as well as the expression of IL-4 receptor-a1 (IL4ra1) and DUOX2 genes. However, there was no change in the level of IL-13 and its downstream gene including IL-13 receptor-a2 (IL13ra2). Moreover, histopathological evaluations showed significant infiltration of lymphocytes and macrophages, fibrosis, as well as vascular and alveolar damages. Treatment with metformin caused suppression of upregulated genes and IL-4 cytokine level, associated with amelioration of pathological changes.
Conclusion: Results of this study showed remarkable pathological damages, an increase in the levels of IL-4, IL4Ra1 and Duox2, while that of IL-13 decreased. Treatment with metformin showed ability to attenuate upregulation of IL-4–DUOX2 pathway and other pathological damages to the lung after exposure to a high dose of IR.

Introduction

Nowadays, cancer treatment using ionizing radiation (IR), also known as radiotherapy, is one of the most common modalities. The aim of radiotherapy is to eradicate all tumor cells with lowest possible damage to the surrounding normal tissues.[1] However, radiation therapy is associated with some side-effects. Early and late side effects of exposure to high doses of radiotherapy may limit the radiation doses delivered.[2] Also, a high dose of radiation may affect the long-term quality of life of cancer patients.[3] lung inflammation and fibrosis is one of the most important late effects of radiotherapy which may appear months or years after

***Corresponding author:** Masoud Najafi, Email: najafi_ma@yahoo.com treatment. These side effects are usually associated with damage to vascular structures, infiltration of immune system cells such as macrophages, lymphocytes and mast cells in addition to oxidative damage and tissue remodeling.[4] Radiation-induced fibrosis develops through long term changes in some biological elements and processes, such as cytokines and growth factors, inflammation, fibroblast differentiation etc.[5]

Several experiments have proposed TGF-β, IL-4 and IL-13 signaling pathways as the most important pathways involved in radiation-induced fibrosis.[6] TGF-β through stimulation of Smad pathway, promotes fibroblast differentiation.[7] IL-4 stimulates both IL-13 and TGF-β. which further amplifies the process of fibrosis. Furthermore, IL-4 and IL-13 stimulate production of free radicals, a long time after exposure, resulting in chronic oxidative stress.[8] It has been shown that IL-4 has a two-fold effect on promotion of fibrosis.[9] Upregulation of Dual oxidase 1 (DUOX1) and DUOX2 by these cytokines play a key role in chronic ROS production, inflammation and fibrosis.[10] Moreover, it has been shown that IL-4 plays a key role in the maintenance of macrophages in lung tissues following exposure to radiation. On the other hand, macrophages are the main source of IL-4 production.[11] It has been suggested that chronic infiltration of macrophages through production of IL-4, plays a central role in the development of pneumonitis and lung fibrosis.[12] Suppressing these genes can ameliorate various side effects induced by IR.

So far, various agents such as herbal compounds, antioxidants etc., have been examined for preventing radiation-induced pneumonitis and lung fibrosis.[13,14] Metformin has shown some radioprotective and antioxidant effects.[15] Moreover, this drug has shown ability to ameliorate fibrosis induced by various toxic agents such as chemotherapy drugs.[16,17] Metformin has been shown to possess antioxidant effect via direct neutralization of ROS and stimulating antioxidant enzymes.[18] However, a major effect of metformin is its stimulatory effect on DNA repair pathways through upregulation of AMP-activated protein kinase (AMPK).[19] AMPK is able to stimulate BER and HR pathways of DNA repair, leading to amelioration of clastogenic agents such as IR.[20,21] Metformin also has a potent inhibitory effect on mitochondrial electron transfer chain 1 (ETC1), leading to attenuation of superoxide production in oxidative stress conditions. In this study, we examined the protective effect of metformin (in a non-toxic dose) on development of radiation-induced inflammation and fibrosis associated with other pathological changes such as vascular damage. In addition, we evaluated its effects on changes in the levels of pro-fibrotic cytokines such as IL-4 and IL-13 and their downstream genes, including IL-4Ra1, IL-13Ra2, DUOX1 and DUOX2.

Materials and Methods

Animal preparation

20 adult male Wistar rats were purchased from Razi institute, Tehran University of Medical Sciences, Tehran, Iran. Rats weighing 200 ± 20 g were housed in accordance to the principles outlined in "The Guide for The Care and Use of Laboratory Animals" prepared by Kermanshah University of Medical Sciences. All rats were kept under controlled conditions, including humidity (60 ± 5%), temperature (25 ± 2°C), as well as 12h light and dark cycle.

Metformin treatment

Metformin powder was prepared by Tehran Chemie Pharmaceutical Company, Tehran, Iran. It was dissolved in distilled water at a concentration of 20mg/ml. Oral administration of the resulting solution was done 4 and 5 consecutive days before and after irradiation, respectively. On the day of irradiation, metformin was administered 30 minutes before irradiation. To obtain a non-toxic drug dose as well as optimum radioprotective effect, a 100 mg/kg dose of metformin was selected based on previous studies.[22]

Irradiation of animals

Before irradiation, animals were anesthetized using intraperitoneal injection of ketamine 10% at a dose of 80 mg/kg and xylazine 2% at a dose of 5 mg/kg. The rats were irradiated on the thoracic region with a ^{60}Co source of gamma rays at a dose rate of 109 cGy/min. A single dose of 15 Gy was selected for inducing lung injury based on previous study by Ghosh et al.[23]

Experimental design

Rats were divided into four groups. Group 1 (control): 5 rats served as controls without any intervention. Group 2 (metformin): 5 rats were treated with metformin for 10 consecutive days. Group 3 (radiation): 5 rats received 15 Gy gamma rays to their chest area. Group 4 (metformin + radiation): 5 rats were treated with metformin for 4 and 5 consecutive days before and after irradiation, respectively. All animals sacrificed 10 weeks after irradiation. Their lung tissues were removed after chest surgery. The right lung tissues were frozen immediately at -80°C for ELISA and real-time analysis, while the left parts were fixed in 10% neutral buffered formalin for histopathological assay.

Real-time PCR

Lung tissues were homogenated and total RNA was extracted. The concentration of total RNA was evaluated by a nanodrop. The extracted RNAs were transcribed to cDNA using cDNA Synthesis Kit (Gene All, South Korea). Afterwards, the expression of IL-4R, IL-13R, DUOX1 and DUOX2 were quantified using Corbett PCR system (USA) and their amplifications were performed with master mix green (Ampliqon). Expression of these mentioned genes was quantified relative to the reference gene and normalized to phosphoglucomutase 1 (PGM1) as the housekeeping gene. The genes' primer sequences were designed using Gene Runner software and BLAST from NCBI. The primer sequences of IL-4R, IL-13R, DUOX1, DUOX2 and PGM1 are shown in Table 1.

Table 1. The primer sequences of genes which were used for real-time PCR.

Gene	Forward sequence	Reverse sequence
IL-4R1	GAGTGAGTGGAGTCCCAGCATC	GCTGAAGTAACAGGTCAGGC
IL-13Ra2	TCGTGTTAGCGGATGGGGAT	GCCTGGAAGCCTGGATCTCTA
DUOX1	AAGAAAGGAAGCATCAACACCC	ACCAGGGCAGTCAGGAAGAT
DUOX2	AGTCTCATTCCTCACCCGGA	GTAACACACACGATGTGGCG
PGM1	CATGATTCTGGGCAAGCACG	GCCAGTTGGGGTCTCATACAAA

Enzyme-Linked Immunosorbent Assay (ELISA)

Lung tissues were homogenated by a homogenizer device. The levels of IL-4 and IL-13 in the lung homogenates were detected by Rat IL-4 and IL-13 ELISA kits (Zelbio, Germany) according to the manufacturer's instructions.

Histopathological evaluation

After sacrificing the rats, their left lungs were removed and fixed in formalin, and then embedded in paraffin. Sections of the removed lungs were cut into 5 μm, stained with hematoxylin and eosin (H and E) and Masson's trichrome (MTC). All pathological analyses were performed at the pathology unit of Imam Khomeini Hospital, Tehran, Iran. The blinded pathological study was performed with a light microscope using a semi-quantitative scoring system for the detection of histological parameters including fibrosis, edema, vascular damage and immune cells infiltration.

Statistical analysis

The results were presented as mean ± standard deviation and $P<0.05$ was considered statistically significant. Data were analyzed using SPSS 16 for Windows, Chicago, USA. Results of real-time PCR were analyzed by t-test while histopathological and ELISA results were analyzed using one-way ANOVA with post-hoc Tukey's HSD.

Results and Discussion

Lung is one of the most radiosensitive but late responding organ to radiotherapy. During radiotherapy for lung cancer or other tumors adjacent to the lung, late effects such as pneumonitis and fibrosis may threaten the life of patients. Moreover, exposing the lungs to radioactive particles after a radiation disaster or during a non-uniform whole body irradiation may cause death due to pneumonitis or fibrosis, months or years after exposure.[24] In recent years, several studies have been conducted to illustrate the molecular mechanisms of radiation injury to the lung. Also, some studies have proposed several agents which inhibit inflammatory and profibrotic pathways to protect or mitigate lung pneumonitis and fibrosis.[25-28] Evidences have shown that inflammatory and profibrotic cytokines play a key role in chronic consequences of exposure to IR in lung tissue.[29] Amongst several cytokines, IL-1, IL-4, IL-6, IL-13, TNF-α and TGF-β are the most effective cytokines in promoting late effects of radiation injury in various organs such as the lung.[24,30] IL-4 and IL-13 are able to induce continuous oxidative stress which mediate chronic inflammation and fibrosis. Studies have shown that IL-4, through its receptor IL-4R1, upregulates the expression of both DUOX1 and DUOX2, while IL-13 can upregulate IL13R and DUOX1.[31,32] This may continue for a long time after exposure to IR, leading to disruption of normal function of tissues and increased risk of carcinogenesis.[30,33] In addition, IL-4 has a key role in infiltration of macrophages in the lung and subsequent consequences such as promotion of fibrosis and inflammation.[34]

Signs of radiation sickness

The results of the survival rates of control, metformin treated, irradiation and irradiation plus metformin, evaluated at the end of the 10th week after local-thorax irradiation showed that rats which received metformin had healthy signs similar to the control group. In addition, those rats which were treated before and after irradiation, did not show any sign of radiation sickness. However, rats which received gamma rays without metformin had signs of reduced weight (possibly because of problems in food and water intake), epilation and ruffling of their hairs.

Real-time PCR

In this study, we aimed to evaluate the level of two important pro-fibrotic cytokines; IL-4 and IL-13, and their downstream genes, including IL4ra1, IL13Ra2, DUOX2 and DUOX1 in rat's lung tissue following exposure to a high dose of radiation. We also examined the radioprotective effect of metformin on development of pneumonitis and fibrosis, infiltration of macrophages and lymphocytes, alveolar and vascular damage, as well as edema and collagen deposition. As shown in Figure 1, the expression of IL4ra1 was significantly increased following exposure to IR when compared to control group (6.55±0.30, p=0.001). However, in metformin treatment group, there was no significant change in the expression of this gene. Treatment with metformin could attenuate the expression of IL4ra1 significantly, compared with IR group (1.91±0.93, p <0.05). Unlike IL4ra1, there was no detectable expression of IL-13ra2 gene in all groups. The expression of DUOX1 increased following exposure to IR when compared to control group (4.83±1.63, p<0.05). Treatment with metformin could attenuate the expression of IL-4r compared to IR group (2.15±0.57, p <0.05). Results of DUOX2 gene expression showed a significant increase for the radiation group compared with control group (4.23±0.57, $p \leq 0.001$). Moreover, its expression was significantly reduced in rats which were treated with metformin (2.09±0.44, $p \leq 0.001$).

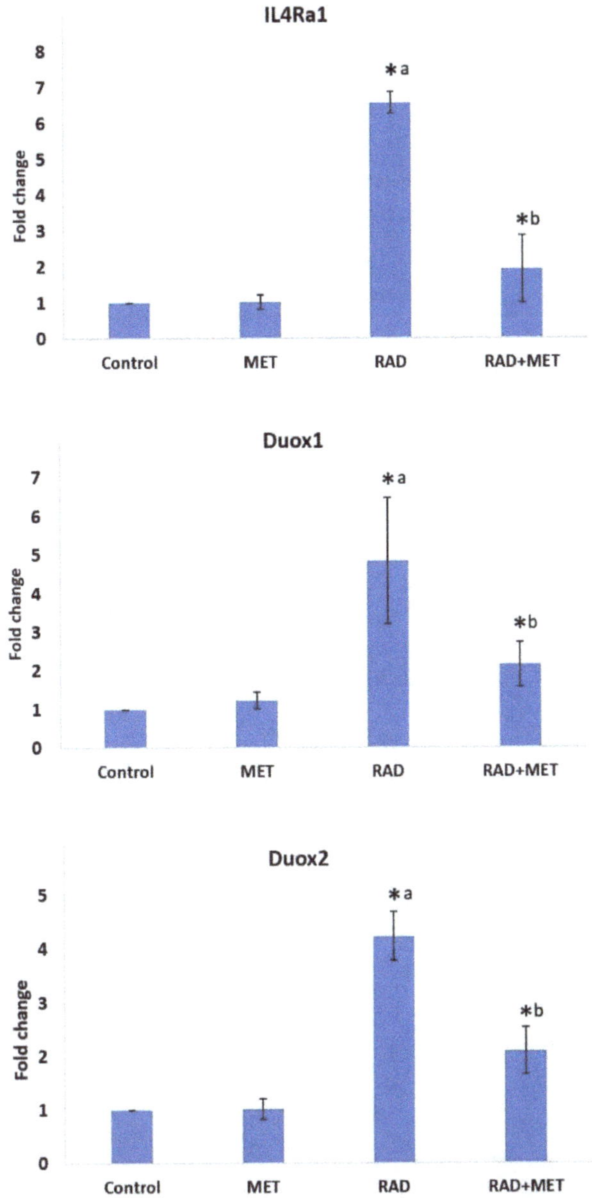

Figure 1. The expression of IL4Ra1, IL13Ra2 and DUOX2 in rat's lung tissues following irradiation, treatment with metformin, and both, (t-test, *$p < 0.05$ is considered a significant difference, a: significant compared to control group; b significant compared to radiation group). RAD=radiation; MET=metformin.

ELISA

IL-4 and IL-13 are among important cytokines that induce ROS production. As earlier mentioned, IL4Ra1 and IL13Ra2 are the main receptors of these cytokines. As upregulation of these genes are involved in chronic oxidative stress and fibrosis, we hypothesized that the increased expression of these genes may be associated with pathological damages to the lung tissue. In addition, we evaluated the levels of IL-4 and IL-13 cytokines as well as pathological changes. Afterwards, we examined the protective effect of metformin on these changes. As shown in Figures 2 and 3, irradiation of lung tissue led to an increase in IL-4 level (640±43 pg/ml vs 413±30 pg/ml). However, treatment with metformin did not cause any change in the level of this cytokine. When rats were treated with metformin before irradiation, the level of IL-4 was suppressed compared to irradiation only group (339±36 pg/ml vs 640±43 pg/ml). In contrast to IL-4, the level of IL-13 was significantly reduced following exposure to IR (243±4 pg/ml vs 215±3 pg/ml), (ANOVA, Tukey's HSD, $p=0.034$). However, no changes were observed for treatment with metformin before and after irradiation compared with IR group (229±14 pg/ml).

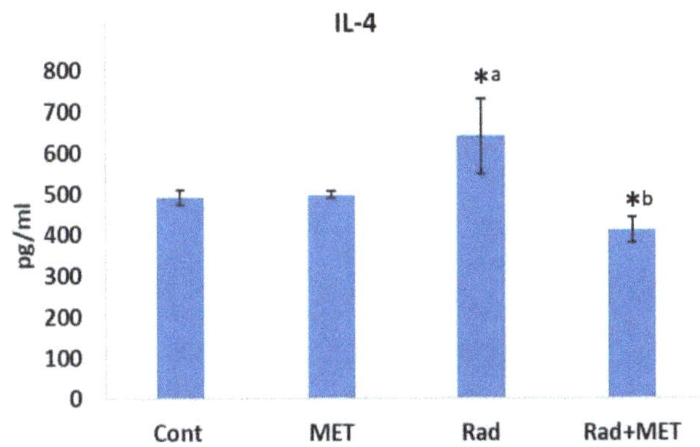

Figure 2. The levels of IL-4 in rat's lung tissues following irradiation or treatment with metformin, or both. a: significant compared to control group; b significant compared to radiation group (ANOVA, Tukey's HSD, $p<0.05$). RAD=radiation; MET=metformin.

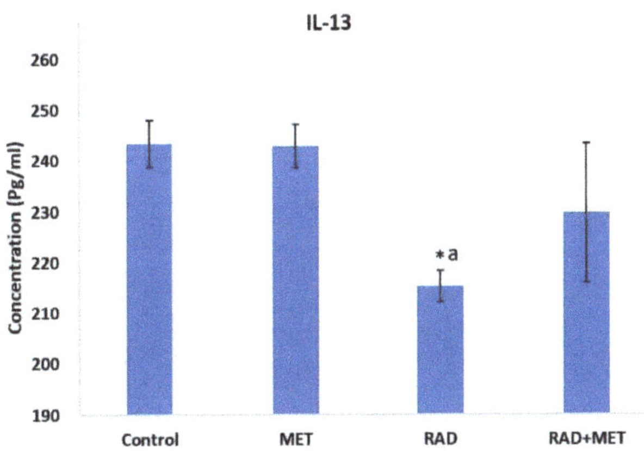

Figure 3. The levels of IL-13 in rat's lung tissues following irradiation of rat's chest area. a: significant compared to control group (ANOVA, Tukey's HSD, $p<0.05$). (ANOVA, Tukey's HSD, $p<0.05$). RAD=radiation; MET=metformin.

Histopathological analyses

As shown in Table 2, irradiation led to an increase in infiltration of macrophages and lymphocytes, thickening of alveolar and vascular endothelium as well as edema and thrombosis. Treatment with metformin led to attenuation of all mentioned factors. In addition, irradiation caused a mild fibrosis, which was suppressed by metformin (Figures 4 and 5). It is well known that macrophages and lymphocytes are able to release large numbers of cytokines that lead to appearance of inflammation and fibrosis. Macrophages and lymphocytes, through some cytokines induce ROS and NO production that have key roles in promotion of pneumonitis and collagen deposition.

Table 2. Results of histopathological evaluation of rat's lung tissues, radiation group was compared to control group while radiation plus metformin group was compared to radiation group (a: significant compared to control group, ANOVA, Tukey's HSD, $p<0.05$).

	Control	Metformin treated	Radiation	Radiation+Metformin
Macrophage infiltration	1.00±00	1.00±00	3.66±0.57^{a}	1.5±0.57^{b}
Lymphocyte infiltration	1.75±0.50	1.00±00	4.00±00^{a}	1.5±0.57^{b}
Neutrophil infiltration	1.25±50	1.00±00	1.00±00	1.25±50
Alveolar thickness	1.00±00	1.00±00	2.66±0.57^{a}	1.25±50^{b}
Vascular thickness	1.00±00	1.00±00	2.00±00^{a}	1.00±00^{b}
Edema and thrombosis	1.00±00	1.00±00	2.00±00^{a}	1.00±00^{b}

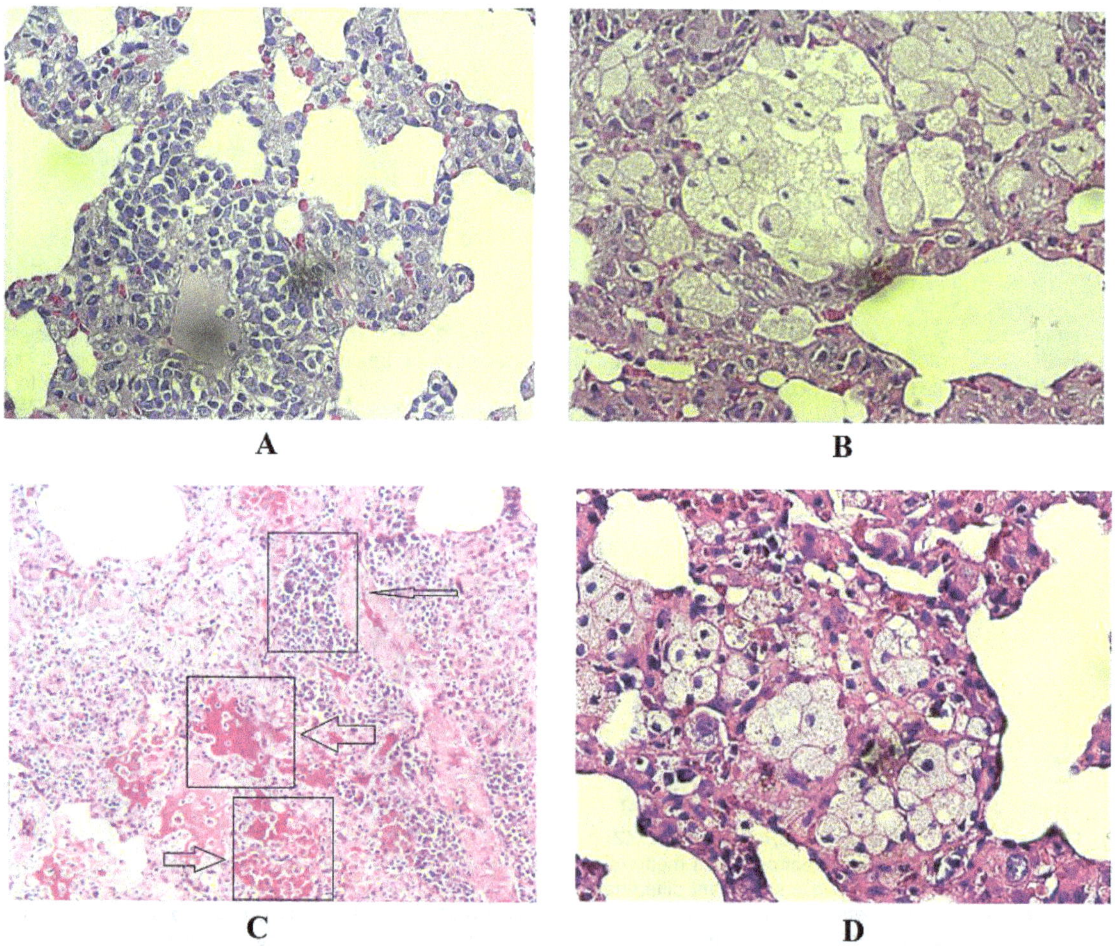

Figure 4. Histopathological effects of irradiation of rat's lungs and protective effect of metformin. A: Normal; B: Radiation; C: Radiation + Metformin. Irradiation caused a mild interstitial infiltration of lymphoplasma, and significant elevation of foam cells. Treatment with metformin before and after irradiation caused suppression of all changes in histological parameters (H&E staining).

Metformin is able to modulate cellular metabolism via inhibition of reduction/oxidation reactions and inflammation. A study by Sato et al. has shown that metformin through inhibition of TGF-β–NOX4 signaling pathway attenuate Smad phosphorylation and myofibroblast differentiation, leading to reduced lung fibrosis.[16] Modulatory effects of metformin have been proposed for protection against radiation injury. It has also shown ability to reduce IR-induced cellular damage as reported in vitro and in vivo studies.[35,36] Metformin has shown reduced cell death and micronucleus formation in human lymphocytes.[35] An in vivo study by Xu et al. has shown that metformin suppresses long term upregulation of NOX4 in mice bone marrow stem cells following irradiation. This was associated with decreased ROS production, DNA damage and apoptosis. Also, metformin could stimulate the activity of antioxidant enzymes such as superoxide dismutase (SOD) and glutathione (GSH).[37]

Targeting IL-4 and IL-13 was proposed for mitigation of radiation injury in the lung.[38] It has been shown that suppression of IL-4 can reduce late effects of radiation in this organ like fibrosis and macrophage accumulation.[34] In this study, we showed that the expression of IL-4 and its downstream genes involved in lung injury after radiation therapy can be potently inhibited by metformin.

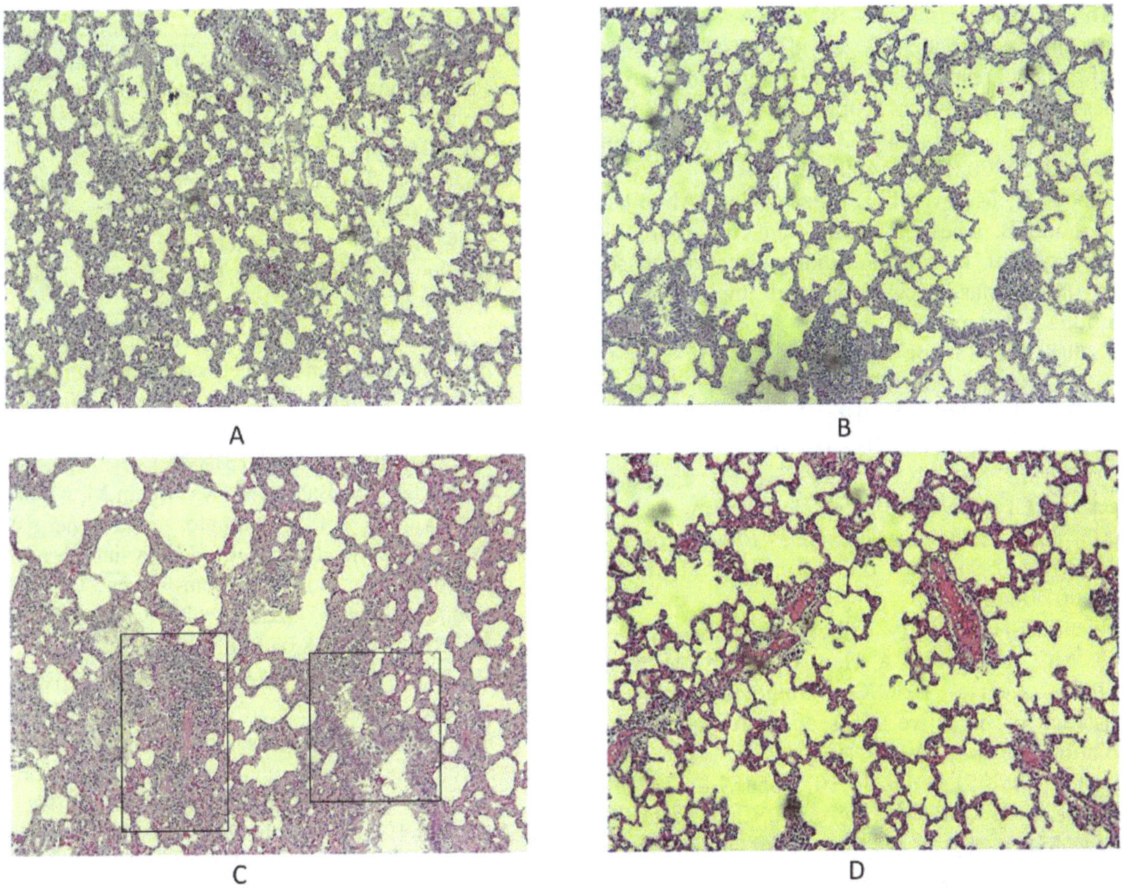

Figure 5. Histopathological effects of irradiation of rat's lungs and protective effect of metformin. Radiation led to mild fibrosis, while metformin reversed it completely. (Massons trichrome staining)

Conclusion

In this study, we showed that irradiation of rat's lung led to upregulation of IL-4–IL-4R1–DUOX2 pathway, associated with inflammation and infiltration of macrophages and lymphocytes. However, there was significant reduction in the level of IL-13. This could be an indication that upregulation of DUOX1 and DUOX2 by IL-4 is involved in lung injury following exposure to IR. Treatment with metformin could suppress pathological damages to the lung such as infiltration of macrophages and lymphocytes after exposure to a high dose of IR. This was associated with a reduction in IL-4 level as well as expression of IL4Ra1, DUOX1 and DUOX2 genes.

Acknowledgments

The authors gratefully acknowledge the research council of Kermanshah University of Medical Sciences (grant number: 3005233) for financial support.

Conflict of Interest

The authors declare that they have no conflict of interest.

References

1. Narmani A, Farhood B, Haghi-Aminjan H, Mortezazadeh T, Aliasgharzadeh A, Mohseni M, et al. Gadolinium nanoparticles as diagnostic and therapeutic agents: Their delivery systems in magnetic resonance imaging and neutron capture therapy. *J Drug Deliv Sci Technol* 2018;44:457-66. doi: 10.1016/j.jddst.2018.01.011
2. Bentzen SM. Preventing or reducing late side effects of radiation therapy: Radiobiology meets molecular

pathology. *Nat Rev Cancer* 2006;6(9):702-13. doi: 10.1038/nrc1950

3. Miller DC, Sanda MG, Dunn RL, Montie JE, Pimentel H, Sandler HM, et al. Long-term outcomes among localized prostate cancer survivors: Health-related quality-of-life changes after radical prostatectomy, external radiation, and brachytherapy. *J Clin Oncol* 2005;23(12):2772-80. doi: 10.1200/jco.2005.07.116
4. Najafi M, Motevaseli E, Shirazi A, Geraily G, Rezaeyan A, Norouzi F, et al. Mechanisms of inflammatory responses to radiation and normal tissues toxicity: Clinical implications. *Int J Radiat Biol* 2018;94(4):335-56. doi: 10.1080/09553002.2018.1440092
5. Yahyapour R, Motevaseli E, Rezaeyan A, Abdollahi H, Farhood B, Cheki M, et al. Reduction-oxidation (redox) system in radiation-induced normal tissue injury: Molecular mechanisms and implications in radiation therapeutics. *Clin Transl Oncol* 2018;20(8):975-88. doi: 10.1007/s12094-017-1828-6
6. Wynn TA, Ramalingam TR. Mechanisms of fibrosis: Therapeutic translation for fibrotic disease. *Nat Med* 2012;18(7):1028-40. doi: 10.1038/nm.2807
7. Gu L, Zhu YJ, Yang X, Guo ZJ, Xu WB, Tian XL. Effect of TGF-beta/Smad signaling pathway on lung myofibroblast differentiation. *Acta Pharmacol Sin* 2007;28(3):382-91. doi: 10.1111/j.1745-7254.2007.00468.x
8. Ameziane-El-Hassani R, Talbot M, de Souza Dos Santos MC, Al Ghuzlan A, Hartl D, Bidart JM, et al. NADPH oxidase DUOX1 promotes long-term persistence of oxidative stress after an exposure to irradiation. *Proc Natl Acad Sci U S A* 2015;112(16):5051-6. doi: 10.1073/pnas.1420707112
9. Di Maggio FM, Minafra L, Forte GI, Cammarata FP, Lio D, Messa C, et al. Portrait of inflammatory response to ionizing radiation treatment. *J Inflamm (Lond)* 2015;12:14. doi: 10.1186/s12950-015-0058-3
10. Kolivand S, Amini P, Saffar H, Rezapoor S, Motevaseli E, Najafi M, et al. Evaluating the radioprotective effect of curcumin on rat's heart tissues. *Curr Radiopharm* 2018. doi: 10.2174/1874471011666180831101459
11. Groves AM, Johnston CJ, Misra RS, Williams JP, Finkelstein JN. Whole-lung irradiation results in pulmonary macrophage alterations that are subpopulation and strain specific. *Radiat Res* 2015;184(6):639-49. doi: 10.1667/rr14178.1
12. Buttner C, Skupin A, Reimann T, Rieber EP, Unteregger G, Geyer P, et al. Local production of interleukin-4 during radiation-induced pneumonitis and pulmonary fibrosis in rats: Macrophages as a prominent source of interleukin-4. *Am J Respir Cell Mol Biol* 1997;17(3):315-25. doi: 10.1165/ajrcmb.17.3.2279
13. Christofidou-Solomidou M, Tyagi S, Tan KS, Hagan S, Pietrofesa R, Dukes F, et al. Dietary flaxseed administered post thoracic radiation treatment improves survival and mitigates radiation-induced pneumonopathy in mice. *BMC Cancer* 2011;11:269. doi: 10.1186/1471-2407-11-269
14. Lee JC, Kinniry PA, Arguiri E, Serota M, Kanterakis S, Chatterjee S, et al. Dietary curcumin increases antioxidant defenses in lung, ameliorates radiation-induced pulmonary fibrosis, and improves survival in mice. *Radiat Res* 2010;173(5):590-601. doi: 10.1667/rr1522.1
15. Najafi M, Cheki M, Rezapoor S, Geraily G, Motevaseli E, Carnovale C, et al. Metformin: Prevention of genomic instability and cancer: A review. *Mutat Res* 2018;827:1-8. doi: 10.1016/j.mrgentox.2018.01.007
16. Sato N, Takasaka N, Yoshida M, Tsubouchi K, Minagawa S, Araya J, et al. Metformin attenuates lung fibrosis development via NOX4 suppression. *Respir Res* 2016;17(1):107. doi: 10.1186/s12931-016-0420-x
17. Zhou W, Kavelaars A, Heijnen CJ. Metformin prevents cisplatin-induced cognitive impairment and brain damage in mice. *PLoS One* 2016;11(3):e0151890. doi: 10.1371/journal.pone.0151890
18. Nna VU, Abu Bakar AB, Md Lazin M, Mohamed M. Antioxidant, anti-inflammatory and synergistic anti-hyperglycemic effects of Malaysian propolis and metformin in streptozotocin-induced diabetic rats. *Food Chem Toxicol* 2018;120:305-20. doi: 10.1016/j.fct.2018.07.028
19. Finley J. Cellular stress and ampk activation as a common mechanism of action linking the effects of metformin and diverse compounds that alleviate accelerated aging defects in Hutchinson-Gilford progeria syndrome. *Med Hypotheses* 2018;118:151-62. doi: 10.1016/j.mehy.2018.06.029
20. Dogan Turacli I, Candar T, Yuksel EB, Kalay S, Oguz AK, Demirtas S. Potential effects of metformin in DNA BER system based on oxidative status in type 2 diabetes. *Biochimie* 2018;154:62-8. doi: 10.1016/j.biochi.2018.08.002
21. Dogan Turacli I, Candar T, Yuksel BE, Demirtas S. Role of metformin on base excision repair pathway in p53 wild-type H2009 and HepG2 cancer cells. *Hum Exp Toxicol* 2018;37(9):909-19. doi: 10.1177/0960327117737145
22. Miller RC, Murley JS, Grdina DJ. Metformin exhibits radiation countermeasures efficacy when used alone or in combination with sulfhydryl containing drugs. *Radiat Res* 2014;181(5):464-70. doi: 10.1667/RR13672.1
23. Ghosh SN, Zhang R, Fish BL, Semenenko VA, Li XA, Moulder JE, et al. Renin-angiotensin system suppression mitigates experimental radiation pneumonitis. *Int J Radiat Oncol Biol Phys* 2009;75(5):1528-36. doi: 10.1016/j.ijrobp.2009.07.1743
24. Mahmood J, Jelveh S, Calveley V, Zaidi A, Doctrow SR, Hill RP. Mitigation of lung injury after accidental

exposure to radiation. *Radiat Res* 2011;176(6):770-80. doi: 10.1667/rr2562.1
25. Cheki M, Yahyapour R, Farhood B, Rezaeyan A, Shabeeb D, Amini P, et al. COX-2 in radiotherapy: a potential target for radioprotection and radiosensitization. *Curr Mol Pharmacol* 2018;11(3):173-83. doi: 10.2174/1874467211666180219102520
26. Medhora M, Gao F, Jacobs ER, Moulder JE. Radiation damage to the lung: Mitigation by angiotensin-converting enzyme (ACE) inhibitors. *Respirology* 2012;17(1):66-71. doi: 10.1111/j.1440-1843.2011.02092.x
27. Haddadi GH, Rezaeyan A, Mosleh-Shirazi MA, Hosseinzadeh M, Fardid R, Najafi M, et al. Hesperidin as radioprotector against radiation-induced lung damage in rat: A histopathological study. *J Med Phys* 2017;42(1):25-32. doi: 10.4103/jmp.jmp_119_16
28. Rezaeyan A, Fardid R, Haddadi GH, Takhshid MA, Hosseinzadeh M, Najafi M, et al. Evaluating radioprotective effect of hesperidin on acute radiation damage in the lung tissue of rats. *J Biomed Phys Eng* 2016;6(3):165-74.
29. Zhao W, Robbins ME. Inflammation and chronic oxidative stress in radiation-induced late normal tissue injury: Therapeutic implications. *Curr Med Chem* 2009;16(2):130-43. doi: 10.2174/092986709787002790
30. Yahyapour R, Amini P, Rezapour S, Cheki M, Rezaeyan A, Farhood B, et al. Radiation-induced inflammation and autoimmune diseases. *Mil Med Res* 2018;5(1):9. doi: 10.1186/s40779-018-0156-7
31. Harper RW, Xu C, Eiserich JP, Chen Y, Kao CY, Thai P, et al. Differential regulation of dual NADPH oxidases/peroxidases, Duox1 and Duox2, by Th1 and Th2 cytokines in respiratory tract epithelium. *FEBS Lett* 2005;579(21):4911-7. doi: 10.1016/j.febslet.2005.08.002
32. Yahyapour R, Amini P, Rezapoor S, Rezaeyan A, Farhood B, Cheki M, et al. Targeting of inflammation for radiation protection and mitigation. *Curr Mol Pharmacol* 2018;11(3):203-10. doi: 10.2174/1874467210666171108165641
33. Yahyapour R, Motevaseli E, Rezaeyan A, Abdollahi H, Farhood B, Cheki M, et al. Mechanisms of radiation bystander and non-targeted effects: Implications to radiation carcinogenesis and radiotherapy. *Current Radiopharm* 2018;11(1):34-45. doi: 10.2174/1874471011666171229123130
34. Groves AM, Johnston CJ, Misra RS, Williams JP, Finkelstein JN. Effects of IL-4 on pulmonary fibrosis and the accumulation and phenotype of macrophage subpopulations following thoracic irradiation. *Int J Radiat Biol* 2016;92(12):754-65. doi: 10.1080/09553002.2016.1222094
35. Cheki M, Shirazi A, Mahmoudzadeh A, Bazzaz JT, Hosseinimehr SJ. The radioprotective effect of metformin against cytotoxicity and genotoxicity induced by ionizing radiation in cultured human blood lymphocytes. *Mutat Res* 2016;809:24-32. doi: 10.1016/j.mrgentox.2016.09.001
36. Wang J, Wang Y, Han J, Mei H, Yu D, Ding Q, et al. Metformin attenuates radiation-induced pulmonary fibrosis in a murine model. *Radiat Res* 2017;188(1):105-13. doi: 10.1667/rr14708.1
37. Xu G, Wu H, Zhang J, Li D, Wang Y, Wang Y, et al. Metformin ameliorates ionizing irradiation-induced long-term hematopoietic stem cell injury in mice. *Free Radic Biol Med* 2015;87:15-25. doi: 10.1016/j.freeradbiomed.2015.05.045
38. Chung SI, Horton JA, Ramalingam TR, White AO, Chung EJ, Hudak KE, et al. IL-13 is a therapeutic target in radiation lung injury. *Sci Rep* 2016;6:39714. doi: 10.1038/srep39714

Mummy Prevents IL-1β-Induced Inflammatory Responses and Cartilage Matrix Degradation via Inhibition of NF-κB Subunits Gene Expression in Pellet Culture System

Fereshteh Morrovati[1], Nahid Karimian Fathi[2], Jafar Soleimani Rad[1], Azadeh Montaseri[1]*

[1] Stem Cell Research Center, Tabriz University of Medical Sciences, Tabriz, Iran.
[2] Biochemistry Department, Faculty of Medicine, Tabriz University of Medical Sciences, Tabriz, Iran.

Article info

Keywords:
- Chondrocyte
- Inflammatory response
- IL-1β
- Pellet culture
- Cartilage

Abstract

Purpose: In Persian traditional medicine, application of Mummy material has been advised since hundred years ago for treatment of different diseases as bone fracture, cutaneous wounds and joint inflammation. Regarding to the claim of indigenous people for application of this material in the treatment of joint inflammation, the present study was designed to evaluate whether Mummy can revoke the inflammatory responses in chondrocytes stimulated with interleukin 1-β (IL-1β).

Methods: Isolated chondrocytes at the second passage were plated in 50 ml conical tubes at density of $1x10^6$ for pellet culture or were plated in T75 culture flasks as monolayer. Cells in both groups were treated as control (receiving serum free culture medium), negative control (receiving IL-1β (10ng/ml for 24 hr)) and IL-1β pre-stimulated cells which treated with Mummy at concentrations of 500 and 1000μg/ml for 72hrs. After 72 hrs, to evaluate whether Mummy can revoke the inflammatory response in chondrocytes, cell in different groups were prepared for investigation of gene expression profile of collagen II, Cox-2, MMP-13, C-Rel and P65 using real-time RT-PCR.

Results: Treatment of chondrocytes with IL-1β (10ng/ml) resulted in a significant increase in expression level of Cox-2, MMP-13, C-Rel and P65 in pellet culture system, while treatment of IL-1β-stimulated choncrocytes with Mummy at both concentrations of 500 and 1000μg/ml inhibited the expression level of above mentioned genes. Compared to the pellet culture, Mummy did not affect expression level of genes in monolayer condition.

Conclusion: The obtained data from this investigation revealed that Mummy can be used as a potent factor for inhibiting the inflammatory responses induced by IL-1β in chondrocytes probably through inhibition of NF-κB subunits activation.

Introduction

Articular cartilage is basically composed of unique cell type named chondrocytes which are trapped in a delicately organized extracellular matrix (ECM).[1,2] Despite of low division activity, chondrocytes are responsible for maintaining the homeostasis in cartilage tissue through regulation of ECM components synthesis and catabolism.[3]

Articular cartilage ECM is particularly formed by macromolecules such as type II collagen, proteoglycans and associated water which provide tensile strength and flexibility for normal function.[3,4]

Due to some constitutional properties such as lack of vessels, nerve and lymphatics and limited proliferative capacity of chondrocytes, articular cartilage has very poor ability for self- regeneration which leads to gradual impairment of joint tissues.

Osteoarthritis (OA) which is the most common debilitating and chronic disorder of synovial joints, is characterized by progressive loss of articular cartilage and involvement of other joint tissues including subchondral bone and synovium.[5,6]

At molecular level, over production of pro-inflommatory cytokines such as IL-1β and TNF-α by stimulated synoviocytes and chondrocytes has a crucial function in osteoarthritis pathogenesis.[7,8] Elevated IL-1β levels upregulates the production of degrading enzymes such as matrix metallopreteinases (MMPs) and downregulates the ECM molecules synthesis by chondrocytes which finally results in degradation of articular cartilage.[7,9] Furthermore, local synthesis and release of IL-1β induces the production of inflammatory pain mediators such as Cox-2 and inducible nitric oxide synthase (iNOS) which leads to clinical symptoms of OA.[10,11]

The biological effects of pro-inflammatory cytokines on chondrocytes such as increased level of Cox-2 and MMPs, are mainly excreted by activation of transcription

***Corresponding author:** Azadeh Montaseri, Email: montaseria@tbzmed.ac.ir factor NF-κB.[7,10] which is the master regulator of several genes involved in inflammation, apoptosis and proliferation.[11,12]

NF-κB is an ubiquitous transcription factor located in the cytoplasm, in its inactive form this molecule is a heterodimer complex consists of two subunits named as P65 and P50 and an inhibitory IκBα subunit.[11] Different stimulants such as pro-inflammatory cytokines can trigger the phosphorylation and subsequent degradation of IκBα which results in translocation of other subunits to the nucleus, where they can bind to the promoter regions of target genes and induce their transcription.[5,13]

In recent decades, transplantation of *in vitro* expanded chondrocytes at the lesion site has been applied to restore damaged cartilage. The drawback for application of chondrocytes is that during *in vitro* expansion, dedifferentiation of these cells occurs which results in loss of phenotype and also ECM components such as type II collagen, glycosaminoglycans and aggrecan. So, it is becoming increasingly believed that transfer of chondrocyte to the pellet culture systems can extend the redifferentiation capacity of these cells.[14]

Conventional options for treatment of OA are non steroidal anti inflammatory drugs (NSAIDs) and Cox-2 inhibitors which can control the symptoms of disease such as pain and stiffness.[9] Even so, due to serious side effects of above mentioned agents, it is of great clinical importance to identify novel natural compounds which can be safely applied as an alternative therapy for OA.[15]

In context of traditional Persian medicine, Mummy which is called also Mumnyae by some indigenous people is being used for hundreds of years for healing of joint inflammation, bone fractures and wound healing.[16] This pitch-like material is dark brown to black in color and formed as a result of oil oxidation in cracks of some caves. Mummy contains different ions including phosphate, calcium, hydrocarbons, polysaccharides and also nitrogen. Recently the potential effects of Mummy for healing of cutaneous wounds, peptic ulcer and bone fractures has been investigated by some researcher in Iran.[16,17] The unpublished data of our research group also revealed that Mummy can promote the proliferation rate of chondrocytes and also up-regulates the expression of some cartilage-specific genes in *in vitro* condition.

In consideration to the Mummy effects for treatment of joint inflammation which is expressed by local people, in the present study we designed to understand if Mummy can suppress the increased amount of MMP-13 and COX-2 in IL-1β-induced chondrocytes and whether Mummy can affect the expression of transcription factor NF-κB in stimulated cells.

Materials and Methods

Cartilage sampling and chondrocyte isolation

Cartilage samples were obtained from patients underwent to the total hip joint replacement surgery due to femoral neck fracture.

Well-preserved cartilage samples were transferred to the culture lab, after washing three times with phosphate buffer saline (PBS)(Cat No: P4417, Sigma-Aldrich, Germany) containing 1% penicillin/ Streptomycin (P/S)(Cat No:ATRA-010, ATOCEL, Hungary), samples were cut into 1x1 mm thickness pieces using sterile scalpel for isolation of chondrocytes, obtained pieces were incubated in pronase 1%(Cat No:10165921001,Roche, Germany) for 60 minutes, further digestion was performed by incubation in collagenase enzyme (Cat No:11088807001,Roche, Germany) at concentration of 0.2% in shaking water bath for 3-4 hours. After enzymatical digestion, undigested particles were removed by filtering through nylon mesh cell strainer (70 μm) and obtained cell suspension was centrifuged at 1500 rpm for 10 minutes. Chondrocytres were counted and seeded in T75 culture flasks containing Dulbecco's Modified Eagle Medium (DMEM)(Lot No:013BS536, biosera, France) supplemented with 10% fetal bovine serum (FBS)(Cat No:10270,Gibco, USA) and 1% P/S. After reaching about 70% confluency cells were passaged using trypsin/ EDTA enzyme.(Cat No:L0940-100, Biowest, France)

Preparation of Mummy

Mummy was purchased from local botanical market in Kermanshah, Iran. The effective concentration of this material on chondroytes has been previously determined using MTT assay technique by our Research group,[18] so in the present study, Mummy was used at concentration of 500 and 1000 μg/ml. Due to the water solubility of this material, Mummy was dissolved in DMEM culture medium and sterilization was done by filtering through syringe filter (0.22 μm).

Experimental design

Chondrocytes at the second cell passage were used for this study. For pellet culture, cells were put at concentration of $1 x 10^6$ in 50ml conical tubes with filtered lids. After centrifugation, cell pellets were formed. Furthermore, monolayer cell culture was also performed by seeding $5 x 10^5$ cells in T75 culture flasks. Chondrocytes in both pellet culture and monolayer condition were cultured in whole culture medium containing 10% FBS for 24hr. To understand the effects of Mummy on inflamed chondrocytes, the cellular events occurred in clinical condition of OA were mimicked by chondrocyte stimulation using IL-1β. For this purpose, chondrocytes in both monolayer and pellet culture were washed with DMEM containing 0.05% FBS before being treated with IL-1β. Serum-starved chondrocytes in both monolayer and pellet culture divided into different groups as below: in the first group (control) cells received only DMEM culture medium (containing 0.05% FBS), in the second group (negative control) cells received DMEM containing 10 ng/ml IL-1β (Cat No: 19401, sigma-Aldrich, USA), cells in the third group received Mummy at concentrations of 500 or 1000μg/ml, and in the fourth group, cells were pre-stimulated for 24 hr using IL-1β (10ng/ml) and then treated with Mummy for additional 72 hrs. After this period, cells in different groups were prepared for further evaluation of gene expression using Real time RT-PCR technique.

Real time RT-PCR for gene expression

The genetic information for type II collagen, Cox-2, MMP-13 and NF-κB subunits including C-Rel and P-65 in all different groups was analyzed using Real time Reverse transcriptase (RT) PCR. For this purpose, firstly the total RNA content was extracted using YTA mini kit (Cat. No: YT9065, Taiwan) based on the manufacture's instruction. Briefly, for cell lysis, RB buffer was added and then obtained mixture was transferred to the collection tube containing filter column. After centrifugation, 70% ethanol was added and then two subsequent washings were performed.

To obtain RNA, in the last step RNase-free dd H_2o was added to samples. About 1000 ng of total obtained RNA was used for CDNA synthesis using cDNA synthesis kit (Cat.No: YT4500, Taiwan). The Real time PCR reactions were performed using PCR Rotor Gene 6000 (Corbett, 010755, Australia) with SYBR green PCR master mix (Takara, RR & 20L, Japan). Different time and annealing temperatures were adjusted for each gene which are listed in Table 1.

Table 1. Primer sequences used in Real Time RT-PCR and related annealing temperature.

Gene	Primer pair sequence (5'→3')	Annealing temperature
hCOL2B	Forward primer AGGGCCAGGATGTCCGGCA Reverse primer GGGTCCCAGGTTCTCCATCT	59°C for 30 sec
COX2	Forward primer CACCGACTACGGCGGACTAA Reverse primer ACGTCAAGGAGTCGCAGGTC	57°C for 30 sec
MMP13	Forward primer CGGCTTAGAGGTGACTGGCA Reverse primer TCAGGAACCCCGCATCTTGG	59°C for 30 sec
c-Rel	Forward primer GAATCAATCCATTCAATGTCCC Reverse primer AAGAGCAGTCGTCAAATTACC	56°C for 30 sec
P65	Forward primer AGCACAGATACCACCAAGAC Reverse primer TCAGCCTCATAGAAGCCATCC	56°C for 30 sec
GAPDH	Forward primer CCATGTTGCAACCGGGAAGG Reverse primer AGGAGCGCAGGGTTAGTCAC	58°C for 45 sec

Statistical analysis

Statistical difference between different groups was determined by Two-Way ANOVA method and followed by t-test post test. The results are shown as the mean ± SD of a representative experiment performed three times. Data shown are representative of three independent experiments.

Results

Mummy enhances the expression of type II collagen by chondrocytes in both monolayer and pellet culture system

To evaluate whether Mummy material can enhance the mRNA expression level of type II collagen, chondrocytes in both monolayer and pellet culture systems were treated with Mummy at concentration of 500 and 1000 μg/ml. Furthermore to understand if Mummy can revoke the effects of IL-1β on chondrocytes, cells were stimulated with IL-1β (24 hr) and then treated with Mummy at above mentioned concentrations.

As it can be found in Figure 1-A, the expression of collagen II in chondrocytes treated with Mummy in both concentration of 500 and 1000 μg/ml elevated significantly compared to the control cells ($p<0.05$), but there isn't any significant difference between expression level of collagen type II in cells treated with IL-1β compared to control cells ($p<0.4$).

Figure 1-B shows the expression level of collagen type II in chondrocytes cultivated as pellet culture. As it can be found, Mummy at concentration of 1000 μg/ml enhanced the level of type II collagen compared to the control cells ($p<0.0005$) but there isn't any significant difference in mRNA expressin level of collagen II between IL-1β treated groups and control cells ($p<0.5$).

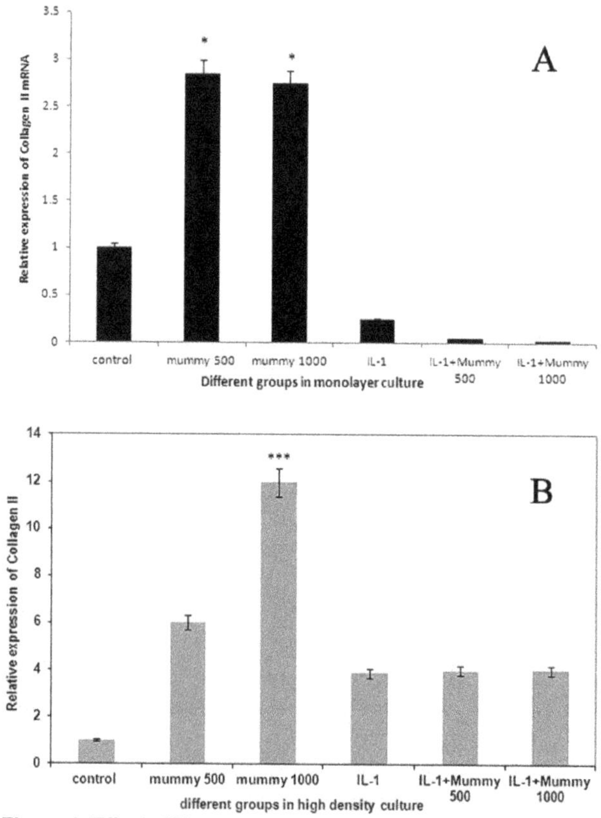

Figure 1. Effect of Mummy material on collagen type II expression level in A) monolayer and B) pellet culture system. as it can be found treatment of chondrocytes with Mummy at 1000mg/ml resulted in a significant increase in expression level of collagen type II gene in both monolayer and pellet culture systems with $^*P<0.05$, $^{***}P<0.0005$, respectively.

Mummy can down regulate the elevated levels of COX-2 and MMP-13 in IL-1β-stimulated chondrocytes

To evaluate whether Mummy can modulate the increased level of COX-2 and MMP-13 in IL-1β-stimulated chondrocytes, at first cells were pre-stimulated with IL-1β (24 hr) and then treated with Mummy (500 and 1000 μg/ml) for additional 72 hrs. As Figures 2-A and C show there isn't any significant difference in COX-2 and MMP-13 expression level between Mummy treated chondrocytes compared to the control cells in monolayer condition ($p<0.6$), also as it can be revealed stimulation of cells with IL-1β didn't affect significantly the COX-2 and MMP-13 expression compared to the control cells or cells treated with Mummy in monolayer culture system ($p<0.9$).

IL-1β pre-stimulation of chondrocytes in pellet culture system resulted in a significant increase of COX-2 expression level compared to the control or Mummy treated cells ($p<0.05$) (Figure 2-B). Furthermore as Figure 2-B reveals Mummy treatment of IL-1β-stimulated chondrocytes revoke the elevated level of COX-2 mRNA expression in pellet culture system ($p<0.05$).

Figure 2-D demonstrates the expression level of MMP-13 in pellet culture cultivated chondrocytes. As it can be understood, Mummy treatment of IL-1β-stimulated cells resulted in a significant down-regulation of MMP-13 compared to the chondrocytes which received only IL-1β ($p<0.4$) (Figure 2-D).

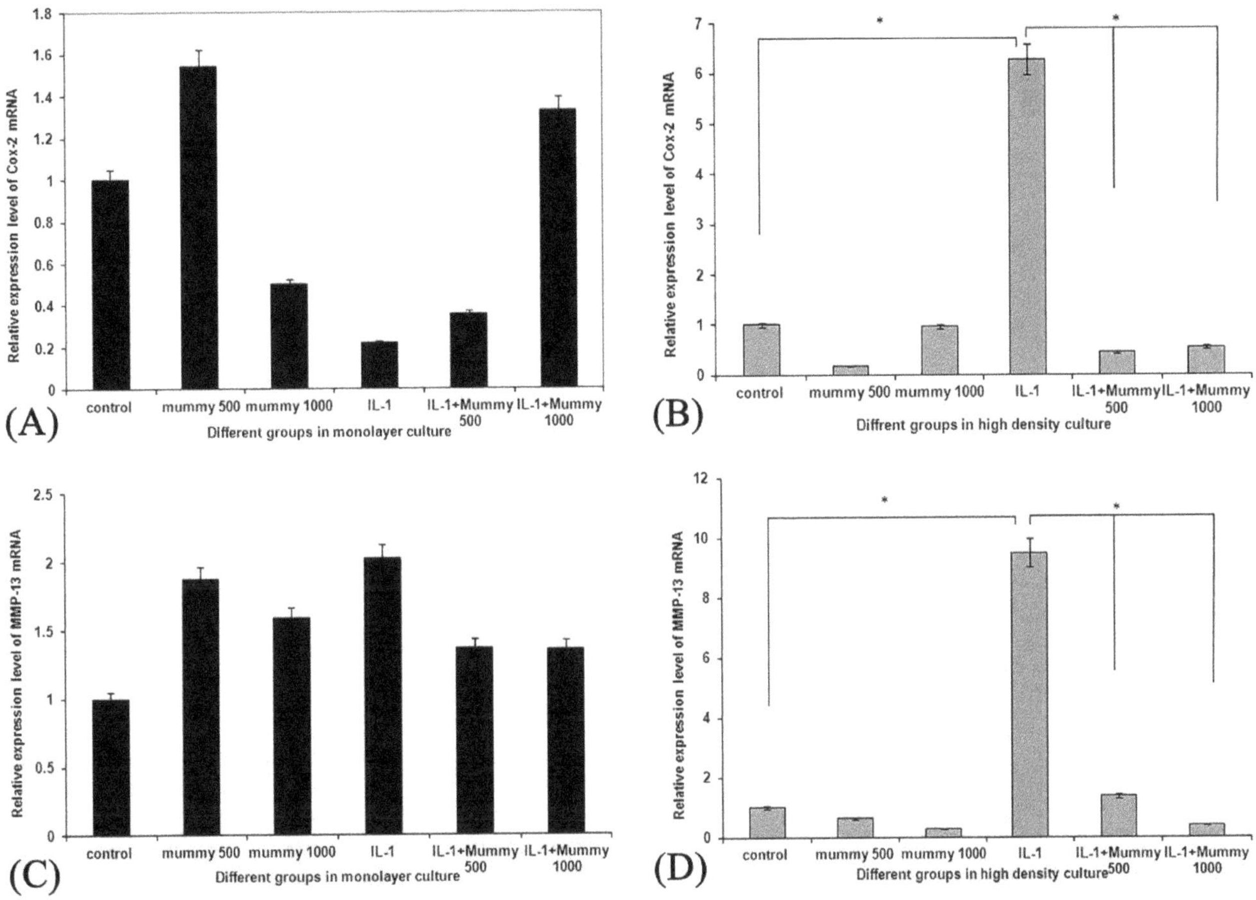

Figure 2. mRNA expression level of Cox-2 gene in A) monolayer and B) pellet culture systems, expression level of MMP-13 mRNA in C) monolayer and D) pellet culture conditions. Treatment of primary chondrocytes in monolayer culture did not affect the expression level of Cox-2 and MMP-13, but as it can be understood from figures 2-B and D, the expression level of both genes in pellet culture decreased significantly after treatment of IL-1β-stimulated chondrocytes with Mummy in both concentrations. *$P<0.05$

Mummy can down regulate the elevated levels of c-Rel and p65 subunits in IL-1β-stimulated chondrocytes cultivated in pellet culture condition

To evaluate whether treatment of chondrocyte with Mummy can change the expression of NF-κB subunits including c-Rel and p65, the mRNA expression level of these genes was assessed in both monolayer and pellet culture conditions.

Figure 3-A shows the expression level of p65 genes in monolayer cultivated cells, as it can be understood stimulation of chondrocytes with IL-1β and also treatment of IL-1β-stimulated chondrocytes with Mummy didn't change the expression level of this gene significantly ($p<0.1$). Additionally the expression level of c-Rel as another subunit of NF-κB decreased significantly after treatment of monolayer-cultivated chondrocytes with IL-1β ($p<0.005$) compared to the control cells and treatment of IL-1β-stimulated chondrocytes with Mummy at both concentrations resulted in a significant change in the expression level of c-Rel compared to control cells

($p<0.001$) but not in comparison with IL-1β-stimulated cells ($p<0.9$) (Figure 3-C).

Figures 3-C and D shows the expression level of both c-Rel and p65 genes in pellet culture of chondrocytes.

As it can be understood stimulation of chondrocytes with IL-1β resulted in a significant increase of both NF-KB subunits compared to the control ($p<0.005$). Furthermore treatment of IL-1β-stimulated chondrocytes with Mummy at both 500 and 1000 μg/ml inhibited significantly the expression level of both c-Rel and p65 genes ($p<0.0005$).

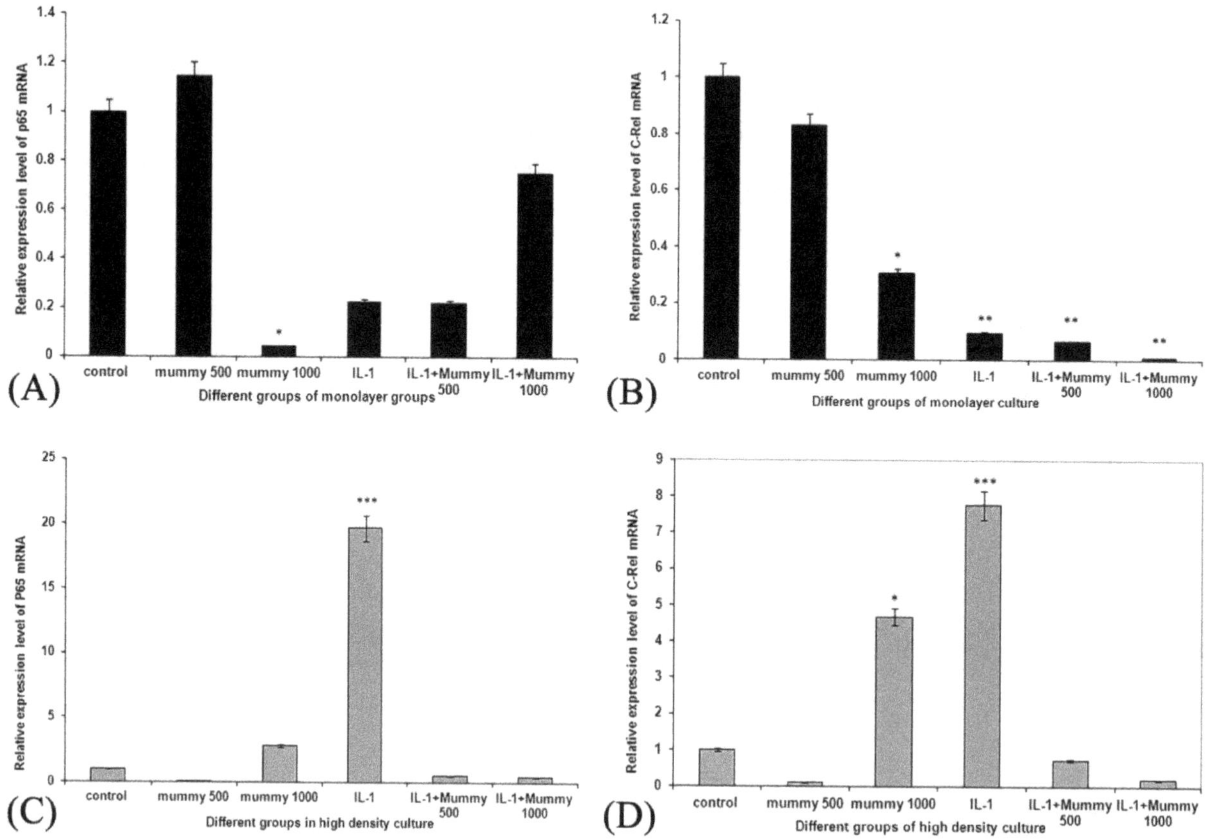

Figure 3. Expression level of P-65 mRNA in A) monolayer and C) pellet culture conditions, and mRNA expression level of C-Rel gene in B) monolayer and D) pellet cultures. As it can be revealed treatment of chondrocytes with IL-1β resulted in a significant increase in expression level of both c-Rel and P65 subunits in pellet culture of cells and treatment of IL-1β-stimulated cells with Mummy at both concentrations decreased the expression level of both mentioned genes significantly. *$p<0.05$, **$p<0.005$, ***$p<0.00053$

Discussion

This study found the following results: 1) Mummy treatment of chondrocytes in monolayer and pellet cultures increased the expression of type II collagen genes, 2) IL-1β stimulation resulted in upregulation of p65 and c-Rel subunits in chondrocytes cultivated in pellet culture which is reversed significantly after treatment with Mummy, 3) Mummy treatment of chondrocytes in pellet culture condition revokes IL-1β-induced upregulation of cox-2 and MMP-13.

One of the most common debilitating diseases affecting large number of elders is osteoarthritis (OA). This active and dynamic disease affects all joint tissues and results in structural and functional impairment of articular cartilage and remodeling of underlying bone. Due to the avascular characteristic of articular cartilage and low proliferative potential of chondrocytes, this tissue has a limited ability for self-regenaration.[11]

Current pharmacologic therapies for treatment of OA usually are alleviative and cannot prevent the progressive degradation of articular cartilage,[19] furthermore long term consumption of these drugs normally is associated with severe side effects.[20] As a consequence, identifying novel complementary medicines with more safety and effectiveness is of great importance.[9]

In Persian traditional medicine Mummy material has been advised since hundreds of years for treatment of different diseases such as joint inflammation, wound healing and bone fractures. Recently, several investigations revealed some pharmacological effects of Mummy such as anti-inflammatory, promoting collagen production at wound site, bone fracture healing and protection of gastric mucosa against ethanol-induced ulcer.[16,17] The molecular mechanisms underlying the therapeutic effects of Mummy in joint inflammation remains unclear, hence this study was designed to evaluate if Mummy can revoke degenerative effects of IL-1β on chondrocytes.

The widely accepted process involved in initiation and advancement of OA includes degradation of articular cartilage, inflammation of synovial membrane and changes in subchondral bone.[8]

Pro-inflammatory cytokines such as IL-1β produced by synoviocytes and chondrocytes are largely participating in OA pathogenesis.[9] Elevated amount of IL-1β results in upregulation of Matrix metaloproteinnases (MMPs), cox-2 and Nitric oxide (NO) which are regulated by the ubiquitous transcription factor, nuclear factor-KB (NF-KB).[5,7]

In unstimulated state, this factor is located in cytoplasm and combined with an inhibitory subunit named as IKBα. Due to IL-1β stimulation, activated NF-κB subunits translocate to the nucleus and bind to the promoter regions of different inflammation-related genes including MMP-1, MMp-9, MMP-13, Cox-2, NO and different types of ADAMTS which finally result in further degradation of cartilage ECM components such as type II collagen and proteoglycans.[10,21]

It has been well accepted that in *in vitro* conditions, stimulation of chondrocytes with IL-1β at concentration of 10 ng/ml can mimic pathological events of OA.[22]

In the present study for understanding the probable effects of Mummy on inflammatory pathway occurred in OA, IL-1β-stimulated chondrocytes were used.

As we found, the gene expression level of two NF-κB subunits including c-Rel and p65 in the presence of IL-1β increased significantly in chondrocytes cultivated in pellet culture system. For evaluating the effects of Mummy, IL-1β-stimulated chondrocytes were treated with Mummy at both 500 and 1000 μg/ml doses. This investigation reveals that the expression level of both c-Rel and p65 subunits decreased significantly after Mummy treatment in IL-1β-pre stimulated chondrocytes. Also, we found that IL-1 stimulation results in upregulation of MMP-13 and Cox-2 genes in pellet culture cultivated chondrocytes and then treatment of IL-1β-stimulated cells with Mummy (500, 1000 μg/ml) inhibit their upregulation. As it has been previously mentioned, due to activation of NF-κB, synthesis of matrix degrading enzymes such as MMPs, Cox-2 and NO levels increase.

In normal conditions, there is a delicately regulated balance in ECM component remodeling through MMP activity and synthesis of new matrix.[7] However, during OA, this equilibrium gets lost and expression of different MMPs such as MMP-13 enhances which plays a crucial role in collagen type II degradation and cartilage destruction.[3]

Our results reveal that Mummy (500 and 1000 μg/ml) inhibited the IL-1β-induced MMP-13 upregulation, so further investigation are necessary to understand the exact underlying mechanism of this material.

Another inflammation-realated gene which its expression is upregulated due to activation of IL-1β, is cox-2.[7] This inflammatory pain mediator exerts excessive catabolic effects through prostaglandinE2 (PGE2) production. In this study we found that IL-1β-induced upregulation of Cox-2 can be revoked by Mummy at both concentrations. It could be suggested that down-regulation of MMP-13 and Cox-2 in Mummy-treated chondrocytes occurs via inhibition of two NF-κB subunits including c-Rel and p65, but for understanding the precise underlying mechanisms, further evaluations are needed.

In this study, the probable effects of Mummy on IL-1β-stimulated chondrocytes were evaluated in both monolayer and pellet culture systems. Our results showed that Mummy exerts its anti-inflammatory effects on chondrocytes cultivated in pellet culture condition, rather than monolayer.

It is well established that monolayer expansion of chondrocytes cannot support their phenotype due to the dedifferentiation process, whereas 3D culture can maintain the chondrogenic potential maybe in part as a result of low oxygen tension which occurred normally in cartilage tissue due to its avascularity.[2]

Taking together, in this investigation we demonstrated that treatment of IL-1β-stimulated chondrocytes can inhibit the expression of inflammation-related genes including MMP-13 and cox-2 probably through down-regulation of NF-KB subunits including c-Rel and p65. Further evaluations are necessary for better understanding the precise underlying mechanisms.

Conclusion

It can be concluded that Mummy can inhibit the inflammatory responses in chondrocytes induced by IL-1β, so it can be introduced as a useful compound with the potential shedding light on advancing the success in cartilage tissue engineering.

Acknowledgments

This article is resulted from the research proposal leading to thesis of Fereshteh Morovvati, M.Sc student of Anatomical Sciences and approved by Stem Cell Research center, Tabriz University of Medical sciences, Tabriz, Iran. The authors gratefully acknowledge the research deputy of Tabriz University of Medical Sciences for financial support.

Conflict of Interest

The authors declare no conflict of interests.

References

1. Cancedda R, Dozin B, Giannoni P, Quarto R. Tissue engineering and cell therapy of cartilage and bone. *Matrix Biol* 2003;22(1):81-91. doi: 10.1016/S0945-053X(03)00012-X
2. Caron MM, Emans PJ, Coolsen MM, Voss L, Surtel DA, Cremers A, et al. Redifferentiation of dedifferentiated human articular chondrocytes: comparison of 2D and 3D cultures. *Osteoarthritis*

Cartilage 2012;20(10):1170-8. doi: 10.1016/j.joca.2012.06.016

3. Greco KV, Iqbal AJ, Rattazzi L, Nalesso G, Moradi-Bidhendi N, Moore AR, et al. High density micromass cultures of a human chondrocyte cell line: a reliable assay system to reveal the modulatory functions of pharmacological agents. *Biochem Pharmacol* 2011;82(12):1919-29. doi: 10.1016/j.bcp.2011.09.009
4. Chung C, Burdick JA. Engineering cartilage tissue. *Adv Drug Deliv Rev* 2008;60(2):243-62. doi: 10.1016/j.addr.2007.08.027
5. Shakibaei M, Csaki C, Nebrich S, Mobasheri A. Resveratrol suppresses interleukin-1β-induced inflammatory signaling and apoptosis in human articular chondrocytes: potential for use as a novel nutraceutical for the treatment of osteoarthritis. *Biochem Pharmacol* 2008;76(11):1426-39. doi: 10.1016/j.bcp.2008.05.029
6. Rufino AT, Ribeiro M, Sousa C, Judas F, Salgueiro L, Cavaleiro C, et al. Evaluation of the anti-inflammatory, anti-catabolic and pro-anabolic effects of E-caryophyllene, myrcene and limonene in a cell model of osteoarthritis. *Eur J Pharmacol* 2015;750:141-50. doi: 10.1016/j.ejphar.2015.01.018
7. Shakibaei M, John T, Schulze-Tanzil G, Lehmann I, Mobasheri A. Suppression of NF-κB activation by curcumin leads to inhibition of expression of cyclo-oxygenase-2 and matrix metalloproteinase-9 in human articular chondrocytes: implications for the treatment of osteoarthritis. *Biochem Pharmacol* 2007;73(9):1434-45. doi: 10.1016/j.bcp.2007.01.005
8. Zheng W, Zhang H, Jin Y, Wang Q, Chen L, Feng Z, et al. Butein inhibits IL-1β-induced inflammatory response in human osteoarthritis chondrocytes and slows the progression of osteoarthritis in mice. *Int Immunopharmacol* 2017;42:1-10. doi: 10.1016/j.intimp.2016.11.009
9. Liu SC, Lee HP, Hung CY, Tsai CH, Li TM, Tang CH. Berberine attenuates CCN2-induced IL-1β expression and prevents cartilage degradation in a rat model of osteoarthritis. *Toxicol Appl Pharmacol* 2015;289(1):20-9. doi: 10.1016/j.taap.2015.08.020
10. Goldring MB, Otero M. Inflammation in osteoarthritis. *Curr Opin Rheumatol* 2011;23(5):471-8. doi: 10.1097/BOR.0b013e328349c2b1
11. Montaseri A, Busch F, Mobasheri A, Buhrmann C, Aldinger C, Rad JS, et al. IGF-1 and PDGF-bb suppress IL-1β-induced cartilage degradation through down-regulation of NF-κB signaling: involvement of Src/PI-3K/AKT pathway. *PLoS One* 2011;6(12):e28663. doi: 10.1371/journal.pone.0028663
12. Haseeb A, Chen D, Haqqi TM. Delphinidin inhibits IL-1β-induced activation of NF-κB by modulating the phosphorylation of IRAK-1(Ser376) in human articular chondrocytes. *Rheumatology (Oxford)* 2013;52(6):998-1008. doi: 10.1093/rheumatology/kes363
13. Jeong JW, Lee HH, Choi EO, Lee KW, Kim KY, Kim SG, et al. Schisandrae Fructus Inhibits IL-1β-Induced Matrix Metalloproteinases and Inflammatory Mediators Production in SW1353 Human Chondrocytes by Suppressing NF-κB and MAPK Activation. *Drug Dev Res* 2015;76(8):474-83. doi: 10.1002/ddr.21283
14. Hassan Famian M, Montazer Saheb S, Montaseri A. Conditioned Medium of Wharton's Jelly Derived Stem Cells Can Enhance the Cartilage Specific Genes Expression by Chondrocytes in Monolayer and Mass Culture Systems. *Adv Pharm Bull* 2017;7(1):123-30. doi: 10.15171/apb.2017.016
15. Zhang Y, Li R, Zhong Y, Zhang S, Zhou L, Shang S. Fuyuan decoction enhances SOX9 and COL2A1 expression and Smad2/3 phosphorylation in IL-1β-activated chondrocytes. *Evid Based Complement Alternat Med* 2015;2015:821947. doi: 10.1155/2015/821947
16. Dehghan M, Faradonbeh AS. The effect of mummy on the healing of bone fractures. *Afr J Pharm Pharmacol* 2012;6(5):305-9. doi: 10.5897/AJPP11.353
17. Abshenas J, Kheirandish R, Salary AR. Gastroprotective effect of mummy on induced gastric ulcer in rats. *Comp Clin Pathol* 2014;23(2):305-9. doi: 10.1007/s00580-012-1610-7
18. Sabetkam S, Soleimani Rad J, Hassan Pour Khodaie S, Roshangar L. Impact of Mummy Substance on Proliferation and Migration of Human Wharton's Jelly-Derived Stem Cells and Fibroblasts in vitro culture system. *Crescent J Med Biol Sci* 2018;5(3).
19. Zhang W, Ouyang H, Dass CR, Xu J. Current research on pharmacologic and regenerative therapies for osteoarthritis. *Bone Res* 2016;4:15040. doi: 10.1038/boneres.2015.40
20. Kanwar JR, Samarasinghe RM, Kumar K, Arya R, Sharma S, Zhou SF, et al. Cissus quadrangularis inhibits il-1β induced inflammatory responses on chondrocytes and alleviates bone deterioration in osteotomized rats via p38 MaPK signaling. *Drug Des Devel Ther* 2015;9:2927-40. doi: 10.2147/DDDT.S77369
21. Buhrmann C, Mobasheri A, Matis U, Shakibaei M. Curcumin mediated suppression of nuclear factor-κB promotes chondrogenic differentiation of mesenchymal stem cells in a high-density co-culture microenvironment. *Arthritis Res Ther* 2010;12(4):R127. doi: 10.1186/ar3065
22. Park K, Hoffmeister B, Han DK, Hasty K. Therapeutic ultrasound effects on interleukin-1β stimulated cartilage construct in vitro. *Ultrasound Med Biol* 2007;33(2):286-95. doi: 10.1016/j.ultrasmedbio.2006.08.009

Effect of Addition of Antifungal Agents on Physical and Biological Properties of a Tissue Conditioner

Pragati Rawat*, Swatantra Agarwal, Siddhi Tripathi

Department of Prosthodontics and Crown & Bridge, Kothiwal dental college and research center, Moradabad, UP-244001, India.

Article info

Keywords:
- Candida albicans
- Viscoelasticity
- Tensile bond strength
- Fluconazole
- Oregano oil
- Virgin coconut oil

Abstract

Purpose: Tissue conditioners are used for healing of abused oral tissues. They may harbour microorganisms causing oral diseases such as candidiasis compromising the health of the patient. Also, addition of antifungal agents into tissue conditioner may alter its properties. This study compares the anti-fungal property and mechanical properties of tissue conditioner containing different antifungal agents.

Methods: Three antifungal agents, one synthetic – fluconazole, and two natural - oregano oil and virgin coconut oil were added into the tissue conditioner (Viscogel) in different concentrations. The antifungal property, tensile bond strength and viscoelasticity of Viscogel containing these antifungal agents were assessed after 24 hours, three days and seven days.

Results: While, the highest antifungal activity was shown by Viscogel containing fluconazole, the maximum tensile bond strength was found to be of Viscogel alone (control). Although Viscogel alone and in combination of fluconazole showed deterioration in viscoelasticity, Viscogel in combination of natural agents showed no significant changes over the period of seven days.

Conclusion: Incorporation of the natural agents in the tissue conditioner can be used as an effective alternative to systemic or topical synthetic antifungal agents.

Introduction

A removable dental prosthesis is one of the commonest mode of treatment in prosthetic dentistry. However, their long term use without rest to underlying oral tissues may lead to adverse effect on their integrity. Both rest and tissue conditioners have been advocated to allow the deformed tissues of the residual ridges to return to normal form. The tissue conditioners are soft, resilient temporary liners that have been widely used in dentistry to manage multitude of patient problems and for various clinical applications.[1] Apart from reducing and evenly distributing stresses on the mucosa of the basal seat[2] they can also be used for temporary relining of immediate dentures etc.[3] However, microbial growth results from the adherence of microbial cells promoted by rough surface, and from adhesive interactions between Candida species and oral bacteria, mostly Candida albicans that may lead to Candidiasis.[4]

The treatment of Candidiasis includes denture repair or replacement, adoption of prophylactic measures by the patient and the prescription of topical and systemic antifungal drugs.[5] However, the success of topical application of drugs in the oral cavity may be compromised by the copious flow of saliva as well as by the lack of patient compliance. Therefore, antifungal agents can be incorporated in tissue conditioners to simultaneous treat injured peri-prosthetic tissues and infection by Candida.[6] More recently, azole antifungal compounds such as fluconazole, which have excellent efficacy-toxicity profiles, have emerged as the principal drugs used in the treatment of candida infections. However, fluconazole produces few side effects: nausea, vomiting and might lead to the development of drug resistance in Candida albicans.[7,8] So, to overcome these unpleasant side effects of chemically synthetic antifungals, herbs with antimicrobial property, especially anti-candida effect are of interest.[9,10] Out of the various natural essential oils such as Oregano oil,[11] Virgin coconut oil[12,13] Melaleuca alternifolia oil,[14] etc incorporated by different researchers in tissue conditioner, origanum oil and coconut oil have been found to exhibit superior antifungal activity. However, their use in dental applications is needed to be investigated more.

The most common problems encountered using soft denture liners are water sorption and solubility which are associated with Candida albicans growth and stresses at the liner/denture base interface leading to reduction in the bond strength.[15] However, no data is available to ascertain the effect of incorporation of fluconazole and virgin coconut oil in the tissue conditioner on it's tensile bond strength to denture base.

Also, the viscoelastic properties of soft denture liners are important since they characterize the ability of the material to exert a cushioning effect on the oral tissues and maintain shape during function.[16] The temporary nature of

***Corresponding author:** Pragati Rawat, Email: rawatpragati@gmail.com these types of materials is because of the leaching of the alcohol and the plasticizer and adsorption of water and saliva which causes loss of viscoelasticity and therefore, compliance.[17] Apart from few studies, there are no studies to comment upon the effect of incorporation of fluconazole, oregano oil and virgin coconut oil in the tissue conditioner on it's viscoelastic properties.

Although, Virgin coconut oil and Oregano oil has been found to provide good anti-fungal protection, scarce investigations has been done for their use in dental applications. Moreover, no conclusive data is available for comparison between anti-fungal property, tensile bond strength and viscoelasticity of tissue conditioners when incorporated with oregano oil, virgin coconut oil and fluconazole. Accordingly, this study was designed to compare and evaluate the aforementioned parameters.

Materials and Methods

Test materials used for the study were divided into following four groups having 10 samples each :

(1) Group I - Visco Gel without any antifungal agents (control)
(2) Group II - Visco Gel + 10 %w/w Fluconazole
(3) Group III - Visco Gel + 60% v/v Oregano Oil
(4) Group IV - Visco Gel + 25% v/v Virgin Coconut oil

Following methodology was employed for the study:

Antifungal property

Candida albicans strain (ATCC NO. 24433) was taken and inoculated in Sabouraud dextrose agar broth which was incubated at 37°C for 24 hours. Standardization was done by diluting with sterile broth to a density visually equivalent to barium sulphate, standard Mc farland tube no. 5. It was then dispensed into a sterile Sabouraud agar plate and was allowed to dry. When the petri dishes had dried, four wells of diameter 6 mm and depth 1 mm were punched using a tissue punch on each of the ten petri dishes such that the wells lie within the lawn culture. Each of the four wells on each petri dish was filled with different test materials. After the materials had set in the wells, the plates were incubated at 37°C. The plates were then taken out after 24 hours, 3 days and 7 days and on each day the Minimum Inhibition Zone (MIZ) was measured using a metallic scale and a divider.[11] Two diametric readings were taken for each sample and their mean was taken as the final reading for that sample

Tensile Bond Strength

For fabrication of test samples, two wax blocks of slightly larger dimensions i.e. 41 mm x 11 mm x 11 mm each were made. Out of the two, one had 3 mm raise borders. These samples were polymerized with heat cure denture base resin using long curing cycle at 74°C for eight hours. The blocks that were obtained were finished and polished. These finished blocks were used to make silicone rubber moulds. These moulds were then used to make 40 more wax blocks which were polymerized and finished in the similar manner to the required dimensions i.e. 40 mm x 10 mm x 10 mm. One side of each block that was having raised border was roughened using 100-grit sandpaper and acrylic trimmer. Test materials in suitable consistency were applied on the side of the block which was roughened then on top of it another block without the raised border was placed as shown in. After setting, the excess material was trimmed and samples were stored in 100 ml distilled water at 37°C.[11] Tensile bond strength was evaluated on Universal Testing Machine (Banbros Engineering Pvt. Ltd., Model no.-WDW-5) at a cross-head speed of 5 mm/min after 24 hours, three days and seven days.

Viscoelasticity

A total of 40 dumbbell shaped moulds measuring 50 mm x 10 mm x 10 mm were prepared using Hydraulic Press. These moulds were placed over a metal platform before the test materials were poured into them. After the material had set, the dumbbell shaped samples were retrieved from the moulds and stored in 100 ml distilled water at 37°C. These specimens were then subjected to stress relaxation tests on Universal Testing Machine (Dak Test Bench, Samruddhi Comercial complex, Model no.- UTB 9052) at a crosshead speed of 20 inches/minute after 24 hours, three days and seven days and a load-deformation curve along with the elastic modulus was obtained for each specimen.[18]

Statistical Analysis

The statistical analysis was done using SPSS (Statistical Package for Social Sciences) Version 15.0 statistical Analysis Software in which the obtained data was subjected to ANOVA and Post-Hoc Tests (Tukey-HSD).

Results

Antifungal property

Group I showed no antifungal activity throughout the tested time period of seven days. Figure 1 shows intragroup wise graphical representation of zones of inhibition. Table 1 illustrates the intergroup comparison.

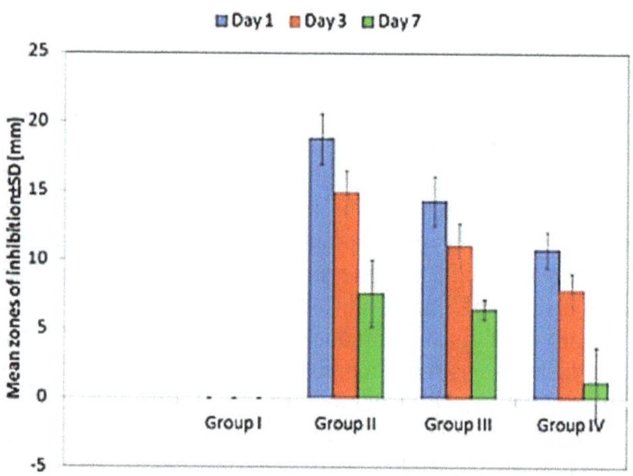

Figure 1. Intragroup wise representation of zones of inhibition

Table 1. Intergroup comparison of Zones of inhibition

Comparison	T1			T2			T3		
	MD	SE	'p-value'	MD	SE	'p-value'	MD	SE	'p-value'
I v/s II	-18.80	0.64	<0.001	-14.90	0.57	<0.001	-7.60	0.80	<0.001
I v/s III	-14.30	0.64	<0.001	-11.10	0.57	<0.001	-6.50	0.80	<0.001
I v/s IV	-10.80	0.64	<0.001	-7.90	0.57	<0.001	-1.20	0.80	0.445
II v/s III	4.50	0.64	<0.001	3.80	0.57	<0.001	1.10	0.80	0.520
II v/s IV	8.00	0.64	<0.001	7.00	0.57	<0.001	6.40	0.80	<0.001
III v/s IV	3.50	0.64	<0.001	3.20	0.57	<0.001	5.30	0.80	<0.001

MD=Mean difference; SE=Standard error; 'p-value'=level of significance

Tensile Bond Strength

An increasing trend in tensile bond strength was noticed in all the groups at all time intervals. Intragroup comparison of tensile bond strength is depicted graphically in Figure 2. Intergroup comparison of tensile bond strength is given in Table 2.

Viscoelasticity

Viscoelasticity of the tissue conditioner having different antifungal agents in various concentrations was tested through measurement of modulus of elasticity through stress relaxation test. The tested groups showed varying results at different time intervals. Figure 3 depicts intra-group representation of modulus of elasticity graphically. Table 3 illustrates intergroup comparison of modulus of elasticity.

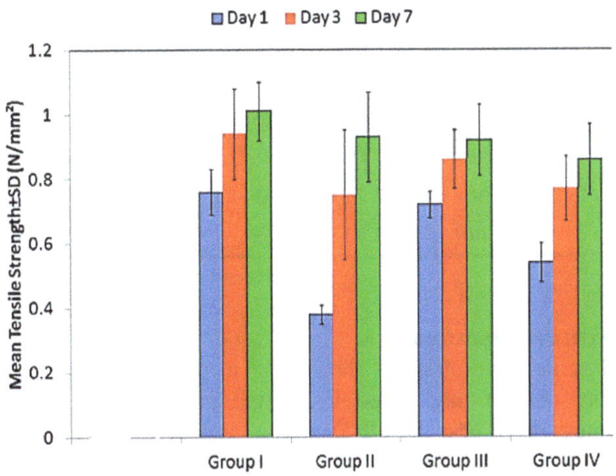

Figure 2. Intra-group representation of tensile bond strength

Table 2. Intergroup comparison of tensile bond strength

Comparison	24 hours			Day 3			Day 7		
	MD	SE	'p-value'	MD	SE	'p-value'	MD	SE	'p-value'
I v/s II	0.39	0.02	<0.001	0.19	0.06	0.018	0.08	0.05	0.408
I v/s III	0.04	0.02	0.245	0.08	0.06	0.597	0.09	0.05	0.298
I v/s IV	0.22	0.02	<0.001	0.17	0.06	0.047	0.15	0.05	0.038
II v/s III	-0.34	0.02	<0.001	-0.12	0.06	0.267	0.01	0.05	0.997
II v/s IV	-0.16	0.02	<0.001	-0.02	0.06	0.980	0.06	0.05	0.606
III v/s IV	0.18	0.02	<0.001	0.09	0.06	0.469	0.05	0.05	0.735

MD=Mean difference; SE=Standard error; 'p-value'=level of significance

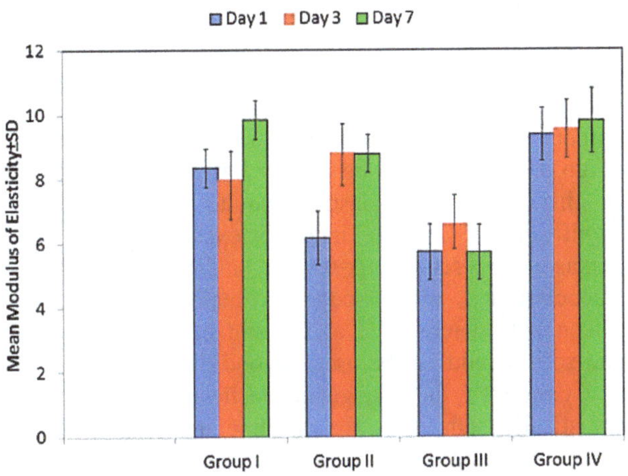

Figure 3. Intra-group representation of modulus of elasticity

Discussion

Antifungal Property

In the present study, when antifungal property was evaluated, it showed a statistically significant decrease during the period of study. This decrease in zones of inhibition at the end of seven days was due to the regrowth of the fungus.[10] Similar decreasing trends in the antifungal activity have also been seen in the studies conducted by Sharma et al,[6] Chopde et al[19] and Falah-tafti et al[20] for fluconazole and Srivastava et al[11] for oregano oil. Although, there are studies confirming the antifungal efficacy of virgin coconut oil as conducted by Ogbolu et al[12] and Kannan et al,[13] studies related to decreasing trend in antifungal activity over a period of time have not been previously reported. Although, the mechanism of action of all the three anti-fungal agents is different from each other and all of them are causing destruction of the fungus cell membrane in one way or the other such as, fluconazole acts by inhibiting the fungal cytochrome P450 enzyme 'lanosterol 14-demethylase' causing impairment in ergosterol synthesis leading to a cascade of membrane abnormalities in the fungus;[8] origanum oil directly inhibits germination and filament formation (the two phases required for tissue invasion) by Candida albicans[21] and virgin coconut oil acts by causing the cell membrane of the fungus to disintegrate[13] but still, fluconazole showed highest antifungal activity amongst all. This is because fluconazole is more potent antifungal agent than the oregano oil and virgin coconut oil which could be supported by the fact that the minimum inhibitory concentration of fluconazole against Candida albicans being reported is 0.25-64 μg/ml,[22] for oregano oil it is 2.5 μg/ml[23] and for virgin coconut oil it is 32 μg/ml.[12]

Table 3. Intergroup comparison of Modulus of Elasticity

Comparison	24 hours			Day 3			Day 7		
	MD	SE	'p-value'	MD	SE	'p-value'	MD	SE	'p-value'
I v/s II	2.18	0.35	<0.001	-0.84	0.44	0.242	1.06	0.35	0.022
I v/s III	2.62	0.35	<0.001	1.38	0.44	0.018	4.14	0.35	<0.001
I v/s IV	-1.03	0.35	0.029	-1.57	0.44	0.006	0.06	0.35	0.998
II v/s III	0.44	0.35	0.604	2.22	0.44	<0.001	3.08	0.35	<0.001
II v/s IV	-3.21	0.35	<0.001	-0.72	0.44	0.374	-0.99	0.35	0.034
III v/s IV	-3.64	0.35	<0.001	-2.94	0.44	<0.001	-4.08	0.35	<0.001

MD=Mean difference; SE=Standard error; 'p-value'=level of significance

Tensile bond strength

Tensile bond strength showed an increasing trend from day one to day seven in all the groups at all time intervals. These results were in accordance with the study conducted by Huddar et al,[24] and Yanikogtlu et.[25] The authors were of the opinion that increase in the bond strength could have occurred because of the leaching out of the plasticizer, which resulted in increased stiffness. This in turn resulted in mechanical bonding and chemical adhesion between soft liner material and acrylic resin.[17,25] According to Srivastava et al,[11] the bond strength of Viscogel alone and in combination with oregano oil after one day was 3.97 ±0.75 MPa and 3.73±0.65 MPa which increased to 5.40 ±0.49 MPa and 5.11 ±0.66 MPa respectively after one week. These results were contradictory to the results of the studies conducted by Mese et al,[26] in which the tensile bond strength of the acrylic resin-based liner (Coe-Soft) decreased over the tested time period from 0.45 MPa after 24 hours to 0.39 MPa after one week because of the swelling and stress formation at the bond interface or from a change in the viscoelastic properties of the liner rendering the material stiffer and better able to transmit external loads to the bond site. On intergroup comparison a statistically significant difference in tensile bond strength was seen after day one ($p<0.001$) and day three ($p=0.014$), but, no statistically significant difference was noted after day seven ($p=0.060$). However, in another study conducted by Srivastava et al no significant difference was seen in tensile bond strength after addition of oregano oil after day one and day seven which indicated that the tensile bond strength of Viscogel was not affected by the addition of oregano oil.[11] Although, antifungal activity of virgin coconut oil has been previously documented by various authors such as Ogbolu et al[12] and Kannan et al,[13] its effect on tensile bond strength of tissue conditioner after getting incorporated into it has not been studied as yet.

Viscoelasticity

On intragroup comparison, statistically significant difference was found in Group I ($p<0.001$), Group II ($p<0.001$) and Group III ($p=0.038$), while Group IV showed no statistically significant difference ($p=0.596$). A higher value of modulus of elasticity which was noted at the end of seventh days in all the groups except Group III denoted increased stiffness of material indicating that the viscoelasticity deteriorated with time. This was in accordance with the studies conducted by Saitoh et al,[27] Mc carthy et al,[18] and Duran et al[28] in which the authors concluded that an increase in the elastic modulus was noted over the tested time period rendering the material stiffer. This change in the viscoelasticity resulted from leaching out of the components contained in the liquid, especially ethyl alcohol which are replaced by water.[3,29] On application of Tukey HSD tests, it was seen that statistically significant increase in elastic modulus was seen for Group I for all time intervals except for day one versus day three ($p=0.596$). This indicated that Viscogel without any antifungal agents got stiffer at the end of seven days and should be replaced after that. For Group II, this increase in elastic modulus was statistically significant for all time intervals except for day three versus day seven ($p=0.999$) indicating that the viscoelasticity of Viscogel containing 10% w/w fluconazole deteriorated at the end of three days only and so it should not be used beyond that. For Group III and Group IV the change in elastic modulus was not statistically significant for all time intervals ($p>0.05$). This implicated that tissue conditioner containing 60%v/v oregano oil (Group III) and 25%v/v virgin coconut oil (Group IV) remained viscoelastic even at the end of seven days and hence, can be used for a longer duration of time. However, studies related to viscoelasticity of the tissue conditioner after addition of fluconazole, oregano oil and virgin coconut oil have not been conducted till now.

The clinical implications of the results of the present study is that the incorporation of various antifungal agents in the tissue conditioner can serve as an alternative to systemic or topical delivery systems of antifungal drug delivery. When mechanical and physical properties were evaluated, oregano oil showed best results amongst all the tested groups. Since, this herbal product have an added advantage of being safe and cost effective, it can be used as an alternative to the synthetic agents that are currently in use.

There are certain limitations in the present study. The present study was aimed at determining the antifungal activity of different antifungal agents incorporated in the tissue conditioner through measurement of zones of inhibition. However, the antifungal potency is also dependent upon the rate of diffusion of these antifungal agents from Viscogel into agar which in turn is affected by it's concentration, molecular size, viscosity and phase (liquid/solid) of the medium which were not evaluated in the present study.[7] Therefore, studies based on these parameters affecting diffusion rate should be used to evaluate antifungal potency of these antifungal agents. Since, the present study was performed under controlled laboratory conditions therefore, in-vivo studies are suggested for more precise results.

Conclusion

Within the limitations of the study, following conclusions were drawn:

- Maximum antifungal activity was shown by Group II followed by Group III and Group IV.
- Group I had the maximum and Group IV had the minimum tensile bond strength at the end of seven days.
- Viscoelasticity deteriorated for Group I and Group II at the end of seven and three days respectively. While, for Group III and Group IV no significant changes were observed for all time intervals.

Conflict of Interest

Authors declare no conflict of interest in this study.

References

1. Zarb GA, Bolender CL, Eckert SE. Prosthodontic treatment for edentulous patients.12th ed. Noida, India: Elsevier India Private Limited; 2004.
2. Jadhav V, Shetty MM, Kalavathy N, Kumar R. Effect of 3 types of antifungal agents on hardness of 2 different commercially available tissue conditioners: An in-vitro study. *SRM J Res Dent Sci* 2013;4(4):150-3. doi: 10.4103/0976-433X.125590
3. Murata H, Hamada T, Djulaeha E, Nikawa H. Rheology of tissue conditioners. *J Prosthet Dent* 1998;79(2):188-99. doi: 10.1016/S0022-3913(98)70215-X
4. Nam KY. In vitro antimicrobial effect of the tissue conditioner containing silver nanoparticles. *J Adv Prosthodont* 2011;3(1):20-4. doi: 10.4047/jap.2011.3.1.20
5. Mutneja P, Raghavendraswamy K, Gujjari A. Antifungal activity of heat cure acrylic resin after incorporating different percentages of silver zinc zeolite- an in-vitro study. *IJCCI* 2012;4(3):49-54.
6. Sharma S, Hegde V. Comparative Evaluation of Antifungal Activity of Melaleuca Oil and Fluconazole when Incorporated in Tissue Conditioner: An In Vitro Study. *J Prosthodont* 2014;23(5):367-73. doi: 10.1111/jopr.12117
7. Guo N, Liu J, Wu X, Bi X, Meng R, Wang X, et al. Antifungal activity of thymol against clinical isolates of fluconazole-sensitive and -resistant Candida albicans. *J Med Microbiol* 2009;58(Pt 8):1074-9. doi: 10.1099/jmm.0.008052-0
8. Tripathi KD. Essentials of Medical Pharmacology. 6th ed. New Delhi: Jaypee Brothers, Medical Publishers; 2008.
9. Choonharuangdej S, Amornvit P, Srithavaj T, Alam MK. In Vitro Anti-Candida Effect of Thai Herbs Supplemented in Tissue Conditioner. *Int Med J* 2014;21(3):331-4.
10. Pinto E, Vale-Silva L, Cavaleiro C, Salgueiro L. Antifungal activity of the clove essential oil from Syzygium aromaticum on Candida, Aspergillus and dermatophyte species. *J Med Microbiol* 2009;58(Pt 11):1454-62. doi: 10.1099/jmm.0.010538-0
11. Srivastava A, Ginjupalli K, Premapalli N, Bhat N, Ballal M. Evaluation of the properties of a tissue conditioner containing origanum oil as an antifungal additive. *J Prosthet Dent* 2013;110(4):313-9. doi: 10.1016/S0022-3913(13)60381-9
12. Ogbolu DO, Oni AA, Daini OA, Oloko AP. In vitro antimicrobial properties of coconut oil on Candida species in Ibadan, Nigeria. *J Med Food* 2007;10(2):384-7. doi: 10.1089/jmf.2006.1209
13. Kannan N, Mohammed A. Comparative evaluation of antifungal activity of Cocos nucifera oil against candida albicans. *Int J Phytother Res* 2014;4(2):27-31.
14. Mertas A, Garbusinska A, Szliszka E, Jureczko A, Kowalska M, Król W. The influence of Tea Tree Oil (Melaleuca alternifolia) on fluconazole activity against fluconazole-resistant Candida albicans strains. *BioMed Res Int* 2015;2015:590470. doi: 10.1155/2015/590470
15. El-Hadary A, Drummond JL. Comparative study of water sorption, solubility, and tensile bond strength of two soft lining materials. *J Prosthet Dent* 2000;83(3):356-61. doi: 10.1016/S0022-3913(00)70140-5

16. Robinson JG, McCabe JF. Creep and stress relaxation of soft denture liners. *J Prosthet Dent* 1982;48(2):135-40. doi: 10.1016/0022-3913(82)90099-3
17. Safari A, Vojdani M, Mogharrabi S, Iraji Nasrabadi N, Derafshi R. Effect of Beverages on the Hardness and Tensile Bond Strength of Temporary Acrylic Soft Liners to Acrylic Resin Denture Base. *J Dent (Shiraz)* 2013;14(4):178-83.
18. McCarthy JA, Moser JB. Mechanical properties of tissue conditioners. Part I: Theoretical considerations, behavioral characteristics, and tensile properties. *J Prosthet Dent* 1978;40(1):89-97. doi: 10.1016/0022-3913(78)90165-8
19. Chopde N, Pharande A, Khade MN, Khadtare YR, Shah SS, Apratim A. In vitro antifungal activity of two tissue conditioners combined with nystatin, miconazole and fluconazole against candida albicans. *J Contemp Dent Pract* 2012;13(5):695-8. doi: 10.5005/jp-journals-10024-1211
20. Falah-Tafti A, Jafari AA, Lotfi-Kamran MH, Fallahzadeh H, Hayan RS. A comparison of the efficacy of nystatin and fluconazole incorporated into tissue conditioner on the in vitro attachment and colonization of Candida albicans. *Dent Res J (Isfahan)* 2010;7(1):18-22.
21. Manohar V, Ingram C, Gray J, Talpur NA, Echard BW, Bagchi D, et al. Antifungal activities of Origanum oil against Candida albicans. *Mol Cell Biochem* 2001;228(1-2):111-7. doi: 10.1023/A:1013311632207
22. Clancy CJ, Yu VL, Morris AJ, Snydman DR, Nguyen MH. Fluconazole MIC and the Fluconazole Dose/MIC Ratio Correlate with Therapeutic Response among Patients with Candidemia. *Antimicrob Agents Chemother* 2005;49(8):3171-7. doi: 10.1128/AAC.49.8.3171-3177.2005
23. Cleff MB, Meinerz AR, Xavier M, Schuch LF, Araújo Meireles MC, Alves Rodrigues MR, et al. In Vitro Activity Of Origanum Vulgare Essential Oil Against Candida Species. *Braz J Microbiol* 2010;41(1):116-23. doi: 10.1590/S1517-83822010000100018
24. Huddar DA, Hombesh MN, Sandhyarani B, Chandu GS, Nanjannawar GS, Shetty R. Effect of Denture Cleanser on weight, surface roughness and tensile bond strength of two resilient denture liners. *J Contemp Dent Pract* 2012;13(5):607-11.
25. Yanikoglu N, Denizoglu S. The Effect of Different Solutions on the Bond Strength of Soft Lining Materials to Acrylic Resin. *Dent Mater J* 2006;25(1):39-44. doi: 10.4012/dmj.25.39
26. Mese A, Guzel KG. Effect of storage duration on the hardness and tensile bond strength of silicone- and acrylic resin-based resilient denture liners to a processed denture base acrylic resin. *J Prosthet Dent* 2008;99(2):153-9. doi: 10.1016/S0022-3913(08)60032-3
27. Saitoh S, Sasaki K, Nezu T, Taira M. Viscoelastic behavior of commercially available tissue conditioners under compression. *Dent Mater J* 2010;29(4):461-8. doi: 10.4012/dmj.2009-130
28. Duran RL, Powers JM, Craig RG. Viscoelastic and Dynamic Properties of Soft Liners and Tissue Conditioners. *J Dent Res* 1979;58(8):1801-7. doi: 10.1177/00220345790580080601
29. Rodrigues S, Shenoy V, Shetty T. Resilient Liners: A Review. *J Indian Prosthodont Soc* 2013;13(3):155-64. doi: 10.1007/s13191-012-0143-8

The Impact of CRISPR-Cas System on Antiviral Therapy

Hadi Bayat[1,2], Fatemeh Naderi[3], Amjad Hayat Khan[4], Arash Memarnejadian[5], Azam Rahimpour[1]*

[1]Department of Tissue Engineering and Applied Cell Sciences, School of Advanced Technologies in Medicine, Shahid Beheshti University of Medical Sciences, Tehran, Iran.
[2]Department of Molecular Genetics, Faculty of Biological Sciences, Tarbiat Modares University, Tehran, Iran.
[3]Department of Molecular Genetics, Tehran Medical Sciences Branch, Islamic Azad University, Tehran, Iran.
[4]Institute for Research in Molecular Medicine (INFORMM), Universiti Sains Malaysia, Penang, Malaysia.
[5]Department of Hepatitis and AIDS, Pasteur Institute of Iran, Tehran, Iran.

Article info

Keywords:
- CRISPR-Cas
- Antiviral therapy
- Genome editing
- Latent viruses
- Delivery system

Abstract

Clustered regularly interspaced short palindromic repeats (CRISPR)-associated protein nuclease (Cas) is identified as an adaptive immune system in archaea and bacteria. Type II of this system, CRISPR-Cas9, is the most versatile form that has enabled facile and efficient targeted genome editing. Viral infections have serious impacts on global health and conventional antiviral therapies have not yielded a successful solution hitherto. The CRISPR-Cas9 system represents a promising tool for eliminating viral infections. In this review, we highlight 1) the recent progress of CRISPR-Cas technology in decoding and diagnosis of viral outbreaks, 2) its applications to eliminate viral infections in both pre-integration and provirus stages, and 3) various delivery systems that are employed to introduce the platform into target cells.

Introduction

The clustered regularly interspaced short palindromic repeats (CRISPR)-associated protein nuclease (Cas) is a prokaryotic antiviral adaptive immune system, which is present in most archaea (~90%) and some bacteria (~50%). The genomic components of the CRISPR system are made up of trans-activating crRNA (tracrRNA), the *cas* operon, a leader sequence and arrays of short direct repeats. These repeats are interspersed by non-repetitive spacer sequences, which are acquired from mobile invasive elements mainly viruses and plasmids (Figure 1). The CRISPR-Cas system confers the organism's resistance against foreign genetic elements that have previously rendered parts of their genome spacer sequences into the CRISPR array. CRISPR-Cas9 system is derived from type II, the simplest and most commonly used system in genome editing approaches.[1] Host codon-optimized Cas9 is recruited on target site by designable guide-RNA (gRNA) and precisely introduces double strand break (DSB) ~3-base pair (bp) upstream of the protospapcer adjacent motif (PAM). Then, the DSB is repaired with either the error-prone non-homologous end joining (NHEJ) or homology-directed repair (HDR) pathways. NHEJ leaves the genome vulnerable to a lethal genomic mutation, by frameshifting an open reading frame (ORF) on the target gene. Giant viruses also have a defense structure reminiscent of the CRISPR-Cas system. The viral defense system known as the mimivirus virophage resistance element (MIMIVIRE) is composed of proteins with both nuclease and helicase activities, representing an adaptive immune system based on nucleic acid against virophages.[2] Over the recent years, CRISPR-Cas technologies have been well-optimized in eukaryotic cells, particularly in human cells.

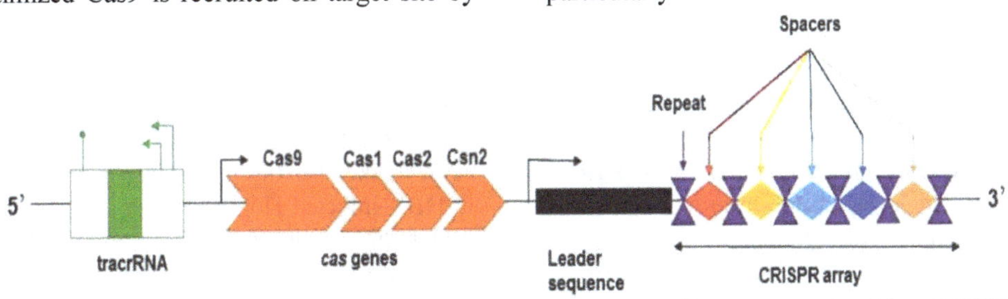

Figure 1. Schematic view of the type II-A CRISPR-Cas system. The components of the CRISPR system ordered from 5' to 3'. tracrRNA: trans-activating crRNA.

***Corresponding author:** Azam Rahimpour, Email: rahimpour@sbmu.ac.ir

Infectious viral diseases are serious global health concerns and despite the huge efforts invested in their eradication, only limited success has been achieved. Establishment of long-term infections leading to chronic disease and also development of antiviral resistant mutants are factors that lead to the persistent viral infections. Novel strategies are required to eliminate even traces of viruses within the host.[3] During the last few years, the applications of CRISPR-Cas9 system have introduced novel antiviral therapeutic options. The advantage of CRISPR-Cas9 technology lies in their ability to directly target the viral DNA or RNA. In this line, the viral infection would be eliminated in the host. CRISPR-Cas systems have shown their efficacy in different viral infections in both pre-integration and provirus stages.[4] Similarly, CRISPR-Cas has generated striking insights for development of novel vaccination strategies in poultry industry. It has been reported that CRISPR-Cas9 system can efficiently modify the genome of duck enteritis virus (DEV) C-KCE strain. The envelope glycoprotein gene and pre-membrane proteins of duck tembusu virus (DTMUV) as well as the hemagglutinin gene of highly pathogenic avian influenza virus (HPAIV) H5N1 were inserted at the suited sites in C-KCE strain to develop a trivalent vaccine that can efficiently prevent the infection of DTMUV, H5N1, and DEV in ducks.[5] In addition to targeting DNA viruses, CRISPR-Cas9 system demonstrated its feasibility and versatility in targeting RNA viruses. Engineered *Francisella novicida* Cas9 (FnCas9) can successfully target positive-sense single strand RNA hepatitis C virus in eukaryotic cells. In contrast to *Streptococcus pyogenes* Cas9 (SpCas9) which needs synthesized PAM-encoding oligomer in targeting RNA *in vitro,* FnCas9 targets the RNA virus PAM-independently. In addition, the ability of FnCas9 to target RNA in cytosol can reduce off-target activity of the system on the host DNA compared to Cas9 which targets DNA in nuclear.[6]

In the current study, we recapitulated the CRISPR-Cas9 system impact on different kinds of viral genomes which can cause either detrimental acute or persistent infection in humans.

Decoding and diagnosis of the obscure viruses

The rapid expansion of human flavivirus infections namely dengue virus (DENV) and Zika virus (ZIKV) have persuaded the research community to devise effective therapies against them. A recent insight about the signaling pathway of flaviviruses, which drives the primary steps of their infection has been successful in providing a schematic diagram of the biology of these viruses. Genome-wide CRISPR-Cas9 screening has identified nine host genes that are involved in flavivirus infectivity. The endoplasmic reticulum (ER) plays an indispensable role in replication, translation, polyprotein processing, virion morphogenesis and consequently, controlling the life cycle of flavivirus.[7] In this line, most of the suspicious genes were associated with ER. Studies have elucidated the unique dependency of flaviviridae on ER-associated signal peptidase complex 1 (SPCS1) proteins. Disruption of SPCS1 processing pathway reduced the infection level of all flaviviridae members.[8] Moreover, orthologous functional genomic CRISPR-Cas9 screening revealed various host factors involved in virus entry (AXL), endocytosis (RAB5C, RABGEF) and transmembrane protein processing and maturation (EMC) which are associated with the infection of the DENV and ZIKV.[9] TLR7/8 agonist R848 strongly restrains ZIKV replication. It is indicated that replication inhibitory effect of R848 is mediated by viperin, an IFN-inducible protein. To confirm this claim, CRISPR-Cas9 genome editing tool was used to knock out (KO) viperin in human MDM cells, as a result, R848 inhibitory effect relieved in KO-cells.[10] The emergent outbreak of ZIKV and the complexities of its infection highlight the need for a low-cost sequence-specific diagnostic platform that can be used in pandemic regions. Likewise, the inferior performance of the detection method based on antibodies and their limitations just as encountering problems with off-targets and gaining false positive results of sequence-based diagnostics; make these conventional methods to meet CRISPR-Cas9 technology, as an alternative strategy.[11] Many strain-specific PAM sites in the Zika strain provide the opportunity to discriminate viral lineages by utilizing a newly established freeze-dried platform termed as 'Nucleic Acid Sequence-Based Amplification (NASBA)-CRISPR'. As part of NASBA reaction 1) the strain-specific PAM sequence, 2) appropriate gRNA, and 3) the double-stranded DNA are produced and subjected to Cas9-mediated split. The presence of a strain-specific PAM leads to the production of truncated RNA product which lacks the sensor H trigger sequence. Contrary to the full-length RNA, the truncated RNA is unable to stimulate the sensor H toehold. Hence, this method could be employed for detecting the strain-specific lineage of the virus without any contamination from other flavivirus types.[12]

The therapeutic application of CRISPR-Cas9 technology to human viruses

Hepatitis B viruses

CRISPR-Cas9 editing tool presents an alternative approach to uproot HBV replication and abolish its latent viral reservoir, i.e. a form of covalently closed circular DNA (cccDNA), in infected cells. Compared to other potential sites, conserved sequences including C, P, S, and X ORFs in HBV genome are more precedent in order to be used as potential targets for designing gRNA. Owing to minor concordance between the conserved sequences of HBV and human genome, the off-target mutations will restrain on host's genome while alleviating viral infections simultaneously. Designed gRNAs have been shown to reduce the HBV DNA level from 77 to 98% in cultured cells.[13] Likewise, designed gRNAs targeting HBV cccDNA in HBV-infected HepG2/NTCP cells has resulted in eight-fold reduction in the expression of HBcAg.[14] Targeting multiple regions of HBV genome by co-transfection of several gRNAs has been reported to increase the effectiveness of the approach.[15] A number of studies have been designed to take advantage of introducing large deletions via CRISPR-Cas9 system in combination with the efficiency of lentivirus mediated gene transfer to effectively prevent the HBV replication.[16] Owing to fact that CRISPR-Cas9 technology can affect the off-target sites, design and characterization of fastidious CRISPR-Cas9 system for more precise targeting of invasive elements should be a matter of focus. In this context, a more accurate form of CRISPR-Cas9 technology, Cas9 nickases (Cas9n), has been proposed for targeting conserved sequences in the S and X ORFs of the HBV genome. This strategy was able to disrupt HBV replication in chronically and *de novo* infected hepatoma cell lines as well as episomal cccDNA and chromosomally integrated HBV target sites.[17] As a proof of concept, it is required to evaluate the antiviral effect of CRISPR-Cas9 system in more pertinent *in vivo* models of HBV infection.

Human immunodeficiency virus

Human immunodeficiency virus (HIV-1) is a major global health problem for which no effectual vaccine is available. The latent reservoir of HIV-1 can persist for as long as 60 years in CD4+ T cells. Purging of HIV-1 reservoirs is the effective cure to obviate the expansion of the virus into healthy cells in patients. Two main strategies are currently followed to cure the HIV-1 infection: 1) a functional cure, in which the viral replication is controlled while latent reservoir still remains; e.g. the impairment of the CCR5 receptors, and 2) a sterilizing cure, in which even viral traces are eliminated from the infected cells.[18] Individuals carrying a 32-bp deletion in their *CCR5* gene (*CCR5Δ32*) are instinctively resistant to HIV-1 infection. By transplanting *CCR5Δ32* hematopoietic stem cells, one can easily devise a sterilizing cure strategy. However, tropism shift to CXCR4 can occur to cope with the impairment of CXCR5. Exploiting CRISPR-Cas9 system can overwhelm this hurdle, because this system has the potential to disrupt CXCR4 without affecting the cell propagation.[19] Introduction of the homozygous CCR5Δ32 mutation in induced pluripotent stem cells (iPSCs) using the combination of CRISPR-Cas9 system and a PiggyBac transposon caused a significant resistance to HIV infection. Also, downstream lineage, the monocytes and the macrophages derived from these engineered iPSCs, represented the same resistance. Therefore, these new established cells could be considered as a source for autologous therapy in HIV infection.[20] To overcome little activity of CRISPR system in $CD4^+$ T cells, it is possible to utilize a dual gRNA approach for inducing biallelic deletion in CCR5 gene and consequently, improve the disruption of CD4+ T cells and $CD34^+$ HSPCs.[21] Recently, Cas9 ribonucleoprotein (RNP) complex has been used to target host factors that are involved in HIV infection. As a result, a tropism-dependent resistance to HIV infection is pointed out in CXCR4 or CCR5 disrupted T-cells. Remarkably, simultaneous targeting of CXCR4 and CCR5 by CRISPR-Cas9 system, significantly decreased tropic-dependent HIV-1 in CXCR4- and CCR5-modifed cells (TZM-bl cells, Jurkat T cells, and human $CD4^+$ T cells) without any cytotoxic effects on cells viability.[22] Moreover, targeting the factors that are involved in later stages of initial HIV infection, such as LEDGF or TNPO3, represented a tropism-autonomous diminution in infected T-cells.[23] Furthermore, CRSPR-based genetic screen discovered that three host dependency factors (*TPST2*, *SLC35B2*, and *ALCAM*) play vital roles in HIV infection in primary $CD4^+$ T cells.[24] In order to target the proviral DNA efficiently, it is utterly crucial to eradicate the viral remnant sequences from cells completely. Long terminal repeat (LTR) is an important element in augmenting transcription of potentially toxic proteins in HIV infectivity. To eliminate the entire viral genome, recruiting Cas9 simultaneously to 5' and 3' LTR will untwist HIV genome from infected cells.[25] Recently, it was reported that HIV-1 genome can be eradicated from the host genome in 2D10 $CD4^+$ T-cells, where CRISPR-Cas9 system was delivered by lentiviral vector to target LTR U3 regions.[26] In a further attempt, recombinant Adeno-associated virus 9 delivery of SaCas9, a shorter variant of Cas9 derived from *Staphylococcus aureus*, was adapted to excise segments of integrated HIV-1 by targeting within the 5′-LTR and the gag gene in transgenic mouse and rat. This was the first report that clarified the promising results of CRISPR-cas9 system for *in vivo* studies.[27]

What would happen if we design gRNAs targeting non-conserved regions in HIV-1 genome? The question was answered recently in $CD4^+$ T cells expressing Cas9 and gRNA ceaselessly. It is elucidated that targeting non-conserved regions resulted in noticeable obstacle of the infection in transient assays but after a variable time all targeted infections came up with a high level of HIV-1 production. Moreover, after a longer time, targeting conserved regions in HIV-1 genome showed an escape as well. Genome sequencing of escaped viruses has disclosed that the gRNA binding site and PAM region in HIV-1 genome were eradicate by some mutations that were introduced by error-prone NHEJ repair pathway.[28] Several approaches can be used to vanquish HIV-1 escape including multiplex targeting by designing strong gRNAs to direct Cas9 on conserved regions,[29] utilizing Cas9 variants that recognize different PAM formats,[30] using CRISPR-like enzyme such as Cpf1 that introduces cut in the distal site of the binding site,[31] and abrogation of NHEJ by chemical drugs for instance SCR7.[32] Table 1 shows CRISPR-Cas9 targeting sites in other virus infections.

Delivery of CRISPR-Cas9 components

Despite investing considerable effort in gene therapy during the last decades, limited success has been achieved due to the shortcomings of existing viral and non-viral gene delivery approaches. Generally, viral delivery systems can be categorized into four main classes 1) adenoviruses, 2) adeno-associated viruses (AAV), 3) retroviruses, and 4) lentiviruses. Lentiviruses are derived from HIV-1 and have the potential to cause undesirable modifications in long-term expression cell lines. Thus, integrase-defective lentiviruses which are replication incompatible or at least single-cycle replicable are more preferred. This preference is more prominent in the case of genome editing that requires long-term expression of the genome editing components and engages an increased risk of unwanted off-target changes.[33] CRISPR-Cas9 system packaged with lentiviral vectors has shown promising results in eliminating latent HIV-1 infection. Moreover, prepackaged Cas9 in a transient form of virus-like particles that target CCR5 represents a reduced off-target effect in target cells.[34] Recombinant AAV vectors have low pathogenicity and low immunogenicity compared to other viral vectors, but their main obstacle is their limited packaging size. The size limitation of AAV vectors can be overcome by exploiting *SaCas9* (3.3 kb) or by using split-Cas9 approaches.[35] *In vivo* genome editing generally requires an effective method to deliver the components of editing tools appropriately. For the first time, it was demonstrated that delivering multiplex saCas9/sgRNA, targeting two LTR sites and two structural proteins, in an all-in-one AAV–DJ/8 vector can be applied to precisely excise HIV-1 proviral from pre-clinical mouse models.[36] This strategy is a promising approach to eradicate even trace of proviral in different organs by simultaneously introducing indels and large deletions at HIV-1 reservoirs. Despite the high productivity of viral vectors, certain limitations such as immunogenicity and random integration of conventional viral vectors led the studies to fluctuate delivery approaches with a view to non-viral gene delivery.[37] So far, different classes of non-viral vectors have been introduced. Non-viral expression plasmid is the most convenient delivery approach that can express CRISPR-Cas system in a safe mode. However, random integration of the plasmids and difficulty in controlling their timeframe expression are the main obstacles. To address these drawbacks, CRISPR mRNA delivery system has been employed, which illustrates great refinement in decreasing the risk of off-target activity by controlling the amount of Cas9 protein and gRNA level.[38] Besides, rapid deterioration of plasmid and mRNA by serum nucleases is another major hurdle that must be resolved. The use of RNPs is another approach to delivering Cas9-gRNA with higher control on editing timeframe. Delivering RNPs by using electroporation method has showed promising results in targeting host factors that are involved in HIV-1 infected $CD4^+$ T cells.[23] However, some complications such as the negative charge of RNAs, flimsy structure, and the large molecular size of proteins limit the diffusion rate of RNPs across the cell membrane. To overcome reduced delivery efficiency of non-viral delivery platforms, positively-charged nano-carriers can be employed as an ideal delivery system. Yarn-like DNA nano-clew is a form of cationic nano-carriers which can be loaded with CRISPR-Cas9 technology to shuttle Cas9-gRNA into the target cell. This method provides stability between binding and discharge of the CRISPR-Cas9 system.[39] Microfluidic membrane deformation (MMD) through the transient disruption of the cell membrane has been exploited as a Cas9-gRNA delivery platform. Similar to microinjection, MMD can deliver payload across different cell types even hard-to-transfect cells, but in an easier manner with a higher yield. Moreover, MMD has portrayed more cell viability than electroporation method. Collectively, MMD seems to warrant a precise and efficient genome editingapproach.[40]

Table 1. CRISPR-Cas9 targeting sites in different virus infections. Applying CRISPR-Cas9 technology to target virus genomes and to find signaling pathways that are involved in virus infections

Virus	Gene target site in virus/Human	Model	Delivery	Reference
EBV	EBNA1, LMP1, EBNA3C	Burkitt's lymphoma cell lines Raji cell	Transfection	41
	BVRF1	Gastric Cancer Cell line, SUN719 and YCCEL1	Transfection	42
	BART5, BART6, or BART16	gastric carcinoma cell line SNU-719	Transduction	43
HTLV1	pX region	ED T-Cell	Transduction	44
	RNF8	HeLa cells	Electroporation	45
JCV	T-antigen	Human oligodendroglioma cell line, primary human fetal glial cells	Transfection	46
	NCCR-a and VP1-b	glial derived SVG-A cells and human fetal kidney derived hTERT transformed HuK(i)G10 cells	Transduction	47
HPV	E6	SiHa and CaSki cells (cervical carcinoma cell lines)	Transfection	48
	E7	SiHa and Caski cells	Transfection	49
	E7	HeLa cells	Nano-micelle	50
HSV	UL8, UL29, and UL52	Vero cells	Transduction	43
	ICP0	HEK293T cells	Transduction	51
	UL7	HEK293T cells, Vero cells and BALB/c mice	Transfection	52
HCV	5′-UTR and 3′-UTR regions	Huh-7.5 cells	Transfection	6
	ISG15	U2OS cells	Transfection	53
	miR-122	Huh-7.5 cells	Transfection	54
	miR-122/hcr locus	hepatoma cells	Transfection	55

EBV: Epstein–Barr virus, HTLV1: Human T-lymphotropic virus 1, JCV: JC virus, HPV: Human papilloma virus, HSV: Herpes simplex virus, HCV: Hepatitis C virus, EBNA1: Epstein–Barr Nuclear Antigen 1, LMP1: Latent Membrane Protein 1, EBNA3C: Epstein–Barr nuclear antigen 3C, BVRF1: DNA packaging tegument protein UL25 of EBV, BART5, BART6, or BART16: BamHI-A rightward transcript 5, 6 or 16, pX region: A region of HTLV1 genome which encodes regulatory and accessory genes, RNF8: Ring Finger Protein 8, T-antigen: Large tumor Antigen, NCCR-a: non-coding control region-a, VP1-b: Viral Protein 1, E6 and E7: Early proteins 6 and 7, UL8, UL29, UL52 and UL7: Unique Long 8, 29, 52 and 7, ICP0: Infected-Cell Protein 0, 5′-UTR and 3′-UTR: 5′ and 3′ Untranslated Region, ISG15: Interferon Stimulated Genes 15, miR-122 : microRNA-122, hcr locus: hepatocellular carcinoma related locus

Conclusion

The versatility and feasibility of the CRISPR-Cas9 system remove some of the impediments that has challenged gene therapy approaches and introduce new opportunities in antiviral therapies. Despite the massive growth spurt of CRISPR-Cas9 technology over the last years, major efforts are needed to address the remaining impediments and develop CRISPR-Cas9 based safe delivery technologies. Further studies are required to investigate the immune responses to exogenously expressed CRISPR-Cas9 system and devise strategies to mask this system and thus reduce their immunogenicity. High-fidelity Cas9 variants introduced their efficacy in the field of genome editing by reducing off-target effects.[1] Application of these variants to eradicate viral infection from host genome may bring forth new perspective. Viral and non-viral delivery systems have their own drawbacks when applied in gene therapy approaches. Recent studies have shown that by combining lipid nanoparticle-mediated delivery of Cas9 mRNA and AAVs encoding gRNA and donor template, efficient *in vivo* restoration of > 6% can be achieved in a mouse model of human hereditary tyrosinemia.[37] The combination of these two conventional delivery methods could pave the way for curing viral infections in clinical settings.

Acknowledgments

Authors wish to thank School of Advanced Technologies in Medicine, Shahid Beheshti University of Medical Sciences for its support.

Conflict of Interest

The authors declare no conflict of interests.

References

1. Bayat H, Omidi M, Rajabibazl M, Sabri S, Rahimpour A. The crispr growth spurt: From bench to clinic on versatile small rnas. *J Microbiol Biotechnol* 2017;27(2):207-18. doi: 10.4014/jmb.1607.07005
2. Levasseur A, Bekliz M, Chabriere E, Pontarotti P, La Scola B, Raoult D. Mimivire is a defence system in mimivirus that confers resistance to virophage. *Nature* 2016;531(7593):249-52. doi: 10.1038/nature17146
3. Kennedy EM, Cullen BR. Bacterial crispr/cas DNA endonucleases: A revolutionary technology that could dramatically impact viral research and treatment. *Virology* 2015;479-480:213-20. doi: 10.1016/j.virol.2015.02.024
4. Chen S, Hou C, Bi H, Wang Y, Xu J, Li M, et al. Transgenic clustered regularly interspaced short palindromic repeat/cas9-mediated viral gene targeting for antiviral therapy of bombyx mori nucleopolyhedrovirus. *J Virol* 2017;91(8). doi: 10.1128/JVI.02465-16
5. Zou Z, Huang K, Wei Y, Chen H, Liu Z, Jin M. Construction of a highly efficient crispr/cas9-mediated duck enteritis virus-based vaccine against h5n1 avian influenza virus and duck tembusu virus infection. *Sci Rep* 2017;7(1):1478. doi: 10.1038/s41598-017-01554-1
6. Price AA, Sampson TR, Ratner HK, Grakoui A, Weiss DS. Cas9-mediated targeting of viral rna in eukaryotic cells. *Proc Natl Acad Sci U S A* 2015;112(19):6164-9. doi: 10.1073/pnas.1422340112
7. Ma H, Dang Y, Wu Y, Jia G, Anaya E, Zhang J, et al. A crispr-based screen identifies genes essential for west-nile-virus-induced cell death. *Cell Rep* 2015;12(4):673-83. doi: 10.1016/j.celrep.2015.06.049
8. Zhang R, Miner JJ, Gorman MJ, Rausch K, Ramage H, White JP, et al. A crispr screen defines a signal peptide processing pathway required by flaviviruses. *Nature* 2016;535(7610):164-8. doi: 10.1038/nature18625
9. Savidis G, McDougall WM, Meraner P, Perreira JM, Portmann JM, Trincucci G, et al. Identification of zika virus and dengue virus dependency factors using functional genomics. *Cell Rep* 2016;16(1):232-46. doi: 10.1016/j.celrep.2016.06.028
10. Vanwalscappel B, Tada T, Landau NR. Toll-like receptor agonist r848 blocks zika virus replication by inducing the antiviral protein viperin. *Virology* 2018;522:199-208. doi: 10.1016/j.virol.2018.07.014
11. Campos Rde M, Cirne-Santos C, Meira GL, Santos LL, de Meneses MD, Friedrich J, et al. Prolonged detection of zika virus rna in urine samples during the ongoing zika virus epidemic in brazil. *J Clin Virol* 2016;77:69-70. doi: 10.1016/j.jcv.2016.02.009
12. Pardee K, Green AA, Takahashi MK, Braff D, Lambert G, Lee JW, et al. Rapid, low-cost detection of zika virus using programmable biomolecular components. *Cell* 2016;165(5):1255-66. doi: 10.1016/j.cell.2016.04.059
13. Ramanan V, Shlomai A, Cox DB, Schwartz RE, Michailidis E, Bhatta A, et al. Crispr/cas9 cleavage of viral DNA efficiently suppresses hepatitis b virus. *Sci Rep* 2015;5:10833. doi: 10.1038/srep10833
14. Seeger C, Sohn JA. Complete spectrum of crispr/cas9-induced mutations on hbv cccdna. *Mol Ther* 2016;24(7):1258-66. doi: 10.1038/mt.2016.94
15. Liu X, Hao R, Chen S, Guo D, Chen Y. Inhibition of hepatitis b virus by the crispr/cas9 system via targeting the conserved regions of the viral genome. *J Gen Virol* 2015;96(8):2252-61. doi: 10.1099/vir.0.000159
16. Kennedy EM, Bassit LC, Mueller H, Kornepati AVR, Bogerd HP, Nie T, et al. Suppression of

hepatitis b virus DNA accumulation in chronically infected cells using a bacterial crispr/cas rna-guided DNA endonuclease. *Virology* 2015;476:196-205. doi: 10.1016/j.virol.2014.12.001
17. Karimova M, Beschorner N, Dammermann W, Chemnitz J, Indenbirken D, Bockmann JH, et al. Crispr/cas9 nickase-mediated disruption of hepatitis b virus open reading frame s and x. *Sci Rep* 2015;5:13734. doi: 10.1038/srep13734
18. Haworth KG, Peterson CW, Kiem HP. Ccr5-edited gene therapies for hiv cure: Closing the door to viral entry. *Cytotherapy* 2017;19(11):1325-38. doi: 10.1016/j.jcyt.2017.05.013
19. Hou P, Chen S, Wang S, Yu X, Chen Y, Jiang M, et al. Genome editing of cxcr4 by crispr/cas9 confers cells resistant to hiv-1 infection. *Sci Rep* 2015;5:15577. doi: 10.1038/srep15577
20. Ye L, Wang J, Beyer AI, Teque F, Cradick TJ, Qi Z, et al. Seamless modification of wild-type induced pluripotent stem cells to the natural ccr5delta32 mutation confers resistance to hiv infection. *Proc Natl Acad Sci U S A* 2014;111(26):9591-6. doi: 10.1073/pnas.1407473111
21. Mandal PK, Ferreira LM, Collins R, Meissner TB, Boutwell CL, Friesen M, et al. Efficient ablation of genes in human hematopoietic stem and effector cells using crispr/cas9. *Cell Stem Cell* 2014;15(5):643-52. doi: 10.1016/j.stem.2014.10.004
22. Liu Z, Chen S, Jin X, Wang Q, Yang K, Li C, et al. Genome editing of the hiv co-receptors ccr5 and cxcr4 by crispr-cas9 protects cd4(+) t cells from hiv-1 infection. *Cell Biosci* 2017;7:47. doi: 10.1186/s13578-017-0174-2
23. Hultquist JF, Schumann K, Woo JM, Manganaro L, McGregor MJ, Doudna J, et al. A cas9 ribonucleoprotein platform for functional genetic studies of hiv-host interactions in primary human t cells. *Cell Rep* 2016;17(5):1438-52. doi: 10.1016/j.celrep.2016.09.080
24. Park RJ, Wang T, Koundakjian D, Hultquist JF, Lamothe-Molina P, Monel B, et al. A genome-wide crispr screen identifies a restricted set of hiv host dependency factors. *Nat Genet* 2017;49(2):193–203. doi: 10.1038/ng.3741
25. Hu W, Kaminski R, Yang F, Zhang Y, Cosentino L, Li F, et al. Rna-directed gene editing specifically eradicates latent and prevents new hiv-1 infection. *Proc Natl Acad Sci U S A* 2014;111(31):11461-6. doi: 10.1073/pnas.1405186111
26. Kaminski R, Chen Y, Fischer T, Tedaldi E, Napoli A, Zhang Y, et al. Elimination of hiv-1 genomes from human t-lymphoid cells by crispr/cas9 gene editing. *Sci Rep* 2016;6:22555. doi: 10.1038/srep22555
27. Kaminski R, Bella R, Yin C, Otte J, Ferrante P, Gendelman HE, et al. Excision of hiv-1 DNA by gene editing: A proof-of-concept in vivo study. *Gene Ther* 2016;23(8-9):690-5. doi: 10.1038/gt.2016.41
28. Wang Z, Pan Q, Gendron P, Zhu W, Guo F, Cen S, et al. Crispr/cas9-derived mutations both inhibit hiv-1 replication and accelerate viral escape. *Cell Rep* 2016;15(3):481-9. doi: 10.1016/j.celrep.2016.03.042
29. Lebbink RJ, de Jong DC, Wolters F, Kruse EM, van Ham PM, Wiertz EJ, et al. A combinational crispr/cas9 gene-editing approach can halt hiv replication and prevent viral escape. *Sci Rep* 2017;7:41968. doi: 10.1038/srep41968
30. Anders C, Bargsten K, Jinek M. Structural plasticity of pam recognition by engineered variants of the rna-guided endonuclease cas9. *Mol Cell* 2016;61(6):895-902. doi: 10.1016/j.molcel.2016.02.020
31. Bayat H, Modarressi MH, Rahimpour A. The conspicuity of crispr-cpf1 system as a significant breakthrough in genome editing. *Curr Microbiol* 2018;75(1):107-15. doi: 10.1007/s00284-017-1406-8
32. Xiong X, Chen M, Lim WA, Zhao D, Qi LS. Crispr/cas9 for human genome engineering and disease research. *Annu Rev Genomics Hum Genet* 2016;17:131-54. doi: 10.1146/annurev-genom-083115-022258
33. Chen X, Goncalves MA. Engineered viruses as genome editing devices. *Mol Ther* 2016;24(3):447-57. doi: 10.1038/mt.2015.164
34. Choi JG, Dang Y, Abraham S, Ma H, Zhang J, Guo H, et al. Lentivirus pre-packed with cas9 protein for safer gene editing. *Gene Ther* 2016;23(7):627-33. doi: 10.1038/gt.2016.27
35. Zetsche B, Volz SE, Zhang F. A split-cas9 architecture for inducible genome editing and transcription modulation. *Nat Biotechnol* 2015;33(2):139-42. doi: 10.1038/nbt.3149
36. Yin C, Zhang T, Qu X, Zhang Y, Putatunda R, Xiao X, et al. In vivo excision of hiv-1 provirus by sacas9 and multiplex single-guide rnas in animal models. *Mol Ther* 2017;25(5):1168-86. doi: 10.1016/j.ymthe.2017.03.012
37. Yin H, Song CQ, Dorkin JR, Zhu LJ, Li Y, Wu Q, et al. Therapeutic genome editing by combined viral and non-viral delivery of crispr system components in vivo. *Nat Biotechnol* 2016;34(3):328-33. doi: 10.1038/nbt.3471
38. Carte J, Wang R, Li H, Terns RM, Terns MP. Cas6 is an endoribonuclease that generates guide rnas for invader defense in prokaryotes. *Genes Dev* 2008;22(24):3489-96. doi: 10.1101/gad.1742908
39. Sun W, Ji W, Hall JM, Hu Q, Wang C, Beisel CL, et al. Self-assembled DNA nanoclews for the efficient delivery of crispr-cas9 for genome editing. *Angew Chem Int Ed Engl* 2015;54(41):12029-33. doi: 10.1002/anie.201506030
40. Han X, Liu Z, Jo MC, Zhang K, Li Y, Zeng Z, et al. Crispr-cas9 delivery to hard-to-transfect cells via

membrane deformation. *Sci Adv* 2015;1(7):e1500454. doi: 10.1126/sciadv.1500454
41. Wang J, Quake SR. Rna-guided endonuclease provides a therapeutic strategy to cure latent herpesviridae infection. *Proc Natl Acad Sci U S A* 2014;111(36):13157-62. doi: 10.1073/pnas.1410785111
42. Kanda T, Furuse Y, Oshitani H, Kiyono T. Highly efficient crispr/cas9-mediated cloning and functional characterization of gastric cancer-derived epstein-barr virus strains. *J Virol* 2016;90(9):4383-93. doi: 10.1128/JVI.00060-16
43. van Diemen FR, Kruse EM, Hooykaas MJ, Bruggeling CE, Schurch AC, van Ham PM, et al. Crispr/cas9-mediated genome editing of herpesviruses limits productive and latent infections. *PLoS Pathog* 2016;12(6):e1005701. doi: 10.1371/journal.ppat.1005701
44. Satou Y, Miyazato P, Ishihara K, Yaguchi H, Melamed A, Miura M, et al. The retrovirus htlv-1 inserts an ectopic ctcf-binding site into the human genome. *Proc Natl Acad Sci U S A* 2016;113(11):3054-9. doi: 10.1073/pnas.1423199113
45. Ho YK, Zhi H, Bowlin T, Dorjbal B, Philip S, Zahoor MA, et al. Htlv-1 tax stimulates ubiquitin e3 ligase, ring finger protein 8, to assemble lysine 63-linked polyubiquitin chains for tak1 and ikk activation. *PLoS Pathog* 2015;11(8):e1005102. doi: 10.1371/journal.ppat.1005102
46. Wollebo HS, Bellizzi A, Kaminski R, Hu W, White MK, Khalili K. Crispr/cas9 system as an agent for eliminating polyomavirus jc infection. *PLoS ONE* 2015;10(9):e0136046. doi: 10.1371/journal.pone.0136046
47. Chou YY, Krupp A, Kaynor C, Gaudin R, Ma M, Cahir-McFarland E, et al. Inhibition of jcpyv infection mediated by targeted viral genome editing using crispr/cas9. *Sci Rep* 2016;6:36921. doi: 10.1038/srep36921
48. Yu L, Wang X, Zhu D, Ding W, Wang L, Zhang C, et al. Disruption of human papillomavirus 16 e6 gene by clustered regularly interspaced short palindromic repeat/cas system in human cervical cancer cells. *Onco Targets Ther* 2015;8:37-44. doi: 10.2147/OTT.S64092
49. Hu Z, Yu L, Zhu D, Ding W, Wang X, Zhang C, et al. Disruption of hpv16-e7 by crispr/cas system induces apoptosis and growth inhibition in hpv16 positive human cervical cancer cells. *Biomed Res Int* 2014;2014:612823. doi: 10.1155/2014/612823
50. Lao YH, Li M, Gao MA, Shao D, Chi CW, Huang D, et al. Hpv oncogene manipulation using nonvirally delivered crispr/cas9 or natronobacterium gregoryi argonaute. *Adv Sci (Weinh)* 2018;5(7):1700540. doi: 10.1002/advs.201700540
51. Lin C, Li H, Hao M, Xiong D, Luo Y, Huang C, et al. Increasing the efficiency of crispr/cas9-mediated precise genome editing of hsv-1 virus in human cells. *Sci Rep* 2016;6:34531. doi: 10.1038/srep34531
52. Xu X, Fan S, Zhou J, Zhang Y, Che Y, Cai H, et al. The mutated tegument protein ul7 attenuates the virulence of herpes simplex virus 1 by reducing the modulation of alpha-4 gene transcription. *Virol J* 2016;13:152. doi: 10.1186/s12985-016-0600-9
53. Domingues P, Bamford CG, Boutell C, McLauchlan J. Inhibition of hepatitis c virus rna replication by isg15 does not require its conjugation to protein substrates by the herc5 e3 ligase. *J Gen Virol* 2015;96(11):3236-42. doi: 10.1099/jgv.0.000283
54. Hopcraft SE, Azarm KD, Israelow B, Leveque N, Schwarz MC, Hsu TH, et al. Viral determinants of mir-122-independent hepatitis c virus replication. *mSphere* 2016;1(1):e00009. doi: 10.1128/mSphere.00009-15
55. Senis E, Mockenhaupt S, Rupp D, Bauer T, Paramasivam N, Knapp B, et al. Talen/crispr-mediated engineering of a promoterless anti-viral rnai hairpin into an endogenous mirna locus. *Nucleic Acids Res* 2016;45(1):e3. doi: 10.1093/nar/gkw805

31

Strategies for Improving siRNA-Induced Gene Silencing Efficiency

Fatemeh Safari[1,2,3]*, Solmaz Rahmani Barouji[4], Ali Mohammad Tamaddon[5]

[1] *Medical Biotechnology Department, Faculty of Advanced Medical Sciences, Tabriz University of Medical Sciences, Tabriz, Iran.*
[2] *Shiraz University of Medical Sciences, Shiraz, Iran.*
[3] *Student Research Committee, Tabriz University of Medical Sciences, Tabriz, Iran.*
[4] *Department of Traditional Medicine, Faculty of Traditional Medicine, University of Medical Sciences, Tabriz, Iran.*
[5] *Center for Pharmaceutical Nanotechnology and Biomaterials, Faculty of Pharmacy, Shiraz University of Medical Sciences, Shiraz, Iran.*

Article info

Keywords:
· RNA Interference
· hTERT
· Gene silencing

Abstract

Purpose: Human telomerase reverse transcriptase (hTERT) plays a crucial role in tumorigenesis and progression of cancers. Gene silencing of hTERT by short interfering RNA (siRNA) is considered as a promising strategy for cancer gene therapy. Various algorithms have been devised for designing a high efficient siRNA which is a significant issue in the clinical usage. Thereby, in the present study, the relation of siRNA designing criteria and the gene silencing efficiency was evaluated.

Methods: The siRNA sequences were designed and characterized by using on line soft wares. Cationic co-polymer (polyethylene glycol-g-polyethylene imine (PEG-g-PEI)) was used for the construction of polyelectrolyte complexes (PECs) containing siRNAs. The cellular uptake of the PECs was evaluated. The gene silencing efficiency of different siRNA sequences was investigated and the effect of observing the rational designing on the functionality of siRNAs was assessed.

Results: The size of PEG-g-PEI siRNA with N/P (Nitrogen/Phosphate) ratio of 2.5 was 114 ± 0.645 nm. The transfection efficiency of PECs was desirable (95.5% ± 2.4%.). The results of Real-Time PCR showed that main sequence (MS) reduced the hTERT expression up to 90% and control positive sequence (CPS) up to 63%. These findings demonstrated that the accessibility to the target site has priority than the other criteria such as sequence preferences and thermodynamic features.

Conclusion: siRNA opens a hopeful window in cancer therapy which provides a convenient and tolerable therapeutic approach. Thereby, using the set of criteria and rational algorithms in the designing of siRNA remarkably affect the gene silencing efficiency.

Introduction

The hTERT (human telomerase reverse transcriptase) gene is a key component of the telomerase catalytic activity, which encodes the reverse transcriptase part of the telomerase complex.[1] The abnormity of hTERT is considered to be associated with tumorigenesis in 85% of various tumors such as breast, prostate, lung, liver, pancreas, and colon cancer.[2] Down-regulation of hTERT has been introduced as a highly attractive approach for cancer treatment.

RNA interference (RNAi) is a sequence-specific gene silencing system which knocks down the gene expression by using double-stranded RNA (dsRNA) homologous to the target gene.[3] The capability of siRNA to induce gene silencing introduces this mechanism as a powerful functional genomic tool.[4] The gene silencing effects of RNAi can be exerted by two different mechanisms. Small interfering RNAs (siRNAs), a sequence containing 21 nucleotides (nt) with two nucleotide overhang, transiently knock down the genes.[5] Short hairpin RNAs (shRNAs) principally provide the stable silencing of genes and are processed by Dicer into siRNAs.[6] The gene silencing mediated by siRNA is started by the direct entrance of siRNA into the RNA induced silencing complex (RISC). The assembling of the guide (antisense) strand with the RISC, activates this complex. The RISC activation induces different mechanisms varying from the repression of translation to the degradation of mRNA which is dependent on the target site of mRNA. Targeting the coding sequence (CDS) with siRNA modulates transcript levels by Argonaute (Ago)2-mediated transcript cleavage. However, targeting 3′untranslated region (UTR) of mRNA by complementary siRNA leads to translational repression which mediated by Ago1, Ago3 and Ago4.[7,8]

The efficiency of siRNA is dependent on various factors including sequence space, target availability, the position of nucleotides, secondary structures of mRNA and intrinsic characteristics of siRNA and target mRNA. Sequence space is the region of a gene which is selected for targeting by siRNA. Recently, regions of the gene

***Corresponding author:** Fatemeh Safari, Email: safarif@tbzmed.ac.ir that are transcribed such as the 5′ and 3′ UTRs and open reading frame (ORF) have been introduced as the appropriate targets. But currently, the regions about 50–100 nucleotides downstream of the start codon in the ORF is recommended. Because in the 5′UTR and sequences close to the start codon, regulatory proteins make space hindrance for RISC and interfere with silencing effect.[9]

At the first step of siRNA designing, the target sequence is searched to find motifs such as 5′-AA(N19)TT, 5′-AA(N21) or 5′-NA(N21). The GC content of the sequence is an important parameter that affects siRNA functionality. It is recommended to choose the sequences with the low to the medium proportion (30–64%) of GC content.[10]

The propensity of a duplex to form internal hairpins and the relative stability are two significant factors of siRNA efficiency which can be estimated by prediction of melting temperatures (Tm).[11] Sequences with the Tm of 20-60 °C is recommended because the siRNAs with this range of Tm are better silencer.[12] Another strong determinant of siRNA functionality is the secondary structures of the mRNA which represents the level of the accessibility to the target site.[13] The asymmetry of siRNA duplex ends is a significant parameter for improvement of siRNA efficacy. This parameter is based on the requirement of less stable 5′end of the antisense strand than 5′end of the sense strand. Achieving this asymmetry needs high A/U content at the 5′end of the antisense strand and high G/C at the 5′end of the sense strand.[14,15] Also, a number of position-specific nucleotide preferences have an influence on the gene silencing efficiency of siRNA (Table 1).[16] The ability of sense and antisense strands to form the duplex has a direct relation with a functionality of siRNA, so any secondary structures may diminish the functionality.

In addition, checking the specificity of siRNA is a crucial issue to reduce the risk of unintended gene silencing which is called off-target effect. Both strands of siRNA must be checked by the BLAST (basic local alignment search tool) online software. The siRNA sequence represents less than 78% query coverage with other genes may be a desirable sequence.[17]

Table 1. A combination of the most important criteria for siRNA designing and scoring system

Criteria	score
GC content 30-52%	1
Up to 5 A/U in position 15-19 of S strand	1 per A/U
Inverse repeat	1
A in position 19	1
A in position 3	1
U in position 10	1
G/C in position 19	1
G in position 13	-1
Relative stability of internal siRNA duplex	1
Internal stability	1

Considering these issues, various rational algorithms have been devised for designing more efficient siRNAs.[15,16,18] Each of these algorithms has focused on the specific dimensions but, sometimes overlap with each other. On the basis of these algorithms, lots of online soft wares have emerged in the area of siRNA designing. Each of these computational tools is in accordance with different parameters to provide an individual scoring system for siRNA designing (Table 2).

Numerous studies have investigated the effects of the rational designing on the gene silencing activity of siRNA. In the study ahead, the effect of these criteria and their priority on the efficiency of siRNA were assessed. Our findings showed that the accessibility to the target site is more important than other criteria. However, in designing an efficient siRNA other parameters such as thermodynamic features and sequence preferences should be observed.

Table 2. Names and addresses of siRNA design computational soft wares

Soft wares	Address
siDirect	http://genomics.jp/sidirect/index.php?type=fc
siDESIGN Center	dharmacon.gelifesciences.com/design-center
siRNA Design Software	http://www.genscript.com/ssl-bin/app/rnai
Block-iT RNAi Designer	https://rnaidesigner.invitrogen.com
siRNA Target Finder	http://www.ambion.com/techlib/misc/siRNA_finder.html
RNAi explorer	www.genelink.com/sirna/siRNAorder.asp

Materials and Methods

Poly (ethylene glycol)-g-polyethylenimine (PEG-g-PEI (PEG; 5 kDa and PEI; 25 kDa)) was synthesized by the pharmaceutics department of the Pharmacy School, University of Medical Sciences (Shiraz, Iran). Human lung adenocarcinoma cell line (A549) was obtained from Pasture Institute (Tehran, Iran). siRNA against hTERT, scramble siRNA, and positive control siRNA sequences were synthesized by Qiagen (Korea). Real-time PCR Kit was purchased from TaKaRa Biotechnology, (Dalian, China). Cell culture medium and fetal bovine serum (FBS) were purchased from GIBCO (Carlsbad, CA, USA).

The in-silico protocol for siRNA designing

The accession number of hTERT (AB085628) was extracted from the national center for biotechnology information (NCBI). Ambion® software (www.lifetechnologies.com) was used for designing of siRNA which provided a list of candidate siRNAs. In the selection, 5′ UTR, 3′ UTR, start codon, introns and splice junctions were avoided.

Analyzing the internal instability, the asymmetry of siRNA duplex and secondary structures of candidate siRNAs were accomplished by Sfold software (http://sfold.wadsworth.org). Melting temperature (Tm) of the siRNA hairpin loop is another thermodynamic feature of siRNA which was predicted by "OligoAnalyzer 3.1" online service (https://eu.idtdna.com/calc/analyzer). BLAST (http://blast.ncbi.nlm.nih.gov) as a worldwide algorithm was used to evaluate the off-target effects. In accordance with the output of soft wares, main sequence siRNA (MS) was selected and synthesized. To confirm the functionality of MS, scramble sequence (SS) as a control negative was designed. Furthermore, the control positive sequence (CPS) was selected from the literature. The sequences of these three siRNAs are listed in Table 3.

Table 3. Sequence of siRNAs. MS: main sequence, CPS: control positive sequence, SS: scramble sequence

Sequences name	strand	Molecular weight	sequences
MS	Sense	13315	GCACUUCCUCUACUCCUCATT
MS	Antisense	13315	UGAGGAGUAGAGGAAGUGCTT
CPS	Sense	13315	UGAUUUCUUGUUGGUGACATT
CPS	Antisense	13315	UGUCACCAACAAGAAAUCATT
SS	Sense	13315	UGAUUUCUUGUUGGUGACATT
SS	Antisense	13315	UGUCACCAACAAGAAAUCATT

Cell Culture

Human lung adenocarcinoma A549 cells were cultured and maintained in RPMI 1641 medium containing 10% fetal bovine serum and antibiotics at 37°C in a humidified atmosphere of 5% CO2.

Synthesis and characterization of PEG-g-PEI nanoparticles for siRNA delivery

The shortcomings of siRNA such as the lack of in vivo stability and the poor permeability of cell membranes propelled the researchers to devise efficient carriers. To this end, PEG-g-PEI nanoparticles have been introduced as an effective tool for siRNA delivery. Therefore, in this study PEG-g-PEI nanoparticles were used as a transfection agent. PEG-g-PEI nanoparticles were synthesized and characterized as previously described.[19]

Preparation of Polyelectrolyte Complex (PECs)

PECs containing hTERT siRNA was prepared by adding appropriate volumes of siRNA (20μM) and PEG-g-PEI solution to deionized water. The mixture was gently blended and incubated for 20 minutes at room temperature.[20] Relay on previous data, N/P (Nitrogen/Phosphate) ratio of 2.5 was chosen as an appropriate ratio for PECs formation.[19]

PECs characterization

The surface charge and diameter of the PECs were determined by measuring of zeta potential and dynamic light scattering (Brookhaven, NY, USA) as previously described.[21] The ability of PEG-g-PEI to condense siRNA into nanoparticles was analyzed by ethidium bromide dye-exclusion assay. The relative stability of PECs was evaluated by measuring the release of siRNA from nanoparticles in the presence of a heparin sulfate.

Transfection Efficiency Assay

Cells (A549 cell line) were seeded in 96 well cell culture plates (1×10^4 cells/well) and incubated for 24 hours prior to treatment. PECs containing FITC-labeled PEG-g-PEI/siRNA and FITC-labeled PEI/siRNA at the N/P ratios of 2.5 were prepared in RPMI. Cell culture media (100 μL) with the final concentration of 200 nM siRNA were added to each well. After 4h incubation, on the basis of previous protocol[20] samples were fixed and the cellular uptake of PECs were assessed by flow cytometry. Finally, data acquisition and analysis was performed by recruiting WinMDI software.

Quantitative Real-time PCR

The attenuation of gene expression mediated by hTERT siRNA was analyzed by quantitative Real-Time PCR. Thereby, 48h after PECs transfection; total RNA was extracted by using TriPure isolation reagent (Invitrogen, Carlsbad, CA, USA) according to the manufacturer's instructions. Reverse transcription and Real-time PCR were performed based on the protocol of SYBR Green-I _ RT-PCR Kit (TaKaRa, China). The list of primers which were used for Real-time PCR is represented in Table 4.

Table 4. Sequence of the primers used in Real Time PCR

Oligonucleotides		Primer sequences	Position	PCR product length
hTERT	Forward	5′ CCGCCTGAGCTGTACTTGT 3′	2156F	198
	Reverse	5' CAGGTGAGCCACGAACTGT 3'	2362R	
Beta-actin	Forward	5′ TCCCTGGAGAAGAGCTACG3′	787F	131
	Reverse	5′GTAGTTTCGTGGATGCCACA3′	917R	

Statistical Analysis Synthesis of and characterization of PEG-g-PEI nanoparticles

Data were expressed as a mean ± standard error (SE). All statistical analyses were performed with SPSS 11.0 software. Analysis of variance (ANOVA) was used, and a P-value ≤ 0.05 was considered as significant.

Results

Characterization of siRNAs

Characters of siRNA sequences including target accessibility score, duplex feature score, duplex thermodynamics score, GC content and, etc were investigated with Sfold online tool. The results of the analysis are shown in Table 5. The Tm of CPS was 38.4°C and MS was 50.4 °C which were in the appropriate ranges. Also, the target accessibility of both MS and CPS sequences are represented in Figure 1. The results of BLAST showed that MS had 100% similarity with hTERT gene and less than 78% homology with the other part of the genome.

Table 5. Individual scores for duplex features and thermodynamic

Duplex features and thermodynamic	Main sequence (MS)	Control positive sequence (CPS)
GC content	0	1
A/U in position 15	0	1
A/U in position 16	0	0
A/U in position 17	1	1
A/U in position 18	0	0
A/U in position 19	1	1
Inverse repeat	1	1
A in position 19	1	1
A in position 3	1	1
U in position 10	0	0
G/C in position 19	0	0
G in position 13	0	-1
Relative stability of internal siRNA duplex	1	0
Internal stability	0	1

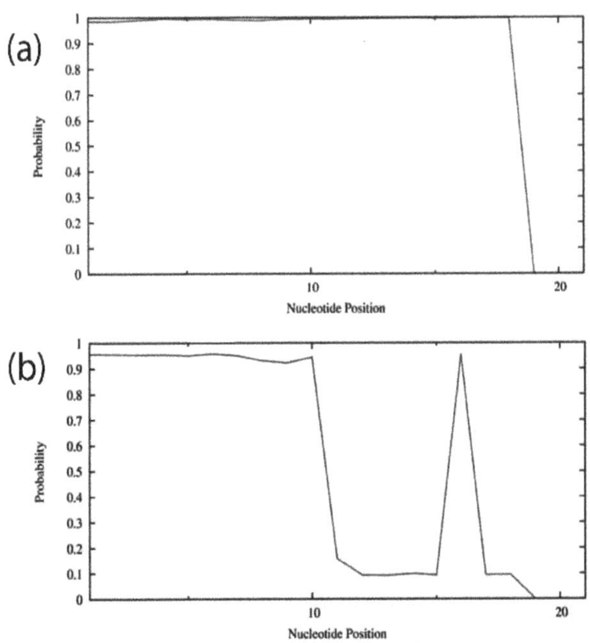

Figure 1. The accessibility to the target site for each nucleotide in the sequence. a: the target accessibility of main sequence (MS). b: the target accessibility of control positive sequence (CPS).

PECs characterization

The size and zeta potential were determined at PEG grafting degree of 0.2 and N/P ratio of 2.5. Size of this nanoparticle was 114 ± 0.645 nm. PEG grafting degree of 0.2 represented negative zeta potential due to charge covering effect of PEG grafting. The findings of ethidium bromide dye-exclusion assay showed that the complexation of siRNA and PEG-g-PEI resulted in decreasing in the intercalating property of ethidium bromide.[19] The results of polyanion competition assays demonstrated that PEG grafting improved the stability of the PECs.[19]

In vitro Transfection Assay

The transfection efficiency of the complexes was evaluated with a flow cytometry. FITC-labeled siRNAs were used to form these complexes. FACs results showed the transfection efficiency of PEI/siRNA was 81 ±2.5 and PEG-g-PEI/siRNA was 95.5% ± 2.4%. PEI/siRNA was used as a control positive. The histogram plots of PEG-g-PEI/siRNA and PEI/siRNA transfection efficiency are represented in Figure 2. Shifting of plot to right side showed that the transfection efficiency of PEG-g-PEI/siRNA is improved in comparison with PEI/siRNA.

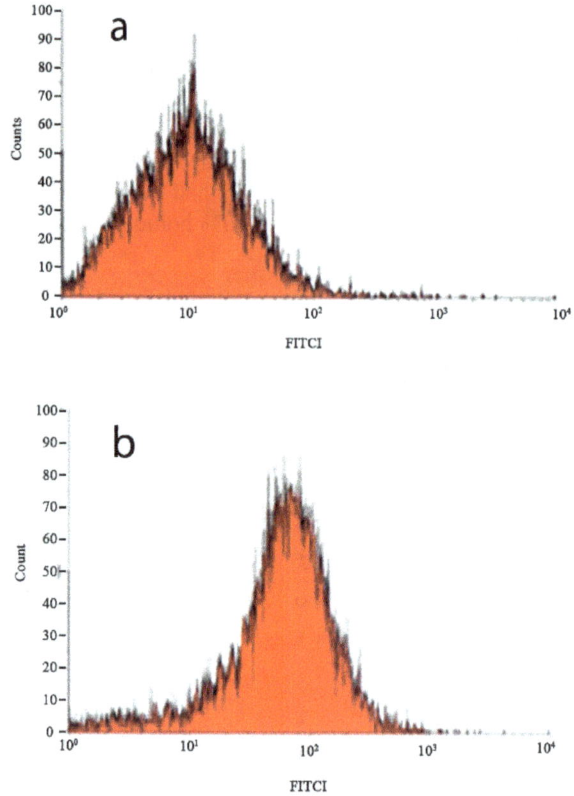

Figure 2. FACS histogram of FITC positive cells after FITC-labeled siRNA transfection. a: PEI/FITC labeled siRNA transfected cells. b: PEG-g-PEI/FITC-labeled siRNA transfected cells.

The Gene Silencing Effect of PECs

Real-time PCR was used to evaluate the potency of MS and CPS to reduce the hTERT mRNA levels respectively. Both MS and CPS reduced the expression of hTERT by targeting its complimentary mRNA. However, attenuation induced by MS was much more than CPS. No obvious changes in hTERT expression of SS, confirmed the results of the other sequences (2−ΔΔCT= 1.27) (Figure 3).

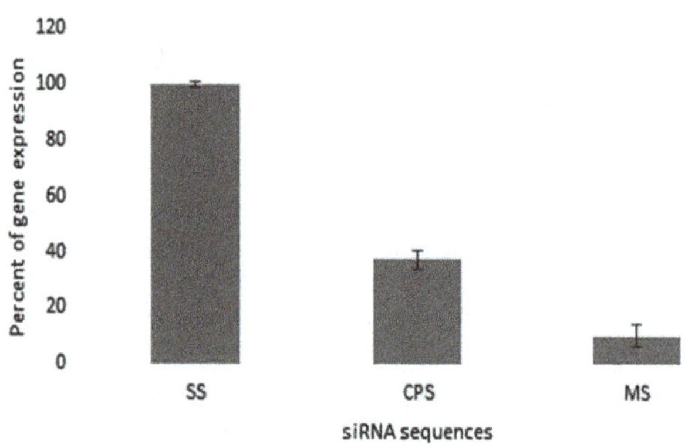

Figure 3. The results of quantitative real-time PCR. (main sequence [MS], control, positive sequence [CPS] and scramble sequence [SS].

Discussion

RNAi-related strategies have become promising methods in various fields of research. Effective gene silencing by the RNAi pathway needs a comprehensive understanding of the criteria that affect siRNA functionality and specificity. Target site, nucleotide content, the accessibility of the target site and thermodynamic features are criteria that influence the functionality of siRNA. Recent experiences showed that siRNAs closer to the start codon are more efficient than farther ones.[22] Based on the algorithm by Reynolds et al., the sequence preferences of the sense strand are influential on the siRNA efficiency. Reynolds studies on the sense strand showed that the presence of A at the third position and U at the tenth position, A at the nineteenth position, besides the absence of G or C at the nineteenth and G at the thirteenth nucleotide potentiate the silencing effect of siRNA.[16] According to Jagla and his research team analysis the presence of at least 3 A/U at position 13–19 increases the efficiency of predicted siRNA.[23] In addition, low internal stability at 5′-end of the antisense strand is required for assembling of the RISC complex.[24] The number of A/U at 5′-end of the antisense strand determines the internal stability.[25] So in the 5′-end of antisense strand, four out of the seven nucleotides must be A or U.[26]

Tm as a thermodynamic parameter affects the functionality of siRNA so that high Tm values give rise to internal hairpin structures and low values lead to high internal repeat stability. Sorting the functional siRNA by Tm revealed that duplexes lacking internal hairpin structures and stable internal repeats were better silencers.

GC content is an important parameter in the efficiency of siRNAs because low GC content gives rise to weak and unspecific binding, while high GC content may impede unwinding the siRNA duplex by RISC complex and helicase. To this end, the different ranges of GC content were suggested by different algorithms such as 31.6-57.9%[18] and 36–52%.[16] Computational modeling suggested that target secondary structure and accessibility are two influential factors which affect the potency of siRNA.[27,28] The target accessibility is necessary for the downstream step of target recognition for gene silencing mediated by RNAi. The importance of target accessibility for RNAi pathway has been approved by the study of HIV. A single point mutation alters the accessibility to the target site and HIV-1 can escape from RNAi pathway.[29] However, the target accessibility is a crucial parameter for functional siRNA but duplex asymmetry is also important and both of them together can greatly improve the efficiency of RNAi.[30]

In this study, the analysis of sequences by OligoAnalyzer and Sfold soft wares showed that nucleotide preferences were more observed in CPS than MS. The GC content of MS was 52.6% and CPS was 36.8%. According to these results, the CPS must be more efficient than MS, but findings of Real-time PCR demonstrated that the gene silencing efficiency of MS (up to 90%) was more than CPS (up to 63%). This controversy is due to the higher target accessibility of MS than CPS which was represented in Figure 1. The local structure of mRNA at the target site determines the level of accessibility of siRNA to target mRNA. The findings of SHAO and his co-workers suggested that, after RISC assembly, the secondary structure of target mRNA plays a crucial role in target binding by the guide of the antisense strand. Thus, to achieve effective silencing by RNAi, the selected siRNAs must have sequence features that facilitate RISC activation, as well as target accessibility that improves target recognition by intermolecular base-pairing.[30]

Poor cellular uptake and hydrolytic sensitivity of naked polyanionic oligonucleotides are the main concerns in current nucleic acid-based therapeutic strategies which lead the researchers to find the efficient and safe delivery systems.[31] Cationic polymers and block copolymers are polymeric condensing carriers for gene delivery due to good stability, simple preparation and easily modified chemical structures.[32] PEI, as a branched or linear cationic polymer, has been used in siRNA delivery because of low immunogenic stimulation and safety issues. In this study, PEI was used as nano-carrier for gene delivery, But to improve the biocompatibility and transfection efficiency, the PEI core was grafted to hydrophilic PEG. In the characterization of PECs, ethidium bromide dye exclusion assay showed that condensation of siRNA by PEG-g-PEI inhibited the intercalating property of ethidium bromide in the siRNA backbone. In addition, heparin competition assay demonstrated that PEG grafting improves the stability of the PECs.[19] The results of transfection efficiency showed that PEG grafting increases the cellular uptake of PEG-g-PEI/siRNA in comparison with PEI/siRNA which is related to the improving of PECs stability.

Conclusion

siRNA-based gene therapies are emerging as a promising novel therapeutic approach for the treatment of various diseases such as cancer. More than 20 RNAi therapeutic agents are currently in clinical trials. Several of these clinically relevant RNAi therapies are in Phase III which represents that the first RNAi therapeutic to be clinically is not so far. Therefore, considering to design efficient and specific siRNAs for clinical uses is so crucial. To this end, various criteria and algorithms have been devised for achieving high functional siRNA. Some of these criteria have the priority than the other so observing these criteria may greatly affect the clinical efficiency of siRNA. However, novel genome editing technologies such as CRISPR revolutionize the gene therapy approaches and comes to the clinic for treatment of the broad spectrum of diseases.

Conflict of Interest

The authors declare no conflict of interests.

References

1. Eissa S, Motawi T, Badr S, Zaghlool A, Maher A. Evaluation of urinary human telomerase reverse transcriptase mrna and scatter factor protein as urine markers for diagnosis of bladder cancer. *Clin Lab* 2013;59(3-4):317-23.
2. Akincilar SC, Tergaonkar V. Long-range chromatin interaction regulates htert expression through epigenetic modifications. *Telomere and Telomerase* 2017;4. doi: 10.14800/tt.1568
3. Fire A, Xu S, Montgomery MK, Kostas SA, Driver SE, Mello CC. Potent and specific genetic interference by double-stranded rna in caenorhabditis elegans. *Nature* 1998;391(6669):806-11. doi: 10.1038/35888
4. Ryoo NK, Lee J, Lee H, Hong HK, Kim H, Lee JB, et al. Therapeutic effects of a novel sirna-based anti-vegf (sivegf) nanoball for the treatment of choroidal neovascularization. *Nanoscale* 2017;9(40):15461-9. doi: 10.1039/c7nr03142d
5. Elbashir SM, Harborth J, Lendeckel W, Yalcin A, Weber K, Tuschl T. Duplexes of 21-nucleotide rnas mediate rna interference in cultured mammalian cells. *Nature* 2001;411(6836):494-8. doi: 10.1038/35078107
6. Paddison PJ, Caudy AA, Bernstein E, Hannon GJ, Conklin DS. Short hairpin rnas (shrnas) induce sequence-specific silencing in mammalian cells. *Genes Dev* 2002;16(8):948-58. doi: 10.1101/gad.981002
7. Rivas FV, Tolia NH, Song JJ, Aragon JP, Liu J, Hannon GJ, et al. Purified argonaute2 and an sirna form recombinant human risc. *Nat Struct Mol Biol* 2005;12(4):340-9. doi: 10.1038/nsmb918
8. Su H, Trombly MI, Chen J, Wang X. Essential and overlapping functions for mammalian argonautes in microrna silencing. *Genes Dev* 2009;23(3):304-17. doi: 10.1101/gad.1749809
9. Elbashir SM, Harborth J, Weber K, Tuschl T. Analysis of gene function in somatic mammalian cells using small interfering rnas. *Methods* 2002;26(2):199-213. doi: 10.1016/s1046-2023(02)00023-3
10. Birmingham A, Anderson E, Sullivan K, Reynolds A, Boese Q, Leake D, et al. A protocol for designing sirnas with high functionality and specificity. *Nat Protoc* 2007;2(9):2068-78. doi: 10.1038/nprot.2007.278
11. Groebe DR, Uhlenbeck OC. Characterization of rna hairpin loop stability. *Nucleic Acids Res* 1988;16(24):11725-35.
12. Reynolds A, Leake D, Boese Q, Scaringe S, Marshall WS, Khvorova A. Rational sirna design for rna interference. *Nat Biotechnol* 2004;22(3):326-30. doi: 10.1038/nbt936
13. Westerhout EM, Berkhout B. A systematic analysis of the effect of target rna structure on rna interference. *Nucleic Acids Res* 2007;35(13):4322-30. doi: 10.1093/nar/gkm437

14. Akbarzadeh A, Mikaeili H, Zarghami N, Mohammad R, Barkhordari A, Davaran S. Preparation and in vitro evaluation of doxorubicin-loaded fe(3)o(4) magnetic nanoparticles modified with biocompatible copolymers. *Int J Nanomedicine* 2012;7:511-26. doi: 10.2147/ijn.s24326
15. Ui-Tei K, Naito Y, Saigo K. Essential notes regarding the design of functional sirnas for efficient mammalian rnai. *J Biomed Biotechnol* 2006;2006(4):65052. doi: 10.1155/jbb/2006/65052
16. Reynolds A, Leake D, Boese Q, Scaringe S, Marshall WS, Khvorova A. Rational sirna design for rna interference. *Nat Biotechnol* 2004;22(3):326-30. doi: 10.1038/nbt936
17. Kim YJ. Computational sirna design considering alternative splicing. *Methods Mol Biol* 2010;623:81-92. doi: 10.1007/978-1-60761-588-0_5
18. Amarzguioui M, Prydz H. An algorithm for selection of functional sirna sequences. *Biochem Biophys Res Commun* 2004;316(4):1050-8. doi: 10.1016/j.bbrc.2004.02.157
19. Safari F, Tamaddon AM, Zarghami N, Abolmali S, Akbarzadeh A. Polyelectrolyte complexes of htert sirna and polyethyleneimine: Effect of degree of peg grafting on biological and cellular activity. *Artif Cells Nanomed Biotechnol* 2016;44(6):1561-8. doi: 10.3109/21691401.2015.1064936
20. Weber ND, Merkel OM, Kissel T, Munoz-Fernandez MA. Pegylated poly(ethylene imine) copolymer-delivered sirna inhibits hiv replication in vitro. *J Control Release* 2012;157(1):55-63. doi: 10.1016/j.jconrel.2011.09.059
21. Merkel OM, Librizzi D, Pfestroff A, Schurrat T, Buyens K, Sanders NN, et al. Stability of sirna polyplexes from poly(ethylenimine) and poly(ethylenimine)-g-poly(ethylene glycol) under in vivo conditions: Effects on pharmacokinetics and biodistribution measured by fluorescence fluctuation spectroscopy and single photon emission computed tomography (spect) imaging. *J Control Release* 2009;138(2):148-59. doi: 10.1016/j.jconrel.2009.05.016
22. Teimoori-Toolabi L, Hashemi S, Azadmanesh K, Eghbalpour F, Safavifar F, Khorramizadeh MR. Silencing the wild-type and mutant k-ras increases the resistance to 5-flurouracil in hct-116 as a colorectal cancer cell line. *Anticancer Drugs* 2015;26(2):187-96. doi: 10.1097/cad.0000000000000175
23. Jagla B, Aulner N, Kelly PD, Song D, Volchuk A, Zatorski A, et al. Sequence characteristics of functional sirnas. *RNA* 2005;11(6):864-72. doi: 10.1261/rna.7275905
24. Sioud M. Rna interference: Mechanisms, technical challenges, and therapeutic opportunities. *Methods Mol Biol* 2015;1218:1-15. doi: 10.1007/978-1-4939-1538-5_1
25. Ui-Tei K, Naito Y, Takahashi F, Haraguchi T, Ohki-Hamazaki H, Juni A, et al. Guidelines for the selection of highly effective sirna sequences for mammalian and chick rna interference. *Nucleic Acids Res* 2004;32(3):936-48. doi: 10.1093/nar/gkh247
26. Hardin CC, Watson T, Corregan M, Bailey C. Cation-dependent transition between the quadruplex and watson-crick hairpin forms of d(cgcg3gcg). *Biochemistry* 1992;31(3):833-41.
27. Kretschmer-Kazemi Far R, Sczakiel G. The activity of sirna in mammalian cells is related to structural target accessibility: A comparison with antisense oligonucleotides. *Nucleic Acids Res* 2003;31(15):4417-24.
28. Luo KQ, Chang DC. The gene-silencing efficiency of sirna is strongly dependent on the local structure of mrna at the targeted region. *Biochem Biophys Res Commun* 2004;318(1):303-10. doi: 10.1016/j.bbrc.2004.04.027
29. Westerhout EM, Ooms M, Vink M, Das AT, Berkhout B. Hiv-1 can escape from rna interference by evolving an alternative structure in its rna genome. *Nucleic Acids Res* 2005;33(2):796-804. doi: 10.1093/nar/gki220
30. Shao Y, Chan CY, Maliyekkel A, Lawrence CE, Roninson IB, Ding Y. Effect of target secondary structure on rnai efficiency. *RNA* 2007;13(10):1631-40. doi: 10.1261/rna.546207
31. van Asbeck AH, Beyerle A, McNeill H, Bovee-Geurts PH, Lindberg S, Verdurmen WP, et al. Molecular parameters of sirna--cell penetrating peptide nanocomplexes for efficient cellular delivery. *ACS nano* 2013;7(5):3797-807. doi: 10.1021/nn305754c
32. Samal SK, Dash M, Van Vlierberghe S, Kaplan DL, Chiellini E, Van Blitterswijk C, et al. Cationic polymers and their therapeutic potential. *Chem Soc Rev* 2012;41(21):7147-94. doi: 10.1039/c2cs35094g

Permissions

All chapters in this book were first published in APB, by Tabriz University of Medical Sciences; hereby published with permission under the Creative Commons Attribution License or equivalent. Every chapter published in this book has been scrutinized by our experts. Their significance has been extensively debated. The topics covered herein carry significant findings which will fuel the growth of the discipline. They may even be implemented as practical applications or may be referred to as a beginning point for another development.

The contributors of this book come from diverse backgrounds, making this book a truly international effort. This book will bring forth new frontiers with its revolutionizing research information and detailed analysis of the nascent developments around the world.

We would like to thank all the contributing authors for lending their expertise to make the book truly unique. They have played a crucial role in the development of this book. Without their invaluable contributions this book wouldn't have been possible. They have made vital efforts to compile up to date information on the varied aspects of this subject to make this book a valuable addition to the collection of many professionals and students.

This book was conceptualized with the vision of imparting up-to-date information and advanced data in this field. To ensure the same, a matchless editorial board was set up. Every individual on the board went through rigorous rounds of assessment to prove their worth. After which they invested a large part of their time researching and compiling the most relevant data for our readers.

The editorial board has been involved in producing this book since its inception. They have spent rigorous hours researching and exploring the diverse topics which have resulted in the successful publishing of this book. They have passed on their knowledge of decades through this book. To expedite this challenging task, the publisher supported the team at every step. A small team of assistant editors was also appointed to further simplify the editing procedure and attain best results for the readers.

Apart from the editorial board, the designing team has also invested a significant amount of their time in understanding the subject and creating the most relevant covers. They scrutinized every image to scout for the most suitable representation of the subject and create an appropriate cover for the book.

The publishing team has been an ardent support to the editorial, designing and production team. Their endless efforts to recruit the best for this project, has resulted in the accomplishment of this book. They are a veteran in the field of academics and their pool of knowledge is as vast as their experience in printing. Their expertise and guidance has proved useful at every step. Their uncompromising quality standards have made this book an exceptional effort. Their encouragement from time to time has been an inspiration for everyone.

The publisher and the editorial board hope that this book will prove to be a valuable piece of knowledge for researchers, students, practitioners and scholars across the globe.

List of Contributors

Khosro Adibkia, Mohammad Barzegar-Jalali and Afshin Shiva
Drug Applied Research Center and Faculty of Pharmacy, Tabriz University of Medical Sciences, Tabriz, Iran

Alireza Mohajjel Nayebi
Clinical Psychiatry Research Center, Tabriz University of Medical Sciences, Tabriz, Iran

Siavash Hosseinzadeh and Saeed Ghanbarzadeh
Students' Research Committee and Faculty of Pharmacy, Tabriz University of Medical Sciences, Tabriz, Iran

Behzad Baradaran
Immunology Research Center, Tabriz University of Medical Sciences, Tabriz, Iran

Mohammad Rahmati-Yamchi and Yasin Ahmadi
Immunology Research Center, Tabriz University of Medical Sciences, Tabriz, Iran
Department of Clinical Biochemistry, Faculty of Medicine, Tabriz University of Medical Sciences, Tabriz, Iran

Nosratollah Zarghami
Department of Clinical Biochemistry, Faculty of Medicine, Tabriz University of Medical Sciences, Tabriz, Iran

Hojjatollah Nozad Charoudeh
Stem Cell Research center, Tabriz University of Medical Sciences, Tabriz, Iran

Mohammad Khalaj-Kondori
Department of Biology, Faculty of Natural Science, University of Tabriz, Tabriz, Iran

Morteza Milani and Abolfazl Akbarzadeh
Liver and Gastrointestinal disease research center, Tabriz University of Medical Sciences, Tabriz, Iran

Maghsud Shaker
Department of Clinical Biochemistry, Faculty of Medicine, Tabriz University of Medical Sciences, Tabriz, Iran

Mohammad Pourhassan-Moghaddam
Department of Medical biotechnology, Tabriz University of Medical Sciences, Tabriz, Iran

Mohammad Reza Mohammad Khani
Department of Pharmacology& Toxicology, School of Pharmacy, Zanjan University of Medical Sciences, Znjan, Iran

Mahdieh Anoush
Department of Pharmacology& Toxicology, School of Pharmacy, Zanjan University of Medical Sciences, Znjan, Iran
Applied Drug Research Center, Zanjan University of Medical Sciences, Znjan, Iran

Simin Sharifi
Department of Pharmaceutical Biotechnology, Faculty of Pharmacy, Tabriz University of Medical Sciences, Tabriz, Iran
Students' Research Committee, Tabriz University of Medical Sciences, Tabriz, Iran

Jaleh Barar
Department of Pharmaceutical Biotechnology, Faculty of Pharmacy, Tabriz University of Medical Sciences, Tabriz, Iran
Research Center for Pharmaceutical Nanotechnology, Tabriz University of Medical Sciences, Tabriz, Iran

Mohammad Saeid Hejazi
Department of Pharmaceutical Biotechnology, Faculty of Pharmacy, Tabriz University of Medical Sciences, Tabriz, Iran
Faculty of Advanced Biomedical Sciences, Tabriz University of Medical Sciences, Tabriz, Iran

Nasser Samadi
Research Center for Pharmaceutical Nanotechnology, Tabriz University of Medical Sciences, Tabriz, Iran
Faculty of Advanced Biomedical Sciences, Tabriz University of Medical Sciences, Tabriz, Iran
Department of Biochemistry and Medical Laboratories, Faculty of Medicine, Tabriz University of Medical Sciences, Tabriz, Iran

Farshad Sadegh Moghanlou, Gity Zareh and Sohrab Rostamkalaei
Department of Pharmaceutics, Faculty of Pharmacy, Mazandaran University of Medical Sciences, Sari, Iran

Jafar Akbari and Majid Saeedi
Department of Pharmaceutics, Faculty of Pharmacy, Mazandaran University of Medical Sciences, Sari, Iran
Pharmaceutical Sciences Research Centre, Mazandaran University of Medical Sciences, Sari, Iran

Hamid Reza Kelidari
Pharmaceutical Sciences Research Centre, Mazandaran University of Medical Sciences, Sari, Iran

Katayoun Morteza-Semnani
Department of Medicinal Chemistry, Faculty of Pharmacy, Mazandaran University of Medical Sciences, Sari, Iran

Jafar Ezzati Nazhad Dolatabadi
Research Center for Pharmaceutical Nanotechnology, Tabriz University of Medical Sciences, Tabriz, Iran
Student Research Committee, Tabriz University of Medical Sciences, Tabriz, Iran

Hamed Hamishehkar
Drug Applied Research Center, Tabriz University of Medical Sciences, Tabriz, Iran

Hadi Valizadeh
Faculty of Pharmacy, Tabriz University of Medical Sciences, Tabriz, Iran

Hamdollah Sharifi
Department of Pharmacology, Faculty of Pharmacy, Urmia University of Medical Sciences, Urmia, Iran

Safar Farajnia
Drug Applied Research Center, Tabriz University of Medical Sciences, Tabriz, Iran

Alireza Mohajjel Nayebi
Drug Applied Research Center, Tabriz University of Medical Sciences, Tabriz, Iran
Department of Pharmacology and Toxicology, Faculty of Pharmacy, Tabriz University of Medical Sciences, Tabriz, Iran

Rasool Haddadi
Department of Pharmacology and Toxicology, Faculty of Pharmacy, Hamadan University of Medical Science, Hamadan, Iran

Hamid Nazarian
Department of Biology and Anatomical Sciences, School of Medicine, Shahid Beheshti University of Medical Sciences, Tehran, Iran

Marefat Ghaffari Novin
Department of Biology and Anatomical Sciences, School of Medicine, Shahid Beheshti University of Medical Sciences, Tehran, Iran
Shahid Beheshti University of Medical Sciences, Infertility and Reproductive Health Research Center (IRHRC), Tehran, Iran

Reza Mirfakhraie
Department of Medical Genetics, School of Medicine, Shahid Beheshti University of Medical Sciences, Tehran, Iran

Akbar Aliasgharzadeh and Farnaz Tavakoli
Faculty of Medicine, Bone Research Center, Tabriz University of Medical Sciences, Tabriz, Iran

Mohammad Khalili
Neurosciences Research Center Tabriz University of Medical Sciences, Tabriz, Iran

Elham Mirtaheri and Bahram Pourghassem Gargari
Department of Biochemistry and Nutrition, Faculty of Nutrition, Tabriz University of Medical Sciences, Tabriz, Iran

Mahdieh Abbasalizad Farhangi
Department of Community Nutrition, Faculty of Nutrition, Tabriz University of Medical Sciences, Tabriz, Iran

Hossein Babaei
Drug Applied Research Center and Faculty of Pharmacy, Tabriz University of Medical Sciences, Tabriz, Iran

Parvin Dehghan
Nutrition research center, Department of Food Science and Technology, Student Research committee, Faculty of Nutrition, Tabriz University of Medical Sciences, Tabriz, Iran

Reza Badalzadeh and Mustafa Mohammadi
Department of Physiology, Faculty of Medicine, Tabriz University of Medical Sciences, Tabriz, Iran

Bahman Yousefi and Shima Mohammadi
Students' Research Committee, Tabriz University of Medical Sciences, Tabriz, Iran

Safar Faranjia
Biotechnology Research Center, Tabriz University of Medical Sciences, Tabriz, Iran

Moslem Najafi
Department of Pharmacology, Faculty of Pharmacy, Tabriz University of Medical Sciences, Tabriz, Iran

Ahmad Reza Jodati and Naser Safaei
Cardiovascular Research Center, Tabriz University of Medical Sciences, Tabriz, Iran

Afsaneh Gharebageri and Danial Fadaei Fouladi
Drug Applied Research Center, Tabriz University of Medical Sciences, Tabriz, Iran

Hossein Babaei
Drug Applied Research Center, Tabriz University of Medical Sciences, Tabriz, Iran
School of Pharmacy, Tabriz University of Medical Sciences, Tabriz, Iran

Yadollah Azarmi and Sahar Fallah
School of Pharmacy, Tabriz University of Medical Sciences, Tabriz, Iran

Sima Lak and Behrooz Nagili
Infectious and Tropical Disease Research Centre, Tabriz University of Medical Sciences, Tabriz, Iran

Alireza Ostadrahimi
Nutrition Research Center, Faculty of Health and Nutrition, Tabriz University of Medical Sciences, Tabriz, Iran

Mohammad Asghari-Jafarabadi
Road Traffic Injury Prevention Centre, Tabriz University of Medical Sciences, Tabriz, Iran

Sanaz Beigzali
Student Research Committee, Faculty of Medicine, Tabriz University of Medical Sciences, Tabriz, Iran

Feridoon Salehi
Burn Center, Sina Hospital, Tabriz University of Medical Sciences, Tabriz, Iran

Roxana Djafarzadeh
Scientific Associate, Global eLearning Academy, Geneva, Switzerland

Shohreh Taziki
Ischemic Disorders Research Center,Golestan University of Medical Sciences, Gorgan, Iran
Students' Research Committee, Faculty of Pharmacy, Tabriz University of Medical Science, Tabriz, Iran

Mohammad Reza Sattari
Department of Pharmacology and Toxicology, Faculty of Pharmacy, Tabriz University of Medical Sciences, Tabriz, Iran
Neurosciences Research Centre, Tabriz University of Medical Sciences, Tabriz, Iran

Siavoush Dastmalchi
Biotechnology Research Center, Tabriz University of Medical Sciences, Tabriz, Iran

Mohammad Ali Eghbal
Drug Applied Research Center, Tabriz University of Medical Sciences, Tabriz, Iran

Javad Tajkey and Bohlol Habibi Asl
Department of Pharmacology, School of Pharmacy, Tabriz University of Medical Sciences, Tabriz, Iran

Alireza Biglari
Department of Genetics and Molecular Medicine, School of Medicine, Zanjan University of Medical Sciences, Zanjan, Iran

Ali Ramazani
Zanjan Pharmaceutical Biotechnology Research Center, Zanjan University of Medical Sciences, Zanjan, Iran

Saeideh Mazloomzadeh
Department of Epidemiology, School of Medicine, Zanjan University of Medical Sciences, Zanjan, Iran

Rasool Haddadi
Department of Pharmacology and Toxicology, Faculty of Pharmacy, Hamadan University of Medical Science, Hamadan, Iran

Shahla Eyvari Brooshghalan and Safar Farajniya
Drug Applied Research Center, Tabriz University of Medical Sciences, Tabriz, Iran

Alireza Mohajjel Nayebi
Drug Applied Research Center, Tabriz University of Medical Sciences, Tabriz, Iran
Clinical Psychiatry Research Center, Tabriz University of Medical Sciences, Tabriz, Iran

Hamdolah Sharifi
Department of Pharmacology, Faculty of Pharmacy, Urmia University of Medical Science, Urmia, Iran

Monir Moradzadeh Khiavi
Department of Oral and Maxillofacial Pathology, School of Dentistry, Tehran University of Medical Sciences, International campus, Tehran, Iran

Ahamd Rostami, Amirala Aghbali and Mahmud Sina
Department of Oral and Maxillofacial Pathology, School of Dentistry, Tabriz University of Medical Sciences, Tabriz, Iran

Hamed Hamishekar, Mehran Mesgari Abassi, Roya Salehi, Bita Abdollahi and Soheila Fotoohi
Drug Applied Research Center, Tabriz University of Medical Sciences, Tabriz, Iran

Prabhanshu Kumar
Amity Institute of Biotechnology, Amity University Uttar Pradesh, Noida, 201301, India

Pawan Kumar Maurya
Amity Institute of Biotechnology, Amity University Uttar Pradesh, Noida, 201301, India
Interdisciplinary Laboratory of Clinical Neuroscience (LINC), Department of Psychiatry, Federal University of São Paulo, São Paulo, Brazil

Subhash Chand
Department of Biochemical Engineering and Biotechnology, Indian Institute of Technology, Delhi, India

Pranjal Chandra
Department of Biosciences and Bioengineering, Indian Institute of Technology, Guwahati, Assam, India

Mohammad Amjadi, Jalal Mohammadi Khoshraj and Mir Reza Majidi
Department of Analytical Chemistry, Chemistry Faculty, Tabriz University, Tabriz, Iran

Behzad Baradaran
Immunology Research Center, Tabriz University of Medical Sciences, Tabriz, Iran

Miguel de la Guardia
Department of Analytical Chemistry, University of Valencia, Valencia, Spain

Ali Golestan
Autophagy Research Center, Shiraz University of Medical Sciences, Shiraz, Iran

Abbas Ghaderi and Zahra Mojtahedi
Institute for Cancer Research, Shiraz University of Medical Sciences, Shiraz, Iran

Sajad Khiali
Department of Clinical Pharmacy, Faculty of Pharmacy, Tabriz University of Medical Sciences, Tabriz, Iran

Afshin Gharekhani and Taher Entezari-Maleki
Drug Applied Research Center, Tabriz University of Medical Sciences, Tabriz, Iran

Soheila Montazersaheb
Stem Cell Research Center, Tabriz University of Medical Sciences, Tabriz, Iran
Molecular Medicine Research Center, Tabriz University of Medical Sciences, Tabriz, Iran
Department of Pharmaceutical Biotechnology, Faculty of Pharmacy, Tabriz University of Medical Sciences, Tabriz, Iran

Mohammad Saeid Hejazi
Molecular Medicine Research Center, Tabriz University of Medical Sciences, Tabriz, Iran
Department of Pharmaceutical Biotechnology, Faculty of Pharmacy, Tabriz University of Medical Sciences, Tabriz, Iran

Hojjatollah Nozad Charoudeh
Anatomical Sciences Department, Faculty of Medicine, Tabriz University of Medical Sciences, Tabriz, Iran

Faezeh Alihosseini
Department of Medical Nanotechnology, Pharmaceutical Sciences Branch, Islamic Azad University (IAUPS), Tehran, Iran

Shirzad Azarmi
Faculty of Pharmacy and Pharmaceutical Sciences, University of Alberta, Edmonton, Alta, Canada
Research Center for Pharmaceutical Nanotechnology, Faculty of Pharmacy, Tabriz University of Medical Sciences, Tabriz, Iran

Solmaz Ghaffari
Department of Medical Nanotechnology, Pharmaceutical Sciences Branch, Islamic Azad University (IAUPS), Tehran, Iran
Young Researchers and Elite Club, Pharmaceutical Sciences Branch, Islamic Azad University, (IAUPS), Tehran, Iran

Setareh Haghighat
Department of Microbiology, Faculty of Advanced Sciences and Technology, Pharmaceutical Sciences Branch, Islamic Azad

Seyed Mahdi Rezayat Sorkhabadi
Department of Medical Nanotechnology, School of Advanced Sciences and Technology in Medicine, Tehran University of Medical Sciences (TUMS), Tehran, Iran
Department of Pharmacology and Toxicology, Pharmaceutical Sciences Branch, Islamic Azad University, (IAUPS), Tehran, Iran

Babak Roushangar Zineh and Mohammad Reza Shabgard
Mechanical Engineering Department, University of Tabriz, Tabriz, Iran

Leila Roshangar
Stem Cell Research Center, Tabriz University of Medical Sciences, Tabriz Iran

Laleh Payahoo
Talented Student Center, Student Research Committee, Nutrition Research Center, Faculty of Nutrition and Food Science, Tabriz
University of Medical Sciences, Tabriz, Iran

Yaser Khajebishak
Student Research Committee, Faculty of Nutrition and Food Science, Tabriz University of Medical Sciences, Tabriz, Iran

Mohammad Asghari Jafarabadi
Road Traffic Injury Research Center, Department of Statistics and Epidemiology, Faculty of Health, Tabriz University of Medical Sciences, Tabriz, Iran

Alireza Ostadrahimi
Nutrition Research Center, Faculty of Nutrition and Food Science, Tabriz University of Medical Sciences, Tabriz, Iran

Neda Roshanravan
Cardiovascular Research Center, Tabriz University of Medical Sciences, Tabriz, Iran

Parina Asgharian
Drug Applied Research Center, Tabriz University of Medical Sciences, Tabriz, Iran
Department of Pharmacognosy, Tabriz University of Medical Sciences, Tabriz, Iran

Hassan Dariushnejad
Department of Medical Biotechnology, Faculty of Medicine, Lorestan University of Medical Sciences, Khorramabad, Iran

Naimeh Mesri Alamdari
Students Research Committee, School of Health, Iran University of Medical Science, Tehran, Iran

Behzad Mansoori and Ali Mohammadi
Immunology Research Center, Tabriz University of Medical Sciences, Tabriz, Iran

Shahriar Alipour
Department of Molecular Medicine, Connective Tissue Disease Research Center, Tabriz University of Medical Sciences, Tabriz, Iran

Meisam Barati
Students Research Committee, Cellular and Molecular Nutrition Department, Shahid Beheshti University of Medical Sciences, Tehran, Iran

Abed Ghavami, Fatemeh Aamazadeh and Alireza Ostadrahimi
Nutrition Research Center, School of Nutrition, Tabriz University of Medical Science, Tabriz, Iran

Vajihe Ghorbanzadeh
Razi Herbal Medicine Research Center, Lorestan University of Medical Sciences, Khorramabad, Iran

Neda Alidadiani, Behzad Mansoori, Vahid Khaze Shahgoli and Behzad Baradaran
Immunology Research Center, Tabriz University of Medical Sciences, Tabriz, Iran

Shahrooz Ghaderi
Immunology Research Center, Tabriz University of Medical Sciences, Tabriz, Iran
Department of Molecular Medicine, Faculty of Advanced Medical Sciences, Tabriz University of Medical Sciences, Tabriz, Iran
Student research committee, Tabriz University of Medical Sciences, Tabriz, Iran

Jafar Soleimani Rad
Department of Anatomy, Faculty of Medicine, Tabriz University of Medical Sciences, Tabriz, Iran

Hamid Reza Heidari
Department of Pharmaceutical Biotechnology, Faculty of Pharmacy, Tabriz University of Medical Sciences, Tabriz, Iran

Nafi Dilaver
Swansea University Medical School, Swansea University, Swansea, UK

Reza Rhabarghazi
Stem cell Research Center, Tabriz University of Medical Sciences, Tabriz, Iran
Department of Applied Cell Sciences, Faculty of Advanced Medical Sciences, Tabriz University of Medical Sciences, Tabriz, Iran

Rezayat Parvizi
Department of Cardiothoracic Surgery, Faculty of Medicine, Tabriz University of Medical Sciences, Tabriz, Iran

Farhad Jahanfar
Biotechnology Research Center and Student Research Committee, Tabriz University of Medical Sciences, Tabriz, Iran
Department of Biochemistry and Clinical Laboratories, Faculty of Medicine, Tabriz University of Medical Sciences, Tabriz, Iran

Akbar Hasani and Mohammad Rahmati
Department of Biochemistry and Clinical Laboratories, Faculty of Medicine, Tabriz University of Medical Sciences, Tabriz, Iran

Dariush Shanebandi
Immunology Research Center, Tabriz University of Medical Sciences, Tabriz, Iran

Hamed Hamishehkar
Drug Applied Research Center, Tabriz University of Medical Sciences, Tabriz, Iran

Rasoul Azmoonfar, Ehsan Khodamoradi and Masoud Najafi
Radiology and Nuclear Medicine Department, School of Paramedical Sciences, Kermanshah University of Medical Science, Kermanshah, Iran

Peyman Amini and Saeed Rezapoor
Department of Radiology, Faculty of Paramedical, Tehran University of Medical Sciences, Tehran, Iran

Hana Saffar
Clinical and Anatomical Pathologist at Tehran University of Medical Science, Imam Khomeini Hospital Complex, Tehran, Iran

Elahe Motevaseli
Department of Molecular Medicine, School of Advanced Technologies in Medicine, Tehran University of Medical Sciences, Tehran, Iran

Mohsen Cheki
Department of Radiologic Technology, Faculty of Paramedicine, Ahvaz Jundishapur University of Medical Sciences, Ahvaz, Iran

Rasoul Yahyapour
School of Medicine, Jiroft University of Medical Sciences, Jiroft, Iran

Bagher Farhood
Departments of Medical Physics and Radiology, Faculty of Paramedical Sciences, Kashan University of Medical Sciences, Kashan, Iran

Farzad Nouruzi
Department of Medical Radiation Engineering, Science and Research Branch, Islamic Azad University, Tehran, Iran

Dheyauldeen Shabeeb
Department of Medical Physics and Biomedical Engineering, Faculty of Medicine, Tehran University of Medical Sciences (International Campus), Tehran, Iran
Department of Physiology, College of Medicine, University of Misan, Misan, Iraq

Ahmed Eleojo Musa
Research Center for Molecular and Cellular Imaging, Tehran University of Medical Sciences (International Campus), Tehran, Iran

Fereshteh Morrovati, Jafar Soleimani Rad and Azadeh Montaseri
Stem Cell Research Center, Tabriz University of Medical Sciences, Tabriz, Iran

Nahid Karimian Fathi
Biochemistry Department, Faculty of Medicine, Tabriz University of Medical Sciences, Tabriz, Iran

Pragati Rawat, Swatantra Agarwal and Siddhi Tripathi
Department of Prosthodontics and Crown & Bridge, Kothiwal dental college and research center, Moradabad, UP-244001, India

Azam Rahimpour
Department of Tissue Engineering and Applied Cell Sciences, School of Advanced Technologies in Medicine, Shahid Beheshti University of Medical Sciences, Tehran, Iran

Hadi Bayat
Department of Tissue Engineering and Applied Cell Sciences, School of Advanced Technologies in Medicine, Shahid Beheshti University of Medical Sciences, Tehran, Iran
Department of Molecular Genetics, Faculty of Biological Sciences, Tarbiat Modares University, Tehran, Iran

Fatemeh Naderi
Department of Molecular Genetics, Tehran Medical Sciences Branch, Islamic Azad University, Tehran, Iran

Amjad Hayat Khan
Institute for Research in Molecular Medicine (INFORMM), Universiti Sains Malaysia, Penang, Malaysia

Arash Memarnejadian
Department of Hepatitis and AIDS, Pasteur Institute of Iran, Tehran, Iran

Fatemeh Safari
Medical Biotechnology Department, Faculty of Advanced Medical Sciences, Tabriz University of Medical Sciences, Tabriz, Iran
Shiraz University of Medical Sciences, Shiraz, Iran
Student Research Committee, Tabriz University of Medical Sciences, Tabriz, Iran

Solmaz Rahmani Barouji
Department of Traditional Medicine, Faculty of Traditional Medicine, University of Medical Sciences, Tabriz, Iran

Ali Mohammad Tamaddon
Center for Pharmaceutical Nanotechnology and Biomaterials, Faculty of Pharmacy, Shiraz University of Medical Sciences, Shiraz, Iran

Index

www.ingramcontent.com/pod-product-compliance
Lightning Source LLC
LaVergne TN
LVHW060528210926
848485LV00005B/1166